THE MODERN MANAGEMENT OF THE MENOPAUSE

A PERSPECTIVE FOR THE 21ST CENTURY

THE INTERNATIONAL CONGRESS, SYMPOSIUM AND SEMINAR SERIES

VOLUME 8

I·C·S·S

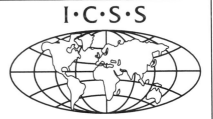

ISSN: 0969-2622

THE MODERN MANAGEMENT OF THE MENOPAUSE

A PERSPECTIVE FOR THE 21ST CENTURY

THE PROCEEDINGS
OF THE VII INTERNATIONAL CONGRESS
ON THE MENOPAUSE
STOCKHOLM, SWEDEN 1993

EDITED BY G. BERG AND M. HAMMAR

The Parthenon Publishing Group

International Publishers in Medicine, Science & Technology

NEW YORK   LONDON

Published in the UK by
The Parthenon Publishing Group Limited
Casterton Hall, Carnforth,
Lancs, LA6 2LA, England

Published in the USA by
The Parthenon Publishing Group Inc.
One Blue Hill Plaza
PO Box 1564, Pearl River,
New York 10965, USA

British Library Cataloguing in Publication Data

The Modern Management of the Menopause: A perspective for the 21st Century.—
(International Congress, Symposium & Seminar Series,
ISSN 0969-2622; Vol. 8)
I. Berg, Göran.   II. Hammar, Mats.   III. Series
612.665
ISBN 1-85070-544-5

Library of Congress Cataloging-in-Publication Data

International Congress on the Menopause (7th : 1993 : Stockholm, Sweden)
    The modern management of the menopause : a perspective for the 21st century /
edited by Göran Berg and Mats Hammar
        p.   cm.—(The International congress, symposium, and seminar series, ISSN 0969-
2622; v. 8)
"The proceedings of the VIIth International Congress on the Menopause, Stockholm,
Sweden, June 1993."
Includes bibliographical references and index.
ISBN 1-85070-544-5
        1. Menopause—Congresses.   I. Berg, Göran.   II. Hammar, Mats.   III. Title.   IV.
Series.
[DNLM: 1. Menopause—congresses. 2. Estrogen Replacement Therapy—congresses.
WP 580 I61m 1994]
RG186.I57   1993
618.1'75—dc20
DNLM/DLC
for Library of Congress   94-1746
                                                                                                                                CIP

First published 1994

Typeset by Lasertext Ltd., Stretford, Manchester
Printed and bound in Great Britain by
Butler and Tanner Ltd., Frome and London

Contents

Contents

Contents

Contents

Preface

Menopause, the very last menstruation, denotes the end of the reproductive period of life and the beginning of a new era with possibilities to look forward to. Many women pass the climacteric period without any psychological or somatic complaints whereas others suffer from a variety of symptoms.

Peri- and postmenopausal women, i.e. women over 50 years of age, are a rapidly growing proportion of the population and in several countries already constitute 15–20% of the population as a whole. These women carry an increasing responsibility within society, in addition to their traditional family roles.

Approaching the next century, women born in the 1940s constitute those who seek advice for menopausal problems. Today's woman – independent, active and well informed – has the right to be offered the latest information and knowledge to enable her to make an informed decision on her future health.

The menopause and women's health are of rapidly growing concern worldwide. The great scientific interest in this field of healthcare and prevention makes it one of the major health issues of our time. During recent years, some areas within the field of the menopause have generated rapidly growing interest. Such areas are the psychosocial aspects of the menopause, neurobiological phenomena in relation to the changing hormonal situation and cardiovascular effects of hormones, with special emphasis on the direct vascular effects of estrogen. This increasing insight together with the growing epidemiological knowledge on differences between hormone users and non-users makes the field of the menopause an extremely interesting and important area in a general health perspective.

Modern clinical studies illustrate the possibility to adapt treatment regimens to the individual woman and her special demands. Such possibilities include the 'spacing' of progestagen administration, giving continuous combined estrogen/progestagen treatment, using an intrauterine progestagen delivering device in order to decrease or avoid bleeding, and utilizing alternative administration systems which make hormonal replacement treatment available for new groups of women.

New possibilities to individualize treatment together with professional and empathic information to the woman are probably the most important means to avoid low compliance among women prescribed hormonal substitution treatment.

In June 1993, clinicians and researchers from several different fields gathered in Stockholm, Sweden, for the VIIth International Congress on the Menopause. The most important lectures from invited speakers are summarized in the Proceedings, which thus give a comprehensive overview of the field. The various contributions have been grouped under a number of section headings which to some extent conform with the main symposia of the Congress.

We hope this compilation will be of interest and help for people who are dedicated to research, health and education within the field of the menopause. Increased knowledge within this field will hopefully, in the end, benefit women during a long and potentially active part of their lives, when they can contribute and enrich people and society with knowledge and experience.

Göran Berg   Mats Hammar
Department of Obstetrics and Gynaecology
University Hospital
Faculty of Health Sciences
Linköping
Sweden

List of principal contributors

T. J. Anderson
Department of Pathology
University Medical School
Teviot Place
Edinburgh
EK8 9AG
UK

T. Aso
Department of Obstetrics and
  Gynecology
Tokyo Medical and Dental
  University
School of Medicine
1-5-45 Yushima Bunkyo-ku
Tokyo 118
Japan

A. Ax:son Johnson
The Axel Johnson Group
Box 26008
10041 Stockholm
Sweden

T. Bäckström
Department of Obstetrics and
  Gynaecology
University Hospital
S-90187 Umea
Sweden

G. Berg
Department of Obstetrics and
  Gynaecology
University Hospital
S-581-85 Linköping
Sweden

H. G. Burger
Prince Henry's Institute of
  Medical Research
PO Box 152
Clayton
Victoria 3168
Australia

L. Cardozo
8 Devonshire Place
London
W1C 1PB
UK

C. Christiansen
Centre for Clinical and Basic
  Research
Ballerup byvej 222
DK 2750 Ballerup
Denmark

A. Collins
Karolinska Intitute
Psychology Division
Punkthuset 6th Floor
Box 50600
104 01 Stockholm
Sweden

E. Daly
Department of Public Health
and Primary Care
University of Oxford
Gibson Building
Radcliffe Infirmary
Woodstock Road
Oxford
OX2 6HE
UK

A. David
Department of Gynecology
105 Ben Gurion Street
Ramat Gan 52396
Israel

L. Dennerstein
Key Centre for Women's Health
in Society
World Health Organization
Collaborating Centre for
Women's Health
The University of Melbourne
209 Grattan Street
Carlton 3053 Victoria
Australia

N. Dusitsin
Institute of Health Research
Chulalongkorn University
5th Floor, Institute Building 2
Chulalongkorn Soi 62, Phyathia
Road
Bangkok 10330
Thailand

M. Ewertz
Danish Cancer Society
Division for Cancer
Epidemiology
Strandboulevarden 49
Box 839
DK-2100 Copenhagen 0
Denmark

M. Flint
Department of Anthropology
Montclair State
Upper Montclair
New Jersey 07043
USA

R. R. Freedman
Department of Obstetrics and
Gynecology and Psychiatry
Wayne State University School
of Medicine
CS Mott Center for Human
Growth and Development
275 East Hancock
Detroit, Michigan 48201
USA

K. W. Gee
Department of Pharmacology
School of Medicine
University of California at Irvine
Irvine
CA 92717
USA

J. Ginsburg
Department of Medicine
The Royal Free Hospital School
  of Medicine
Pond Street
Hampstead
London
NW3 2QG
UK

I. F. Godsland
Wynn Institute for Metabolic
  Research
21 Wellington Road
London NW8 9SQ
UK

J. Haarbo
Center for Clinical and Basic
  Research
Ballerup Byvej 222
DK-2750 Ballerup
Denmark

G. Hall
Department of Rheumatology
St. Thomas' Hospital
Lambeth Palace Road
London
SW6 5AX
UK

M. Hammar
Department of Obstetrics and
  Gynaecology
University Hospital
S-581-85 Linköping
Sweden

G. Heytmanek
1st Department of Gynecology
  and Obstetrics
University of Vienna
Spitalgasse 23
A-1090 Vienna
Austria

A. Holte
Psykologsektionen
University of Tromsö
N-9037 Tromsö
Norway

G. Holzer
Department of Orthopedics
University of Vienna
Waehringer Guertel 18-20
A-1090 Vienna
Austria

J. Huber
I Department of Obstetrics and
  Gynecology
University of Vienna
Spitalgasse 23
A-1090 Vienna
Austria

B. S. Hulka
Department of Epidemiology
School of Public Health
University of North Carolina
CB # 7400, McGavran-
  Greenberg Hall
Chapel Hill
North Carolina 27599-7400
USA

M. S. Hunter
Unit of Psychology
Medical School, Guy's Hospital
London Bridge
London
SE1 9RT
UK

P. A. Kaufert
Department of Community
  Health Sciences
Faculty of Medicine
University of Manitoba
750 Bannatyne Avenue
Winnipeg
Manitoba R3E 0WE
Canada

H. Kuhl
Division of Endocrinology
Department of Obstetrics and
  Gynecology
JW Goethe University
Theodor-Stern-Kai 7
D-6000 Frankfurt am Main
Germany

F. Kuttenn
Department of Endocrinology
  and Reproductive Medicine
Faculte de Medicine Necker
  Enfants Malades
Universite Rene Descartes
Hôpital Necker
149 rue de Sèvres
75015 Paris
France

M. Lachowsky
17 rue Carducci
75019 Paris
France

B.-M. Landgren
Department of Obstetrics and
  Gynaecology
Karolinska Hospital
S-104 01 Stockholm
Sweden

K. A. Matthews
Department of Psychiatry
University of Pittsburgh
3811 O'Hara Street
Pittsburgh
PA 15213
USA

L.-Å. Mattsson
Associate Professor
Department of Obstetrics and
  Gynaecology
East Hospital
University of Göteborg
S-416 85 Göteborg
Sweden

N. L. McCoy
1807 St Louis Drive
Honolulu
HI 96816-1932
USA

B. S. McEwen
Laboratory of
    Neuroendocrinology
The Rockefeller University
1230 York Avenue
New York
NY 10021-6399
USA

M. Metka
I Department of Obstetrics and
    Gynecology
University of Vienna
Spitalgasse 23
A-1090 Vienna
Austria

J. H. J. M. Meuwissen
Department of Gynecologi
St Joseph Hospital
PO Box 7777
5500 MB Veldhoven
The Netherlands

L. E. Nachtigall
251 East 33rd Street
New York
New York 10016
USA

M. Notelovitz
Women's Medical and
    Diagnostic Center and The
    Climacteric Clinic, Inc.
222 S.W. 36th Terrace, Suite C
Gainesville
Florida 32607
USA

J. O'Leary Cobb
President
A Friend Indeed Publications,
    Inc.
3575 Boul. St-Laurant, No. 402
Montreal
Quebec, H2X 2T7
Canada

C. M. Oakley
Clinical Cardiology
Department of Medicine
Hammersmith Hospital
The Royal Postgrad School,
Duncane Road
London
W12 0NN
UK

T. Ohkura
Department of Obstetrics and
    Gynecology
Koshigaya Hospital
Dokkyo University School of
    Medicine
2-1-50 Minami-Koshigaya
Koshigaya
Saitama 343
Japan

A. Oldenhave
Academic Hospital Utrecht
Department of Obstetrics and
  Gynecology
Heidelberglaan 100
3584 CX Utrecht
The Netherlands

I. Persson
Cancer Epidemiology Unit
University Hospital
S-751 85 Uppsala
Sweden

P. M. Sarrel
Department of Obstetrics and
  Gynecology
Division of Mental Hygiene
Box 1505-A
Yale Station
New Haven, Connecticut 06520
USA

W.-B. Schill
Department of Dermatology and
  Andrology
Justus Liebig University
Gaffkystrasse 14
D-35385 Giessen
Germany

J. Sciarra
Department of Obstetrics and
  Gynecology
North Western University,
  Medical School
Room 490
333 East Superior Street, Suite
  490
Chicago, Illinois 60611
USA

B. B. Sherwin
Department of Psychology and
  Obstetrics and Gynecology
McGill University
1205 Dr Penfield Avenue
Montreal
Quebec H3A 1B1
Canada

S. K. Smith
MD MRCOG
Department of Obstetrics and
  Gynaecology
University of Cambridge
Rosie Maternity Hospital
Cambridge
CB2 2SW
UK

S. S. Smith
Department of Anatomy
Institute of Neuroscience
Hahnemann University
Broad and Vine
Philadelphia
PA 19102-1192
USA

G. Tang
Department of Obstetrics and
  Gynaecology
University of Hong Kong
Queen Mary Hospital
Pokfulam Road
Hong Kong

J. A. Tieffenberg
President
Association for Health Research
  and Development
ACINDES
Soler 4829
Buenos Aires (1425)
Argentina

P. Topo
National Research and
  Development Centre for
  Welfare and Health
PO Box 220
SF 00531 Helsinki
Finland

E. Valverius
Experimental Oncology Section
The Radium Home
The Karolinska Institute
S-171 76 Stockholm
Sweden

H. J. J. Verhaar
Research Group for Geriatrics
  and Bone Metabolism
PO Box 85500
3508 GA Utrecht
The Netherlands

A. Vermeulen
Endocrine Department
Medical Clinic
University Hospital
De Pintelaan 185
9000 Gent
Belgium

S. Wasti
Department of Obstetrics and
  Gynaecology
Sultan Qaboos University
  College of Medicine
PO Box 35
Al-Khod Code 123
Muscat
Sultanate of Oman

B. Weiss
1165 Park Avenue
New York
NY 10128
USA

M. Whitehead
Department of Obstetrics and
  Gynaecology
King's College School of
  Medicine
Bessemer Road
London
SE5 9PJ
UK

O. Ylikorkala
Department II Obstetrics and
  Gynecology
University Central Hospital
Haartmaninkatu 2
SF-00290 Helsinki
Finland

1

The Pieter van Keep Memorial Lecture

INTRODUCTION

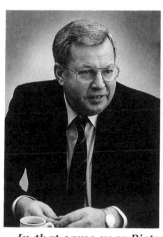

On 17 June, 1991 Dr Pieter A. van Keep, then President of the International Menopause Society passed away at the age of 58. During his whole professional career, his main interest was the menopause and the study of all aspects of the climacteric in women. Together with Bob Greenblatt, he organized – in 1976 and 1978 – the first and the second International Congresses on the Menopause and following that second meeting, Pieter van Keep, together with some of his dear friends who shared his ideas, founded the International Menopause Society.

In that same year Pieter van Keep made another important contribution to the advancement of science in the field of the climacteric by launching a new journal, Maturitas. *This was to provide a multidisciplinary approach to the menopause and the climacteric, and he became the founding editor. Since the inception of the Society, almost 15 years ago now, both the knowledge about, and the recognition of the climacteric syndrome, and the role of hormone replacement therapy, have increased tremendously. In addition, life expectancy around the world is rising which means that a rapidly increasing number of women will spend an important part of their lives in the 'Golden Age'. It was Pieter's aim, and it is one of the aims of the Society, that this 'Golden Age' for women becomes a happy, healthy age; not only devoid of short- and medium-term complaints such as hot flushes and*

1

urogenital symptoms, but also free from osteoporosis, and optimally protected against cardiovascular disease. Like many of you here, I was with Pieter at the last Menopause congress in Bangkok, a congress which he helped organize and which he enjoyed tremendously, both scientifically and socially. I know that he was really looking forward to this World Meeting in Stockholm where he would have seen all his old friends again and certainly have made new ones.

As Pieter's successor at Organon, I had very long discussions with him during the last month of his life on almost all of his activities. Pieter remained interested in the well-being of the International Menopause Society and he was very happy that a man whom he loved and trusted, Malcolm Whitehead, would replace him as President of this Society. He also remained interested in the psychosocial well-being of women during and after their climacteric. And it is for these reasons I know that Pieter van Keep would share my tremendous pleasure and honor now to open the scientific session of this International Menopause Congress and invite Mr Malcolm Whitehead to present the opening lecture, the first Pieter van Keep Memorial Lecture.

Hans Vemer

THE PIETER VAN KEEP MEMORIAL LECTURE

It is an honor to be asked to give the first Pieter van Keep Memorial Lecture. As you know Pieter died in June 1991. Those of you who did not know him perhaps may not fully appreciate the enormous, pivotal role that he held in this Society – the keystone of the Society – and therefore may not fully appreciate why we should honor his memory in this way. If it had not been for Pieter van Keep there would not be an International Society as it now stands, and without an International Society it is, of course, unlikely, that we would all be here in Stockholm today.

About a third of what I'm about to say relates exclusively to Pieter and my talk today is in many ways like a curate's egg. This doesn't really exist, but is an expression in English which is often used to describe something that is perhaps good, and also bad in parts. You may approve, or disapprove of some of what I have to say. I am going to concentrate, initially, by talking about Pieter, his early years, his psychosocial interests, and his relationship with the International Health Foundation and the International Menopause Society.

Our story begins on 14 August, 1932 in Ginniken, which was then a small town outside of Breda in The Netherlands. There Pieter was born into a Catholic family and it is a shining example of the liberal Dutch tradition that a Catholic could become so interested in gyne-endocrinology and contraception because, throughout his working life, Pieter wore two hats: contraception and the menopause. As a small boy, like all small boys perhaps, he thought of becoming a soldier or a sailor, but by the age of 22 he had decided that he was going to pursue a medical career. He graduated in medicine in 1958 at the University of Utrecht. And at that time, of course, like all Dutch young men, he was called up to do national service which he did between 1958 and 1960.

In 1960, Pieter joined Organon, and was to remain with them from 1960 until 1969. It was during this decade that he was first 'bitten by the bug' of psychosocial issues – a good friend at that time, Laszlo Jaszmann, was setting up cross-cultural and cross-sectional studies on psychosocial issues in the Dutch town of Ede.

By 1969, Pieter had decided that he wanted to spend more time doing research and spreading the message of gyne-endocrinology in women's issues and, therefore, he left Organon and moved to Geneva as the first Director General of the International Health Foundation. Also in 1969, Jaszmann published some of his cross-sectional data and Pieter, in Geneva, wasted no time commissioning a study from a professional opinion poll organization. He asked the poll organization to sample 2000 women, 400 in each of five western European countries. Each patient was interviewed for a minimum of 30 minutes by a professional pollster. What Pieter had in mind was to look, within western Europe, at how cross-national differences might influence and affect attitudes towards menopause. I know Pieter was impressed by Marcha Flint's early work which reported that Rajput Indians did not experience hot flushes at menopause. Clearly there were many cross-cultural differences which at that time were waiting to be identified and elucidated. Pieter had thought, 'Well let's have a look in western Europe,' and showed that in terms of the question, 'Is it good to be free from periods or menstruation?' the percentage of women who agreed in these five countries – Belgium, France, Great Britain, Italy, and West Germany – was remarkably similar.

For other questions, however, there were really quite profound differences which had not been reported previously. Asked whether the menopause marks the beginning of old age, 60% of Italian women said yes, but only 25% of women in Great Britain replied affirmatively. Today, I think we would regard these data as being somewhat 'soft' but they were an early attempt to look at cross-cultural and cross-national differences 23 years ago.

Similarly, asked whether the menopause meant the end of attractiveness to men, only 9% of British women agreed with this view, whereas 34%

of West German women agreed. It has been suggested, of course, that British women were so negative in their responses to these potentially disadvantageous questions because British women, at that time, didn't really understand what the menopause was. The bottom line of this 1970 survey was that there were going to be differences between nations within Europe.

1971 saw the publication of the second volume of *Frontiers of Hormone Research*. The first volume had been on thyroid disease, and the second was to be on estrogens and aging. It was published by Karger and was the result of a Workshop Conference – Ageing and Estrogens, held in Geneva, October 5th and 6th, 1972 (sponsored by the International Health Foundation), which Pieter co-organized and co-chaired. Some of the more senior members of this Society, in the audience today, I know were at this meeting. Jaszmann presented some of his cross-sectional data from a huge study; 6500 women were sent questionnaires, and the response rate was in the order of 71%.

Jaszmann's data showed that the percentage of women reporting particular psychosomatic symptoms or complaints varied with biological age (from pre- through to late postmenopause). As might be predicted, there were clear increases in incidence for some symptoms (e.g. hot flushes and perspiration) in the early perimenopause which were maintained through to late postmenopause. Jaszmann also reported that, for other types of symptoms (headache and irritability) there was almost a doubling in incidence in the early perimenopause and it was suggested that certain psychological symptoms might be related to changes in ovarian status and to fluctuations in endogenous ovarian activity. This was, as far as I can see, one of the first reports linking psychological changes to ovarian activity and we have spent much of the last 20 years trying to confirm or refute this link.

All the data presented at this Workshop Conference were interesting, and there was clearly a lively discussion between the presentations. The comments about Jaszmann's paper were particularly interesting. Pieter was aware, as long ago as 1972, that there were methodological problems and that different methodologies could give different responses. Pieter had repeated Jaszmann's work in Zurich, but used a semi-structured interview, and found that the results were different for some symptoms from those obtained in Ede.

So, it was realized that the type of methodology might affect the results. I sometimes think it rather strange that we forget that the debate about methodology with psychosocial issues which is still continuing really starts back in the late 1960s and early 1970s.

There were of course, other interesting comments from participants at this meeting. Of Jaszmann's results, Mattson from Copenhagen asked 'Does PMT, whatever PMT is, influence menopausal symptoms?' and Hans Kopera from Austria who is still serving the Society as one of its Editors-in-Chief of *Maturitas*, said that his interpretation of Jaszmann's study was that low income and educational levels were associated with more complaints. Thus, sociodemographic issues appeared to affect the reporting of climacteric complaints. Differences between European and Mexican women were commented upon. Zárate Trevino who had worked with Pieter said, 'Yes, but at home in Mexico it's different – the higher the social class, the more the symptoms'. This meeting really exposed numerous problems which we still face in terms of how social class and income, for example, influence cultural attitudes and influence the reporting of symptoms. These are not new developments; they have been with us right from the early days.

Pieter then teamed up with Jean Kellerhals and in 1975 published data in *Acta Obstetricia Gynecologica Scandinavica*. I can give you, in the time permitted, no more than a flavor of this work. Their survey asked, amongst other things, about the effects of children being at home or having left home on psychological symptom reporting. In women whose children had left home, they showed that there was more reporting of symptoms (almost twice as much) in the premenopausal age group, but this finding was not present in older women. This was one of the first studies to suggest that the 'empty nest' syndrome – the fact that the children had left home, might influence reporting of symptoms during the climacteric. The effects of social class, already commented on by Jaszmann, again showed lower social classes reporting more symptoms in the early 40s and again in the late 50s age groups.

Largely, I suspect, because of Pieter's interest, *Maturitas* has always published extensively on the scientific and psychosocial issues of the climacteric. Anyone with any interest in this field has only to read the recent edition of the Journal to know this is so. This issue begins with a review by Jerry Greene of early cross-sectional data and this is followed by four different chapters, each by the lead author of groups worldwide who have done what are now called the longitudinal studies. At the end, there is an overview by Jerry Greene.

Before we consider the longitudinal studies. I thought it would be appropriate to review some of the cross-sectional data with you. My comments are based upon the review of Jerry Greene, to whom I make due acknowledgement. His review subdivided the cross-sectional data from 1965 through to 1979, and from 1980 through to 1990. There are,

I think, three important points to be made from the cross-sectional studies:

(1) For the most part, the studies report that there is a clear relationship between loss of ovarian function and the incidence of vasomotor symptoms;

(2) It is much less clear whether other symptoms increase in incidence during the climacteric and through into the early postmenopausal period. There is no consistency across the studies;

(3) The number of women who seem to be really distressed by psychological symptoms arising during the climacteric is, in fact, remarkably small if the general population studies are considered.

Greene's review also looked at the effects of sociodemographic and psychosocial factors. In these cross-sectional studies on symptom reporting during the climacteric years it is evident that sociodemographic factors, such as low socio-economic status, low income, low educational level, unemployment or unskilled employment, increase the reporting of climacteric symptoms. In terms of the psychosocial issues, negative attitudes have a similar influence. If the individual believes that menopause is going to be 'bad news' for any reason – perhaps because an elder sister or their mother had problems – if you have a negative attitude, then you are more likely to have problems. Poor social networking, poor marital relations, stressful life events, and recent bereavement are all associated with increased reporting of symptoms during the climacteric. All these data have been available from cross-sectional studies for some years but there is an important caveat; the cross-sectional studies are all, to a greater or lesser extent, flawed. Sample-size, statistical analyses and sampling methods are often inadequate and menopausal status criteria are often appallingly defined. There are problems with measurement of dependent and independent variables. Thus, the cross-sectional studies provide interesting but not definitive answers.

It is appropriate at this time to move back to Pieter. We left him in Geneva in 1975 and, as Hans Vemer has already mentioned, 1976 saw Pieter together with Bob Greenblatt and Michel Albeaux-Fernet organizing the first International Congress on the Menopause in La Grande Motte, France. Two things must be noted: firstly, the meeting was run under the auspices of the American Geriatric Society and the University of Montpellier, because the International Society had still to be founded; and secondly the Proceedings of that meeting (attended by about 130 menopause-mad freaks), still holds what I believe is a world record for sales. It was translated, as far as I know, into five languages selling 120 000 copies. I spoke to David Bloomer, who was responsible for its publication in 1976, and who is still associated, I am pleased to say, with this Society. If only writing text books today could achieve anything like those sales!

1978 saw the second International Congress on the Menopause, again held under the auspices of the American Geriatric Society, organized by Pieter, David Serr (who is the immediate past President of the Society), and by Bob Greenblatt. This second Congress went very well, and a group of delegates decided to play midwives and oversee two 'births'. Firstly, this group, the 'menopause club', had to have its own journal; late in 1978 Pieter became the founding editor of *Maturitas*. The second birth was that of the society. On November 25th 1978, at the International Health Foundation in Brussels, papers were signed which brought the International Menopause Society into existence. The signatures were those of Bob Greenblatt, David Serr, Pieter van Keep, Stuart Campbell, Herman Schneider, Regine Sitruk-Ware (still serving on the Executive Committee of the Society), and Jos Thijssen who has given the Society such tremendous help and support as auditor to its accounts over the last few years.

I really got to know Pieter very well during the summer and autumn of 1978. Pieter was Dutch – it goes without saying that I'm English – and for the most part England and Holland have enjoyed good relationships for the last 200 years. However, around 1670 or 1680 we were, for a time, at war. I'm afraid to say that the Dutch had much the better of some of the fights and skirmishes. The painting by Willem van de Velde the younger depicts the Battle of Texel. This was fought at sea and the *Golden Landy*, the Dutch flagship, fought with the *Charles*, the English flagship. Sadly, the Dutch won the day. In another skirmish, the *Royal Charles*, shown in the painting by Ludolf Bakhuizen was towed away into Dutch waters. This led the great English essayist, diarist, and political commentator, Samuel Pepys, to say – and I think it's a mark of great English literary talent to take a few words to express an entire nation's sentiments – 'The devil shits Dutchmen'. In later years Pieter often came to London to meetings with our Committee on Safety of Medicines, and if he had had a good day, he'd go and have a drink in the evening and would say 'Tonight Samuel Pepys has woken from his grave and he is sitting there saying, "the devil is shitting Dutchmen again."'

I will comment but briefly on Pieter's contraception career. In 1981 he was awarded the 9th Annual Gregory Pincus Lectureship for his work on oral contraceptive formulations and that, I know, made Pieter immensely proud. In 1984, Pieter left the International Health Foundation (which, by this time, had moved its headquarters to Brussels) and returned, as International Medical Director, to Organon.

I would now like to review the five major longitudinal psychosocial studies with you. But before we do that, I'd like to go back to Ede where Laszlo Jaszmann, supported and encouraged by Pieter in the mid 1960s, had started off his cross-sectional studies. The 1967 study from Ede was repeated in 1977 and then repeated again in 1987 by Anna Oldenhave. The data from these three studies spanning the 20-year period appear in *Well-being and Sexuality in the Climacteric*. I will just draw, if I may, two sets of information from it. Up to now in this Memorial Lecture, we have considered women as though they were all intact (i.e. with intact ovaries) but clearly some women will have undergone hysterectomy. The effect of hysterectomy on reporting of symptoms and how it affects them, not only during the climacteric but at other times, must be considered.

Over this 20-year period of investigation, if they had undergone hysterectomy, the Ede data showed that women from their late 30s to early 60s report more moderate and severe flushes.

In terms of severe aches and atypical complaints (a compilation of 21 different symptoms, including restlessness, irritability, etc.) it was found that from the age of 40 through to 60, 'hysterectomized' women do less well than apparently non-hysterectomized women and that their problems predated the hysterectomy. This led Anna Oldenhave to conclude that women who eventually come to surgery have long-standing problems and make more use of medical resources, eventually ending up with a gynecologist who, because he/she has no other alternative, offers a hysterectomy. This really doesn't help because their problems continue thereafter. We will return to this later on.

Now, back to the longitudinal studies. Four of these studies are reviewed by their first authors in the recent edition of *Maturitas*; the principal authors are Holte from Norway, Hunter from England, Kaufert from Manitoba and McKinlay from Massachusetts. The fifth study is by Matthews and colleagues from Pittsburg, Pennysylvania

I can only give you a flavor of these studies. I am briefly going to show what I think are the more interesting data from each of these studies. Beginning with Arne Holte's data – the climacteric was associated with an increase in vasomotor complaints, vaginal dryness, palpitations, and social dysfunction, a reduction in headaches and breast tenderness, and no change in depression, anxiety, and irritability.

Myra Hunter, working in the southeast of London, reported that the climacteric was associated with vasomotor symptoms and sleep problems. And factors which predicted vasomotor symptoms were premenopausal flushes (25% of the variance) and previous premenstrual tension (PMT) (12% of the variance). Although she reported an increase in depressed mood during peri- and postmenopause, this was not really related to changes in ovarian status. Depressed mood was best predicted by premenopausal depression, a negative stereotype, low employment status, and low social class.

We will now cross the Atlantic to Manitoba, and to Patricia Kaufert and co-workers and then to Massachusetts and Sonia McKinlay and her group. I must say that I think that all of these groups have made huge contributions to our understanding of these issues. Patricia Kaufert, in this article in *Maturitas*, concentrated on relationships between menopause and depression and concluded that the individual's health coupled with shifts and stress in the family life during menopausal years are more likely to trigger depression than hormonal changes. She also confirmed what Anna Oldenhave had reported previously; that of the four categories of menopausal status – pre, peri-, postmenopausal and hysterectomy, only one was linked to depression, and that was hysterectomy. Again, the explanation is not that hysterectomy *per se* causes depression. There is a relationship due to a greater risk of surgery in patients with pre-existing depression, and sadly these patients continue to have depression postoperatively.

Sonia McKinlay's huge study confirmed that menopausal age is profoundly affected by smoking (bringing menopause forward by 1.8 years). It reported for the first time that the perimenopause transition lasts almost 4 years, and again that there is a transitory relationship between reporting of symptoms and menopause with the exception of vasomotor symptoms. Interestingly, this study reported the highest rate of medical consultations in women with the longest perimenopausal transitions, which perhaps is to be expected.

The fifth longitudinal study that I could find in the literature is not reviewed within this edition of *Maturitas* but was published in the *Journal of Consulting Clinical Psychology*. Matthews and colleagues described an increased reporting of flushes and decreased reporting of introspectiveness during the climacteric period. Natural menopause did not have negative mental health consequences. I found the data here difficult to interpret because women with hypertension, with diabetes, and other long-term diseases, and women on psychotropic medication were not, in fact, included but were deliberately excluded from this investigation. It is not clear whether this selection bias influenced the results. However, far be it for me to criticize any of the longitudinal studies. Arne Holte, in his review of his and the other work, did so and said that with all the longitudinal studies we must remember that, although they are much better than the cross-sectional studies, although they are prospective, and although the methods of statistical analysis are far improved, some of them still have problems with small numbers, short follow-up periods, and perhaps less than ideal criteria for definition of menopause.

So, how do these longitudinal data assist us in an interpretation of what is and what is not closely related to changes in ovarian status as women go through the climacteric years? It seems to me that Patricia Kaufert and Sonia McKinlay have investigated these possible relationships from a sociological and epidemiological viewpoint, whereas Arne Holte and Myra Hunter have used more of a psychological viewpoint. The answer may well depend on from which point of view you look at the data. If you are a sociologist or an epidemiologist, you may say that the data stand, as they clearly do, in their own right and that nothing more needs to be said; that would be one point of view. I would like to think that, as a clinician and also perhaps if I were a psychologist, that I would use these data as a springboard for asking other questions which may help to improve the quality of medical services on offer to our climacteric and early postmenopausal patients. Despite some limitations and anxieties about methodology, there is a consensus that in a general population only vasomotor symptoms are associated with the climacteric and that there are sociodemographic and psychosocial issues that will predict symptom reporting. Also, in a general population, few women actually have significant distress.

However, as clinicians, whether in primary care in the community, or in secondary or tertiary care in hospital, we need to know how the women who sit in front of us at a menopause consultation differ from women within the general population. Increasingly in western Europe and in the United States, the so-called developed countries, clinicians and the pharmaceutical industry are going to have to justify more and more the expenditure on hormone preparations to relieve menopausal symptoms. If I was to be asked by a government accountant or minister, 'How do your menopause clinic women, in terms of symptoms, differ from the general population? Give me a list of references.' I would actually find that there are scant data in the literature to help provide an answer. Within the peri- and postmenopausal population, as I have said, I think it's clinically and psychologically useful, and increasingly economically important, to identify women who are susceptible to high rates of symptom reporting and use of medical services.

If we turn to the literature, there is only one study that I can find that actually reports a comparison between a general population and a

10

menopause clinic population in the same locality – the study of Susan Ballinger published in *Maturitas* in 1985. I know many gynecologists will be surprised to hear that between the general population and the menopause clinic attenders, there was no difference in reporting of hot flushes and vaginal dryness. When comparisons of menopause clinic attenders and women in the general population were made, the clinic patients suffered more from psychosocial stress, clinical depression, anxiety, and vulnerability. It was the psychological reporting that brought the patients to the menopause clinic.

Myra Hunter is conducting a similar study in southeast England. Some of these data have already been published in 1988, again looking at the group of women Myra and I had previously studied in 1986. Factors predicting menopause clinic attendance in southeast London were investigated and five variables correctly classified three out of four women who were attending a menopause clinic. These were depressed mood; flushes and sweats; a conviction that menopause was a disease; difficulties in coping with symptoms, and anxiety. It was this type of symptom clustering that was making women request a menopause clinic appointment.

Later this week, one of my research fellows, Michael Marsh, will present some data from a recently completed study in which we have tried to go one step further back than Susan Ballinger. We have compared women in the general population who have made it clear that they are not going to seek HRT and women in the general population who have made a decision to seek HRT. Menopause clinic attenders may, of course, be a biased and selective group, and previously symptomatic women who have been adequately treated by primary care physicians will not appear in a menopause clinic. By going direct to the general population, we have tried to minimize these types of selection bias.

When we looked at the women in the general population who were not going to seek HRT and the women in that population who said they were going to request HRT, we found no differences between the groups for frequency or severity of flushes or vaginal dryness. What separated the two groups were differences in reporting of depression and somatic symptoms such as 'butterflies' in the stomach, and palpitations. So, if we consider an imaginary woman of about 55 years of age in the general population, who has decided against HRT, we can say that for the most part she will experience flushes and sweats which are related to a change in ovarian status. If we consider her equally imaginary twin sister, who is going to attend for a menopause consultation and request HRT, she will attend not so much because she has the flushes and sweats but because of (and our data are absolutely consistent with those of Myra Hunter and those of Susan Ballinger), anxiety, irritability, depressed mood, and certain somatic symptoms. It is these which differentiate the clinic attenders and clinic non-attenders.

So, in 1993, which treatments should we be offering menopause clinic attenders? The gynecologists are going to say, 'Give these women hormones', whereas the psychiatrists are going to say, 'Give these women psychotrophic medication'. I'm sure that many of you have been exposed to these arguments. The gynecologist insists, 'You should not poison women with psychotrophic medication,' and the psychiatrist retorts, 'You should not poison them with hormones.' What we need, of course, are some good prospective placebo-controlled studies to try to untangle these issues. We need studies where we have some sort of psychological therapeutic intervention, with one group of women receiving that plus estrogen and another group receiving that plus a matching placebo. It is only if we do those studies that we will be able to determine which strategy is more effective.

What else, in 1993, might we clinicians be able to learn from the social scientist? Women are increasingly requesting some sort of treatment to prevent osteoporosis and fractures, yet there are remarkably few data in the literature about psychosocial consequences of osteoporotic fractures. Fortunately, *Maturitas*, and Pieter's influence as founding editor, are there to make sure that the social scientists have a platform for publication of good data.

And then there is the other major consequences of ovarian failure, which you will hear of much during the next four days, which is arterial disease. We have a fair amount of data on psychosocial issues, on smoking, and on type A behavior in men with arterial disease, but where are the comparable data for women? The database is so scant as to be transparent.

This will be the first symposium, the first International Menopause Symposium, that Pieter will not have attended. There are aspects of Pieter which do not come across in a formal portrait and which I would like to leave you with in terms of a thought. When Pieter knew he was dying, he took to himself this text, these few words from Kanzatzakis the Greek Nobel Laureate as expressed through the mouth of Zorba the Greek, 'I do not fear anything, I do not expect anything, and I am free'. I'm sure Pieter's spirit will be with us over the next four or five days – his humor, his humanity, his humility, his drive, his enthusiasm, and his kindness as well. I think that, of all his achievements, it was the establishment of this Society that gave him the greatest pleasure.

Malcolm Whitehead

12

SOURCES

Jaczmann, L. (1973). Epidemiology of climacteric and post-climacteric complaints. *Frontiers of Hormone Research*, Vol. 2, *Ageing and Estrogens*, pp. 22–34. (Basel: Karger)

van Keep, P. A. (1970). A study of attitudes to menopause across Western Europe. International Health Foundation, Geneva

van Keep, P. A. and Kellerhals, J. (1975). The ageing woman: about the influence of some social and cultural factors on the change in attitudes and behaviour that occur during and after menopause. *Acta Obstet. Gynecol. Scand.,* Suppl. 51, 17–27

Greene, J. G. and Visser, A. Ph. (1992). The cross-sectional legacy: an introduction to longitudinal studies of the climacteric. *Maturitas*, 14, 2, 95–101

van Keep, P. A., Greenblatt, R. B. and Albeaux-Fernet, M. (1976). *Consensus on Menopause Research: a Summary of International Opinion.* (Lancaster: MTP Press)

van Keep, P. A., Serr, D. M. and Greenblatt, R. B. (1979). *Female and Male Climacteric: Current Opinion 1978.* (Lancaster: MTP Press)

Willem van de Velde the Younger. *The Battle of the Texel, 11th–21st August 1673.* Greenwich National Maritime Museum

Ludolf Bakhuizen. *The Royal Charles carried into Dutch Waters, June 1667.* Greenwich National Maritime Museum

Oldenhave, A. (1991). *Well-being and Sexuality in the Climacteric: a Survey Based on 6622 Women.* (Dissertation). (Leidschendam: Drukkerij Excelsior)

Holte, A. (1992). Influences of natural menopause on health complaints: a prospective study of healthy Norwegian women. *Maturitas*, 14, 2, 127–41

Hunter, M. (1992). The South-East England Longitudinal Study of the Climacteric and Postmenopause. *Maturitas*, 14, 2, 117–26

Kaufert, P. A., Gilbert, P. and Tate, R. (1992). The Manitoba Project: a Re-examination of the Link between Menopause and Depression. *Maturitas*, 14, 2, 143–55

McKinlay, S., Brambilla, D. J. and Posner, J. G. (1992). The Normal Menopause Transition. *Maturitas*, 14, 2, 103–15

Matthews, K. A., Wing, R. R., Kuller, L. H. *et al.* (1990). Influences of natural menopause on psychological characteristics and symptoms of middle-aged healthy women. *J. Consult. Clin. Psychol.,* 58, 345–51

Ballinger, S. E. (1985). Psychosocial stress and symptoms of menopause: a comparative study of menopause clinic patients and non-patients. *Maturitas*, 7, 315–27

Hunter, M. (1988). Psychosocial aspects of the climacteric and postmenopause. In Studd, J. W. and Whitehead, M. I. *The Menopause*, pp. 55–64. (Oxford: Blackwell)

Section 1

A global aspect
on the menopause – symptoms,
work and social life

2

Menopause – the global aspect

M. Flint

BACKGROUND

Several aspects of the menopause are universal, shared by all women from all parts of the globe. One of these is a mean age at which this reproductive phenomenon is achieved. This does not mean that all women have their menopause at around the age of 50, the traditional age given for modern Western women. Quite the contrary, the mean age is population-specific, with a range from the early 40s, in Yucatan Mayan women[1] to the early 50s for the Ede population in the Netherlands[2].

Furthermore, the notion that each culture's menopausal age would be unchangeable is no longer tenable. Flint's suggestion that there may have been a secular trend in menopausal age in European cultures, as there had been in the United States[3], and that this trend might continue, was based on the belief that this trend had been seen in Western cultures, with menarcheal age. Flint also naïvely stated that Western cultures might have reached an age limit with a 'universal' mean of about 50 years, which would be followed in other cultures as they became more westernized, with diets richer in protein and fat, better health care and better education. This was modified as recently as 1989, when Brambilla and McKinlay[4] noted that for a population of women in the state of Massachusetts, the mean age of menopause was 51.3 years. This is far later than the age of 49.7, reported by MacMahon and Worcester in 1966[5]. Can we then conclude that a secular trend appears to be continuing, at least in the United States? Will it also hold for other cultures? Only more longitudinal research into secular trends in age of menopause in non-Western cultures will be able to answer this question.

Table 1 Age at menopause in various populations

Culture	Age
Indonesians in Central Java	
educated[12]	50.2
rural	46.0
Indonesians in West Sumatra	
educated[12]	48.7
rural	47.5
Karachi, Pakistan[22]	47.0
Netherlands (Ede)[2]	51.4
Rajputs	
state of Rajasthan[8]	48.9
state of Himachal Pradesh[8]	47.3
United States – Massachusetts[4]	51.3
Yucatan Mayan[1]	42.0

The range of ages is quite varied, culture to culture. We do not yet know whether this is due to genetic or environmental factors, both physical and cultural, or to methodological differences in attaining these ages. Some examples of age at menopause are presented in Table 1. These ages were derived by probit analysis and, therefore, have statistical validity. Menopausal age is, particularly for non-Western cultures, usually derived from data that are retrospective and have poor statistical reliability and validity. Further, this age information comes from small samples or populations with non-random selection, or both. Until a concerted effort is made to use probit analysis, random sampling and large sample size in studies of menopausal age in non-Western cultures, we need to look at the ages given for these cultures with some concern.

Another global aspect of menopause is the physiological dimension of this event. Whatever else is known about menopause, whatever it may be called and however it may be acknowledged, there is a universal recognition by all women of the physiological cessation of menstrual periods at a specific time, if not a specific age. There is not, however, a universal set of symptoms associated with menopause that we can say all women cognitively share.

Even those purely physiological symptoms noted by Utian and Serr[6] – hot flashes, profuse perspiration and atrophic vaginitis – which are due to estrogen loss in the menopause, are not cognitively known or acknowledged by many women in different cultures. Many authors[1,7–10] attest to a lack of these symptoms in the various cultures they have studied. In fact, both Lock[7], studying Japanese women, and Wright[9], studying the Navaho Indians, claim that there are no words for menopause or hot flash in the vocabularies of these respective cultures.

Wilbush[11] has emphasized the fact that 'no woman of another culture, unaffected by Western medical attitudes has been known to complain of climacteric disturbances'. He explains this by noting that there is a dichotomy between what Western medicine views as symptoms associated with the menopause, whether they be physiological, psychological or psychosomatic and what he calls 'semeions'. The former he defines as spontaneous complaints of an ailing person, often non-verbal, that have low reliability, are strongly affected by culture and draw attention to the plight of the sufferer. The latter are defined as subjective sensations, largely verbal, usually elicited by a physician which gives information about discomforts and are relatively culture-free. He advocates using both of these definitions in defining the menopausal physiological symptoms experienced by women, particularly in non-Western cultures.

Prior to Flint and Samil's[12] menopausal research, using physicians as interviewers of urbanized, and therefore more Westernized Indonesian women, as well as rural and migratory urbanized rural women, Wilbush's[11] dichotomy might have been supported. It would certainly be one explanation of why some populations of women do not have any climacteric complaints – are we asking non-Western women for their symptoms (Western defined) or semeions (individually described sensations)? However, whether we are describing symptoms or semeions, Indonesian women do complain of hot flashes, atrophic vaginitis, profuse perspiration and fatigue, among their most common disturbances.

A final global aspect shared by all women is their culture's influence on the cognition of the meaning of the menopause itself, not just its physiological symptomatology. Each individual woman has been raised in her own culture, with its belief systems, attitudes and values about all facets of life, including the menopause. In order for her to have established a cognitive map of responses to the menopause, both physiological and emotional, she would have had to have learned what is culturally relevant about the menopause, throughout her life. If she is a member of a culture in which being stoic, suffering in silence and not complaining about menopausal symptoms is valued, such as Davis[13] found among Newfoundland women, then she will try to be that during her premenopausal, perimenopausal and postmenopausal years. If she is in a culture in which her status becomes elevated after menopause and her life is made easier, as is true in many cultures such as those of the Basuto[14], Iteso[15], Ibo[16], the Moroccans[17] and the Homa[18], then expectations and behaviors will adhere to these cognitions. If she is in many Western cultures, conversely,

Table 6 Factors influencing the age at menopause

Menopause vs. parity	$p < 0.05$
Menopause vs. age at menarche	NS
Menopause vs. smoking	NS
Menopause vs. oral pills	NS
Menopause vs. nutritional status	NS

NS, not significant

Table 7 Menopausal symptoms. Figures are percentages

	Menstruating women		Menopausal women ($n = 1327$)
	Regular ($n = 735$)	Irregular ($n = 292$)	
No complaints	49.4	25.7	53.4
Vasomotor symptoms			
Hot flushes	10.3	22.3	5.7
Night sweats	6.5	17.5	5.2
Psychosomatic symptoms			
Dizziness	23.1	45.7	22.2
Palpitation	18.4	34.2	15.0
Irritability	23.7	41.1	17.3
Headache	22.6	36.3	18.0
Insomnia	16.6	34.2	16.4
Depression	2.7	8.7	2.2

Some women reported more than one symptom

taken into account. Higher parity seemed to show a statistically significant correlation with a later than average menopause (Table 6).

Climacteric symptoms

In one of our studies using interviews of women between 45 and 59 years of age, climacteric symptoms were observed before the actual menopause (Table 7). About 50% of women who were still having more or less regular periods experienced one or more climacteric manifestations. When periods became irregular, 75% of the women experienced symptoms, and about half still experienced symptoms 1 year after menstrual cessation. These symptoms varied a great deal from person to person with respect to number, intensity and duration. Women with irregular menstruation seemed to complain of a greater number and intensity of symptoms.

Table 8 Urinary problems in 534 women

	n	%
No symptom	228	42.7
Occasional but very slight	248	46.4
Occasional and quite disturbing	19	3.6
Often and most unpleasant	39	7.3

Table 9 Vaginal dryness in 511 women

	n	%
No symptom	201	39.3
Sometimes, but very slight	237	46.4
Sometimes, and quite embarrassing	39	7.6
Often and most unpleasant	31	6.1
Often, but not unpleasant	3	0.6

Urinary complaints

In a study of women with college education aged between 45 and 60 years, 11% complained of disturbing urinary symptoms such as urgency, frequency and/or incontinence (Table 8). These symptoms were rarely, if ever, sought by examining physicians and were equally rarely mentioned by the patients. Several resigned themselves to these disturbing symptoms, accepting them as a part of the change of life.

Genital manifestations

In the same group of college educated women, 13% reported significant vaginal dryness (Table 9). The implication of this complaint was not, however, exactly clear to the investigators.

The frequency of sexual intercourse was rather low in this group of women, currently married and living with their husbands (Table 10). This tendency for decreased libido was somewhat substantiated by their attitudes (Tables 11 and 12). A similar pattern of sexual attitude was found in another group of women, who were housewives with up to grade 6 schooling, currently married and living with their spouses and were at least 1 year into their menopause (Tables 13 and 14).

Table 10 Time since last sexual intercourse in 452 women

	n	%
Within the last week	160	39.8
About 15 days ago	88	21.9
About 1 month ago	52	12.9
About 2–3 months ago	27	6.7
About 3–6 months ago	15	3.7
>6 months ago	60	14.9

Table 11 Preferred frequency of sexual intercourse in 394 women[1]

	n	%
Far more frequently	2	0.5
Rather more frequently	20	5.1
As often as you do now	178	45.2
Rather less frequently	122	30.9
Much less frequently	71	18.0
None at all	1	0.3

Table 12 Attitude towards sexual intercourse in 493 women[1]

	n	%
At my age sex is no longer of great importance	234	47.5
At my age, I am done with sex	22	4.5
At my age sex is still important	235	47.7

Table 13 Sexual intercourse in 1192 menopausal housewives of lower education[2]

	n	%
Sexual intercourse		
Yes	467	39.2
With dyspareunia	67	5.6
Without dyspareunia	400	33.6
No	725	60.8

Association between the wives' menopause and human immunodeficiency virus (HIV) infection in men

The decline of libido during the menopausal period may be a direct influence of the ebbing estrogen on the female psyche, or an indirect

Table 14 Sexual desire in menopausal housewives of lower education[2]

	n	%
Sexual desire after menopause	1147	
No sexual desire	681	59.4
Decreased	315	27.5
Same as before	147	12.8
Increased	4	0.3

result of dyspareunia caused by an atrophic vagina. Occupational and/or domestic responsibilities may also have a negative effect on libido. If this is the case, the effect of the menopause on the sexual behavior of the spouses can only be conjectured. Some of the husbands may possibly be accommodating to their wives' loss of libido and come to accept it in time. A number of them, however, may be obliged to seek gratification for their sexual need away from home.

Thailand is one of a few countries in Asia that has a major HIV epidemic. Most cases are infected through heterosexual contacts, and the number of HIV-positive individuals was estimated at >500 000 up to May 1993. Studies in two districts in Chiangmai, where HIV-positive rates are among the highest in the country, revealed an interesting biphasic pattern of prevalence rates in Thai males (Figure 1). The first peak is probably not difficult to understand: these young men, many of whom are army recruits and college freshmen, and many unmarried, seek pleasure and sexual adventure from commercial sex workers. Many of them drink before visiting brothels, fail to take proper precautions and do not use condoms. The second peak is, however, quite disturbing. Could it be that these middle-aged men, who were mostly married, became victims of HIV because their wives had reached the menopause and could not gratify them sexually? Could hormonal replacement therapy (HRT) and sexual counselling be helpful for such middle-aged couples?

Coronary heart disease (CHD) and osteoporosis

There have been some clinical studies on CHD and osteoporosis in Thailand, but good epidemiological data are scarce and often unsatisfactory. The available statistics reported by the Ministry of Public Health are probably grossly under-reported.

The menopause can be rightly regarded as a biological change due to the waning of ovarian hormones. Biological changes are further modified

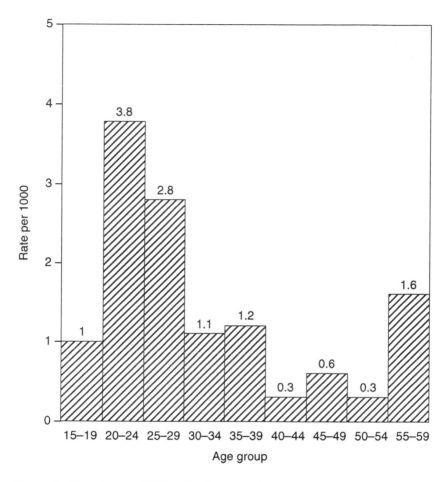

Figure 1   Prevalence of HIV antibody seropositivity per 1000 population of San Pa Tong District, Chiangmai Province. Source: monitoring of male patients attenting out-patient department, San Pa Tong Hospital, Nov. 90–Dec. 91 (V. Poshyachinda, personal communication)

by lifestyles adopted by the women. Therefore it can only be assumed that as Thailand is becoming more and more industrialized, the prevalence rates for CHD and osteoporosis will increase proportionally, as in the case of the Hong Kong Chinese[3].

The pill generation

There is an emerging new generation of women in developing countries who have either been satisfied acceptors of hormonal contraception and/or are well educated. They are often career women who are usually health conscious. Some of them subscribe to health clubs or fitness centers. This new generation of women, usually eager to discuss frankly various subjects, including those related to sexual problems during the perimenopause, are prospective acceptors of HRT with long-term compliance.

THE CONCERNS

The United Nations' Agencies have many good health programs, with particular emphasis on women in developing countries. There are programs for children carried out by UNICEF, and many WHO programs for different periods in life, including maternal and child health, the adolescents, the child-bearing period and geriatrics. However, there seems to be a big gap in a woman's life between 45 and 60 years of age, during which there is virtually no supporting program for her at all. Although a monograph was compiled by WHO experts[4], relevant to the health of women during this critical period, it is now over 10 years old and none of its 13 expert recommendations has ever been implemented. This is rather disappointing when one considers that many victims of the menopause are probably at their best as far as personal endeavors are concerned and have reached the peak of maturity or the top of their career ladders, both in government and private sectors, and even in politics. Even if they are just housewives, many are important breadearners for their families and play a major role in taking care of their children. Yet many of them live miserable lives, all because of their declining ovarian function. Without the leadership of WHO, developing countries, as member states of WHO, will not be able to place health issues of perimenopausal women at a high enough priority to draw adequate government support to establish relevant health care services.

A large number of women in the third world are enduring the passage through the menopause phase of their lives without attention. This is a denial of their rights to health care and services which would enable them to attain 'true health' as defined by the World Health Organization. Health and social equity demands that steps be taken to end this unfortunate situation for this large segment of society.

The success of family planning programs in developing countries has been attributed mainly to women: men have only contributed a small complementary role in the effort. Women may be likened to brave soldiers who fight determinedly the war against population explosion. These women are not only practising family planning, but thousands of them around the world have participated as volunteers in the development of new contraceptives. In clinical trials some have suffered fatal complications, although fortunately this is very rare, and many may have been left with varying degrees of morbidity. After all they have done, they are dismissed with little or no concerns about their future health, just because they are no longer needed, having passed their fertile period. How can we be sure that there will not be any long-term post-contraceptive effects from hormonal agents and tubal ligation, for instance.

We do not seem to be interested in the mid-life crisis that follows contraceptive discontinuation. Some women in their fifties have refused to stop taking oral contraceptive pills because they would experience untoward symptoms of estrogen deficiency. These women have come to realize their health needs in the perimenopausal period from self-observation. Family planning programs in developing countries should perhaps be extended a little longer into the perimenopausal years to cover those needs, together with proper counselling and clinical services.

HORMONAL REPLACEMENT THERAPY IN THAILAND

The VIth International Congress on the Menopause held in Bangkok in November 1990, attended by 150 Thai participants, mostly gynecologists, can rightly be regarded as an important milestone for the HRT program in Thailand.

Since that Congress, there have been regular educational opportunities for the public, including three television programs arranged by the Royal Thai College of Obstetricians and Gynecologists and numerous talks using private forums such as Lions and Rotary Clubs. People in the field of education have been made to understand the problems posed by the menopause, thereby lessening the fear of HRT. and its complications. Pharmaceutical companies have been very supportive in this attempt and have sponsored numerous symposia and lectures for members of the medical profession, taking advantage of world renowned experts passing through the region. Many articles on the menopause and HRT have been published in daily newspapers and popular women's magazines.

In our Menopause Clinic at Chulalongkorn University Hospital, inter-specialty referrals have been increasing. Dry eyes, dry skin, joint pains and urinary complaints are some of the problems being referred to us.

Lately, psychiatrists have also been referring their patients for hormonal evaluation and subsequent HRT, an unprecedented practice. Earlier this year, a small survey by telephone followed by short questionnaires was made to colleagues in Obstetrics and Gynecology Departments of major hospitals around the country. It is very interesting to discover that the Congress had made considerable impact on their attitude to the menopause and HRT. Several well-known opponents of HRT have become fervent supporters. Several larger hospitals now run menopause clinics. In the past, if the patient was over 40 years of age, bilateral salpingo-oophorectomy was routinely performed during abdominal hysterectomy. As a rule, no HRT or only short-term hormonal therapy was offered after such surgical menopause. From the small survey mentioned earlier, most of the gynecologists interviewed would now leave the ovaries alone unless the patient is over 45 years of age. The majority now advocate long-term HRT postoperatively.

It is difficult to obtain accurate figures on drug sales related to HRT since they are closely guarded commercial secrets. It is, however, estimated that drug sales increased by about 50% in 1992 compared to those in 1990. The annual increase is now about 20% with total annual sales worth more than US$ 600 000.

Last but not least, while the pattern of HRT in Bangkok and other large urban areas would be rather similar to that in developed countries, the picture in the rest of the country is entirely different. The Family Health Division of the Ministry of Public Health, the agency responsible for our National Family Planning Program, is now undertaking studies to develop a more appropriate model for menopause counselling and HRT. A model to suit the lifestyles of the majority of women who live outside Bangkok and in rural areas is urgently needed and hopefully it will also be a cost-effective one. This program will eventually be an extension of our present family planning program.

REFERENCES

1. Dusitsin, N., Yamarat, K. and Havanond, P. K. A. P. Studies on HRT in college educated Thai women aged 45–60. In press
2. Chompootweep, S., Tankeyoon, M., Yamarat, K., Poomsuwan, P. and Dusitsin, N. (1993). The menopausal age and climacteric complaints in Thai women in Bangkok. *Maturitas,* **17**, 63–71
3. Lau, E. M. C., Cooper, C., Wickham, C., Donnan, S. and Barker, D. J. P. (1990). Hip fracture in Hong Kong and Britain. *Int. J. Epidemiol.,* **19**, 1191
4. Report of a WHO Scientific Group. (1981). *Research on the Menopause.* WHO Technical Report Series 670

4

Characteristics and perceptions of menopause in a Pakistani community

S. Wasti, R. Kamal and S. C. Robinson

INTRODUCTION

Population growth is a major problem which the country is facing. The population of Pakistan is 120 million. If the assumptions underlying the median variant projection of the World Bank[1] are correct, then by the year 2025, the total population of the country will be 250 million. Twelve percent of the female population will be postmenopausal. At present, menopause is a neglected life-cycle milestone. Health resources are directed towards combating female health issues of the reproductive age group. Will menopause be thought to present a major physiological and psychological change in a female's life and will it be associated with an increase in morbidity and health care utilization? As very little information was available concerning this event in Pakistan, we undertook to collect information on the age, features and perceptions of menopause in three socioeconomic groups of urban Karachi. Our aim was also to verify the findings of our earlier study[2].

MATERIALS AND METHODS

Using a female interviewer who was familiar with Urdu (the national language of Pakistan), candidates did answer questions quite readily. Interview surveys were conducted from 1st November 1991 to 30th June 1992 in three socioeconomic groups of urban Karachi, as socioeconomic status has been demonstrated to influence health, nutrition and education.

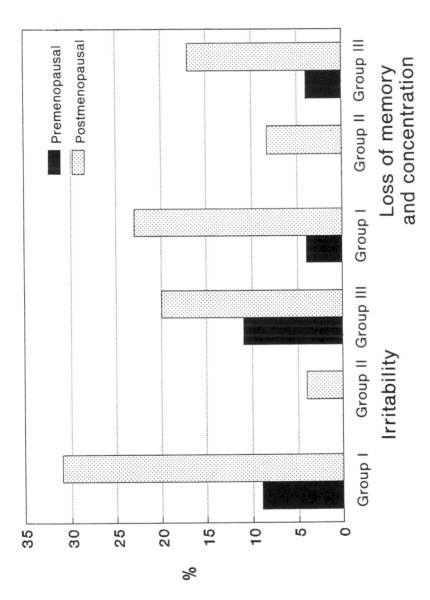

Figure 3a Psychological symptoms

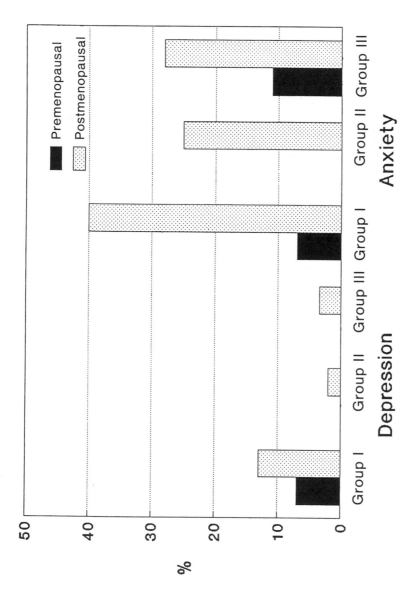

Figure 3b Psychological symptoms

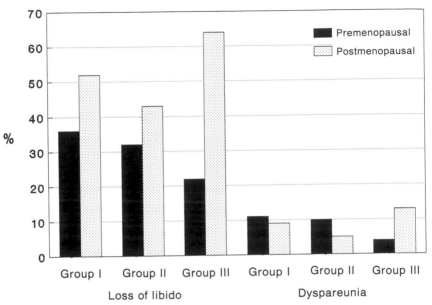

Figure 4 Sexual problems

women and 29% of postmenopausal women in Group I. In Group II only 7% of postmenopausal women experienced difficulty in sleeping and in Group III 2% and 15% of pre- and postmenopausal women, respectively, reported such problems. Figure 3 represents psychological symptoms such as anxiety, depression, irritability and loss of memory and concentration. The frequency of the symptoms was associated with menstrual status. Loss of libido and dyspareunia were also assessed. A total of 36% of premenopausal women and 52% of postmenopausal women in Group I experienced loss of libido. In Group II, 32% of premenopausal and 43% of postmenopausal women reported this complaint and 4% of premenopausal and 64% of postmenopausal women in Group III. Dyspareunia was reported by 11% and 9% in pre- and postmenopausal women, respectively, in Group I, 10% in premenopausal and 5% in postmenopausal in Group II, and 4% and 13% in pre- and postmenopausal women in Group 3. This problem did not show intergroup variance. Table 2 illustrates urinary symptoms and Table 3 shows the frequency, nature of treatment and advice taken for problems related to the menopause. The table includes the different health care providers that were used by women of the three groups.

Table 2 Percentage distribution of urinary symptoms in women of three socioeconomic groups ($n = 606$)

	Group I		Group II		Group III	
	Pre.	*Post.*	*Pre.*	*Post.*	*Pre.*	*Post.*
Incontinence	0	17	3	14	0	12
Urgency (<5 min)	2	15	10	12	3	9
Frequency (>7 times/day)	4	10	3	8	2	8
Nocturia >twice/night	2	4	2	6	3	6
Dysuria	4	6	3.2	8	2	8

Pre. = premenopausal; Post. = postmenopausal

Table 3 Percentage of women taking advice and treatment

	Group I (32%)	Group II (20%)	Group III (8%)
Nurses	—	2	2
TBA	—	2	2
Homoeopath	—	7	6
Family doctor	31	25	20
Gynecologist	4	10	0
Psychiatrist	3	0	0
Orthopedics	4	2	6

DISCUSSION

The mean age of menopause was found to be 47 ± 3.65 years. This figure correlates with that reported in our earlier study[1]. The median age was 48 years. Socioeconomic status had no bearing on the age of menopause. Mean and median age of menopause was the same in the three socioeconomic groups. There is evidence that menopause may be delayed in women of high parity. Stanford and colleagues[3] reported that women with five or more children had a median age at menopause 2 years later than nulliparous females. In our study, the mean parity was five and did not seem to have an effect on the age of menopause.

In Karachi, except for loss of libido and dyspareunia, women belonging to the lower socioeconomic status had less symptoms. We can only speculate on the reason for this. Women facing problems due to socioeconomic deprivation may tend to overlook minor problems. This is in contrast to the work done by Green and Cooke[4]. In their study, no relationship was found between vasomotor symptoms and social class status, but there was a marked association between the latter and other symptoms. A differential relationship between socioeconomic status and mean symptom was found in a study of a general population of Italian women by Campagnoli and co-workers[5]. This study found that socioeconomic status was unrelated to vasomotor symptoms but women of low status tended to report more severe psychological symptoms than did women of high status.

In our study, dyspareunia had no intergroup variance in the postmenopausal women. However, loss of libido occurred in 62% of postmenopausal women in socioeconomic Group III, 43% of postmenopausal women in socioeconomic Group II and 52% of the most affluent postmenopausal women. This could be due to our sociocultural milieu, where sexuality is associated with younger age and a female above 40 years is considered old in the middle and lower socioeconomic strata of the society. Two or more generations may share the same housing unit, thus having an inhibitory influence on sexuality.

Treatment sought was found to be related directly to socioeconomic status; 32% in Group I, 20% in Group II and 8% in Group III taking advice and treatment. The family doctor was consulted by 31% in Group I, 25% in Group II and 20% in Group III. A gynecologist was consulted by 4% of women in Group I, 10% in Group II and 1% in Group III. A psychiatrist was only approached by 3% of women in Group I for psychological symptoms. Customs, tradition, cost, availability perceptions and awareness may influence the decision to seek advice.

Sixty percent of women interviewed perceive menopause as a natural physiological phenomenon and were happy that they were getting more time to pray, had a feeling of well being and felt clean. There was general relief at no longer having children and freedom from worry about contraception. Menopause was welcomed if the family size was complete. In our society, as a female ages she gains considerable importance in the family. Her opinion and advice is sought and she is respected more than ever. Daughter and daughter-in-laws take over the household chores and grandchildren become a great source of pleasure. These factors could influence their perceptions of the menopause. Forty percent felt some change in sexual life, and only 5% regretted the change in body image and felt old and unhappy.

CONCLUSION

This study confirms the findings of our previous work[1]. The mean age of menopause was 47 years in three socioeconomic groups of urban Karachi. Except for symptoms related to urogenital atrophy, women of the lower socioeconomic groups had fewer symptoms than the affluent groups. Treatment sought for the symptoms of menopause was found to be directly related to socioeconomic status. Women belonging to higher socioeconomic groups are more educated and travel more. They are subjected to Western medical and advertizing pressure concerning menopause and related symptoms. In addition, menopause is now discussed frequently and women's groups organize lectures and seminars on this topic. It may be that this may generate interest in hormone replacement therapy. Early age of menopause could result in related complications affecting more of the aging populations. As resources are limited, through education and simple programs, cost-effective benefits may be achieved. Efforts should be directed towards increasing awareness of the management of menopause among medical personnel so as to improve the quality of life in the aging female.

ACKNOWLEDGEMENTS

We would like to thank Jawad Iqbal Quereshi and Dory P. Cahanding for preparing the manuscript.

REFERENCES

1. United Nations Population Division: World Population Prospects: Estimates and Projections as Assessed in 1982, to be issued as a United Nations Publication; data reproduced in the *Review and Appraisal of the World Population Plan of Action; Report of the Secretary General, United Nations International Conference on Population, Mexico City, August 1984*; E/Conf. 76/4 Corr. 1.26, July 1984, pp.29–30
2. Wasti, S., Robinson, S.C., Akhtar, Y., Khan, S. and Badaruddun, N. (1993). *Maturitas*, **16**, 61–9
3. Stanford, J., Hartge, P., Brinton, L., Hoover, R. and Brookmeyer, R. (1987). Factors influencing the age at natural menopause. *J. Chron. Dis.*, **40**, 995–1002
4. Green, and Cooke, D.J. (1980). Life stress and symptoms at the climacteric. *Br. J. Psychiatry*, **136**, 486–91
5. Compagnoli *et al.* (1981). Climacteric symptoms according to body weight in women of different social economic groups. *Maturitas*, **3**, 279–87

Table 1 Age distribution. Numbers in parentheses are percentages

Age	*Hospital patients*	*Well Woman Clinic*	*Factory workers*	*Professional women*
40–45	237 (55.5)	270 (60.5)	264 (61.8)	90 (53.9)
46–50	130 (30.4)	112 (25.2)	101 (23.7)	42 (25.1)
>51	60 (14.1)	64 (14.3)	62 (14.5)	35 (21.0)
Total	427 (100)	446 (100)	427 (100)	167 (100)

Well Woman Clinic, a gynecology ward in a public hospital and professional women's clubs. Recruitment took into consideration socioeconomic factors, women's health conscious behavior, the effect of non-malignant gynecological diseases and the accessibility of the interviewers to these women. It was clear from the outset that the study sample could not be said to be representative of the total population of women in Hong Kong, but the information gathered will enhance the understanding of menopause in a large proportion of Chinese women.

Three interviewers were each responsible for one group of women in the face-to-face interview. All women between the age group of 40 and 55 years were asked to participate in the study. There were no refusals in women from the optics factory, clients of the Well Woman Clinic of Kwong Wah Hospital and women admitted into Queen Mary Hospital for non-malignant gynecological disorders. It was difficult to conduct face-to-face interviews with professional women who could not be reached as easily as the others. They belonged to different professional clubs, and it was not feasible for the interviewer to travel to their various work places to carry out the interviews. It was resolved that since the questionnaire was a simple one, the professional women would be able to fill it out themselves. Women of the appropriate age were sent explanatory notes regarding the study, requests to participate and questionnaires with return envelopes.

RESULTS

In this cross-sectional study, 1467 women were recruited: 427 factory workers, 446 women from the Well Women Clinic and 427 women from the hospital. Of 500 questionnaires sent to professional women's clubs, 167 were returned and were suitable for analysis (response rate 33%).

The age distribution was similar in the four groups (Table 1). Women in the Well Woman Clinic, hospital and factory had similar levels of education: half of them had primary and half of them had secondary

Table 2 Educational level. Numbers in parentheses are percentages

	Hospital patients	Well Woman Clinic	Factory workers	Professional women
≤ Primary	214 (50.1)	240 (53.9)	173 (40.5)	—
Secondary	180 (42.2)	192 (43.0)	242 (56.7)	13 (7.8)
Tertiary	33 (7.7)	14 (3.1)	12 (2.8)	154 (92.2)
Total	427 (100)	446 (100)	427 (100)	167 (100)

Table 3 Marital status. Numbers in parentheses are percentages

	Hospital patients	Well Woman Clinic	Factory workers	Professional women
Single	15 (3.5)	1 (0.2)	5 (1.2)	21 (12.6)
Married	379 (88.8)	419 (94.0)	397 (92.9)	133 (79.6)
Separated	6 (1.4)	0 –	5 (1.2)	4 (2.4)
Divorced	14 (3.3)	12 (2.7)	2 (0.5)	7 (4.2)
Widowed	13 (3.0)	14 (4.2)	18 (4.2)	2 (1.2)
Total	427 (100.0)	446 (100.0)	427 (100.0)	167 (100.0)

Table 4 Parity. Numbers in parentheses are percentages

	Hospital patients	Well Woman Clinic	Factory workers	Professional women
*0	26 (6.3)	16 (3.6)	10 (2.4)	17 (11.6)
1	55 (13.3)	45 (10.1)	31 (7.4)	36 (24.7)
2	124 (30.1)	178 (40.0)	108 (25.6)	72 (49.3)
3	109 (26.5)	110 (24.7)	147 (34.8)	16 (10.9)
4	47 (11.4)	56 (12.6)	82 (19.4)	3 (2.1)
>5	51 (12.4)	35 (7.9)	44 (10.4)	1 (0.7)
Missing	0 –	5 (1.1)	0 –	1 (0.7)

*single women excluded

education. As expected, almost all women in the professional group had had tertiary education. The small number of women who only had secondary education were in professions such as stocks and shares (Table 2). Over 60% of the hospital and Well Woman Clinic groups and over 90% of professional women and factory workers were working. Less than 5% of women were single, except for the professional group which contained 12.6% single women (Table 3).

The professional women were relatively 'subfertile' (Table 4): 11.6% of those who were married had no children and 49.3% of those with children

Table 5 Contraceptive methods. Numbers in parentheses are percentages

	Hospital patients	Well Woman Clinic	Factory workers	Professional women
Oral contraception	1 (0.3)	5 (1.4)	8 (2.3)	7 (6.0)
Intrauterine device	18 (5.0)	20 (5.8)	35 (10.3)	7 (6.0)
Condom	95 (26.6)	94 (27.2)	85 (25.1)	45 (38.8)
Female sterilization	138 (38.6)	138 (39.9)	85 (25.1)	23 (19.8)
Male sterilization	4 (1.1)	4 (1.2)	4 (1.2)	1 (0.9)
Safety period	23 (6.4)	31 (9.0)	23 (6.8)	1 (0.9)
Spermicide	10 (2.8)	5 (1.4)	8 (2.4)	0 –
Others†	8 (2.2)	8 (2.3)	17 (5.0)	13 (11.2)
Nil	61 (17.0)	41 (11.8)	74 (21.8)	19 (16.4)
Total	358 (100.0)	346 (100.0)	339 (100.0)	116 (100.0)

†Missing cases and not applicable cases excluded

Table 6 Distribution of women by menstrual status. Numbers in parentheses are percentages

	Hospital patients	Well Woman Clinic	Factory workers	Professional women
Premenopausal	148 (34.7)	260 (59.5)	236 (55.2)	93 (59.2)
Perimenopausal	225 (52.7)	96 (22)	108 (25.3)	27 (17.2)
Postmenopausal	54 (12.6)	81 (18.5)	83 (19.5)	37 (23.6)
Total	427 (100)	437* (100)	427 (100)	157* (100)

*Some cases are excluded

had only two. On the other hand, 20–30% of women in the other three groups had four or more children. Contraceptive use (Table 5) was worthy of note. Very few women (1.8%) were using oral contraceptives at the time of the study. Condoms were used by similar proportions in the four groups. Female sterilization was the most common contraceptive method, except for the professional group.

The distribution of women according to menstrual status is shown in Table 6. Premenopause means that the woman is still having her usual cycles, perimenopause means that the woman is having more and more irregular cycles and menopause means that the woman has not menstruated for 1 year. The distribution is similar.

The presence of menopausal symptoms is listed in Table 7. Between 58 and 88% of women had symptoms, and women attending the Well Woman Clinic had the highest symptom-reporting rate. When menopausal symptoms were examined against menstrual status (Table 8), the greatest symptom-reporting period was in the perimenopause, except for the

Table 7 Presence of vasomotor and neurosis symptoms. Numbers in parentheses are percentages

	Hospital patients	*Well Woman Clinic*	*Factory workers*	*Professional women*
Present	288 (67.4)	391 (87.7)	249 (58.3)	115 (68.9)
Absent	139 (32.6)	46 (10.3)	178 (41.7)	42 (25.1)
Missing	0 –	9 (2.0)	0 –	10 (6.0)
Total	427 (100.0)	446 (100.0)	427 (100.0)	167 (100.0)

Table 8 Presence of menopausal symptoms vs. menstrual status. Numbers are percentages

	Menstrual status		
	Premenopausal	*Perimenopausal*	*Postmenopausal*
Hospital patients	66.2	67.1	72.2
Well Woman Clinic	90.0	97.9	77.8
Factory workers	53.8	73.1	51.8
Professionals	68.8	88.8	73.0

hospital group, which in fact had a relatively similar level of symptom reporting in the three menstrual periods. This finding is different from those reported for Caucasian women, who have most symptoms at the menopause.

With regard to the menopausal symptoms, hot flushes and night sweats (10–25%) were the least reported symptoms in all the four groups of women. This finding is very different from surveys of Caucasian women. The psychological component of menopausal symptoms, such as nervousness, irritability, headache, depression and insomnia, was relatively more common (70%). Most women reported only one or two symptoms, except those recruited from the Well Woman Clinic. These women had the highest symptom-reporting rate as well as experiencing a greater number of symptoms.

Although there was a high rate of symptom reporting, the proportion of women who had ever sought treatment was low: 11.9% for the factory workers, 11.6% for those attending a Well Woman Clinic, 20.6% for those admitted to hospital and 13.2% for professional women. A variety of medications had been used: hormonal therapy was used by less than 3% of the total consulting women. This therapy was used more often in

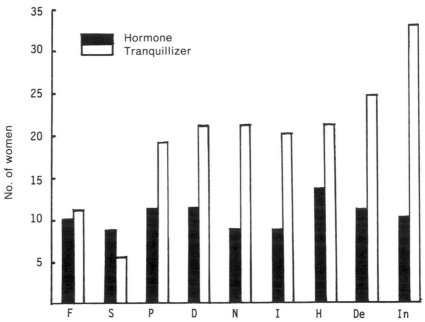

Figure 1 Distribution of symptoms vs. treatment. F, hot flushes; S, sweating; P, palpitation; D, dizziness; N, nervousness; I, irritability; H, headache; De, depression; In, insomnia

women who complained of hot flushes and night sweats (Figure 1). Tranquillizers were used when the symptoms were of the nervous type, particularly for insomnia.

Women were asked about their interpretation of what the menopause is and whether they had any fear about it. Multiple responses were allowed. 'A period of menstrual alteration' was the most frequent answer (22–38%). Up to 20% of women indicated that this period was associated with menopausal symptoms similar to those mentioned in the questionnaire. A comparable proportion of responses came from women who had no menopausal symptoms. 'A period of mood changes' was mentioned by 18% of women from the Well Woman Clinic, a percentage which is three to four times higher than the other three groups. 'A period of health changes' was mentioned by 16% of the factory workers, a proportion two to three times higher than the rest. The risks of osteoporosis and coronary heart disease were mentioned by less than 0.5% of women. Even the highly educated professional women did not make special reference to these two health hazards.

Between 68 and 84% of symptomatic women were not afraid of the menopause: some 70% said that it was a natural process. Only four women in the professional group thought that the menopause was a blessing that freed them of menstrual problems. The premenopausal women were asked if they would anticipate problems during their menopause: 40% of hospital and professional groups of women said 'no'. Surprisingly, 83% of the Well Woman Clinic group, though having the highest symptom-reporting rate, did not anticipate problems.

DISCUSSION

This cross-sectional study is the first attempt to examine the menopause in different socioeconomic and educational groups of Chinese women. Women from the hospital, Well Woman Clinic and factory environments represent the lower to middle classes and the professional women represent the upper class. Although the number of professional women was only half of that of the other groups, the distribution of symptoms reported by them was similar.

Hot flushes were under-reported, compared with their prevalence in Western studies, such as in the Massachusetts Women's Health study[4] and the West Germany Study[3], in which the symptom was reported by up to 74% of women. This finding of a low rate of hot flushes is consistent with the experience in clinical practice: castrated Chinese women are not found to report many hot flushes. There is no explanation for this phenomenon except to say that a 'symptom' may be present, but the extent of its effect on a person could be very variable. The effect could be so small as not to be reportable.

Women attending the Well Woman Clinic had the highest symptom rate. These women are probably more health conscious and hence are more able to recall symptoms. These symptoms to them do not seem to carry a connotation of 'illness', as only 11.6% of them had ever sought treatment. It is also interesting that these women have more mood-related symptoms and at the same time also felt the menopause as 'a period of mood changes'. One does not know why these women had so many mood-related symptoms, and such symptoms may influence how they feel about the nature of the menopause. Women of the hospital group who had a similar background did not have the same presentation with nervous symptoms.

Hunter[5] reported that women who were hypochondriacal, lacking in regular exercise and holding negative stereotypic beliefs about the menopause, suffered more from depression. Our Chinese women largely felt that menopause was a 'natural process' and hence could be regarded as having a positive view of this change in their life. Such an attitude could explain why so few women were ever treated and why they did not consider 'symptom' equivalent to suffering.

Osteoporosis and coronary heart disease do not appear to be of major concern to these women, even those professionals who are expected to be more knowledgeable. These two health problems have been much emphasized in the context of hormonal therapy, which was used by < 3% of the population studied. The author feels that it is not surprising for women not to be concerned by problems which do not give rise to symptoms in their 40s and 50s. Institution of hormonal therapy in a population of women who consider the menopause to be a natural process and who have so few estrogen-dependent symptoms of hot flushes would probably fail. The discontinuation rate would be high. Nevertheless, education on this aspect is important and health measures can be taken to minimize these two health hazards. Hormonal therapy should not be instituted without thorough exploration showing that women realize the need of such treatment.

It was the belief of the author that professional women would have more menopausal problems since they are more likely to be exposed to information. The data so far obtained, though not comparable in number, do not seem to suggest a substantial difference between this group of women and the middle–lower class groups in their experience, feeling and thinking regarding the menopause. It could be argued that women with severe symptoms would not respond to the questionnaire. Equally, it could also be said that only those with symptoms would be interested in responding. It is important to study this group further in such a way that selection bias can be eliminated.

CONCLUSION

This study shows the difference in menopausal symptoms in Chinese women living in Hong Kong. There is more reporting of psychological symptoms than of vasomotor symptoms. The use of hormone therapy in these women was low. While there is a need to give information regarding the healthcare of women in the menopause, over-enthusiasm should not make this natural process into a disease.

ACKNOWLEDGEMENT

This study was supported by the International Health Foundation.

REFERENCES

1. Boalet, M. J. and Visser, A. Ph. (1993). A study of the Hong Kong Chinese women in the menopause and the climacteric in seven Asian countries. *International Health Foundation,* 20–5
2. Utian, W. H. (1980). *Menopause in Modern Perspective: a Guide to Clinical Practice,* pp. 105–19. (New York: Appleton-Century-Crofts)
3. Van Keep, P. A., Utian, W. H. and Vermeulen, A. (1981). The controversial climacteric. *Proceedings of the Third International Congress on the Menopause,* pp. 9–19. (Casterton: Parthenon)
4. McKinlay, S. M., Brambilla, D. J. and Posner, J. G. (1992). The normal menopause transition. *Maturitas,* **14**, 103–15
5. Hunter, M. (1992). The South-East England longitudinal study of the climacteric and postmenopause. *Maturitas,* **14**, 117–26

6

Socio-economic and quality-of-life analysis in postmenopausal Argentine women

J. A. Tieffenberg

We propose a model to assess the socioeconomic impact of introducing health technology innovations for the care of patients with chronic conditions. Our study focused on examining the influence of consumer satisfaction (physicians and patients) on the effectiveness of treatment. The management of menopause was considered to be a good case-study, since women ≥ 45 years old will comprise about 12% of the world population by the year 2000[1]. In 1989 35% of women in Argentina were > 40 years old, and comprised 17.8% of the total population[2].

The increase in women's life expectancy has consequences for women and health care systems: the problem is not only medical but also economic. Evaluation of the efficiency of available health care resources and therapies is therefore of increasing interest to decision-makers in health services. This requires analysis of costs and benefits of treatment. According to current medical consensus, hormonal replacement therapy (HRT) is recommended for most menopausal women on a continued, long-term basis. During the last few years, clinical and epidemiological evidence of the benefits of HRT on symptoms and problems such as osteoporosis and fractures, coronary heart disease (CHD) and stroke, improving life expectancy and quality-of-life, have been published world-wide.

To assess the impact on costs and expected outcomes of consumer satisfaction with different treatment choices, a multicenter prospective

Table 1 Clinical inclusion and exclusion criteria

Inclusion criteria
(1) Menopausal women age 45–65.
(2) Women age < 45 years with early or surgical menopause (these women will receive only estrogens).
(3) At least 6 months of menses cessation.
(4) Follicle stimulating hormone (FSH) > 30 IU, and/or menopausal Pap smear.

Table 2 Treatment groups

Group	n	%	Treatment
Transdermal	85	41.5	17β-estradiol + progesterone 10 mg
Other hormonal	41	20.0	6 patients: estradiol 2 mg + progestin 0.5 mg
			4 patients: micronized 17β-estradiol,
			2 mg + progestin 5 mg
			24 patients: conjugated estrogens, USP 0.625,
			7 patients with USP 0.315 mg + progesterone
Non-hormonal	79	38.5	symptomatic or no medication
Total	205	100.0	

study was undertaken on a sample of normal menopausal women, with no other health problems and on no other medication.

PROSPECTIVE STUDY

The medical records of 272 women, aged 45–65 from six different clinic services in Buenos Aires, were chosen randomly for the study. Of these, 19 refused to participate, and 48 failed to meet the inclusion criteria (Table 1). The remaining 205 were divided into three treatment groups, statistically controlled for age, time since cessation of menses and type of menopause (Table 2). A total of 85 women were randomly assigned to transdermal HRT; 41 received other HRT treatments, and 79 received no HRT but symptomatic medication, or no treatment at all. Of the initial 205 women, 30 (14.6%) were lost to follow-up and 175 (85.4%) completed the study; of these, 29 (14.2%) changed or abandoned the prescribed treatment.

Methodology

We assumed no increased risk of endometrial cancer in these women, as all were treated with combined estrogen/progestin therapy[3]. Breast

58

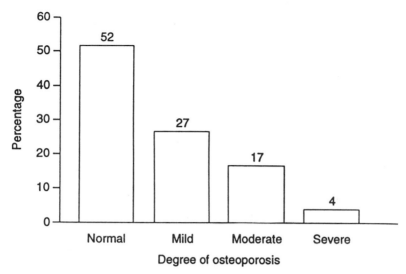

Figure 1 Distribution of bone mineral density used to establish the risk of osteoporosis and fractures

cancer risk was not considered, as the most recent epidemiological studies suggest no relationship between duration of therapy and number of breast cancer cases, and relative risks are not clearly defined[4,5].

Osteoporosis and fracture risk

The actual distribution of bone mineral density (BMD) in the study sample was used to establish the risk of osteoporosis and fractures (Figure 1). Life-time fracture risk was determined according to the formula developed by Melton and colleagues relating age and BMD (g/cm^2)[6].

Coronary heart disease (CHD) and stroke risk

The lipid blood levels determined in the study population (Figures 2–4) were comparable with those obtained in the USA in 1986[7] and with the distribution of expected cases of infarction, sudden death and angina according to Lerner and Kannel[8]. In the same way, the expected cases of stroke were estimated according to matching incidence rates published by Wolf in the USA[9].

The CHD incidence rate reported by Levy and Lafarge[10] was used to project the number of expected cases for our population, as that number

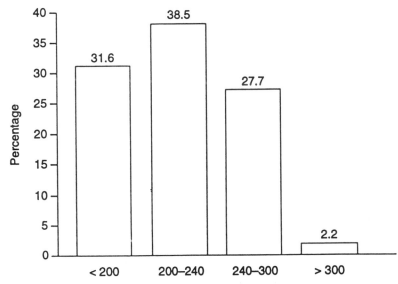

Figure 2 Total cholesterol levels in the study population

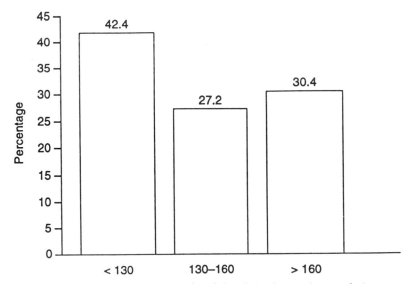

Figure 3 Low-density lipoprotein (LDL) levels in the study population

matches the 1986 estimates for France, and less than 5% of the total women population of France was receiving estrogen therapy, as is the case in our country.

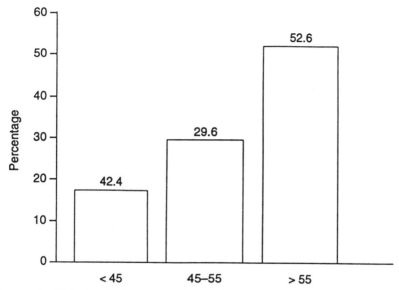

Figure 4 High-density lipoprotein (HDL) levels in the study population

Drug expenditures

The drug expenditure hypothesis was based on the frequency and distribution of prescriptions according to diagnosis and therapeutic class, obtained from 1988 Argentine data (INTE survey)[11]. The products were valued based on market prices and number of products sold (PMA survey)[12].

Physician visits

The number of consulting patients and number of visits for all causes per year was estimated, based on data covering 17 000 women $\geqslant$ 50 years of age, from the National Home Survey, health services and utilization module[13]. Women of this age make an average of 10–12 physician visits each year. The number of visits attributed to menopause was then calculated based on the diagnosis distribution of those visits obtained from a 1-year sample of 600 medical records of menopausal patients. The number of visits that could be avoided by HRT was estimated from the rate of symptom reduction as reflected in the Kupperman Index. These 'avoidable visits' were estimated to be about 22–25% of the annual total

Table 3 Probability of gain: HRT vs. non-hormonal treatment

| | *Hormonal vs. non-hormonal* | | | |
	p	σ^2	*Hormonal*	*Non-hormonal*
Satisfaction Index	0.76	0.0022	85	66
Kupperman Index	0.74	0.0025	77	57

From reference 15

(four per woman). The same type of calculation was used to estimate the reduction in unnecessary use of drugs.

Kupperman Index

For many years, physicians have used the 'Kupperman Index' to monitor the success of therapy[14]. It is a well-known standardized measure, weighting the intensity and frequency of symptoms present at follow-up clinical visits. The physician's and the woman's perception of treatment success or failure constitute a good measure of 'consumer satisfaction'. To complement the Kupperman Index we developed a 'Satisfaction Index' based on the analysis of 36 symptoms recorded at home visits performed four times during the study. This index excluded symptoms present in less than 25% of the cases, while grouping and weighting the rest in the same way as in the Kupperman Index. We then used the values obtained to weight the results of therapy.

Probability of therapeutic success (or failure)

This probability, based on the proportion of women who did or did not show improvement (gain) with the treatment being considered, was determined using the Kupperman Index and the women's own Satisfaction Index. The 'probability of gain' is a measurement developed by Laird and Mosteller[15] that estimates the odds that a random subject from an experimental group performed better than a random subject from a control group. Thus, estimates have a fairly high power, depending on the statistical significance of the difference, assessed by the Mann–Whitney–Wilcoxon statistic test (Table 3). This method avoids potential biases linked to design difficulties frequently associated with epidemiological research, since it is based on the direct recording of the assessment of each treatment, made independently by physicians and patients, as a function of their satisfaction with the therapeutic results in terms of

Table 4 Total public expenditure ($US) for the
health care of menopausal women without HRT

Drugs	398 337 000
Physician visits	342 808 680
Coronary heart disease	181 696 595
Osteoporosis	103 968 802
Strokes	76 239 357
Total	1 103 050 434

Table 5 Costs and years of life saved according to treatment and coverage

Population coverage (%)	Total costs transdermal (US$ (millions))	Years of life saved	Total costs other hormonal (US$ (millions))	Years of life saved
5.0	17 068	49 690	16 679	26 450
25.0	19 445	248 445	17 501	132 245
50.0	22 417	496 885	18 528	264 440
75.0	25 389	745 330	19 555	396 740
84.3	26 494	837 750	19 937	445 930

symptom reduction. Continuity of treatment and compliance can be
predicted, if other important factors (e.g. socioeconomic status and price)
are controlled, since this analysis is carried out from a societal point of
view. This probability was used to weigh the results obtained, which will
obviously affect both the effectiveness and costs.

Costs

Costs were estimated using expenditure estimates for osteoporosis, CHD,
stroke, physician visits and pharmaceutical drugs. The figures used were
those obtained from the public sector (Table 4); private sector estimates
may increase that figure by US$ 500 million.

The data were obtained from registries of health care utilization in
Buenos Aires, assuming a higher standard of medical care quality and then
projecting the results to the rest of the country. For example, to determine
costs for CHD, the following items were considered: hospitalization;
revascularization procedures; and outpatient services. To follow the
example, in the case of hospitalization for infarct, the costs considered
were: 8 days intensive care unit, 7 days hospital bed and 1 coronary
arteriography, with a unit cost of US$ 2817 and a total cost of US$
40 874 670 for 14 510 expected cases.

Table 6 Changes in Kupperman and Satisfaction indices

	Kupperman index* (%)	Satisfaction index† (%)
Worse		
hormonal	1.3	2.4
non-hormonal	12.3	44.1
No change		
hormonal	20.5	31.8
non-hormonal	56.1	29.4
Better		
hormonal	78.2	65.9
non-hormonal	31.6	26.5

*$\chi^2 = 30.715$; †$\chi^2 = 43.707$; $p < 0.0000$

Effectiveness

The population studied was analysed according to age, educational level, marital status, socioeconomic level and ethnicity. It is of interest that the intensity of symptoms showed inverse correlation with socioeconomic level and education (higher socioeconomic level and education corresponded to lower Kupperman Index scores). The same inverse relationship was seen with social and physical activities. Those women who recalled having intense symptoms at the beginning of their fertile life, or had more symptoms associated with their menses, had higher Kupperman Index scores.

Symptomatic suppression

To monitor treatment efficacy, we used the physician's Kupperman Index and the women's Satisfaction Index. HRT was clearly superior to non-hormonal treatment (Table 6). The Satisfaction Index showed similar but smaller decreases in symptoms, suggesting that women felt that the impact of therapy, even though positive, was less important than indicated by physicians. The changes observed in the Kupperman Index and the Satisfaction Index with the three treatments (transdermal, other hormonal and non-hormonal) are shown in Table 7. Based on these differences, the probability of therapeutic success was used to predict the probability of abandoning treatment. This probability was used in turn to weight the

Table 7 Changes in Kupperman and Satisfaction indices

	Kupperman Index* (%)	Satisfaction Index† (%)
Worse		
transdermal	0.0	3.8
other hormonal	4.3	0.0
non-hormonal	12.3	44.1
No change		
transdermal	10.2	26.4
other hormonal	47.8	44.0
non-hormonal	56.1	29.4
Better		
transdermal	89.8	69.8
other hormonal	47.8	56.0
non-hormonal	31.6	26.5

*$\chi^2 = 38.514$; †$\chi^2 = 42.843$; $p = 0.0000$

theoretical results of therapy, in order to obtain outcome values more close to the real life situation.

Years of life saved

The years of life saved by HRT were estimated using the calculated reduction in the relative risk of death from osteoporosis and fractures, CHD and stroke in each age bracket, assuming 25 years of therapy, according to the life expectancy of women > 50 years of age. Alternative treatments showed remarkable differences in effectiveness, as high as 50%.

Cost-effectiveness

Assuming the current medical recommendation of maximizing therapeutic benefits with continuous administration of HRT for the rest of a woman's life, a model of cost-effectiveness analysis (CEA) is outlined (Figure 5). HRT for 25 years, as proposed, would save 370 675 fractures, 117 250 CHD and 56 500 stroke cases, and 641 850 years of life. The HRT savings based on reduced costs of treatment amount to approximately US$ 100 million/year of treatment during the 25 years.

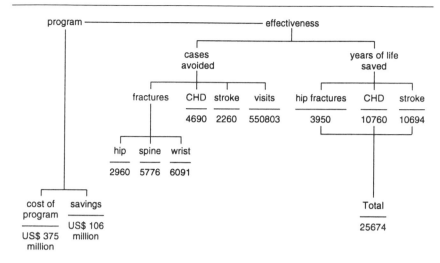

Figure 5 Lifetime hormonal replacement therapy (annualized)

Table 8 Cost per year of life saved according to therapy and population coverage

Population	Cost per year of life saved (US$)	
coverage (%)	Transdermal	Other hormonal
5.0	343 492	630 593
25.0	78 268	132 336
50.0	45 115	70 051
75.0	34 064	49 289
84.3	31 625	44 708

Cost per year of life saved

The cost per year of life saved decreased as the proportion of population treated increased, and the results also varied according to the type of treatment considered (Table 8).

With transdermal HRT, both the number of cases avoided and the years of life saved increased by about 30%, while savings amounted to US$ 138 million/year of treatment. When other hormonal replacement alternatives were considered, effectiveness and savings dropped about 50%.

Marginal costs and benefits

In planning a health investment it is important to look for the alternative that will maximize the investment return in terms of additional years of

Table 9 Marginal (incremental) cost-effectiveness: proportion of population treated, years of life saved (YLS), costs and effectiveness of treatments

	Coverage	Transdermal	Other hormonal
Female population 50–79 years of age under lifetime HRT (%)	100% of target (theoretical goal)	YLS 1 106 650	YLS 1 106 650
	84.3% of target (real goal)	YLS 932 906	YLS 932 906
Effectiveness transdermal therapy	75.7% of target effectively treated (probability of abandoning treatment values)	YLS 837 734	—
Effectiveness other hormonal treatment	40.3% of target effectively treated (probability of abandoning treatment values)		YLS 445 980
Costs ($US)	84.3% of target	26 494 134 125	19 936 771 156
	Cost/YLS	31 625	44 708

life gained for each additional dollar spent. For example (Table 9), if the decision is made to treat all menopausal women, decision-makers will probably look for the cheapest alternative to minimize the cost of treating all. However, this alternative will only achieve 40.3% of the target population, because of the poor effectiveness of the treatment considered, at a cost of US$ 44 708 per year of life saved. Instead, the preferred form of treatment (even though more costly because it is a technological innovation) will reach 75.7% of the target, with a cost of US$ 31 625 per year of life saved. Funds will be best invested choosing this alternative.

Quality of life

Quality of life changes with therapy were investigated in home surveys. The questions were related to socio-emotional factors, and levels of physical as well as intellectual activity. In six of seven questions, women on transdermal therapy noticed improvements after therapy, while women on other hormonal therapies gave negative answers in five out of seven (Table 10). Of the women receiving transdermal therapy during the follow-up study, 69 were interviewed again at 6 months, and asked about their preferences regarding treatment, and their willingness to pay. If they changed treatments, the reasons were recorded, as was the kind of health insurance that they had. Results showed that 37.7% were still on

Table 10 Quality of life analysis

Variable	Treatment		
	Transdermal	*Other hormonal*	*Non-hormonal*
Visits and outings			
Outings	34.0	4.8	23.1
Receiving visitors	28.0	4.8	18.5
Visiting	18.4	14.3	13.8
Psychosocial			
Personal activity	44.0	19.0	21.5
Depression	44.0	4.8	15.4
Concentration	43.7	14.3	24.6
Enjoyment	43.0	15.0	24.6

Table 11 Utility analysis in menopause: preference among treatment alternatives. Mean values – Scale: 0–10

Preference	Current treatment			
	Transdermal	*Other hormonal*	*No treatment*	*Total*
No treatment	0.5	1.9	2.6	1.7
Treatment	9.5	8.9	7.7	8.6
Non-hormonal	2.0	2.1	4.0	2.9
Other hormonal	3.9	7.6	5.2	5.1
Hormonal	9.4	8.4	7.3	8.3
Transdermal	9.3	6.9	6.0	7.4

transdermal therapy, 40.6% were in no treatment, and 15.9% were on other HRT. A total of 45 questions was constructed with a 'Lickert-type' scale-scoring system. Women were asked to indicate their preferences for therapy in numerical terms.

Preferences

When considering the preferences according to the patients' treatment at the time of the interview, most women favored some kind of treatment, and transdermal HRT was preferred to non-transdermal alternatives. The women not receiving therapy scored 7.3 for HRT, and 4 for favoring no-HRT therapy (Table 11), while 23.2% dropped transdermal therapy because of unwanted side-effects and 9.3% did so because of fear of cancer. Almost 70% of transdermal drop-outs were due to changes in prescriptions, indications by physicians or cost considerations.

Willingness to pay

Nearly 75% of women were willing to pay up to US$ 20/month for transdermal therapy (approximately the market price at the time of the study). Of women not receiving HRT, 52.4% would be willing to pay that amount. Nearly half of the women on HRT would pay US$ 40 (twice the market value) for the transdermal alternative. The fact that the health coverage is poor (only 35.4% had 50% or more coverage) significantly affected these results. For example, women with coverage were willing to pay a much higher amount than those without it. Of those women not covered, 41% would not pay more than US$ 17 for the transdermal therapy, while 96% of those insured would be willing to pay more than that.

CONCLUSIONS

Socioeconomic analysis is helpful in making rational investment decisions in health technology innovations. Life-time HRT is cost-effective in menopause; cost-effectiveness ratios improved as duration of treatment and the number of women treated increased. HRT may increase costs without affording additional benefits in terms of years of life saved, improved quality of life and reduction in health care costs, if it is administered for short periods and in inadequate or erratic dosages. Quality of life analysis is useful to help in making women's preferences known, and to improve the chances of them influencing medical and health policy decision-making.

REFERENCES

1. Diczfalusy, E. (1986). Menopause, developing countries and the 21st century. *Acta Obstet. Gynecol. Scand.,* Suppl. **134**, 45–7
2. Ministerio de Salud y Acción Social de la República Argentina. Organización Panamericana de la Salud. Organización Mundial de la Salud. (1985). *Argentina: Descripción de su situación de salud.* Buenos Aires, Octubre, 1985. (Spanish)
3. Paterson, M., Wade-Evans, T., Sturdee, D. W., Thomas, M. H. and Studd, J. W. W. (1980). Endometrial disease after treatment with oestrogens and progestogens in the climacteric. *Br. Med. J.,* **96**, 1–8
4. Wingo, P., Layde, P., Lee, A., Rubin, G. and Ory, N. (1987). The risk of breast cancer in postmenopausal women who have used estrogen replacement therapy. *J. Am. Med. Assoc.,* **257**, 209–15
5. Colditz, G., Stampler, M., Willet, W. C., Hennekeus, C. H., Rosher, B. and Speizer, F. E. (1990). Prospective study of estrogen replacement therapy and

risk of breast cancer in postmenopausal women. *J. Am. Med. Assoc.,* **264**, 2648–53

6. Melton, J., Kan, S., Warner, H. and Riggs, B. L. (1988). Lifetime fracture risk: an approach to hip fracture risk assessment based on bone mineral density and age. *Am. J. Epidemiol.,* **41**, 985–94

7. Wynder, E. L., Field, F. and Haly, N. J. (1986). Population screening for cholesterol determination: a pilot study. *J. Am. Med. Assoc.,* **256**, 2841

8. Lerner, D. J. and Kannel, W. B. (1986). Patterns of coronary heart disease morbidity in the sexes: a 26 year follow-up of the Framingham population. *Am. Heart J.,* **112**, 383–90

9. Wolf, P. A. (1990). An overview of the epidemiology of stroke. *Stroke,* **21**, Suppl. II, 4–6

10. Levy, E. and Lafarge, H. (1987). *Le Cout de la Menopause non Traittée. Une Evaluation pour la France 1986/7.* (Université Paris – IX, Dauphine). (Report)

11. INTE (1989). *Indice de Terapéutica y Enfermedades* (Survey of Therapeutics and Diseases, Annual Report, INTE) (Spanish)

12. *Encuesta de venta de Medicamentos PMA* (1988). (National Sales Survey of Pharmaceutical Drugs – Annual Report, PMA) (Spanish)

13. Ministerio de Salud y Acción Social de la República Argentina. Dirección de Estadísticas de Salud y Acción Social y Dirección de Encuesta Permanente de Hogares y Otras Encuestas Especiales del INDEC. (1990). Programa Nacional de Estadísticas de Salud, y Encuestas a la Población: *Módulo de Utilización y Gasto en Servicios de Salud,* Serie 10 No. 2. (Spanish)

14. Kupperman, H. S., Blatt, M. H. G., Wiesbader, H. and Filler, W. (1953). Comparative clinical evaluation of estrogenic preparations by the menopause and amenorrheal indices. *Endocrinology,* **13**, 688–703

15. Laird, N. M. and Mosteller, F. (1990). Some statistical methods for combining experimental results. *Int. J. Tech. Assess. Health Care,* **6**, 5–30

7

Experience of symptoms during transition to menopause: a population-based longitudinal study

A. Collins and B.-M. Landgren

INTRODUCTION

The transition to menopause is frequently associated with an increase of physical as well as psychological symptoms. Vasomotor and atrophic symptoms are widely recognized as being associated with estrogen deficiency[1,2]. There is much more debate about the etiology of psychological complaints, such as depressed mood, tension, irritability or difficulty concentrating, and whether they can be attributed to hormonal changes or whether they are mainly affected by other factors such as expectations, stressful life events or cultural and socioeconomic factors[3-5].

While there is general agreement among clinicians about the beneficial effects of estrogen treatment for vasomotor symptoms and for prevention of osteoporosis and heart disease, researchers continue to argue about the value of estrogen treatment for psychological symptoms[6]. In recent years, many social scientists have pointed out that selection factors may influence the use of hormone replacement therapy (HRT). Women using HRT are better educated, consume more alcohol and are more likely to smoke than non-users. They also tend to be more depressed and have a lower self-esteem than non-users[7-10]. These differences should be considered when assessing compliance with and the effectiveness of HRT.

Much of the controversy regarding menopausal symptoms and their treatment stems from methodological problems associated with research in this area. Earlier studies vary in terms of sample size, sampling

71

method, criteria for menopausal status, measurement of dependent and independent variables as well as statistical analysis. As Holte[11] and Greene[12] have pointed out, most of our current knowledge about menopause is based on small samples of women attending menopausal clinics for their symptoms or women who have had a surgical menopause, and we do not know whether these findings apply to the general population of middle-aged women. There is, therefore, a great need for prospective, population-based research with a follow-up of women over several years.

The aim of this study was to examine reproductive health, use of estrogen, life-style, and experience of menopausal symptoms in a population-based sample of healthy perimenopausal women.

SUBJECTS AND METHODS

The data reported here were collected as the first part of a prospective, longitudinal study of a population-based sample of premenopausal women, focusing on the interaction between hormonal and psychosocial changes that characterize the transition to menopause. The postal survey, which was cross-sectional in design, formed the first part of the project and was carried out in Stockholm county in the catchment area of the Karolinska Hospital. All 48-year-old women in that district ($n = 2011$) were contacted by obtaining their names and addresses through the Swedish population register.

The women received a letter including a stamped envelope for returning a completed questionnaire covering four different areas:

(1) Sociodemographic variables such as marital status, age, number of children born, number of children living at home, education, occupation and type of residence. Also, questions about life-style and health behaviour were asked, such as smoking, intake of medication and physical exercise.

(2) Questions regarding work role and social roles, such as degree of autonomy on the job, stress associated with work, satisfaction with work, and social support.

(3) Questions concerning health and gynecological history such as contraception, miscarriages, abortions and gynecological treatment and surgeries. Also included were questions about current menopausal status, regularity of menstrual bleeding or cessation of menses and the date of the last menstrual period.

(4) A 20-item symptom rating scale adapted from Rosseau and col-

leagues[13]. Each item had to be rated from 1 to 7, corresponding to 'never' and 'very frequently'.

RESULTS

A total of 1399 women returned the questionnaire after one postal reminder, giving a response rate of 70%.

Sociodemographic background and health behavior

The majority of the women were married (75%), while 17% were never married, 7% were divorced and 1% were widowed. Ninety-four percent of the women had children and 6% were childless. Thirty-five percent had a primary education, 35% had a secondary education and 30% had college or university education. The level of education in our sample corresponds to the levels reported by the National Bureau of Statistics for women of this age group residing in Stockholm. Seventy-three percent were employed full time and 27% were employed part time. Only 1% were housewives or students without paid work.

As for life-style and health behaviors, 33% of the women reported being smokers, and 67% were non-smokers. Forty-four percent said they participated in regular physical exercise while 56% reported not participating in sports or physical exercise on a regular basis. Some medication was currently being taken by 32%.

Menopausal development and gynecological characteristics

Seventy-three percent of the women were premenopausal, 6% were perimenopausal, and 21% were postmenopausal. The classification was based on the women's report of presence and regularity of their menstrual bleeding. Absence of menstrual bleeding for a minimum of 6 months was used as the criterion for postmenopausal status. The use of hormonal replacement therapy was 7.5%, this proportion being divided between premenopausal (3.7%), perimenopausal (0.3%) and postmenopausal women (3.5%). The majority were taking sequential estrogen treatment combined with progestin. The majority of the women (93%) reported a history of regular menstrual cycles and only 7% had a history of irregular cycles. Hysterectomy had been performed in 8.6% of the women, 5% had undergone unilateral oophorectomy and 2.5% bilateral oophorectomy. With regard to breast surgery, 2.5% had undergone unilateral and 0.3%

had undergone bilateral mastectomy. One percent had had radiation treatment.

Symptom dimensions

Factor analysis of the symptom ratings is described in detail elsewhere[14]. The first factor was a negative moods factor including tension, feeling depressed and spells of crying. The second factor included vasomotor symptoms such as hot flashes, excessive sweating and waking up sweating. The third factor concerned decreased sexual desire combined with vaginal dryness and life experienced as less pleasurable. The fourth factor was a positive well-being factor including vitality, happiness and harmony. Factor scores were calculated for each individual and each factor and the scores were compared between the three different groups: premenopausal and postmenopausal women and those receiving hormonal treatment. The postmenopausal group included surgically menopausal women, since *t*-tests showed that they did not differ significantly from the naturally menopausal women on any of the symptom dimensions. Analysis of variance showed that there were significant overall differences between the three groups of women for negative moods ($p < 0.001$), vasomotor symptoms ($p < 0.001$) and decreased sexual desire ($p < 0.001$), the premenopausal group scoring lowest and the hormonally treated group the highest. There were no significant differences between the groups for scores on the well-being factor, although the hormonally treated group had the lowest ratings.

Women on HRT did not differ from the other women on any of the sociodemographic variables such as level of education, occupation, type of residence, smoking, exercise or intake of other medication.

Physical exercise

Forty-four percent of the women reported participating in sports or physical exercise at least once a week. Comparison of the women who reported exercising regularly and those who did not, using χ^2 tests for trends, showed that women who exercised were better educated ($p < 0.001$), had a higher occupational status ($p < 0.001$), tended to live in a house rather than an apartment ($p < 0.001$), and tended to have both husband and one or more children living at home rather than living just with the husband or alone ($p < 0.05$). They were less likely to smoke ($p < 0.001$). They rated their jobs to be more demanding ($p < 0.01$) but also felt more satisfied with the way they divided work and leisure time

($p < 0.001$). They had more social contacts and received more social support at work ($p < 0.01$) and perceived themselves to be more in control of the content of their work ($p < 0.05$).

Two-way analysis of variance showed that both menopausal status and physical exercise contributed significantly to symptom experience and well-being. Women who exercised on a regular basis had significantly fewer vasomotor symptoms ($p < 0.02$), a lesser degree of negative moods ($p < 0.001$), a lesser degree of decreased sexual desire ($p < 0.01$) and significantly higher well-being scores ($p < 0.001$) compared to women who did not exercise.

CONCLUSIONS

There were significant differences in experience of adverse symptoms between pre- and postmenopausal woman as well as those receiving hormonal therapy. The hormonally treated group had the highest scores on negative moods and vasomotor symptoms as well as decreased sexual desire. The premenopausal women had the lowest scores. There were no significant differences in well-being scores between the three groups. Our data suggest that menopausal status is related to incidence of not only vasomotor but also psychological symptoms, such as negative moods and decrease in sexual desire. These results are supported by those of Hunter[15] who found an increase of depressed mood and sexual problems during the transition to menopause. On the other hand, the results are at variance with those of McKinlay and co-workers[16], who found no association between menopausal status and increased psychological symptoms.

It is interesting that the hormonally treated group had the highest symptom ratings in terms of vasomotor symptoms, negative moods and reduced sexual desire, despite their treatment. These findings suggest that hormonal treatment is not effective for all symptoms, but they could also indicate that the women had even more intense symptoms before treatment. The notion based on earlier findings that women who use HRT differ in life-style and sociodemographic background was not supported in the present study. The use of HRT was unrelated to level of education, marital status and occupational status, type of residence, smoking or intake of other medication.

The rate of HRT use was relatively low, thus contradicting the notion of the menopause as being excessively medicalized. The low rate is probably partly due to the fact that the majority of the women were still premenopausal, but these figures correspond closely to the national

Swedish figures based on epidemiological studies[17], and they are low even for postmenopausal women when compared to rates in other countries[14].

Physical exercise is an important contributor to well-being at all ages. The results showed that postmenopausal women exercised significantly less than premenopausal women. Notelowitz[18] has shown that physical activity is related to increased well-being and a lesser degree of adverse menopause-related symptoms. A study by Hammar and colleagues[19] showed that postmenopausal women who exercised had fewer vasomotor symptoms. These authors pointed out that regular physical exercise is known to increase central opioid activity and may therefore reduce the incidence of hot flashes. Exercise seems to be a life-style variable which is strongly related to level of education and occupational status. The results suggest that women who exercise on a regular basis and who have a higher education and a more autonomous job and who are living with both husband and children are less likely to suffer from symptoms associated with menopause. Further studies are needed to confirm these results.

REFERENCES

1. Utian, W. H. (1972). The true clinical features of postmenopause and oophorectomy and their response to oestrogen therapy. *S. Afr. Med. J.*, **46**, 732–7
2. Greene, J. G. (1984). *The Social and Psychological Origins of the Climacteric Syndrome.* (Aldershot: Gower)
3. Hunter, M. (1988). Psychosocial aspects of the climacteric. In Studd, J. and Whitehead, M. (eds.) *The Menopause*, pp. 55–64. (Oxford: Blackwell)
4. Hällström, T. (1973). *Mental Disorder and Sexuality in the Climacteric.* (Copenhagen: Scandinavian University Books)
5. Kaufert, P., Gilbert, P. and Tate, R. (1992). The Manitoba project: a re-examination of the link between menopause and depression. *Maturitas*, **14**, 143–55
6. Hunter, M. (1990). Emotional wellbeing, sexual behaviour and hormone replacement therapy. *Maturitas*, **12**, 299–314
7. Palinkas, L. A. and Barrett-Connor, E. (1992). Estrogen use and depressive symptoms in postmenopausal women. *Obstet. Gynecol.*, **80**, 30–6
8. Egeland, G. M., Matthews, K. A., Kuller, L. H. and Kelsey, S. F. (1988). Characteristics of noncontraceptive hormone users. *Prev. Med.*, **17**, 403–11
9. Cauley, J., Cummings, S. R., Black, D. M., Mascioli, S. R. and Seeley, D. G. (1990). Prevalence and determinants of estrogen replacement therapy in elderly women. *Am. J. Obstet. Gynecol.*, **163**, 1438–44
10. Topo, P., Klaukka, T., Hemminki, E. and Uutela, A. (1991). Use of hormone-replacement therapy in 1976–1989 by 45–64-year-old Finnish women. *J. Epidemiol. Commun. Health*, **45**, 277–80

11. Holte, A. and Mikkelsen, A. (1991). Psychosocial determinants of climacteric complaints. *Maturitas,* **13**, 205–15
12. Greene, J. G. (1992). The cross-sectional legacy: an introduction to longitudinal studies of the climacteric. *Maturitas,* **14**, 95–101
13. Rosseau, M. E., Maxure, C. and Sarrel, P. (1987). Use of a quantitative instrument to assess symptoms before and after hormonal replacement therapy. In *Proceedings of the 5th International Congress of Menopause*, Sorrento. (Carnforth: Parthenon)
14. Collins, A. and Landgren, B. M. (1993). Reproductive health, use of estrogen and experience of symptoms in perimenopausal women: A population-based study. *Obstet. Gynecol.,* in press
15. Hunter, M. (1992). The South-England longitudinal study of the climacteric and postmenopause. *Maturitas,* **14**, 117–26
16. McKinlay, J., McKinlay, S. and Brambilla, D. (1987). The relative contribution of endocrine and social circumstances to depression in mid-aged women. *J. Health Soc. Behav.,* **28**, 345–63
17. Persson, I., Adami, H. O. and Lindberg, B. S. (1983). Practice and patterns of estrogen treatment in climacteric women in a Swedish population. *Acta Obstet. Gynecol. Scand.,* **62**, 289–96
18. Notelowitz, M. (1989). Exercise and cognitive function in the menopause. In Demers, L. M., McGuire, J. L., Phillips, A. and Rubinow, D. (eds.) *Premenstrual, Postpartum and Menopausal Mood Disorders*, pp. 205–12. (Baltimore: Urban & Schwarzenberg)
19. Hammar, M., Berg, G. and Lindgren, R. (1990). Does physical exercise influence the frequency of postmenopausal hot flushes? *Acta Obstet. Gynecol. Scand.,* **69**, 409–12

8

Climacteric hormone therapy use and women's employment in Denmark, Finland and Norway

P. Topo, A. Holte, A. Køster, E. Hemminki and A. Uutela

INTRODUCTION

In Scandinavia, most middle-aged women work outside the home, either full- or part-time[1]. The possible effect of climacteric symptoms on the functioning of women at work has been little researched. The few studies done so far suggest that climacteric symptoms lower women's capability of functioning at work[2].

The aims of the present study were to compare the use of hormone therapy during the climacterium and postmenopause in Finland, Denmark and Norway, and to investigate whether the use of hormone therapy was related to women's employment and their position at work.

MATERIAL AND METHODS

The study was based on sales figures of menopausal and postmenopausal hormones in Scandinavia, collected by the Nordic Council on Medicines[3-7], and on three questionnaire surveys conducted in Norway, Denmark and Finland in the 1980s.

The Norwegian survey was undertaken in 1981 in the municipality of Oslo on a random sample of 1997 women aged 45–55 years. The response rate was 94%[8,9]. The Danish survey was performed in 1987 as part of a prospective health study of the cohort born in 1936 and living in the county of Copenhagen. The number of the women was 597, and the response rate was 88%[10]. The Finnish study took place in 1989 on a random sample of all Finnish women aged 45–64 years. The number of women was 2000, and the response rate was 86%[11].

In all these surveys women were asked questions on the climacterium, employment, occupation and the use of hormone therapy. The results for the Finnish sample, which included women from a larger age range, and the whole country, were adjusted for age and place of residence, as these two variables are related to both hormone use and employment. Results from the capital area of Finland were quite similar to those from the whole country. Only the results from the whole of Finland are presented.

RESULTS

According to the sales figures, the use of hormone therapy was low in Norway in the 1980s and in the beginning of the 1990s and then increased slowly. In Finland the use increased rapidly in the 1980s, and early in the 1990s it passed the level for Denmark. In Denmark the sales have been high for the whole study period.

In Norway in 1981, 9% of the women aged 45–55 years reported current hormone use[8]. In Denmark in 1987, 22% were current hormone users[10] and 2 years later among Finnish women aged 45–64 the proportion of users was also 22%.

Most of the women sampled were working. In Norway and Denmark[10] part-time work was common, but in Finland part-time work was very rare. In every country, most of the working women were doing lower-level white-collar work.

In Norway and Denmark, employed women were using hormones as often as those not in the labour force, but in Finland their use was more common among employed women. There was no difference between full-time and part-time workers. Furthermore, the use in Finland was more common among white-collar workers than blue-collar workers. No such difference was found in Norway or Denmark.

DISCUSSION

The finding from Norway and Denmark that labour force participation is not related to hormone use agrees with the findings from Massachusetts, USA, and from Canada[12,13]. In the Finnish survey, employment was positively related to hormone therapy, which accords with a study from France[14]. Thus, even if hormone use was on the same level in Denmark and Finland, the relationship between employment and hormone use was different. Hormone use was not related to women's occupational status in Norway or Denmark, but in Finland it was.

What could explain these contradictory results? More common part-time work in Denmark and Norway than in Finland does not explain the differences. Innovation diffusion theories[15] offer another explanation. According to the innovation diffusion theories, the first groups using a new innovation are often members of the highest socioeconomic groups. When the innovation is widely accepted and stabilized at a certain level, the first people to stop its use often belong to the highest socioeconomic groups. A third explanation for the contradictory results could be varying cultural factors.

REFERENCES

1. International Labour Office (1988). *Yearbook of Labour Statistics 1988*, 48th issue, pp. 39–48. (Geneva)
2. Sarrell, P. M. (1991). Women, work, and menopause. In Frankenhaueser, M., Lundberg, U. and Chesney, M. (eds.) *Women, Work, and Health*, pp. 225–37. (New York: Plenum Press)
3. Nordic Council on Medicines (1982). *Nordic Statistics on Medicines 1978–1980,* p.120. (Uppsala)
4. Nordic Council on Medicines (1986). *Nordic Statistics on Medicines 1981–1983,* p. 133. (Uppsala)
5. Nordic Council on Medicines (1988). *Nordic Statistics on Medicines 1984–1986,* p. 35. (Uppsala)
6. Nordic Council on Medicines (1990). *Nordic Statistics on Medicines 1987–1989,* p. 64. (Uppsala)
7. Nordic Council on Medicines. *Nordic Statistics on Medicines 1989–1991.* (Manuscript)
8. Holte, A. and Mikkelsen, A. (1982). Menstrual coping style, social background, and climacteric symptoms. *Psychiatry Soc. Sci.,* 2, 41–5
9. Holte, A. (1991). Prevalence of climacteric complaints in a representative sample of middle-aged women in Oslo. *J. Psychosom. Obstet. Gynaecol.,* 12, 303–17
10. Køster, A. (1990). Hormone replacement therapy: use patterns in 51-year-old Danish women. *Maturitas,* 12, 345–56
11. Topo, P., Klaukka, T., Hemminki, E. and Uutela, A. (1991). Use of hormone replacement therapy in 1976–1989 by 45–64 year old Finnish women. *J. Epidemiol. Commun. Health,* 45, 277–80
12. Hemminki, E., Brambilla, D. J., McKinlay, S. M. and Posner, J. G. (1991). Use of estrogens among middle-aged Massachusetts women. *DICP, Ann. Pharmacotherapy,* 25, 418–23
13. Kaufert, P. (1986). The menopausal transition; the use of estrogen. *Can. J. Publ. Health,* 77 (Suppl. 1), 86–191
14. Ringa, V., Ledesert, B., Gueguen, R., Schiele, F. and Breat, G. (1992). Determinants of hormone replacement therapy in recently postmenopausal women.

Eur. J. Obstet. Gynecol. Reprod. Biol., **45**, 193–200

15. Banta, D. (1990). Empirical work on technology diffusion. In Adreasen, P. B. and Lund, A. B. (eds.) *Life-cycles of Medical Technologies.* (Fredriksberg: Academic Publishers)

9

From workplace to community: an educational support program for menopause in transition

B. Weiss

INTRODUCTION

Health care reform has become the focus of intense national discussion and debate in the United States. Cost containment and universal health care coverage for all Americans are the core issues to be resolved. These dual concerns demand that the traditional medical model of health care expands beyond the treatment of acute illness to include preventive care. Simply, wellness is less expensive than illness.

Women's health, specifically relating to the menopause and the peri-menopausal years, provides an excellent opportunity to develop a preventive approach to health care and well-being. As with any effort aimed at prevention, success depends to a great extent on the effective education of the public. What do women need to know in order to better understand the biological, psychological and social effects of the significant transitional period of their lives preceding and following the menopause?

AUSPICE

The Mount Sinai Medical Center, a tertiary health care institution located in New York City, is a sprawling complex of 10 buildings extending over four city blocks. The medical center is a 1200-bed facility with a combined staff of over 26 000 people. In 1992, Mount Sinai provided ambulatory, in-patient and clinic services to approximately 450 000 patients.

Table 1 Menopause: an educational support program in the workplace

Sessions
(1) Definitions and information
(2) Health care concerns
(3) Hormone replacement therapy and alternatives
(4) Stress management: recognition and techniques
(5) Nutrition
(6) Exercise
(7) Female sexuality and sexuality at midlife
(8) Review and open discussion

PILOT PROGRAM

The Employee Wellness Program, a component of the Employee Assistance Program at the medical center, initiated a series of educational support programs for menopause in June 1991. The programs, advertised in the Weekly Bulletin, attracted groups of self-selected women from all parts of the medical center who were motivated to obtain information about the menopause and related concerns. The results of this pilot project, conducted in the highly structured medical center community of professionals and ancillary personnel, were presented at the annual meeting of the North American Menopause Society held in Cleveland, Ohio, USA, in September 1992.

Each program ran for 8 consecutive weeks at the lunch hour and addressed areas of greatest interest and concern to women approaching the menopause (Table 1). Teams of interdisciplinary health care professionals addressed the specialized areas of nutrition, exercise, sexuality and stress management. A physician and nurse/clinician spoke on the medical aspects of the menopause and the perimenopausal years, discussing the current therapeutic approaches, such as hormone replacement therapy and some of the alternatives. Educational materials were provided to each group participant, creating a Menopause Resource Book. Each meeting included time for group interaction, creating an atmosphere of comfort which encouraged an exchange of experience and ideas. Based on the success of this series of programs, the Wellness Program received funding to develop comparable programs in the local community of East Harlem.

COMMUNITY CHARACTERISTICS AND NEEDS

East Harlem is located in the northeastern section of Manhattan in New York City. Mount Sinai Medical Center is situated in the southwest corner

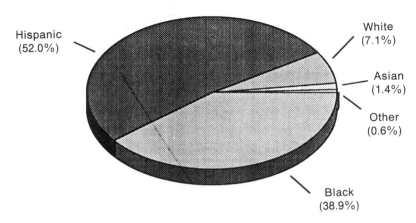

Source: 1990 Census Data

Figure 1   East Harlem residents: ethnic profile

of East Harlem and serves as a primary health care facility for many East Harlem residents.

According to 1990 Census Data, the population of East Harlem is 110 508 or 7.4% of Manhattan's total population of 7.4 million people. Life in East Harlem is characterized by poverty, high unemployment, crime, poor education and single parent households, mainly headed by women. There is a conspicuous absence of men due to the problems of drug addiction, crime and illness, such as AIDS. Consequently, women bear the burden of organizing community and family life, often caring for several generations of family members – their parents, their own children and perhaps their grandchildren, as many adult children are not able to carry out this responsibility. The ethnic and cultural diversity of East Harlem (Figure 1) becomes an uneasy mix against this subculture of poverty, crowding, and disadvantage.

East Harlem is one of the least affluent communities in Manhattan. This is reflected in the 1990 Census data which reported that the median household income in East Harlem was $8305, compared to a median household income of $20 000 in Manhattan as a whole. Forty-eight percent of East Harlem residents live below the federal poverty level and 34.1% receive public assistance, which is a package of medicaid – public health insurance for the medically and financially needy – food stamps and cash assistance, targeted at providing subsidy for housing.

Table 2 Program goals

(1) Provide educational support for midlife and menopause to low income minority women residing in the East Harlem community
(2) Promote wellness and disease prevention using group interaction and health education
(3) Adapt program to cultural context

PROGRAM DESIGN

Adapting a successful educational support program for menopause to a cultural context of hardship and profound deprivation posed a great challenge. The stated purpose of the newly funded program was to reach desperately poor women living on the edges of society, frequently isolated from health care systems, and lacking the motivation or habit of seeking information, much less making lifestyle changes compatible with good health.

How could information be presented in an understandable way, given the minimal educational levels of women in this community? How could these women become their own advocates for better health care and well-being? The program goals were ambitious but essential to address the unmet health care needs of the women we hoped to engage in our program (Table 2).

A public housing project located across the street from the Medical Center was selected as the first site for the pilot project. A social service drop-in center which links residents with services in the community, hosted our program. As the Mount Sinai Medical Center provides many of the health care services to community residents, the program proposal proved interesting to the administration of the housing project, as well as to the community representatives. There was enthusiastic support expressed to begin planning the new program.

The process of transition of the program from the Mount Sinai work-place to the community began with a luncheon at the Medical Center for the staff members of Mount Sinai and the Public Housing Project who would be working together. By that time we had recognized the need for a cultural liaison – an ambassador – to bridge the distance between the worlds of the medical center and East Harlem. We looked outside the medical center and selected an African–American woman who is both a social worker and an ordained minister with a parish of her own, and with a great deal of experience in working minority women's issues.

At our first meeting, 'Reverend Julia', as she came to be called by the group members, said that menopause was viewed as a middle class

Table 3 Midlife concerns for women:
a new healthy outlook

Sessions

(1) Welcome and introduction
(2) Stress management
(3) Menopause: Part I
(4) Menopause: Part II
(5) Nutrition
(6) Exercise
(7) Outdoor walk and yoga
(8) Midlife sexuality
(9) Access to health care systems

problem, meaning a white middle class problem, and a program focused on menopause alone would never attract low income minority women beyond one or two meetings, if at all.

'The changes' as menopause is called, are viewed as a normal part of life and not as anything requiring special attention. Together, we developed an inviting approach, broader in scope, with menopause as only part of the content to be offered.

The Educational Support Group for Menopause became Midlife Concerns For Women – A New Healthy Outlook. This became the first major transformation in adapting the original program to a new cultural context.

After many planning sessions, and outreach carried out by the coordinators of the drop-in center, the Midlife Concerns Group began a nine session program which extended over 4 months to allow time off for school vacations and holidays. All sessions were held in the familiar setting of the community drop-in center.

PROGRAM DESCRIPTION

The following is a brief description of each of the nine sessions of the *Midlife Concerns* program (Table 3).

Session 1: We opened our first meeting by introducing ourselves, the program and its goals. All the women were invited to introduce themselves as well, say why they had come to the program and what they hoped to learn.

Session 2: Stress management followed, to give the participants an opportunity to share some of the many stresses of their lives. This session was led by 'Reverend Julia' and a clinician, expert in techniques of stress recognition and reduction.

Session 3: The first session on menopause included some basic teaching about female reproductive life with supporting educational materials. Large diagrammatic pictures of the female reproductive system were provided and a discussion of the events leading to puberty and menstruation took place. Many of the women had had no idea what the female reproductive system looked like, much less how it functioned.

Session 4: Menopause Part II was led by a health educator who had previously conducted a program on gynecologic and breast health in this setting. Appropriately, material from the previous program was repeated and information was added relating to the physiological effects of the menopause. Hormone replacement therapy was explained and alternative therapies were discussed.

Session 5: Two registered dieticians from the medical center discussed nutrition and brought a selection of ethnic food stuffs to discuss in terms of the widespread problems of overweight, hypertension and diabetes that afflict women in this group.

Session 6: Mount Sinai offers a walking program to employees each spring and fall. This session on exercise was led by the gentleman who developed that program. He explained the health benefits of walking, and made suggestions about to how to begin to exercise.

Session 7: On a beautiful spring morning in late April, the Midlife Group met for a health walk in Central Park. This activity was led by a health educator, together with an African–American woman who is a certified yoga instructor. Following the walk, there was instruction in simple yoga techniques for relaxation and stress reduction. A healthful lunch ended the morning.

Session 8: Midlife sexuality discussed sexual activities as well as education on 'safe sex'. This was a primary concern for these women, as an increasing number of women over age 50 in this population are becoming HIV positive. Clearly there is a myth that after 'the changes' sexually transmitted diseases are no longer a threat. The urgency of safe sex was re-emphasized.

Session 9: The closing session of the program was perhaps the most important to many of the women in the group. The focus was on gaining access to the helping systems, and acknowledged the obstacles, both real and perceived, that low-income minority women frequently encounter when seeking help. The director of patients' rights and entitlements at the hospital answered many questions about getting help and made herself available to group members on an ongoing basis. A festive farewell dinner followed with healthfully prepared ethnic food served by The Mount Sinai staff to group members.

Child care was available throughout the program to encourage attendance and refreshments were always served. Bi-weekly meetings were held for the staffs of both the medical center and the housing project to monitor the group's progress. The community representatives critically evaluated the program at each meeting. Their suggestions were often incorporated into the style and content of the program with the result that the Midlife Group developed a sense of ownership of their group.

PROGRAM EVALUATION

The program reached a total of 25 women, all residents of public housing. Although the greatest age concentration was 41–50, women of ages 20–74 attended, and as one woman commented 'As a younger woman, I'm not afraid any more of being over 40'.

What made our program work?

(1) Consistent participation by Mount Sinai staff, who became group members and familiar to the residents;

(2) Mutual sharing and the recognition of the common bonds of womanhood;

(3) Adapting the program to the needs of the community and presenting the educational material in understandable ways; and

(4) Above all, our cultural ambassador, Reverend Julia.

We learned that the successful 'Educational Support Program for Menopause' at Mount Sinai had little meaning to low income minority women living in the community, who are preoccupied with survival issues. Menopause and midlife became, for this group, a unique opportunity to

Table 4 The future: women of high horizons

Program objectives
Safe sex
Crime prevention
Survival skills
Domestic violence
Recycling program
Plant a vegetable garden

value themselves as individuals and begin to consider ways of improving their lives.

Thanks to Reverend Julia, who spoke the language of both worlds, the spirit and content of the program became meaningful to the group members. The women were able to take in the program and reshape it to meet their own needs. At the conclusion of the formal program, The Midlife Concerns Group decided to continue as *Women of High Horizons* (Table 4).

CONCLUSION

While the program agenda may not be explicitly about menopause and health care, it is certainly about overcoming the immense difficulties of daily living which come before other considerations. The spirit of preventive care is emerging for this group. Good health begins with self-esteem and feelings of self worth. Health care professionals and health educators have a responsibility to convey knowledge that is understandable to others, support its application and help to remove the barriers that frequently stand between low income minority women and the help that they seek to improve their lives and the lives of their families.

10

Work, social life and health in women during transition to menopause

B.-M. Landgren and A. Collins

In Sweden, the mean age of menopause is 51.5 years. The last menstruation is an indicator of the end of reproductive life and the beginning of aging. In the developed countries women can expect to live one-third of their lives after the menopause. The perimenopausal years indicate the transition from reproductive life to postmenopausal life and thus represent a period of important physiological events for middle-aged women.

Some researchers consider vasomotor symptoms such as sweating, hot flushes and vaginal dryness as the only true climacteric symptoms. There is still controversy whether other somatic and psychological symptoms which have been described in the perimenopausal years may be related to other factors such as negative life events, employment and socio-economic factors[1-4].

In order to further investigate the somatic, hormonal and psychosocial factors affecting women's work, health and social life during the transition to menopause, we initiated a longitudinal analysis of a representative sample of normal, healthy women from Stockholm who will be followed from the age of 48 years until they all are postmenopausal.

STUDY DESIGN

The study was carried out in two stages. The first stage consisted of a cross-sectional postal survey which included 2000 women, aged 48 years when the background data were collected. The sample, representative of the whole female Stockholm population born in 1942, was recruited through the population register. Each woman received a letter and questionnaire covering three different areas:

(1) Sociodemographic background, such as marital status, level of education, employment, number of children, smoking habits and physical exercise.

(2) Health and gynecological history including questions about the menstrual cycle, dysmenorrhea, previous treatment and contraceptive use.

(3) Questions about the occurrence of vasomotor climacteric symptoms such as sweating, hot flushes, vaginal dryness and mood.

The second stage of the study involved 150 of those women who had responded to the survey. The sample was random and proportional to the levels of education and parity/non-parity of the original sample of 1400 subjects. These women were invited to participate in a longitudinal study including gynecological and general health screening, physiological measurements, hormonal characterization and bone density measurements once yearly until they are postmenopausal. Inclusion criteria for these women were a history of regular cycles, intact uterus, intact ovaries and no hormonal replacement therapy. They had no chronic illnesses nor an earlier history of psychiatric disease.

RESULTS

A total of 1400 women returned completed questionnaires, a response rate of 70%. The results showed that 27% of the women were postmenopausal; 8% of these had had a hysterectomy and 7% an oophorectomy, and 7.5% of the women received hormonal replacement therapy.

Marital status

The background data showed that 75% of the women were married, 17% were divorced and 8% widowed or never married. Eleven per cent of the women were living alone, 26% lived with husband or partner and 46% lived together with husband or partner and children. Six percent of the women were childless, 94% had borne one to six children. Twelve per cent of the women had consulted a doctor for infertility.

Table 1 Medication reported by women at baseline

Blood pressure lowering and anticoagulants	24.8%
Thyroid substitution	19.6%
Antihistamine	17.1%
Insulin	3.4%
Antidepressives	6.9%
Analgesics	5.5%
Sedatives	3.2%
Migraine medication	2.8%
Anti-inflammatory	6.0%
Nutritional supplementation	12.3%
Antifibrinolytics	1.9%
Cytostatics	1.3%

Employment

Ninety-eight per cent of the women were employed: 73.3% worked full-time and 26.7% worked part-time. Concerning occupation, 10% were higher professionals, 26% lower professionals, 55% were working in service or clerical jobs and 8% had unskilled occupations, while only 1% of the women were housewives.

Education

Thirty-five per cent of the women had primary school, 35% secondary school and 30% had college or university education.

Lifestyle

Twenty-three per cent of women were smokers. When asked about physical exercise, 57% reported that they took exercise at least once a week, whereas 43% reported not taking any exercise at all. Thirty-two per cent were on current medication (Table 1).

Menstrual cycle

In the group of 1400 women, 51% reported having mainly regular menstrual cycles, whereas 49% had mainly irregular cycles. Eighty per cent of the women reported having experienced some changes in their menstrual cycle, length or bleeding pattern during the preceding 12 months; 32.4% reported having experienced premenstrual symptoms and

48% dysmenorrhea; 32% were currently using contraceptives, 59% did not use any contraceptives and 8% were sterilized.

Two and a half per cent of the women had had unilateral mastectomy, 0.3% bilateral mastectomy and 1% radiation therapy for breast disease.

With respect to climacteric symptoms, 47% reported having experienced sweating or hot flushes and 31% vaginal dryness; 56% were suffering from depression, sleep disturbances or difficulty in concentrating.

In the second subgroup of 150 women 22% were postmenopausal and 78% premenopausal. Contraceptive use was as follows: none 49%, regular use 46% and occasional use 15%. The methods used were coitus interruptus 15%, periodical 5%, barrier 29%, intrauterine device 23%, combined pills 0%, low-dose gestagen 2% and 12% of the women were sterilized. Forty three percent had experienced hot flushes or sweating and 37% vaginal dryness; 49% were suffering from depression, insomnia and concentration difficulties. Fifty two percent had experienced stress incontinence and 39% had had this problem often.

When hormonal levels were compared between postmenopausal and premenopausal women, levels of luteinizing hormone (LH) and follicle stimulating hormone (FSH) were significantly higher in the postmenopausal women ($p < 0.0001$). Testosterone levels were significantly lower in postmenopausal compared to premenopausal women ($p < 0.0001$). Estradiol levels were significantly lower in the postmenopausal group ($p < 0.001$).

When hormone levels were compared between women suffering from climacteric symptoms and those lacking symptoms, significantly higher FSH and LH levels were found in those experiencing symptoms ($p < 0.001$). No difference was found between the two groups in the other hormones (estradiol, prolactin and testosterone).

Although these results only reflect the situation for Stockholm women during transition to menopause, they represent data from a group of normal middle-aged women and not, as most earlier studies, from women seeking medical help for symptoms. Therefore it will be interesting to follow this group of women until they all are postmenopausal.

REFERENCES

1. Voda, A. M. and Eliasson, M. (1983). Menopause: a closure of menstrual life. *Women Health,* **8**, 137–56
2. Ballinger, C. B. (1990). Psychiatric aspects of the menopause. *Br. J. Psychiatry,* **156**, 773–87

3. Hunter, M. (1988). Psychological aspects of the climacteric and the postmenopause. In Studd, J. and Whitehead, M. (eds.) *The Menopause*, pp. 55–64. (Oxford: Blackwell)
4. Collins, A. (1990). Psychosocial aspects of the menopause. In Beerman, B. and Strandberg, K. (eds.) *Pharmacological Treatment of Climacteric Symptoms*, Vol. 3, pp. 57–70. (Stockholm: Swedish National Board of Health and Welfare)

11

Female leadership in Sweden

A. Ax:son Johnson

I had a dream last night. It was a delightful dream, a precious dream ...
The room was large with crystal chandeliers. The meeting table was set
up with flags in front of each seat, flags from all the nations of the world.
On the table lay an agenda, which had seven items:

(1) My children,
(2) Our family,
(3) Economy and economic development,
(4) The good society,
(5) Environment,
(6) Peace, and
(7) The world.

Into the room came the leaders of the world. Wise and decisive. Clear in
their objectives yet willing to learn. Intellectually of the highest wit yet
practical in their approach. Humble in face of their task – to outline a
program for the survival, the development and the balance of our earth.

The world leaders were all women. They varied in age and experience,
in color and religion. Together they had set the agenda for their
deliberations. Their work started ... and I woke up, my mind full of
questions about the outcome and maybe an answer or two.

I think it was a Midsummer Night's Dream! On my desk lies a copy of
a businessman's weekly magazine with a cover story on power in Sweden.
Of the 200 most influential people of power, 26 are women. The prime
ministers of the Community had their group photo taken in Copenhagen
this week – not one is a woman.

In the business world, the world I know, women may be managers, but they are not at the very top of influence. Approximately two-thirds of the employees in Swedish industry, which is traditionally raw material-based, heavy industry, are men. A typical Swedish manufacturing company has no more than 2–5% women managers. Some companies, typically in retailing or services (banking) may have more, but not at the top. I must admit that even our group of companies, the Axel Johnson Group, is not proud to announce its figures. Being a private company, owned by a woman, with some 25 000 employees, mainly in trade, wholesaling and retailing, we should be able to show different results. We brag about our women managers that make up some 20–25% of all leadership. But in the top 100 maybe three to five are women.

Sweden is an organized country. It is also a country with a long-standing and rich social welfare structure. Our traditions are those of the peasant collectives, the villages, the group, rather than that of individualists. We share, we guard the righteous division of wealth, we sometimes jealously watch the welfare of others and protect our own. Thus we have built a system of sharing and of support which has been, for many years, a model for other countries.

This system has formed a structure which should bring out many women leaders. Maternity leave with full pay, day-care centers, job security, a fine public school system, health care – all are dreams or hopes in other countries. We have had it all. Yet we lack. The question remains: why?

I will share with you some possible reasons I have found within our companies. I cannot say whether they are representative of Swedish organizations or even of all Swedish corporations, but they come from some 25 years of experience in the business world.

First, our social welfare system is theoretical or even mythical. Some 85% or more of Swedish women work. The support system is in place, yet true sharing of family responsibilities is still far off. Women still bear the greatest burden and responsibility for their homes – both in terms of administration and practical tasks. The men support, the women work. The delights of child-bearing naturally belong to womanhood, but the 'main' parent over many years is still the mother. Until deep-rooted attitudes change, women will be trapped in overload; this has been shown in many recent studies.

Second, in Swedish companies women are isolated and feel lonesome (67% men, 33% women). The corporate world is still a world of men. Men *see* men, men *choose* men, men *speak* men's language. This is natural, if not acceptable. Men work and live in hierarchies, women work in social networks. Women need other women. Good companies need more women, at all levels and in all parts of business. In our company we have decided to build a 40/60 balance. But rather than to start from the top with a couple of 'symbolic' women we have started from below. Better balance brings better decisions which, in turn, brings more profit.

Third, men and women have different life, age and career cycles. Most Swedish organizations are built for the life- and career-cycle of men. Men are trained, start to work and build a career, charge ahead with definite goals, and retire to less operational positions after the age of 50. Women are trained, start to work and build a career but then break off for maternity leave, fit into jobs with less travel, that take less time, then charge ahead sometimes only to find themselves caught between teenage children and aging parents. When women return to a full-time career with time, energy, wisdom and perspective they – or we – are middle-aged, and are often considered, by the rules of the game, old, tired or out-of-date. I feel that unless business people are willing to build organizations that cater for families rather than to 'men only' and create specific careers for individuals, men and women, rather than creating male careers, our companies will falter.

Finally, the question of female leadership of course has to do with attitudes. Attitudes of others – and of ourselves.

This year I reach middle-age, with mixed feelings. I am a typical product of the 1940s (now being disputed and questioned by the 1960s generation), with a housewife mother and career daughters. Has it been too easy for many of us to abdicate as business women and career women? Have we had too many excuses? Attitudes are definitely shifting, albeit slowly, towards a defined need for women's specific values in all parts of our global society.

For the agenda of the future, this congress on the menopause is a valuable statement and a contribution to change others' attitudes towards us and our attitudes towards ourselves. Thank you for helping my Midsummer Night's Dream come closer to being realized.

Section 2

Reproductive endocrinology and physiology with relevance to the menopause

12

Reproductive hormone measurements during the menopausal transition

H. G. Burger

INTRODUCTION

The pituitary–ovarian axis can in some ways be considered as a type of biological clock, characterized by a monthly cycle of various phenomena, including those of ovulation and menstruation. These phenomena in turn reflect the successful recruitment of a cohort of follicles, from which one is normally selected to become the dominant ovulatory follicle, giving rise to the corpus luteum. Follicle stimulating hormone (FSH) is generally taken as one of the endocrine markers of that clock. The secretion of FSH is stimulated by gonadotropin releasing hormone (GnRH) but has a constitutive component, independent of GnRH, in contrast to luteinizing hormone (LH) which is highly dependent on GnRH input. FSH is under dual feedback control from the ovary both by estradiol and by the gonadal peptide hormone, inhibin. It is well known that after the menopause, in the absence of both of these feedback factors, FSH levels rise 10- to 15-fold compared with their follicular phase concentrations in mid-reproductive life, whereas the levels of LH rise only 3- to 5-fold, reflecting mainly a loss of steroidal, rather than non-steroidal, feedback.

A number of studies have shown that the population of primordial follicles in the normal ovary declines slowly during reproductive life until about the fortieth year when the decline becomes much steeper, so that by the time of the menopause itself few, if any, follicles remain in the ovary[1]. Because follicles are the source of both estradiol and inhibin, it is not surprising that FSH levels may become elevated prior to the final menstrual period, even in women who continue to cycle regularly.

The present study examines the evidence for the phenomenon of rising FSH levels in regularly cycling older women and in those who have started to experience some cycle disturbance. Evidence is presented that FSH levels in such women may fluctuate quite abruptly and that these fluctuations are generally associated with changes in the opposite direction in the levels of estradiol and inhibin. It is shown that while FSH may be a marker of the functioning of the biological clock constituted by the pituitary–ovarian axis, it cannot be taken as a reliable indicator of potential reproductive status, i.e. potential fertility.

FSH LEVELS IN REGULARLY CYCLING WOMEN

Several representative studies can be cited to provide evidence for an often selective rise in serum FSH levels in older, regularly cycling women.

Sherman and colleagues[2] studied a group of eight regularly cycling women aged 46–56 years and compared hormone measurements throughout the menstrual cycle with those found in a control group of women aged 18–30. FSH levels in the older women were frequently well above the normal younger follicular phase range, whilst LH and progesterone levels were generally normal. Estradiol levels were frequently below the young normal range, averaging 339 pmol/l in the older group, and 552 pmol/l in the younger. These investigators postulated that one factor leading to the selective increase in serum FSH levels was a declining secretion of the ovarian hormone inhibin, at that time not yet isolated and characterized[3].

Lee and associates[4] studied three groups of women, ranging in age from 36 to 40 ($n = 19$), 41 to 45 ($n = 18$) and 46 to 50 ($n = 16$), and compared reproductive hormone levels with those in a control group of 41 women aged 24–35 years. As age increased, early follicular and mid-cycle levels of FSH progressively rose and were threefold higher than the young normal range in the oldest group of women studied. Only a minor change in serum LH was noted in the oldest group, and there was no change in the two younger groups compared with the controls. Interestingly in this study, no change was seen in the circulating concentrations of estradiol and progesterone. Clearly, selective deficiency of inhibin secretion from the older ovary would provide a satisfactory explanation of this selective rise in serum FSH.

MacNaughton and colleagues[5] obtained blood samples on days 4–7 of the menstrual cycle from volunteers who were grouped by age (20–29, 30–39, 40–44, 45–49) with nine to ten subjects in each group. All were cycling regularly at the time of the study. Mean follicular phase levels of immunoreactive inhibin were significantly lower in the 45–49-year-olds compared with the younger age groups, while mean FSH levels were significantly higher in that oldest group, being more than twice those of the younger age groups. Mean estradiol levels in the oldest group were also significantly lower than those in the 30–39-year-olds but not when compared with the 20–29 and 40–44 age groups. LH levels did not differ significantly across age groups. Furthermore, there was a significant negative correlation between serum immunoreactive inhibin and FSH ($r = -0.45$, $p < 0.05$) and between estradiol and FSH ($r = -0.35$, $p < 0.05$). There was a significant negative relationship between immunoreactive inhibin and age ($r = -0.46$, $p < 0.05$). Analysis of the data indicated that average FSH levels remained unchanged until the age of 43 years and then rose significantly as a function of increasing age, while estradiol levels remained steady until the age of 38 years and then decreased significantly with increasing age. Inhibin levels fell linearly with increasing age. It was postulated that the results were consistent with a role for serum immunoreactive inhibin, in addition to estradiol, in the regulation of FSH during the follicular phase of the menstrual cycle, as a function of increasing age. This was suggested to reflect diminished folliculogenesis as age increased.

PREVALENCE OF INCREASED FSH AND DECREASED ESTRADIOL AND INHIBIN IN THE COMMUNITY

In an attempt to obtain further data on the significance of increased FSH levels, serum FSH, LH, estradiol and inhibin were measured in 484 women, participating in the first stage of a longitudinal study of the menopausal transition and the menopause in Melbourne, Australia. For an initial cross-sectional study of the significance of the menopausal transition, 1897 women were recruited, using telephone numbers selected randomly from a computerized data base of the Melbourne telephone directory[6]. Of these, 484 women agreed to volunteer for a longitudinal study which would involve annual interview and blood sampling. All continued to cycle at the time of recruitment for this phase. Single blood samples were obtained on days 5–8 when a regular menstrual cycle was still occurring. Of 105 women who had not yet experienced any change in cycle frequency or flow, seven (6.7%) had serum FSH levels above the lower limit of normal found in postmenopausal women. A further 60 (39%) of 236 women in whom a change of frequency or flow had been noted in the preceding 12 months had similar FSH levels, whereas 75% of women who had not bled for 3 months but had had a bleed within the preceding 12 months, had postmenopausal FSH levels. Furthermore, levels of FSH elevated above the normal follicular phase range for young women were found in 41 of 105 who were still cycling quite regularly (39%) and in 87 of 236 with a change in frequency or flow (37%), whereas 18% of the 45 who had had no bleed for at least 3 months had FSH levels which were elevated but below the postmenopausal range.

Estradiol concentrations < 100 pmol/l were found in 9% of those with no change in cycle frequency or flow and inhibin was undetectable in 28% of these. In 233 subjects who had had a change in frequency or flow estradiol levels were low in 48, while inhibin was undetectable in 97.

PERIMENOPAUSAL PATTERNS OF GONADOTROPINS, IMMUNOREACTIVE INHIBIN, ESTRADIOL AND PROGESTERONE

To gain some insight into the dynamics of reproductive hormone secretion during the time of menstrual irregularity preceding the menopause, three normal volunteers who had begun to develop cycle irregularity at the age of 45–46 years were studied, by intermittent blood sampling[7]. Abrupt changes were observed, with transient elevations of FSH and LH and decreases of inhibin and estradiol into the postmenopausal range, followed by levels more characteristic of women of reproductive age. In one subject, for example, normal reproductive age levels of FSH, LH, estradiol and inhibin were found in the middle of the normal luteal phase. She menstruated 5 days later and a follicular blood sample was obtained on day 6 of the succeeding cycle. An FSH level in the postmenopausal range (23.9 IU/l) was found with a marginally elevated LH level and postmenopausal range values for estradiol and inhibin. Despite these findings the cycle length was again 28 days. The following cycle was, however, prolonged to 47 days. Despite the hormonal findings, this subject, and the other two similar subjects, reported no menopausal symptoms.

SUMMARY AND CONCLUSIONS

Several studies have demonstrated increasing FSH levels in regularly cycling women of increasing age. The prevalence of raised FSH and low estradiol and inhibin increases as cycle irregularity becomes manifest in some women. Changes in reproductive hormones may occur abruptly at the time of declining ovarian function.

It is concluded that the rise in FSH seen in regularly cycling older women reflects decreased ovarian feedback from a declining pool of follicles. The finding of postmenopausal FSH levels in regularly cycling or irregularly cycling women invalidates FSH measurement as a reliable marker that menopause has occurred or that further fertility is not possible.

REFERENCES

1. Richardson, S. J., Senikas, V. and Nelson, J. F. (1987). Follicular depletion during the menopausal transition: evidence for accelerated loss and ultimate exhaustion. *J. Clin. Endocrinol. Metab.*, **65**, 1231–7
2. Sherman, B. M., West, J. H. and Korenman, S. G. (1976). The menopausal transition: analysis of LH, FSH, estradiol, and progesterone concentrations during menstrual cycles of older women. *J. Clin. Endocrinol. Metab.*, **42**, 629–36
3. Sherman, B. M. and Korenman, S. G. (1975). Hormonal characteristics of the human menstrual cycle throughout reproductive life. *J. Clin. Invest.*, **55**, 699–706
4. Lee, S. J., Lenton, E. A., Sexton, L. and Cooke, I. D. (1988). The effect of age on the cyclical patterns of plasma LH, FSH, oestradiol and progesterone in women with regular menstrual cycles. *Hum. Reprod.*, **3**, 851–5
5. MacNaughton, J., Bangah, M., McCloud, P., Hee, J. and Burger, H. G. (1992). Age related changes in follicle stimulating hormone, luteinizing hormone, estradiol and immunoreactive inhibin in women of reproductive age. *Clin. Endocrinol.*, **36**, 339–45
6. Dennerstein, L., Smith, A. K. A., Morse, C., Burger, H., Green, A., Hopper, J. and Ryan, M. (1993). *Med. J. Aust.*, **159**, 232–6
7. Hee, J., MacNaughton, J., Bangah, M. and Burger, H. G. (1993). Perimenopausal patterns of gonadotrophins, immunoreactive inhibin, oestradiol and progesterone. *Maturitas*, in press

13

The aging ovary – the changes in the vascular system of the ovary in perimenopausal periods

T. Aso, T. Kubota, S. Obayashi, S. Sakamoto, Y. Shimizu,
M. Tada, T. Yaguchi, H. Azuma and S. Sato

INTRODUCTION

The beginning of the biological activities of the ovaries causes characteristic physiological changes in menarche, which corresponds to the start of reproductive life. The initiation of this process in man arises mainly as the consequence of functional maturations in the central nervous system. Throughout the reproductive period, the ovaries ovulate regularly and are the major source of sex steroid hormones. During this period, a number of follicles mature in each menstrual cycle, but in most cycles, only one reaches ovulation, the rest becoming atretic. A rough estimate indicates that the overwhelming majority of follicles undergoes atresia, < 400 reaching maturity.

By 20 weeks of gestation, the fetal ovary contains 6–7 million germ cells; however, oocyte depletion by atresia begins at approximately 15 weeks of gestation. The newborn female infant bears approximately 2 million oocytes; this number decreases continually until menopause, when the store is finally exhausted.

During the approach to menopause, the twilight of reproductive life, various physical and mental alterations are commonly observed as the result of aging of ovarian functions. As extensive studies have demonstrated, oocyte depletion is the ultimate background of the aging process of the ovary. During this process, extremely accelerated oocyte depletion has been observed in the perimenopause, especially between 41 and 45 years of age. The observable involution of ovarian size and decrease of steroidogenic capacity are also essential changes in this stage of reproductive life.

In an attempt to understand the mechanisms governing the specific changes in ovarian functions in the perimenopausal period, structural and functional alterations in the vascular system perfusing and draining the ovary were studied.

MATERIAL AND METHODS

The mechanical responses to vasoactive substances in transverse strips of ovarian arteries obtained from pre- and postmenopausal women were investigated using the Magnus apparatus. The details of the method have been reported elsewhere[1,2]. In brief, ovarian artery specimens were obtained at hysterectomy. The specimens were removed within 10 min after clamping the bilateral ends of 3 cm segments of ovarian artery contained in the infundibulo-pelvic ligament. The removed strips were dissected free from surrounding connective tissue. Special care was taken to avoid stretching or otherwise injuring the specimens during handling. One end of the strip was secured to the bottom of an organ bath, and the other end was attached to a force-displacement transducer. Isometric changes in tension were recorded on a pen oscillograph. After 60 min of equilibration with bathing solution, 10^{-6} mol/l of acetylcholine was given, while contraction was induced by 10^{-6} mol/l of norepinephrine to confirm the functional capacity of endothelium. Subsequently, the cumulative concentration–relaxation curves were constructed under the influence of each substance and enzyme inhibitor. The concentration of the substances and enzyme inhibitors were: bradykinin 10^{-10}–10^{-7} mol/l, sodium nitroprusside 10^{-9}–3×10^{-6} mol/l, calcium ionophore (A23187) 10^{-6} mol/l, indomethacin 10^{-5} mol/l, L-nitroarginine 10^{-4} mol/l, and OKY-046 10^{-6} mol/l. The duration of reincubation with enzyme inhibitors was 20 min. Simultaneously, part of the specimen was processed for morphological examination.

Ovarian tissues were obtained from premenopausal (40–45 years of age) and postmenopausal (55–60 years of age) women undergoing surgery. Some specimens were obtained from the same patients as the ovarian arteries. Wangison-elastica staining and preparation for electron microscopic observation were conducted by conventional methods. Frozen ovarian tissue was cut using cryosection and the immunohistochemical localization of endothelin was studied by the ABC method using

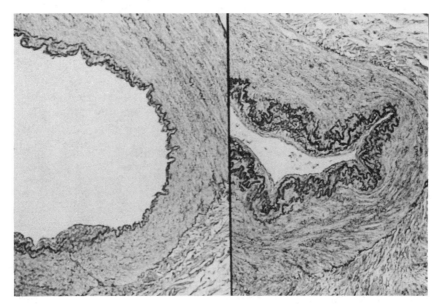

Figure 1 Microscopic features of ovarian arteries in premenopause (left) and postmenopause (right). Wangison elastica double staining ($\times$ 100)

the antisera raised against human endothelin-1, supplied by Peptide Institute, Osaka, Japan.

RESULTS

Physicomechanical studies on the ovarian arteries in peri-menopausal women

Cross-section views of ovarian arteries obtained from pre- and postmeno-pausal women are shown in Figure 1. Wangison-elastica double-stained microscopy showed marked thickening of the intima layer in the wall of postmenopausal ovarian arteries. Scanning electron microscopy showed that endothelial cells covering the inner surface of premenopausal ovarian arteries had a vivid and active appearance with regular and smooth arrangement (Figure 2). In contrast, the surface of postmenopausal arteries was covered with numerous platelets, from which protruded a fibrin-like substance adhering to the endothelium (Figure 3).

The cumulative concentration–relaxation curves of the ovarian arteries obtained from pre- and postmenopausal women were constructed using

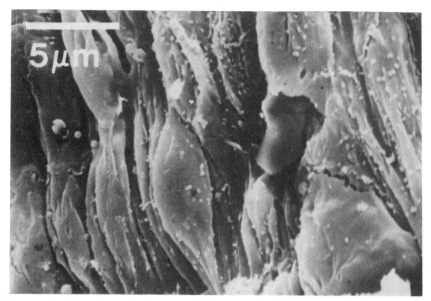

Figure 2 Scanning electron microscopical finding of the inner surface of a premenopausal ovarian artery

three different vaso-relaxants. As depicted in Figure 4, the degree of relaxation induced by bradykinin in premenopausal arteries was significantly greater than that in postmenopausal arteries. Sodium nitroprusside and A23187 produced no difference in the relaxation response in pre- and postmenopausal arteries.

The effects of pretreatment with two endothelium-derived vasoactive prostanoid inhibitors, indomethacin and OKY-046, are shown in Figures 5 and 6. Preincubation with the cyclo-oxygenase inhibitor indomethacin, which inhibits both prostaglandin I2 and thromboxane A2 production in the endothelium, had no significant influence on the magnitude of bradykinin-induced relaxation in the specimens obtained from either pre- or postmenopausal women (Figure 5). Incubation with OKY-046, which only blocks thromboxane A2 synthase, apparently enhanced the magnitude of bradykinin-induced relaxation in postmenopausal arteries; no such response could be detected in premenopausal arteries (Figure 6).

The effect of enzyme inhibitors on the maximum relaxation induced by A23187 is summarized in Figure 7. It is obvious that the inhibition induced by L-nitroarginine in premenopausal arteries was greater than that in postmenopausal specimens. Indomethacin suppressed and OKY-046 enhanced the maximum relaxation in postmenopausal ovarian arteries.

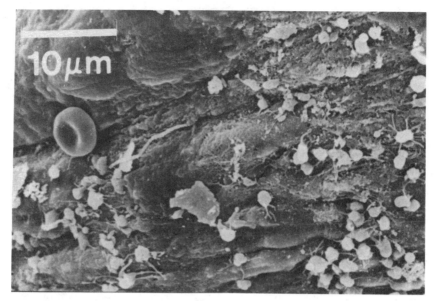

Figure 3 Scanning electron microscope of the inner surface of a postmenopausal ovarian artery

The ultrastructure of blood vessels in ovarian tissue obtained from pre- and postmenopausal women

In tissue slices containing both cortical and medullary portions of ovarian tissues (Figure 8), the number and size of the lumen of the arterioles were apparently greater in premenopause ovaries than in the postmenopausal ovaries. A close-up view (Figure 9) revealed more collagenous fibers surrounding the postmenopausal arterioles. In a premenopausal ovary, the lamina elastica interna layer of arteriole wall could be traced with partial and slight irregularity and interruptions; extremely advanced degenerative changes were seen in the postmenopause ovaries.

Electron microscopy of the arterioles in the medulla of premenopause ovaries (Figure 10) indicated that the structure of the endothelium and basal layer is maintained with slight degeneration, and the amount of collagenous fibers in the intercellular matrix is obviously increased. Postmenopaual ovaries showed endothelial atrophy, basal layer hypertrophy, decreased smooth muscle cells, and a marked increase in collagenous fibers.

The blood vessels of the cortex of premenopause ovaries were filled with red blood cells (Figure 11). Collagenous fibers regularly proliferated

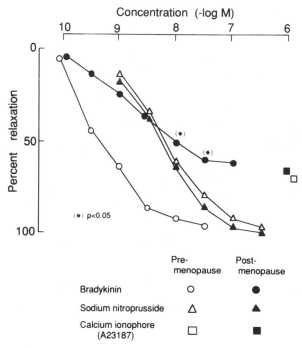

Figure 4 The patterns of mean relaxation response to bradykinin, sodium nitroprusside and calcium ionophore in pre- and postmenopausal ovarian arteries

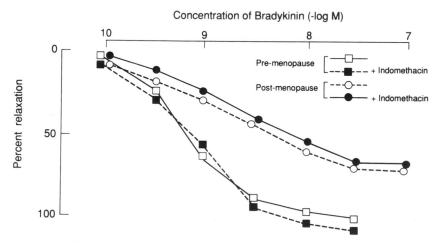

Figure 5 The influence of indomethacin on bradykinin-induced relaxation in pre- and postmenopausal ovarian arteries

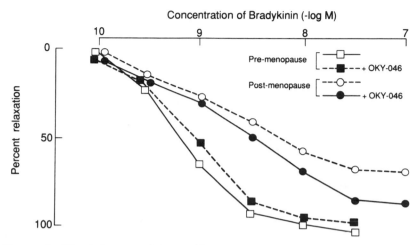

Figure 6 The influence of OKY-046 on bradykinin-induced relaxation in pre- and postmenopausal ovarian arteries

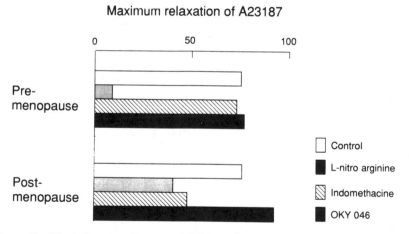

Figure 7 The influence of enzyme inhibitors (L-nitroarginine, indomethacin and OKY-046) on the maximum relaxation induced by calcium ionophore (A23187)

around the vessels. Two different types of stromal cells, large cells with a round nucleus and spindle form cells, were seen. The endothelium of postmenopausal arterioles was atrophic and vacuole formation could be observed. Only spindle form stromal cells were observed around the vessels.

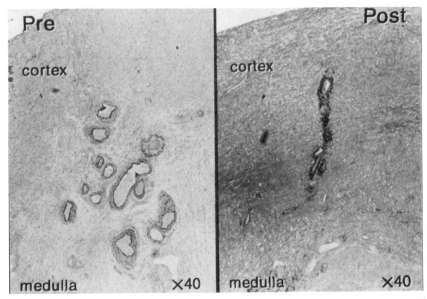

Figure 8 Microscopical findings of the ovarian slice including cortex and medulla obtained from a premenopausal (left) and a postmenopausal (right) woman. Wangison elastica double staining

The localization of endothelin in pre- and postmenopausal ovarian tissues

Immunoreactive endothelin was positively stained in the hyalinized portion of postmenopausal ovarian tissue. As shown in Figure 12, the endothelin-positive cells were located on the wall of arterioles scattered in hyalinized ovarian tissue.

DISCUSSION

Contraction and relaxation of the arterial wall is controlled by various chemical and vasoactive substances, including endothelium-derived relaxing factor (EDRF), the role of which in the relaxation of the smooth muscle surrounding the arterial walls has been studied extensively[3,4]. In endothelial cells, nitric oxide synthase is activated by bradykinin, which converts L-arginine to EDRF through a receptor-mediated mechanism[5]. Subsequently, EDRF stimulates guanylate cyclase in the smooth muscle to induce muscle relaxation.

One of the significant differences in the physicomechanical response

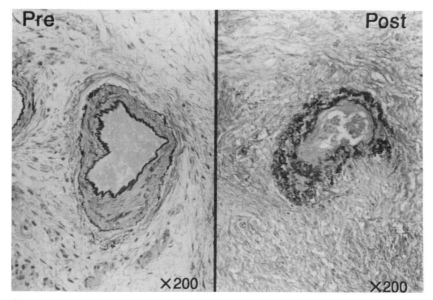

Figure 9 Close-up view of arterioles in pre- (left) and postmenopausal (right) ovaries

of pre- and postmenopausal ovarian arteries was detected on stimulation by bradykinin. However, ovarian arteries from these two periods exhibited the same responses to both sodium nitroprusside, which acts directly on the smooth muscles and is a non-endothelium-derived substance, and A23187, which increases the intracellular calcium concentration in a non-receptor-mediated manner. These results indicate that impairment of the EDRF-related relaxation mechanism is the major alteration in post-menopausal ovarian arteries, but that the non-EDRF-mediated relaxation capacity of endothelium and the function of smooth muscle cells are reversed.

Prostanoids, including prostaglandin I_2 and thromboxane A2, have been postulated to be involved in the mechanism of smooth muscle relaxation and contraction[6]. The simultaneous block of prostaglandin I_2 and throm-boxane A2 synthesis by indomethacin did not affect the bradykinin-induced relaxation of pre- or postmenopausal ovarian arteries. Treatment with OKY-046, which only blocks thromboxane A2 synthesis, produced a pattern of response in postmenopausal arteries different from that of premenopausal arteries. The results of experiments investigating the effect of enzyme inhibitors on A23187-induced relaxation provided further information concerning the specific changes in the endothelium of pre-

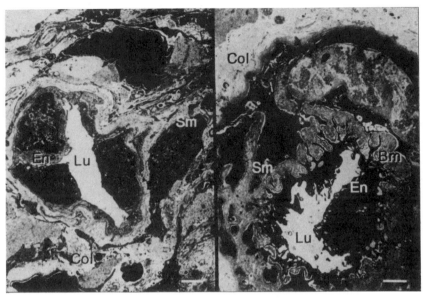

Figure 10 Electron microscopic findings of arterioles in pre- (left) and post-menopausal (right) ovaries. En, endothelium; Lu, lumen; Sm, smooth muscle; Bm, basal membrane; Col, collagenous fiber (bar = 5 μm)

and postmenopausal ovarian arteries. In premenopausal arteries, the greatest inhibition was induced by L-nitroarginine, an inhibitor of EDRF synthesis, but suppression by indomethacin and OKY-046 was not detected. On the other hand, in postmenopausal arteries, the suppressive effect of L-arginine was relatively less than that seen in the premenopause. The biological significance of EDRF may, therefore, be relatively less in causing relaxation of postmenopausal ovarian arteries. It is also obvious that indomethacin and OKY-046 exhibit different effects on the A23187-induced relaxation of pre- and postmenopausal ovarian arteries. As mentioned above, this indicates that a decrease in EDRF synthesis is one of the essential changes in postmenopausal endothelium. Whereas the contribution of prostanoids to the relaxation of premenopausal ovarian arteries is limited, their roles on arterial wall relaxation becomes dominant in the postmenopause.

The structural changes of arterioles in postmenopausal ovaries are striking. Disappearance of the lamina elastica interna, hypertrophy of the basal layer, and an increase in intercellular collagenous fibers reduce the elasticity of the arterial wall and narrow the lumen of the arteries. The distinct atrophic and degenerative alterations in endothelium are

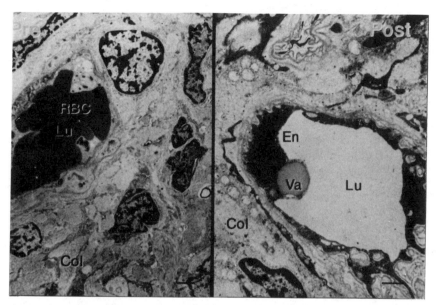

Figure 11 Electron microscopic findings of arterioles in pre- (left) and post-menopausal (right) ovaries. RBC, red blood cell; En, endothelium; Lu, lumen; Col, collagenous fiber; Va, vacuole formation (bar = 5 μm)

compatible with the changes in mechanical response of the ovarian arteries.

The perivascular localization of endothelin, which has been reported to be a potent endothelium-derived contracting factor[7], in the hyalinized ovarian tissue, strongly indicates its involvement in the local control mechanism of vascular tone. Previous studies showed that contractions of the blood vessel wall induced by endothelin can only be reversed by EDRF[8], and the production and/or release of endothelin is suppressed by EDRF[9]. In addition to the effects on vascular tone, EDRF was also reported to prevent platelet adhesion and aggregation[10]. Thus, the decrease in EDRF release is one of the crucial factors in the initiation and promotion of the sequence of events in the perimenopausal vascular system. The cumulative alterations in the blood vessels which result from these events seem ultimately to contribute to the overall aging process of ovaries.

ACKNOWLEDGEMENTS

This study was supported by the Research Grant of Japan Ministry of Education (# 04670992), and Akaeda Medical Research Foundation.

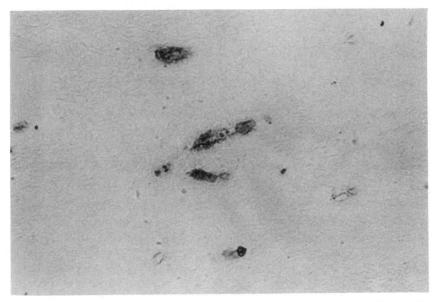

Figure 12 Immunohistochemical finding of endothelin-positive cells on the walls of the hyalinized portion of intra-ovarian blood vessels (× 40)

REFERENCES

1. Azuma, H., Niimi, Y. and Hamasaki, H. (1992). Prevention of intimal thickening after endothelial removal by a nonpeptide angiotensin II receptor antagonist, losartan. *Br. J. Pharmacol.*, **106**, 665–71
2. Tujii, T., Azuma, H. and Oshima, H. (1992). A possible role of decreased relaxation dedicated by β-adrenoreceptors in bladder outlet obstruction by benign prostatic hyperplasia. *Br. J. Pharmacol.*, **107**, 803–7
3. Furchgott, R. F. and Zawadzki, J. V. (1980). The obligatory role of endothelial cells in the relaxation of arterial smooth muscle by acetylcholine. *Nature (London)*, **288**, 373–6
4. Palmer, R. M. J., Ferrige, A. G. and Moncada, S. (1987). Nitric oxide release from the biological active endothelium-derived relaxing factor. *Nature (London)*, **327**, 524–6
5. Palmer, R. M. J., Ashton, D. S. and Moncada, S. (1988). Vascular endothelial cells synthesize nitric oxide from L-arginine. *Nature (London)*, **333**, 664–6
6. Steinleitner, A., Stanczyk, F., Levin, J. H., d'Ablaing, G. III, Vijod, M. A., Shahbazian, V. L. and Lobo, R. A. (1989). Decreased *in vitro* production of 6-keto-prostaglandin F by uterine arteries from postmenopause women. *Am. J. Obstet. Gynecol.*, **161**, 1677–81
7. Yanagisawa, M., Kurihara, H., Kimura, S., Tomobe, Y., Kobayagshi, M., Mitsui, Y., Yasaki, Y., Goto, K. and Masaki, T. (1988). A novel potent vasoconstrictor

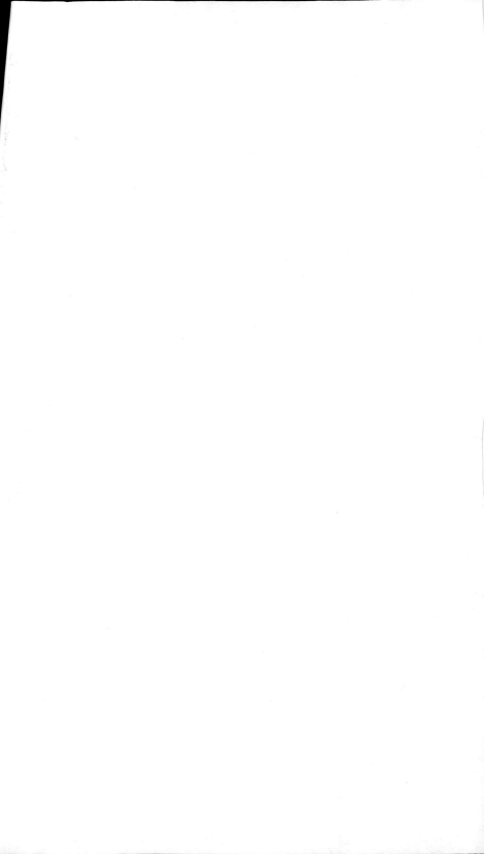

peptide produced by vascular endothelial cell. *Nature (Lona* 411–15

8. Vanhoutte, P. M., Auch-Schwelk, W., Boulanger, C., Janssen, P. A. Z. S., Komori, K., Miller, V. M., Shini, V. B. and Vidal, M. (1989). Does er. 1 mediate endothelium-dependent contractions during anoxia? *J. Cai Pharmacol.*, **13**, S124–8

9. Boulanger, C. and Luscher, T. F. (1990). Release of endothelin fr porcine aorta. *J. Clin. Invest.*, **85**, 587–90

10. Azuma, H., Ishikawa, M. and Sekizaki, S. (1986). Endothelium-dep(inhibition of platelet aggregation. *Br. J. Pharmacol.*, **88**, 411–15

14

The menopausal hot flush: facts and fancies

J. Ginsburg and P. Hardiman

Apart from Hippocrates' statement on the absence of gout in menstruating women[1], there are apparently no references in Greek medical literature to symptoms peculiar to those in whom the menses have ceased. Indeed Saronus, a Roman physician, commented in 100 AD[2] 'the fact that they do not menstruate any more does not affect the health of women past their prime'. At the same time, however, he noted 'one must take care that the stoppage of menses does not occur suddenly', since 'that which is unaccustomed is not tolerated but is like some unfamiliar malaise'. Unfortunately the precise form of this malaise was not stated. Thereafter and for some 1500 years, there was little interest in gynecological problems in general. The first reference to a menopausal complaint is probably by Willis in 1683[3], of 'convulsions in the stomach'. The first description of a menopausal hot flush is nearly 30 years later, in 1712, when Lawrence Heister[4] described the symptoms of the Dowager Lady Rieden at Kornburg in Germany. This lady, aged 40, and still menstruating, albeit irregularly, complained of an intermittent 'commotion in the blood' starting in the stomach and accompanied by great heat and facial redness and also often by sweating. Subsequently, many authors both in England and in France, described typical hot flushes. The French physician Chauffe, coined the term 'bouffées de chaleur' (puffs of heat), a name still used by the French when referring to menopausal flushing. By the middle of the nineteenth century, recommendations for the treatment of hot flushes laid particular emphasis on avoidance of large gatherings and heated rooms[5]. A detailed study was made by Tilt (1858)[6], who noted that the frequency of this symptom was nearly 50% (244 women) in his series of 500 women. He observed that menopausal women, in general, seemed to generate more heat and tended to leave windows and doors wide open. Although many gynecologists recognized the distress caused by hot flushes, and that they were specific complications of the menopause, a considerable body of opinion (not just confined to the medical profession) then, as now, viewed hot flushes at the menopause as analogous to the wayward maiden's blush – an emotional reaction to stress.

Hence, although the hot flush is conventionally considered the characteristic clinical manifestation of the climacteric, occurring in around 70% of menopausal women[7] and sufficiently severe in at least half for them to seek medical help, they may still be fobbed off with sedatives and advised to avoid stressful situations. Germaine Greer's claim[8] regarding the mechanism of the hot flush, that 'the process that causes the blood vessels in the surface of the skin to dilate is similar to the mechanism that makes some of us feel hot with embarrassment and go red' is little different from that of Victorian doctors in numerous texts of the time, as are her recommendations for hydrotherapy! But the menopausal hot flush, as we have shown[9], is not the same as the blush although both may be precipitated or exacerbated by stress.

One of the problems in studying the hot flush is its extreme variability. It may start at any age. The onset may be in the perimenopausal phase in a woman who is still menstruating and can be very severe at that stage. More often, however, it is first noticed with the onset of the menopause, the most striking example being the sudden occurrence of drenching and debilitating hot flushes in women subjected to hysterectomy and oophorectomy in their 40s, at a time when they are still menstruating. On the other hand, a woman may cease menstruating and enter the menopause without a hint of a flush, only to be confronted with devastating symptoms 10 or even 20 years later. The length of time for which flushes last is also variable. Some women have flushes for a few months, some for years on end. Some women never flush at all. The intensity and frequency of flushing can vary in the same woman, flushes being slight one year but severe and frequent another year.

There is also variation with social class and marital status. Professional women and those in social classes I or II tend on the whole to be less affected; single women were reported to suffer more than married women[10]. There are differences according to race and also within races, modified by sociological factors, in particular by the view of a society on the woman's role with the advent of the menopause – whether this is positive or negative may affect the frequency and intensity of flushing[11].

Hard facts about the flush have been scarce until the last three decades. Indeed it is a mere 12 years since we made the first quantitative measurement of what actually happens during the hot flush[12]. Before that, in view of the thermal accompaniments of the phenomenon, attempts to find out what happens during the flush were confined to skin temperature measurements. The classic paper is that of Molnar in 1975[13], who used thermocouples inserted into various orifices – rectum, vagina, tympanum, and esophagus – as well as cutaneous temperature probes, during flushing episodes. His paper is based on recordings of flushing episodes in one woman studied naked in different temperatures and during the application of various stimuli! Bearing in mind the number of orifices into which these thermocouples were inserted, one can but marvel at the compliance of the subject until one appreciates that the lady was Molnar's wife. He showed that a rise in skin temperature occurred *after* the flush itself, generally around 8 min after the onset of symptoms but with no corresponding rise in core temperature; in fact this fell. There was also a disturbance of the baseline electrocardiographic record, a phenomenon confirmed by Sturdee[14]. The pattern of change in skin temperature associated with flushing episodes has subsequently been studied by many workers, mainly in North America, and particularly in California[15].

Skin temperature measurements were heralded as an objective record of what happens during the hot flush and used in the evaluation of drug effects. They have been assumed to reflect what happens during the hot flush, particularly changes in blood flow. This assumption is not justified. Of itself, a skin temperature measurement has very limited use and inferences from changes in skin temperature must be made with caution. It is generally forgotten that cutaneous temperature reflects the difference between the heat lost to the environment by convection evaporation, radiation and conduction and that conveyed to the skin by the incoming arterial blood. Hence if a rise in skin temperature is to be considered a valid index of the rate of blood flow, the amount of heat lost to the environment must not change. Sweating is, however, frequent during the hot flush. This increases evaporation from the skin and thus alters skin temperature. Even if there is no sweating, an increase in blood flow to a local area of skin will then increase heat lost by radiation.

Furthermore, skin temperature reaches a maximum long before that of skin blood flow, so that no increase in surface temperature is then recorded with any further increase in cutaneous flow. At high rates of blood flow and with rapid fluctuations in flow, skin temperature is thus an insensitive and unreliable indicator of changes in the local circulation. Moreover, changes in skin temperature provide no indication of what is happening to the circulation in tissues deep to the skin, such as muscle. The foregoing explains why the temporal relation between a rise in skin temperature and the symptoms of a flush is poor. In Meldrum's[15] series for example, only 28 of 41 temperature elevations (69%) were associated with symptomatic flushes reported by the woman. On the other hand, a woman might say she felt a flush but no change in surface temperature was recorded. At best, surface temperatures provide a retrospective, qualitative indication of the approximate frequency of flushes.

The apparatus required for skin temperature measurement is, however, relatively simply and can be used throughout the 24 h, even with the woman ambulant. By this means, it has been shown that increased fluctuations in skin temperature occur in menopausal women but not in those before the menopause or in menopausal women whose flushes have been abolished by estrogen therapy.

Since the hot flush is essentially a vascular phenomenon, if we want to know what is happening during the flush, it is obviously essential to measure what is happening to blood flow directly. We therefore measured hand and forearm flow during hot flushes, either spontaneous or evoked by stressful mental arithmetic, in menopausal women[12]. The onset of symptoms of the hot flush is associated with an immediate and rapid increase in hand blood flow (Figure 1). This reaches a peak within $2\frac{1}{2}$ min and remains elevated for some 2 min after the sensations of the hot flush have subsided before falling to control values over a further 2 min. Forearm flow and pulse rate rise at the same time, but to a lesser extent, and both fall to control values before hand blood flow. These circulatory changes, it must be emphasized, occur before the reported rise in surface temperature after the flush.

There is, however, no change in blood pressure during the period of altered peripheral blood flow and pulse rate. This excludes the release of a circulating generalized vasodilator causing widespread vasodilatation during the hot flush; if this were the case blood pressure would fall. From studies using strain gauge plethysmography we concluded further that the increase in forearm flow is essentially due to vasodilatation in the vessels of forearm skin. Indeed, if significant vasodilatation occurred in a major vascular bed during the hot flush, blood pressure would only be maintained constant if vasoconstriction occurred simultaneously elsewhere.

The circulatory phenomena observed during the menopausal hot flush are not, however, specific to the female. After orchidectomy[16] or the administration of a gonadotropin releasing hormone (GnRH) agonist[17], men may also flush, and their symptoms can be as severe as those in

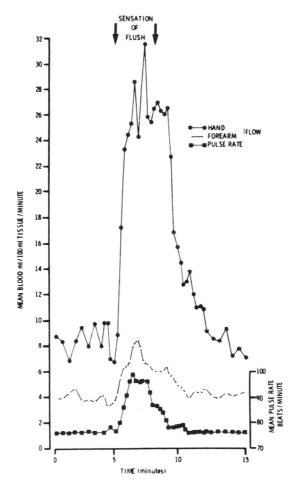

Figure 1 Mean hand and forearm blood flow (ml/100 ml tissue/min) and pulse rate (beats/min) in six women before, during, and after a menopausal hot flush. (Reproduced with permission from reference 12)

menopausal women. Our investigation of a man who flushed frequently and severely after orchidectomy for carcinoma of the prostate[16] showed an identical circulatory change to that reported in the female – a rapid and marked increase in hand blood flow, with a lesser but nevertheless significant rise in both forearm flow and pulse rate.

The pattern of circulatory change observed during the flush is similar to that recorded during indirect body heating. The mechanisms for heat dissipation are therefore activated during the hot flush, but in the absence of any rise in core temperature. This inappropriate inactivation of the mechanisms for heat loss is a reflex phenomenon which differs from that observed in response to stress such as stressful mental arithmetic or during the emotional blush. During the former, whilst forearm flow rises, hand flow may fall and blood pressure is significantly elevated. Similarly with the emotional flush, forearm flow rises significantly but there is no overall change in hand flow. Blood pressure also increases during the blush.

The menopausal flush is thus a specific, well defined, reflex response characterized by an increase in hand and blood flow and also, although to a lesser extent, in pulse rate, but which is not associated with a change in systemic blood pressure. The pattern of circulatory change during the menopausal flush is in turn quite different from that recorded in the emotional blush and also from the cardiovascular response to stress, as illustrated by that of stressful mental arithmetic. A flush is therefore not a blush and the flush is not a response to stress *per se* although hot flushes may be precipitated or exacerbated by stress.

Women who flush frequently seem to be more intolerant of heat than women who do not flush. Heat intolerance is present even when they are not actually flushing. They are hot when they are doing housework, they are hot at night and they may even sleep on top of the bed covers. It has also been claimed that women who flush frequently tend to have higher blood pressures than those who do not[1]. We therefore compared various cardiovascular parameters in women who flushed frequently with those in a group of women who did not. We found forearm flow to be higher in flushing women than in non-flushers[19] (Figure 2). This elevation in forearm flow was sustained during stressful mental arithmetic and also in response to administration of the catecholamines or noradrenaline. We have therefore provided objective evidence of a difference in the functioning of the peripheral vasculature in women who complain of hot flushes compared with those who do not experience such symptoms. The control of blood flow through the periphery in women who experience flushes thus differs from that of their asymptomatic peers. Differences in the response of the heart to catecholamines were also apparent, with a greater alteration in pulse rate observed during the infusion of adrenaline and a greater fall in pulse rate during infusion of noradrenaline in 'flushers' compared to that in asymptomatic women. This indicates a change in various aspects of cardiovascular function in flushing women outside the episodes of flushing themselves. The flush itself may be only one manifestation of a more widespread disturbance in cardiovascular function after the menopause. In order for flushes to

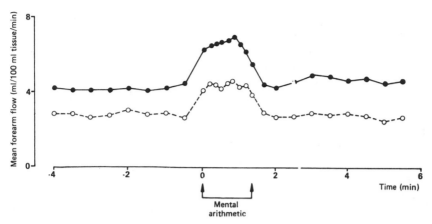

Figure 2 Mean forearm blood flow (ml/100 ml tissue/min) before, during, and after stressful mental arithmetic in 15 menopausal women who had hot flushes (●) and 13 who did not (○). (Reproduced with permission from reference 19)

occur, changes in peripheral vascular control and blood flow in the extremities may therefore be an essential prerequisite.

Because the menopause is characteristically a time of major endocrine change, attempts have been made to invoke hormonal change in the genesis of flushing. Unfortunately, no one hormone has been shown to be responsible either for the initiation of a flush or as an essential background to their occurrence.

Whilst there is no doubt that the advent of the menopause is associated with hypo-estrogenicity and the concurrent elevated gonadotropin levels set the background, so to speak, for the appearance of hot flushes, it has not been possible to link changes in either estrogen or gonadotropins with the onset of individual flush episodes. Thus there are no acute changes in estrogen levels before or during the flush itself. It is, however, of interest that women with gonadal dysgenesis do not flush until after they have been treated with estrogens and therapy is withdrawn for a while.

There was great excitement when a temporal relationship was claimed between pulsatile luteinizing hormone (LH) release and individual hot flushes[20]. Unfortunately, however, these studies used skin temperature elevations to indicate flush episodes, which, as already discussed, are poor indicators of menopausal flushing. Furthermore, the peak of the LH pulse occurred several minutes after both the symptoms of the hot flush and any temperature elevation. Again, the temporal correlation between the LH pulse and a hot flush as indicated by a rise in skin temperature, was poor: Tataryn[21] found that only 76% of 31 LH peaks were associated with a rise in skin temperature. Similarly Casper and colleagues[20] found that only 55 of 66 LH peaks were accompanied by a flush; in the remaining 11 an LH peak occurred in the absence of a flush. The fact that the increase in LH occurs considerably after the onset of symptoms indicates that it is not responsible for the flush but is merely a "para"-phenomenon'. In any case, estrogen therapy may relieve hot flushes in a dose which is insufficient to effect a significant reduction in gonadotropin levels. Furthermore, when we injected GnRH in order to evoke release of LH, we failed to evoke the symptoms of a hot flush or induce changes in peripheral blood flow or pulse rate[12]. The fact that administration of a GnRH agonist, which abolishes LH pulsatility, may evoke flushes does not imply a causal relation between GnRH and menopausal flushes. We do not know that the flushes evoked in these circumstances are necessarily the same as those which occur spontaneously after the menopause. The fact that estradiol does not alleviate the flushes occurring after administration of a GnRH agonist depot preparation, although clonidine may abolish such flushes (van Leusden personal communication), suggests that the 'flushes' may not be identical in the circumstances. Other conditions in which the circulating level of LH is low, such as after hypophysectomy, may also be associated with the occurrence of 'flushes'.

Increased circulating LH is therefore not causally responsible for the initiation of hot flushes, nor is it related to the occurrence of the individual flush episodes. Nevertheless, an increase in gonadotropin levels is a characteristic feature of the menopause. That a peak of LH may be observed some time after an individual flush suggests that the appearance of this inappropriate reflex response may have, as a secondary consequence, an accompanying alteration in LH pulsatility. A change in LH levels may therefore accompany the controlling trigger disturbance but is not in itself the responsible agent.

Several workers have investigated the possibility that adrenergic hormones are involved in flushing. Casper[20] found no change in either noradrenaline or adrenaline after a hot flush whilst Lightman[22] reported a slight but non-significant fall in noradrenaline. Most of these measurements were, however, made after the hot flush and since the half life of adrenaline is at most 2–3 min, one would need to sample earlier and more frequently in order to detect any change in circulating catecholamines during or immediately before the flush. This aspect was examined by Kronenberg[23] who reported a significant elevation in plasma adrenaline and a significant decrease in noradrenaline during the flush. The fall in noradrenaline would fit with what we observed – a marked rise in hand blood flow during the flush – since control of blood flow through the hand is essentially, if not exclusively, through variations in vasoconstrictor tone; it has not been possible to demonstrate any vasodilator fibers to the skin of the hand. A decrease in constrictor tone could thus be related to some aspects, at least, of menopausal flushing. The release of adrenaline during the hot flush, as suggested by Kronenberg's work, would, however, constrict hand blood flow and also change blood pressure. Other mechanisms must therefore be responsible. And even if an adrenergic mechanism is involved in the initiation of individual flushes, it is not a simple 'cause and effect' as suggested by a rise in circulating adrenaline and a fall in noradrenaline.

From the clinical point of view, β-blockers have proved disappointing as therapy for menopausal flushing and do not reduce the frequency or intensity of hot flushes. Clonidine, an α-agonist, has been used to relieve the vasomotor accompaniments of the climacteric, its presumed mechanism of action being through a central effect of the drug on α-adrenergic mechanisms. However, while we found that clonidine does not affect the basal level of peripheral blood flow, it reduces peripheral vasodilator effects of the catecholamines noradrenaline, adrenaline and also angiotensin. Additionally, the drug exerts a direct influence on vascular reactivity in the forearm, reducing the vasodilatation induced by anoxic forearm exercise[24].

A major difficulty for investigators of the menopausal hot flush is the lack of a suitable animal model. Those which have been used for studying the pathogenesis of hot flushes have little, if any, relevance to events in menopausal women. Infusion of naloxone, for example, induces variations in tail skin temperature in the morphine-addicted rat, associated with a progressive fall in rectal temperature and an increase in LH[25]. The latter, however, occurs at varying times in relation to the change in tail skin temperature, an increase in LH preceding the temperature rise in some animals but being coincidental in others. Without proof that this model could in any way reflect events during the hot flush in menopausal women, it has been suggested that this study supports the presence of opioid neurones which tonically inhibit LH secretion and affect body temperature. Spontaneous elevations in tail skin temperature in aging female rats have also been assumed to exemplify menopausal flushing[26]. These fluctuations apparently occur in 100% of the animals in anestrous and in 40% of those in constant estrous. The relevance of this to human flushing is, however, obscure, since the estradiol level is persistently elevated in rats in constant estrous or anestrous, whereas estradiol levels are low in the human menopausal female. Furthermore, ovariectomy abolishes the temperature fluctuations in the tail skin of the rat, whereas ovariectomy in the human female would precipitate temperature fluctuations. There is, therefore, no evidence that the aging female rat can be used as a model for menopausal flushing. In all animals where spontaneous temperature peaks occur, their relationship to levels of circulating estrogens differs from that observed in the human.

None of the theories proposed to account for menopausal flushing provide a satisfactory explanation either of its initiation or of the episodic nature of the phenomenon. In the light of the 'hard facts' described thus far, it is reasonable to conclude that the altered autonomic activity which produces the peripheral manifestations we demonstrated during the hot flush, probably results from a disturbance of thermoregulatory mechanisms. Normally the hypothalamic thermoregulatory center responds by promoting heat loss (peripheral vasodilatation and sweating) if body temperature exceeds a 'preset' level. Alternatively, if body temperature falls below the preset level, heat conservation mechanisms (vasoconstriction and shivering) are set in motion. Since there is no evidence that body temperature rises before the flush – on the contrary core temperature falls after the flush – it is possible that the center is given false information about body temperature or that the preset temperature level is suddenly reduced. Body temperature is then presumed to be excessive and heat dissipating mechanisms such as peripheral dilatation are activated. It is of interest that some women can predict the onset of the hot flush by an 'aura', often an unpleasant sensation, sometimes originating in the thorax or abdomen.

What is responsible for any such alteration in the body thermostat which then triggers off the flush? Because of the presumed association between LH pulses and flush episodes, it has been suggested that there is a link between the central neuroendocrine mechanisms that initiate episodic GnRH neuronal activity and those determining the onset of flush episodes[15,20]. The fact that the thermoregulatory center and GnRH neurones are anatomically close has been considered evidence in support of a neuroendocrine theory[27]. We have already pointed out, however, the imperfection of the association between LH and the flush and the lack of evidence that LH release or GnRH activity could be the trigger mechanism[28]. Anatomical contiguity of controlling mechanisms is no proof of a linkage between two disparate physiological responses. There are several contiguous centers in the brain and elsewhere in the body which behave independently of one another. Nevertheless, a variety of neuronal mechanisms have been suggested as responsible for initiation of the flush. The three systems suggested, according to the transmitter substance released – noradrenaline, dopamine or endogenous opioid peptide (EOP) – are purportedly supported by data from animal studies, which, as already discussed, bear little if any relation to events in the menopausal woman. That infusion of opioid peptides provoked flushing in men has been cited as evidence of the involvement of the EOP system in the pathogenesis of the menopausal flush![29]. A claim that naloxone infusion reduced the frequency of menopausal flushing and LH peaks[22] was not confirmed by subsequent workers[30]. In any case, none of the studies concerned with linking the flush with blood levels of various hormones or neurotransmitters or the administration of their antagonist, has used circulatory parameters as evidence of the occurrence of a flush. The studies depend either on the statement of the woman regarding her symptoms or an elevation in skin temperature which, as we have discussed above, occurs after the flush and may correlate poorly with the woman's actual perception of the event. Until and unless we can use a specific objective indicator of the flush, such as the change in peripheral blood flow that we demonstrated, the various theories proposed must remain a matter for speculation.

It is indeed surprising that no theory proposed thus far to explain the mechanism of hot flushes, has taken into account the fact that men also may flush. Whilst one might speculate that the mechanism of flushing in men differs from that in women, so that they flush for a different reason, it is much more likely that the male after orchidectomy and the woman after ovarian failure, flush for the same reason. If this is so, then the initiator may be neither estrogen nor androgen but a substance common to both gonads and in whose absence, the activity of the thermoregulatory center is disturbed. But this still fails to explain why the process is episodic and why some women never flush.

CONCLUSION

The menopausal hot flush is characterized by the rapid onset of a marked elevation in hand blood flow which remains elevated for 2 min after symptoms have abated. Forearm blood flow and pulse rate also increase but to a lesser extent, and both fall to control levels while hand flow is still elevated. There is no change in blood pressure during this period.

The pattern of circulatory change during the flush is similar to that observed with indirect body heating, indicating inappropriate activation of heat dissipating mechanisms.

A flush is not a blush. The circulatory response during emotional blushing is similar to that evoked in response to emotional stress, with a slight increase in hand flow, a marked elevation in forearm flow and a significant rise in blood pressure.

None of the theories proposed to explain the mechanism of menopausal flushing provide a satisfactory explanation for the initiation of the phenomenon, its episodic nature and the fact that men also may flush.

ACKNOWLEDGEMENTS

We would like to thank our colleagues, in particular Dr B. O'Reilly, and our patients for their co-operation. The work was supported by the British Heart Foundation and the Stanley Johnson Foundation to whom we also express our thanks.

REFERENCES

1. Hippocrates. *Aphorisms. Section VI.* Number 29
2. Soranus, C. (100 AD). *Gynaecology,* translated by Temkin, O. (1956, Baltimore)
3. Willis, E. (1684). In Thompson, J. (1979) The effect of oestrogen treatment on sleep, mood, anxiety and hot flushes in perimenopausal women. MD Thesis (Edinburgh)
4. Heister, L. (1712). *Medical, Chirurgical and Anatomical Cases and Observations,* translated by Wirgman, G. (1755)
5. Colombat de L'Isére (1845). *Diseases of Women,* translated by Meigs, C. D.
6. Tilt, E. J. (1858). *The Change of Life in Health and Disease. A Practical Treatise on the Nervous and other Affections Incidental to Women at the Decline of Life.* (London: S. Churchill)
7. McKinley, S. M. and Jeffreys, M. (1974). The menopausal syndrome. *Br. J. Prev. Soc. Med.,* **28**, 108–15
8. Greer, J. (1991). *The Change: Women, Ageing and the Menopause.* (London: Hamish Hamilton)
9. Ginsburg, J. and O'Reilly, B. (1987). Are blushes the same as flushes? *Clin. Sci.,* **72** (suppl. 16), 65
10. Barnett, L., Cullis, W., Fairfield, L. and Nicholson, R. (1933). An investigation of the menopause in one thousand women. *Lancet,* **1**, 106–8
11. Willbush, J. (1987). The female climacteric. PhD Thesis, University of Oxford
12. Ginsburg, J., Swinhoe, J. and O'Reilly, B. (1981). Cardiovascular responses during the menopausal hot flush. *Br. J. Obstet. Gynaecol.,* **88**, 925–30
13. Molnar, G. W. (1975). Body temperature during menopausal hot flashes. *J. Appl. Physiol.,* **1**, 499–503
14. Sturdee, D. W., Wilson, K. A., Pipili, E. and Crocker, A. D. (1978). Physiological aspects of menopausal hot flush. *Br. Med. J.,* **2**, 79–80
15. Meldrum, D. R., Shamonkki, I. M., Frumar, A. M., Tataryn, I. V. and Chang, R. J. (1979). Elevations in skin temperature as an objective index of postmenopausal hot flashes; standardization of the technique. *Am. J. Obstet. Gynecol.,* **135**, 713–17

16. Ginsburg, J. and O'Reilly, B. (1983). Climacteric flushing in a man. *Br. Med. J.,* **287**, 262
17. Linde, R., Doelle, G. C., Alexander, N., Kirchner, F., Vale, W., Rivier, J. and Rabin, D. (1981). Reversible inhibition of testicular steroidogenesis and spermatogenesis by a potent gonadotropin releasing hormone agonist in normal men: an approach toward the development of a male contraceptive. *N. Engl. J. Med.,* **305**, 663–7
18. Hoffman, C. H. (1965). Das Verhalten des diastolischen Blutdrucks bei Frauen mit klimakterischen Wallungen im stehund Belasturguersuch (Inaugural Dissertation). Wurtzburg University
19. Ginsburg, J., Hardiman, P. and O'Reilly, B. (1989). Peripheral blood flow in menopausal women who have hot flushes and in those who do not. *Br. Med. J.,* **208**, 1488–90
20. Casper, R. F., Yen, S. S. C. and Wilkes, M. M. (1979). Menopausal flushes: a neuroendocrine link with pulsatile luteinizing secretion. *Science,* **205**, 823–5
21. Tataryn, I. V., Meldrum, D. R., Frumar, A. M. and Judd, H. L. (1979). LH, FSH and skin temperature during the menopausal hot flash. *J. Clin. Endocrinol. Metab.,* 49, 152–4
22. Lightman, S. L., Jacobs, H. S., Maguire, A. K., McGarrick, G. and Jeffcoate, S. L. (1981). Climacteric flushing: clinical and endocrine response to infusion of naloxone. *Br. J. Obstet. Gynaecol.,* **88**, 919–24
23. Kronenberg, F., Cole, L. J., Linkie, D. M., Dyrenfurth, I. and Downey, J. A. (1984). Menopausal hot flushes: thermoregulatory, cardiovascular and circulating catecholamine and LH changes. *Maturitas,* **6**, 3–43
24. Ginsburg, J., O'Reilly, B. and Sinhoe, J. C. (1985). Effect of oral clonidine on human vascular responsiveness: a possible explanation of the therapeutic action of the drug in menopausal flushing and migraine. *Br. J. Obstet. Gynaecol.,* **92**, 1169–75
25. Simpkins, J. W. and Katovich, M. J. (1986). An animal model for pharmacologic evaluation of the menopausal hot flush. In Notelwitz, M. and van Keep, P. (eds.) *The Climacteric in Perspective: Proceedings of the Fourth International Congress on the Menopause,* pp. 213–51. (Lancaster: MTP Press)
26. Simpkins, J. W. (1984). Spontaneous skin flushing episodes in the ageing female rat. *Maturitas,* 269–78
27. Gambonne, J., Meldrum, D. R., Lauffer, L., Chang, R. J., Liu, J. H. K. and Judd, H. L. (1984). Further delineation of hypothaiamic dysfunction responsible for menopausal hot flashes. *J. Clin. Endocrinol. Metab.,* **51**, 179–81
28. Ginsburg, J. and Hardiman, P. (1991). What do we know about the pathogenesis of the menopausal hot flush? In Sitruk-Ware, R. and Utian, W. H. (eds.) *The Menopause and Hormonal Replacement Therapy,* pp. 15–46. (New York: Marcel Dekker)
29. Stubbs, W. A., Jones, A., Edwards, C. R. W., Delitala, G., Jeffcoate, W. J., Ratter, S. J., Bloom, S. R. and Alberti, K. G. M. M. (1978). Hormonal and metabolic responses to an enkephalin analogue in normal men. *Lancet,* **2**, 1225–7
30. De Fazio, J., Verheugen, C., Chetowski, R., Nass, T., Judd, H. L. and Meldrum, D. R. (1984). The effects of naloxone on hot flashes and gonadotropin secretion in post menopausal women. *J. Clin. Endocrinol. Metab.,* **58**, 578–8

15

Hormonal regulation of the normal breast – an update

T. J. Anderson, S. Battersby and W. R. Miller

Encouragement to understand the factors and mechanisms regulating the normal breast derives from the evidence that physiological influences have a major effect on the risk of developing breast cancer. Menstrual cycles, the influence of parity and the effects of exogenous hormones through use of oral contraceptives (OC) or hormone replacement therapy (HRT) feature strongly in the list of events which would be considered to have an effect on this disease risk. Efforts have been made in the last quarter of the twentieth century to define more clearly the nature of these influences on breast tissue. Such studies have focused on morphological, biochemical and molecular biological characteristics, but these have all resulted in controversy due to the different interpretations which are drawn from the observations. The following comments attempt to put these in a modern context with the addition of some recent findings.

MORPHOLOGICAL CHANGES

It was natural to assume that the breast, like the endometrium, would respond to the cyclical fluctuations of the sex steroids estrogen and progesterone, while fully recognizing that for lactational differentiation the addition of prolactin was essential. Claims were made[1,2] and denied[3,4] for the recognition of specific histological or ultrastructural features in the terminal duct lobular unit (TDLU) that characterized different phases of the menstrual cycle, the two most recent being in 1981 and 1986. The report of 1981[5] commented on features of epithelial cell cytoplasm and nucleus, as well as interstitial patterns of the TDLU, that were used to define five major phases of the menstrual cycle. The claim was made for consistent 'blind' identification of the precise (or adjacent) actual menstrual cycle phase, although these findings have not so far been independently corroborated. The report of 1986[6] compared changes in breast and endometrium at medico-legal autopsies, emphasizing similarities and differences of cyclical variation, but these have not found practical use.

Around that time there were also comments made on the epithelial proliferative response of TDLU, judged either by radioactive thymidine labelling[7] or by direct counting of mitoses[5,8], which prompted the first major controversy over whether maximal response was in the first or second half of the natural cycle. This has now been resolved, with general agreement that it occurs late in the second half and is, furthermore, associated with an increased frequency of apoptotic cell death[8–10]. There were, however, major variations in the level of proliferation between cases at any given time of the cycle, which were accounted for, in part at least, by the heterogeneity of breast response to the endocrine fluctuations of the cycle. Nevertheless, attainment of pregnancy both further increased and sustained the proliferative response until at least the third trimester[11]. In other words, using the analogy of a motor cycle, the resting breast received a 'kick-start' with each menstrual cycle but only became a 'running machine' if pregnancy ensued. The role of estrogen and/or progesterone as the stimulus for this effect was implied, but could not be considered established.

In the 1980s there was also the controversy over the effects of OC on the breast, in particular the influence on cancer risk[12], but it was not until the latter part of that decade that reports with sufficient case numbers were able to provide any valid comment on the response of breast tissue to OC use[13,14]. Here again the maximum proliferative response occurred in the late part of the (artificial) cycle and was indeed greater than that of the natural cycle, with a dose effect being suggested for estrogen but not progesterone[13]. This 'delayed' response to exogenous estrogen and progesterone in combination was difficult to explain on the same basis as that used to account for endometrial responses to endo- or exogenous sex steroid hormones and was a further indicator that these two 'end-organs' could no longer be considered comparable in the manner of their responses to estrogen and progesterone. This point has considerable relevance to the pharmaceutical industry, but leaves the academic issue of 'what, where and how' of breast parenchymal response somewhat unfulfilled. Was it estrogen or progesterone alone, or both (or neither) that was responsible for regulating breast responses? What contributions were available from the biochemical front?

STEROID BIOCHEMICAL CHANGES

The commercial production of antibodies to the receptors for estrogen (OR) and progesterone (PR) dramatically altered the feasibility of specifically localizing the cells within TDLU that were likely to be sensitive to these hormones. Positive immunohistochemical reactions were obtained by several workers[14-18], but there was no understanding of the threshold level for detection or whether the receptor was occupied or unoccupied, or indeed biologically viable. Simple 'positive or negative' reaction charts lacked the sensitive discrimination of biochemical quantitation and did not seem appropriate (or informative[19]). However, with the application of the same scoring system, combining the proportion and intensity of cell staining, that was used to validate the immunohistochemistry of breast cancers against the standard biochemical radioligand assays[20], the results from over 150 samples from premenopausal women were illuminating[21]. Two patterns of immunohistochemical reactivity for OR were observed, one uniform and the other sporadic among the epithelial cells within TDLU. It was evident that only the latter pattern significantly reduced in the second half of the natural cycle, in confirmation of the recognized down-regulation effect of cell response to progesterone. PR did not vary significantly across natural cycles, but increased steadily through OC cycles. Another immunohistochemical direction was to look for fatty acyl synthetase as a marker for progesterone response in cells of TDLU[22]. We have recently been able to explore the reactivity of 140 samples of resting breast tissue with the antibody OA-519 (Chektec Corp.) believed to react with fatty acyl synthetase (G. R. Pasternack, personal communication). Only ten samples showed staining accepted as specific, and these did not correlate with proliferative status.

These studies helped to clarify areas of disagreement arising from previous immunohistochemical studies for OR and PR with smaller case numbers[15,16,17,22] and highlighted the critical importance of adequate case numbers to enable multivariate analysis to be performed for the interpretation of normal breast responses. This latter approach has convincingly shown that the interval since pregnancy is an independent significant factor for both OR and PR presence[21]. Thus, phase of cycle, type of cycle, parity status and age were all factors which affect TDLU response. Instead of becoming simpler with more extended analysis it is now evident that systems regulating breast response to menstrual cycles, exogenous hormones and parity operate at an altogether different level of complexity than that which is applicable to the endometrium. To be more precise, it is necessary to recognize influences not only at endocrine, but also autocrine and paracrine levels[19,23]. The issue has now devolved down to investigating other intracellular pathways of response.

BIOCHEMICAL RESPONSE MEDIATORS

We have chosen to investigate two other pathways in breast tissue with respect to variability of response in differing physiological states. These pathways reflect the mechanism of signal transduction, one at the level of the cell membrane and the other in the cytoplasm. In this latest series of studies, over 100 normal breast tissue samples were assessed, taken not only from women undergoing natural and artificial cycles, that were parous and nulliparous, but also including the states of pregnancy, lactation and involution. The groups were chosen to maximize the contrasting physiological states of responsiveness. First, the pattern and levels of protein phosphorylation in cell membrane extracts were evaluated. Differences between groups were observed and were to some extent predictable on the basis of differentiated function and cellular stimulation, but there was considerable overlap in the range of values obtained. Two bands of interest were located around 180 and 44 kDa, one of which (44 kDa) correlated with resting breast proliferative activity, suggesting that pathways other than the direct nuclear switch action of OR and PR[24] are involved in mediating breast epithelial responses. Second, levels of the different isoforms of the cytoplasmic binding protein for cyclic AMP-dependent protein kinase – a well-recognized cytoplasmic second messenger system – were found to vary, and indeed did so according to predictions based on known associations of the isoforms with either differentiation or proliferation[25]. In particular, the variation in resting breast mirrored closely the pattern already found for epithelial proliferation across the menstrual cycle, a feature that had never been demonstrable for steroid hormone[14,21] or epidermal growth factor receptors (S. Battersby and T. J. Anderson, unpublished observations). These two studies are thus compatible with the concept that the cellular mechanisms involved in regulating breast epithelial responses – in this instance proliferation – are detached in both temporal and mechanistic senses from the direct actions of estrogen and probably also progesterone.

In summary, we have continued to pursue the aim of illuminating the mechanism of normal breast response to menstrual cycles, both natural and artificial, and to parity. Whilst breast epithelial tissues undoubtedly possess the specific mechanisms of reactivity to the steroid hormones, estrogen and progesterone, they alone are not adequate to account for the modulation of the various responses of which the breast is capable. Our current studies have implicated other pathways in at least the control of epithelial proliferation, but the equally important aspect of involution should not be forgotten. It is now necessary to consider and explore other dimensions of multisystem inter-relationships within the breast.

REFERENCES

1. Ingleby, H. and Gershon-Cohen, J. (1960). *Comparative Anatomy, Pathology and Roentgenology of the Breast*, pp. 35–7. (Philadelphia: University of Pennsylvania Press)
2. Fanger, H. and Ree, H. J. (1974). Cyclic changes of human mammary gland epithelium in relation to the menstrual cycle – an ultra structural study. *Cancer Res.*, **34**, 574–9
3. Haagensen, C. D. (1986). The normal physiology of the breast. In *Diseases of the Breast*, 3rd edn, pp. 50–1. (Philadelphia: WB Saunders)
4. Waugh, D. and Van der Hoeven, E. (1962). Fine structure of the human adult female breast. *Lab. Invest.*, **11**, 220–8
5. Vogel, P. M., Georgiade, N. G., Fetter, B. F., Vogel, F. S. and McCarty, K. S. Jr. (1981). The correlation of histologic changes in the human breast with the menstrual cycle. *Am. J. Pathol.*, **104**, 23–34
6. Longacre, T. A. and Bartow, S. A. (1986). A correlative morphologic study of human breast and endometrium in the menstrual cycle. *Am. J. Surg. Pathol.*, **10**, 382–93
7. Meyer, J. S. (1977). Cell proliferation in normal breast ducts, fibroadenomas and other ductal hyperplasia measured by nuclear labelling with tritiated thymidine. *Hum. Pathol.*, **8**, 67–81
8. Anderson, T. J., Ferguson, D. J. P. and Raab, G. M. (1982). Cell turnover in the 'resting' human breast: influence of parity, contraceptive pill, age and laterality. *Br. J. Cancer*, **46**, 376–82
9. Going, J. J., Anderson, T. J., Battersby, S. and MacIntyre, C. C. A. (1988). Proliferative and secretory activity in human breast during natural and artificial menstrual cycles. *Am. J. Pathol.*, **130**, 193–204
10. Potten, C. S., Watson, R. J., Williams, G. T., Tickle, S., Roberts, S. A., Harris, M. and Howell, A. (1988). The effect of age and menstrual cycle upon proliferative activity in the normal human breast. *Br. J. Cancer*, **58**, 163–70
11. Battersby, S. and Anderson, T. J. (1988). Proliferative and secretory activity in the pregnant and lactating breast. *Virchows Arch. [A]*, **413**, 189–96
12. Pike, M. C., Henderson, B. E., Krailo, M. D., Duke, A. and Roy, S. (1983). Breast cancer in young women and use of oral contraceptives: modifying effect of formulation and age at use. *Lancet*, **2**, 926–9
13. Anderson, T. J., Battersby, S., King, R. J. B., McPherson, K. and Going, J. J. (1989). Oral contraceptive use influences resting breast proliferation. *Hum. Pathol.*, **20**, 1139–44
14. Williams, G., Anderson, E., Howell, A., Watson, R., Coyne, J., Roberts, S. A. and

Potten, C. S. (1991). Oral contraceptive (OCP) use increases proliferation and decreases oestrogen receptor content of epithelial cells in the normal breast. *Int. J. Cancer,* **48**, 206–10

15. Carpenter, S., Georgiade, G., McCarty, K. S. Sr. and McCarty, K. S. Jr. (1989). Immunohistochemical expression of oestrogen receptor in normal breast tissue. *Proc. R. Soc. Edinburgh,* **95B**, 59–66

16. Peterson, O. W., Hoyer, P. E. and van Deurs, B. (1987). Frequency and distribution of oestrogen receptor-positive cells in normal nonlactating human breast tissue. *Cancer Res.,* **47**, 5748–51

17. Markopoulos, C., Berger, U., Wilson, P., Gazet, J. C. and Coombes, R. C. (1988). Oestrogen receptor content of normal breast cells and breast carcinomas throughout the menstrual cycle. *Br. Med. J.,* **296**, 1349–51

18. Jacquemier, J. D., Hassoun, J., Torrente, M. and Martin, P. M. (1990). Distribution of estrogen and progesterone receptors in healthy tissue adjacent to breast lesions at various stages immunohistochemical study of 107 cases. *Breast Cancer Res. Treat.,* **15**, 109–17

19. Anderson, T. J. and Battersby, S. (1989). The involvement of oestrogen in the development and function of the normal breast: histological evidence. *Proc. R. Soc. Edinburgh,* **95B**, 23–32

20. McCarty, K. S. Jr., Miller, L. S., Cox, E. B., Konrath, J. and McCarty, K. S. (1985). Estrogen receptor analyses. Correlation of biochemical and immunohisto-chemical methods using monoclonal antireceptor antibodies. *Arch. Pathol. Lab. Med.,* **109**, 716–21

21. Battersby, S., Robertson, B. J., Anderson, T. J., King, R. J. B. and McPherson, K. (1992). Influence of menstrual cycle, parity and oral contraceptive use on steroid hormone receptors in normal breast. *Br. J. Cancer,* **65**, 601–7

22. Joyeux, C., Chalbos, D. and Rochefort, H. (1990). Effects of progestins and menstrual cycle on fatty acid synthetase and progesterone receptor in human mammary glands. *J. Clin. Endocrinol. Metab.,* **70**, 1438–44

23. Bates, S. E., Valverius, E. M., Ennis, B. W., Bronzert, D. A., Sheridan, J. P., Stampfer, M. R., Mendelsohn, J., Lippman, M. E. and Dickson, R. B. (1990). Expression of the transforming growth factor/epidermal growth factor receptor pathway in normal human breast epithelial cells. *Endocrinology,* **126**, 596–607

24. King, R. J. B. (1992). Effects of steroid hormones and related compounds on gene transcription. *Clin. Endocrinol.,* **36**, 1–14

25. Beebe, S. J. and Corbin, J. D. (1986). Cyclic nucleotide dependent protein kinases. In Boyer, P. D. and Krebs, E. G. (eds.) *The Enzymes Vol. XVII Control by Phosphorylation Part A,* pp. 43–111. (London: Academic Press)

16

Hormonal regulation of the normal breast: current understanding and research issues

E. Valverius

The growth and development of the normal breast and breast cancer are governed by many different factors, most of which are poorly or incompletely understood or difficult to study appropriately. Based on epidemiological observations, there is evidence for important influential roles of heredity, age, geographical localization and hormonal exposure[1]. Diet, alcohol and exposure to environmental toxins have also been implicated. In the last decade, a large amount of data have been published showing important roles for various oncogenes, repressor genes, and growth factors and their receptors[2]. From the point of view of the gynecologist, the role of hormonal factors is evidently of the greatest interest for the consideration of prescription of oral contraceptives (OC) or hormonal replacement therapy (HRT). It is, however, crucial to remember that the role of hormones in the normal and pathological development of the breast is incompletely understood and that a great number of other factors also contribute in ways which may be parallel to, but not dependent upon, the hormonal balance.

Bearing this complexity in mind, it is not surprising that research on the hormonal effects on breast cells, using both *in vivo* histopathology and *in vitro* experiments, have produced conflicting results. It has been proposed that extended estrogen exposure increases the risk for development of breast cancer[3], since epidemiological studies indicate that among the risk factors are early menarche, late menopause, late first pregnancy and lactation[1]. However, epidemiological studies on the effects of OC and HRT have been inconclusive: some reports indicate increased risk for breast cancer while others do not. *In vitro* data from various research groups have also indicated diverse results, especially concerning the cellular growth response to progesterone. Some groups report increased cell proliferation[4-6], others have seen growth inhibition, particularly progesterone inhibition of estrogen-stimulated growth[7,8].

In an extensive review, Clarke and Southerland[9] present a number of explanations for the different observations on progesterone action *in vivo* and *in vitro*. They also propose a hypothetical cell cycle model that could accommodate the reported differences. Very simplified, in this model, cell cycle progression is governed by two hypothetical genes called START and STOP, both localized in early G1 phase. The START gene product regulates the rate of cell cycle progression and has in its promoter region response elements for estrogen, progesterone, and various serum factors, all of which have been shown to stimulate cell proliferation. The STOP gene precedes START very early in the G1 phase, however. The STOP promoter region contains only a progesterone-responsive element. Thus, the response of a cell to progesterone would depend on where in the cycle the cell is when exposed to the hormone. If the cell is in G1 between STOP and START, progesterone would stimulate the promoter of START and the cell would continue through the cycle including cell division. As the cell again enters G1, progesterone would stimulate the promoter of STOP and the cell would thus stop its cell cycle progression. In this way, progesterone could cause either growth stimulation (albeit limited to one round of the cell cycle) or inhibition. The model also explains the antiestrogenic effect of progesterone on cell proliferation. Stimulation of the estrogen-responsive element of the START promoter would initiate proliferation. Estrogen would have no effect on STOP since there is no estrogen-responsive element in the STOP promoter, but progesterone would turn on STOP expression. Differential expression of START and STOP could explain the reported different effects of progesterone on different target cells and tissues.

This is obviously a hypothetical model, which needs to be corroborated by extensive research. While candidate genes can be proposed for both START (cell cycle division genes, proto-oncogenes, growth factor genes) and STOP (genes of terminal differentiation), they need to be identified and experimentally tested. There still remain many other questions to answer concerning the action of progesterone in the breast: which cells are actually growth-stimulated by progesterone? Can progesterone cause sustained proliferation of these cells? Are these the only cells that express the progesterone receptor? Does progesterone have a direct or indirect paracrine action in stimulating cell proliferation? Is a transient proliferative stimulus a prerequisite for progesterone's induction of differentiation?

The panel in this Special Interest Group represented different viewpoints on the effect of progesterone in the human breast. An overview of the precise controversial issues was given by Dr Regine Sitruk-Ware.

Dr Thomas Anderson gave a summary of recent research concerning the morphological and steroid biochemical changes in the breast in response to estrogen and progesterone. Dr Anderson reported results from his studies on protein phosphorylation in cell membrane extracts, indicating that pathways other than the direct nuclear switch action of estrogen and progesterone receptors are involved in mediating breast epithelial responses to the hormones. Dr Anderson also showed that levels of the different isoforms of the cytoplasmic binding protein for cyclic AMP-dependent protein kinase vary in the resting breast in a similar fashion to the pattern already found in epithelial proliferation in the menstrual cycle. Such variation has not been found to follow upon hormonal stimulation. He writes: 'These two studies are thus compatible with the concept that the cellular mechanisms involved in regulating breast epithelial responses – in this instance proliferation – are detached in both temporal and mechanistic senses from the direct actions of oestrogen and probably also progesterone'.

Dr Frédérique Kuttenn presented data from *in vivo* studies of cultured normal human breast epithelial cells. The progestin promegestone (R5020) was found to have opposite effects to estradiol on the ultrastructural characteristics of the cells as seen in scanning and transmission electron microscopy, on cell growth, evaluated by daily cell counting and DNA assessment, on induction of estradiol dehydrogenase activity, on expression of estrogen and progesterone receptors and on expression of the c-*myc* oncogene.

Dr Anne Gompel correlated immunohistochemical data on normal breast tissue biopsies with the hormonal status of the women at the time of sampling. Ki67 antibody staining, indicating proliferative activity in cells, was greatest at mid-cycle or luteal phase. Staining for the epidermal growth factor receptor (EGFR) and the related c-*erb*B2 gene product showed cyclical variation and differential tissue localization: EGFR was predominant in the stroma and basal epithelial and myoepithelial cells whereas c-*erb*B2 positivity was never seen in the stromal cells.

Dr Bruno de Lignières presented data on 'influences of estradiol and progesterone on the epithelial cell cycle in normal breast tissue'. A gel containing either placebo, estradiol, progesterone, or both hormones was applied topically for at least 10 days prior to breast surgery in pre- and postmenopausal women. Surgery was performed in midcycle for premenopausal women. Mitoses were counted, or proliferating cell nuclear antigen labelling was used as a proliferation marker, in the breast biopsies. Progesterone reduced the proliferation induced by 17β-estradiol in normal breast epithelial cells after 10–13 days of topical application to the breast.

Dr Bo von Schoultz and Dr Gunnar Söderqvist reported results from two studies using fine needle aspiration biopsies of breast tissue obtained from healthy female volunteers. In the first study, immunohistochemistry was used to detect estrogen receptor (ER) and progesterone receptor (PR) variations during the menstrual cycle. ER levels showed cyclical variation, while PR remained essentially unchanged throughout the cycle. Thus, in contrast to the endometrium, down-regulation of PR during the luteal phase does not occur in normal breast epithelial cells. In the second study, the metabolism of estrone sulfate to estrone and the metabolically active 17β-estradiol was assessed. Lowest levels of metabolism were found in postmenopausal women, and metabolism was suppressed in premenopausal women using oral contraceptives (OC). Thus, these results refute the proposal by other researchers that OC could promote estrogen-dependent breast cancer by increasing the metabolism of estrone sulfate.

In conclusion, the members of the panel were asked whether they would prescribe both estrogens and progestogens as hormone replacement therapy, based on the presented studies. Some said they would include progestogens and some said they would not. Clearly, differences in research findings and in interpretation of results prevail, and there remains a need for much more research on the effects of progestogens on the normal and pathological growth and development of the human breast.

REFERENCES

1. Kelsey, J. L. and Berkowitz, G. S. (1988). Breast cancer epidemiology. *Cancer Res.*, **48**, 5615–23
2. Valverius, E. M. (1990). The role of growth factors and oncogenes in growth regulation of normal, non-neoplastic and malignant human mammary epithelial cells. *Thesis*, Uppsala University
3. Davidson, N. E. and Lippman, M. E. (1989). The role of estrogens in growth regulation of breast cancer. *Crit. Rev. Oncogenesis*, **1**, 216–23
4. Braunsberg, H., Coldham, N. G., Leake, R. E., Cowan, S. K. and Wong, W. (1987). Actions of a progestogen on human breast cancer cells: mechanisms of growth

stimulation and inhibition. *Eur. J. Cancer Clin. Oncol.,* **23**, 563–71

5. Simon, W. E., Albrecht, M., Trams, G., Dietel, M. and Holzel, F. (1984). *In vitro* growth promotion of human mammary carcinoma cells by steroid hormones, tamoxifen, and prolactin. *J. Natl. Cancer Inst.,* **73**, 313–21
6. Hissom, J. R., Bowden, R. T. and Moore, M. R. (1989). Effects of progestins, estrogens and antihormones on growth and lactate dehydrogenase in the human breast cancer cell line T47D. *Endocrinology,* **125**, 418–23
7. Sutherland, R. L., Hall, R. E., Pang, G. Y. N., Musgrove, E. A. and Clarke, C. L. (1988). Effect of medroxyprogesterone acetate on proliferation and cell cycle kinetics of human mammary carcinoma cells. *Cancer Res.,* **48**, 5084–91
8. Vignon, F., Bardon, S., Chalbos, D. and Rochefort, H. (1983). Antiestrogenic effect of R5020, a synthetic progestin in human breast cancer cells in culture. *J. Clin. Endocrinol. Metab.,* **56**, 1124–30
9. Clarke, C. L. and Southerland, R. L. (1990). Progestin regulation of cellular proliferation. *Endocrine Rev.,* **11**, 266–301

Section 3

Psychosocial aspects of the menopause

17

In pursuit of happiness: well-being during the menopausal transition

L. Dennerstein

INTRODUCTION

Throughout history philosophers and governments have considered happiness to be of the highest good and ultimate motivation for human action[1].

> What is the highest of all goods achievable by action?...both the general run of man and people of superior refinement say that it is happiness...but with regard to what happiness is they differ. (Aristotle, *Nicomachean Ethics*, Book 1, Chapter 4)

The pursuit of happiness was considered amongst the most important of human rights and nominated in the Declaration of Independence.

> We hold these truths to be self-evident – that all men are created equal; that they are endowed by their Creator with certain unalienable rights; that among these are life, liberty, and the pursuit of happiness. (Declaration of Independence)

Happiness is the simple emotion underlying well-being, just as the simple emotion underlying depression is sadness[2]. Despite universal acceptance of the World Health Organization's definition of health as 'a state of complete physical, mental and social well-being and not merely the absence of disease or infirmity', few studies positively measure health and well-being. Most medical research focuses on ill-health or morbidity and mortality indices. Research on the menopause has had an overwhelming focus on pathology and medical treatments, with portrayal of the menopausal woman in much Western medical literature as depressed, anxious and low in self-esteem[3]. Surveys which have drawn their samples from general populations rather than menopause clinics contradict assertions that the menopause has a negative effect on mental health[4]. No increase in the incidence of major depression associated with the natural menopause transition has been demonstrated[5]. Some studies suggest an increase in psychological symptoms in the premenopausal years[6–8], while in others no perimenopausal change was evident[9,10] or the increase was not significant[11].

Few studies have addressed psychological well-being during the menopausal transition. Journal article titles may be misleading so that articles purporting to measure well-being in fact address illness measures. Only one of the published studies reviewed included a measure of well-being, and this measure was used only during the pilot phase of the study[3]. This pilot study of 148 women patients of a family practitioner found no significant changes in well-being assessed by the Bradburn Index of Well-being[2] in women of differing menopausal status.

It is not clear why there has been so little attention paid to the assessment of well-being. A major reason indicated above is the focus of the medical model on pathology. Humanistic psychologists have maintained that concern with psychopathology ignores the positive aspects of life. Perhaps there would be more attention paid to happiness if it was classified as a psychiatric disorder as proposed recently by Bentall[12].

Despite the inattention of medical research to well-being as a useful and valid health indicator, a large literature has accumulated in the social sciences. In 1973 Psychological Abstracts International began listing happiness as an index term. By 1974 the journal Social Indicators Research was founded with a large number of articles devoted to subjective well-being (SWB). A comprehensive bibliography of SWB was published by Diener and Griffin in 1984[13].

This paper will summarize for menopause researchers and clinicians what is known of the history, concepts, measurement and factors predicting subjective well-being. The SWB results of a population sample of midlife women will be used to examine the effects of the menopausal transition on SWB and the results compared with those from the social science literature on SWB.

WHAT IS HAPPINESS?

Concepts of well-being and happiness can be grouped into three categories[1]. First, well-being may be defined by external criteria such as virtue or holiness: that is, happiness is not thought of as a subjective state but rather as possession of some quality desired by an observer. For example Aristotle wrote that happiness is gained by leading a virtuous life. A second concept has been that of life satisfaction. Chekola[14] describes happiness as the harmonious satisfaction of one's desires and goals. A third meaning of happiness comes closer to the way it is used in everyday discourse – denoting a preponderance of positive affect over negative affect[2]. This definition of subjective well-being stresses pleasant emotional experiences and could be thought of as occurring both as a state and a trait.

Subjective well-being has three hall-marks[1]: it is within the experience of the individual, it includes positive measures; and it usually includes a global assessment of aspects of a person's life over a certain time frame.

Measures

Single item survey questions have been used frequently. Single item scales are less reliable over time than are multiple item scales. Scores tend to be skewed, there is a possible response bias, and a single item cannot cover all aspects of SWB. A number of multi-item scales have been devised. Some measures emphasise the emotional side of happiness (feeling in a good mood) while others emphasize the cognitive side – satisfaction with life. Satisfaction with life can be subdivided into specific areas or domains such as work, marriage, health and one's own competence.

Kammann and colleagues[15] examined the intercorrelations and factor structures of 13 well-being scales and found that there were many plausible scales available, but that some of these were better than others in measuring general well-being. The Kammann and Flett scale[16] (the Affectometer) had a high convergence with other SWB scales (an average of 0.70). Most measures have adequate temporal reliability and internal consistency[1]. Scales of depression, anxiety and the dimension of neuroticism appear to be measuring the negative region of an overall well-being spectrum, but well-being could not necessarily be inferred from scales which measured negative mood only[2]. Bradburn[2] found that positive and negative affect scales were independent of each other. When frequency of feeling is included in the scale[16] positive and negative scales are negatively correlated ($r = -0.58$) as it is hard to feel happy and unhappy at the same time. However, the intensities of emotions are positively related[17].

Methodological problems identified by Diener[1] include:

(1) The extent to which the measure is influenced by momentary mood at the time of recording. There is evidence that both current mood and long-term affect are reflected in SWB measures.

(2) Validity of self-report. None of the scales show high social-desirability effects. Scales relate with non-self-report data such as demographic variables, and measures of smiling/laughing during the interview[1].

(3) Most studies are cross-sectional, so the direction of causality is impossible to determine.

Influences on subjective well-being

Philosophers have postulated many causes of happiness[1]. Rousseau suggested as sources of happiness a good bank account, a good cook, and good digestion. Thoreau, his follower, wrote that happiness comes from activity. The ascetics maintained that attitudes and activities that reflect detachment from the world lead to well-being.

Domains that are closest and most immediate to people's personal lives are those that most influence SWB[18]. Happiness is increased by the presence of certain social relationships and depressed by losing these and by other stressful life events[19].

Positive affect correlates with extraversion, education, employment, social participation, positive life events, satisfying leisure and exercise[1], while negative affect correlates with neuroticism[2], anxiety, worries, low social status, unemployment, women, poor health, low self-esteem and stressful life events[19].

SWB correlates with high self-esteem, an internal locus of control, income and with marriage[1]. Glen and Weaver[20] found that marriage was the strongest predictor of SWB even when education, income and occupational status were controlled. Satisfaction with family and marriage were the strongest predictors of SWB in many studies. On the other hand, most studies find either negligible or negative effects of having children on SWB. Love has been found to be an important correlate of SWB in many studies. SWB has also been found to correlate with self-rated health and with satisfaction with health. The relationship between health and SWB is strongest for women.

Gender

Warr and Payne[21], using a random sample of the UK adult population

(1964 men, 1113 women), found that there were no gender differences in the reports of feeling very pleased with things yesterday. However, the reported cause of pleasure yesterday differed. Family features are significantly more likely to be cited by women (43%) than by men (34%). Two studies have reported an interesting interaction with age in that younger women are happier than younger men, and older women are less happy than older men with the cross-over occurring around age 45.

In summary, it is evident that a large number of factors influence SWB.

MELBOURNE WOMEN'S MID-LIFE HEALTH PROJECT

Data presented here are drawn from the base-line cross-sectional phase of the Melbourne Women's Mid-life Health Project. This phase involved a survey during 1991 of a random sample of 2000 Melbourne women. Subjects eligible to enter the study were those women who were Australian born, and aged between 45 and 55 years inclusive at the time of interview. They were contacted by random selection of telephone numbers from the Melbourne White Pages. Subjects completed a 20–25 min interview by telephone, conducted by trained interviewers.

Measures

Psychological well-being

A validated measure of psychological well-being was used – the Affecto-meter 2[16]. Affectometer[16] provides three measures of psychological well-being, a measure of positive affect, a measure of negative affect, and an overall measure of well-being which was the difference between the positive affect and negative affect scales. Positive affect and negative affect are inversely correlated on this scale ($r = -0.66$). Each scale contains 10 adjectives, with the score being the mean of responses. In the current study women are asked whether in the last week they had felt that way most of the time, often, sometimes or hardly ever. This differs from Kammann and Flett[16] who described five possible responses to each question.

Explanatory variables

The Melbourne research team were allowed access to a questionnaire[22] carefully constructed by Kaufert and McKinlay, used with a sample of 2500 Manitoba women[22] and as the basis for a study of 8050 women in Massachussets[23]. The variables used in the Melbourne study were

Table 1 Percentage of the sample who experienced particular feelings 'most of the time'

Positive adjectives	%	Negative adjectives	%
Satisfied	61.4	Lonely	4.0
Relaxed	45.0	Helpless	2.9
Clear-headed	72.0	Impatient	8.4
Useful	68.4	Depressed	3.9
Loving	55.5	Hopeless	15.4
Optimistic	51.4	Withdrawn	2.2
Enthusiastic	43.5	Discontented	4.6
Good-natured	70.5	Confused	3.6
Confident	57.8	Tense	11.4
Understood	60.4	Insignificant	4.2

demographic, menopausal status[24] (pre-, peri-, natural, surgical), self-rated health, symptoms, chronic conditions, use of medication, premenstrual complaints, body mass index, lifestyle factors (smoking, alcohol consumption, exercise), interpersonal stress and attitudes to aging[3] and to menopause[3,24,25].

Statistical analysis

Each of the three measures obtained from the Affectometer (positive affect, negative affect and overall well-being) was subjected to separate analysis of variance. The results are described in detail in Dennerstein and co-workers[26].

Women who were using the oral contraceptive pill were excluded from the analysis. Respondents who were using hormone replacement therapy were assigned a separate menopausal status and were treated separately in the analyses carried out in the present study.

Results

The response rate among those women eligible and available for the study was 70.6%.

Table 1 indicates the percentage of the sample answering for each adjective that they had felt that way 'most of the time' in the last week. It is evident that the majority of women report experiencing many positive feelings most of the time. The only positive feelings not experienced by the majority of women most of the time were 'relaxed' and 'enthusiastic'. In contrast, only a small number of women report experiencing negative feelings most of the time. The number of complete responses eligible for analysis of variance was 1503 individuals.

Positive affect was significantly associated with being married or living with a partner, having few symptoms, no history of premenstrual complaints, better self-rated health, low interpersonal stress, exercise and fewer worries about aging or menopause.

Negative affect was significantly related to not living with a partner, presence of more symptoms, history of premenstrual complaints, self-rated health worse than most of peers, increased interpersonal stress, current smoking, not exercising and increased worries about aging and menopause.

Overall well-being was significantly related to being married or living with a partner, few symptoms, no history of premenstrual complaints, better self-rated health, low interpersonal stress, not smoking, exercising and few worries about aging or menopause.

DISCUSSION

Happiness appears to be enjoyed by the majority of Australian-born women in the mid-life years. The results of this population-based study contradict negative stereotypes of mid-aged and menopausal women. The findings of this study confirm the earlier report of Kaufert and Syrotuik[3] that menopausal status is not associated with well-being. With regard to the negative affect measure, the present study concurs with the results of other population studies of mid-aged women which have found that depression was associated with poor self-rated health, symptomatology, interpersonal stress, negative attitudes to menopause[5,11,24], and to prior 'menstrual coping style'[10]. Results of the present study are in accord with the SWB literature in finding that positive affects and well-being are associated with marriage (or live-in relationships), exercise and better health and that negative affect was associated with poor health, stress and worries.

In conclusion, in this cross-sectional population study well-being was not related to menopausal status but was related to health status, psychosocial and lifestyle variables. Information from the longitudinal phase of the Melbourne study will help to further elucidate the etiology of mood and well-being in mid-life and to determine the effects of happiness.

ACKNOWLEDGEMENTS

The Melbourne Women's Mid-life Health Study is funded by the Victorian Health Promotion Foundation. Telephone interviewing for this study was carried out by the Roy Morgan Research Center, Melbourne, Australia. Project Director was Dr Carol Morse. Statistical analysis of the data was carried out by Dr A. Smith and Dr J. Shelley. We are indebted to Drs Sonja and John McKinlay of the New England Research Institute, Boston, for their advice and access to methodologies and the questionnaires developed for the Massachusetts Women's Health Study.

REFERENCES

1. Diener, E. (1984). Subjective well-being. *Psychol. Bull.,* **95**, 542–75
2. Bradburn, N. M. (1969). *The Structure of Psychological Well-being.* (Chicago: Aldine)
3. Kaufert, P. and Syrotuik, J. (1981). Symptom reporting at the menopause. *Soc. Sci. Med.,* **15E**, 173–84
4. Ballinger, C. B. (1990). Psychiatric aspects of the menopause. *Br. J. Psychiatry,* **156**, 773–87
5. Kaufert, P. A., Gilbert, P. and Tate, R. (1992). The Manitoba project: a re-examining of the link between menopause and depression. *Maturitas,* **14**, 143–56
6. Jazsmann, L., van Lith, M. D. and Zaat, J. (1969). The perimenopausal symptoms: the statistical analysis of a survey. *Med. Gynecol. Sociol.,* **4**, 268–77
7. Ballinger, C. B. (1975). Psychiatric morbidity and the menopause: screening of a general population sample. *Br. Med. J.,* **3**, 344–6
8. Bungay, G. T., Vessey, M. P. and McPherson, C. K. (1980). Study of symptoms in middle life with special reference to the menopause. *Br. Med. J.,* **2**, 181–3
9. Greene, J. G. and Cooke, D. J. (1980). Life stress and symptoms at the climacterium. *Br. J. Psychiatry,* **136**, 486–91
10. Holte, A. and Mikkelsen, A. (1982). Menstrual coping style, social background and climacteric symptoms. *Psychiatry Soc. Sci.,* **2**, 41–5
11. McKinlay, J. B., McKinlay, S. M. and Brambilla, D. (1987). The relative contributions of endocrine changes and social circumstances to depression in mid-aged women. *J. Health Soc. Behav.,* **28**, 345–63
12. Bentall, R. P. (1992). A proposal to classify happiness as a psychiatric disorder. *J. Med. Ethics,* **18**, 94–8
13. Diener, E. and Griffin, S. (1984). Happiness and life satisfaction: a bibliography. *Psychol. Doc.,* **14**, 11
14. Chekola, M. G. (1975). The concept of happiness. (Doctoral dissertation, University of Michigan, 1974). *Dissertation Abstracts International,* **35**, 4609a. (University microfilms No. 75-655)
15. Kammann, R., Farry, M. and Herbison, P. (1984). The analysis and measurement of happiness as a sense of wellbeing. *Soc. Indic. Res.,* **15**, 91–115
16. Kammann, R. and Flett, R. (1983). Affectometer 2: a scale to measure current level of general happiness. *Aust. J. Psychol.,* **35**, 259–65

17. Diener, E., Larsen, R. J., Levine, S. and Emmons, R. A. (1985). Intensity and frequency: dimensions underlying positive and negative affect. *J. Personality Social Psychol.,* **48**, 1253–65
18. Andrews, F. M. and Withey, S. B. (1976). *Social Indicators of Well-being: America's Perception of Life Quality.* (New York: Plenum Press)
19. Argyle, M. (1987). *The Psychology of Happiness.* (New York: Methuen)
20. Glen, N. D. and Weaver, C. N. (1981). The contribution of marital happiness to global happiness. *J. Marriage Fam.,* **43**, 161–8
21. Warr, P. and Payne, R. (1982). Experiences of strain and pleasure among British adults. *Soc. Sci. Med.,* **16**, 1691–7
22. Kaufert, P. (1984). Women and their health in the middle years: a Manitoba project. *Soc. Sci. Med.,* **18**, 279–81
23. McKinlay, S. M. and McKinlay, J. B. (1984). Health status and health care utilisation by menopausal women. In Notelovitz, M. and Van Keep, P. A. (eds.) *The Climacteric in Perspective,* pp. 59–75. (Lancaster: MTP Press)
24. Avis, N. E. and McKinlay, S. M. (1991). A longitudinal analysis of women's attitudes toward the menopause: results from the Massachusetts Women's Health Study. *Maturitas,* **13**, 65–79
25. Neugarten, B. L., Wood, V., Kraines, R. J. and Loomis, B. (1963). Women's attitudes toward the menopause. *Vit. Hum.,* **6**, 140–51
26. Dennerstein, L., Smith, A. M. A. and Morse, C. (1993). Psychological well-being, mid-life and the menopause. *Maturitas,* in press

18

Menopause and depression: a sociological perspective

P. A. Kaufert

INTRODUCTION

One of the more intriguing dilemmas in menopause research is that different people from different disciplines at different points in time have asked the same question about the relationship between menopause and depression, and have returned with quite different answers. Such apparent inconsistency can be explained quite simply by the use of different research methods and designs, although it is the theories and assumptions which guide both the processes of research and the interpretation of its results which are equally, if not more, responsible. Rather less obviously, much depends on who is asking the question and exactly why they are interested in the relationship between changing estrogen levels and negative mood.

I want to look first at what sociological research has had to say about the relationship between menopause and depression, then discuss what is particular to this perspective relative to that of the clinical researcher. For convenience, I will use my own work in Manitoba and that of Sonja and John McKinlay and Nancy Avis in the Massachusetts Women's Health Study. Much of what I have to say, however, could equally have been based on the work of other social scientists, such as Arne Holte[1], Myra Hunter[2], or Lorraine Dennerstein[3].

MENOPAUSE AND DEPRESSION: SOCIOLOGICAL PERSPECTIVES

The initial linkage between the Massachusetts and Manitoba studies was based on an agreement to match certain elements in the design of the two cross-sectional surveys. These included the selection of women from general rather than clinical population sources, the use of common measures of the same variables and a decision to share data and collaborate on their analysis. (One of the products of this agreement was the paper presented at this Congress by Sonja McKinlay[4] in which she compared data dealing with symptom patterns and health characteristics taken from the two surveys.)

Women who were 45 and over and still menstruating when they took part in the cross-sectional surveys were then asked to participate in longitudinal studies. In the Manitoba longitudinal study, 505 women accepted the invitation (87% of those eligible)[5]; 2565 women took part in the Massachusetts study[6]. Each study collected data on women's health, their symptoms, their use of medication, their chronic health problems, their experience of gynecological surgery and their menstrual status. The same measure of depression was used in each study, the Centre for Epidemiological Studies Depression scale (CES-D)[7]. Questions on the menopause included items on their menstrual history, their symptoms and whether they were using hormone replacement therapy, but also on their attitudes towards menopause, towards becoming themselves menopausal, towards aging. Women were also asked about changes in the structure of family life (such as children leaving home, marriage, divorce, illness, retirement, death) and current areas of stress in their relationships with family or other kin, or connected with their employment or economic situation.

The scale of the Massachusetts study is much larger; 2565 women in Massachusetts relative to 505 in Manitoba. Women in Massachusetts were interviewed six times at 9-month intervals; the number of interviews in Manitoba was the same, but the interval between each interview was only 6 months. The CES-D was included in five of the six interviews in Manitoba, but women in the Massachusetts study completed the CES-D only twice during their six interviews with an interval of approximately 27 months between each completion.

Detailed, albeit separate, analyses of the data from the Manitoba and Massachusetts studies have been published or are in press[8,9]. Direct comparisons of the data on depression, as we have undertaken with the symptom data from the cross-sectional surveys, are made more difficult because of these differences in the number of times depression was measured and in the spacing between interviews. Nevertheless, a rough comparison of the conclusions to each study is both possible and informative.

The data are remarkably similar. The convention when using the CES-D is to treat a score of ≥ 16 as indicative of depression; the percentage of women with this score fluctuates almost imperceptibly, ranging between 9% and 11% across the five data collection points in the Manitoba study and the two collection points in the Massachusetts data. Depression may be a more common experience, however, than suggested by these figures; a quarter of the women taking part in the Manitoba study had a score of ≥ 16 on at least one of the five interviews. Being depressed was the strongest predictor in both these studies that a woman would be depressed the next time interviewed. Chronic depression, however, insofar as that could be measured by having the same depression score on the CES-D at four or more interviews in the Manitoba study, was rare and afflicted the lives of only 4% of women[8].

In neither the five interviews of the Manitoba study nor the two in Massachusetts was a woman's menopausal status at the time she was interviewed significantly related to her score on the CES-D scale[8,9]. Looked at longitudinally, neither study found that a change between interviews from one menopausal status category to another predicted that a woman would be depressed at her next interview. In the Manitoba data, however, the likelihood of a woman being depressed at two interviews in succession was slightly higher among perimenopausal relative to pre- and postmenopausal women, although not significantly so. Women from Massachusetts, who were perimenopausal when first completing the CES-D and still perimenopausal 27 months later, were significantly more likely to be depressed when completing the scale a second time[9].

These results are intriguing, although leaving open the question of whether perimenopausal women are at greater risk of depression while their menstrual patterns are irregular, or during the 12 months elapsing between their last menstrual period and becoming defined as postmenopausal. In other words, is it the fluctuations in their hormonal levels which put this particular set of women at risk, or is it the sharp fall in estrogen levels coming at the end of the perimenopause? If hormonal changes are related to depressed mood, this seems to happen only in a relatively small group of women and is of short duration. Depression does not seem to persist into the postmenopause phase and the re-establishment of a form of hormonal equilibrium.

While women may be at the same time both menopausal and depressed, the general conclusions to both these studies suggest that the triggers of their depression more often lie in the social context of their lives and their general health rather than in their menopause *per se.* Table 1 shows the results from an analysis of the Manitoba data which included a wider array of social and health status variables (such as changes in family

Table 1 Relative odds of being depressed: adjusted rates

	Adjusted relative odds	95% confidence interval	Probability
Not depressed			
Health (good, fair, poor)	0.52	0.3, 0.8	0.001
Problems with husband or children	3.23	1.6, 6.5	0.001
Problems with other relationships	2.8	1.5, 5.4	0.002
Hysterectomy	0.62	0.4, 1.0	0.03
Depressed			
Age	1.15	1.0, 1.3	0.03
High blood pressure	0.38	0.2, 0.9	0.04
Thyroid problems	5.61	1.4, 22.1	0.01
Number of health problems	0.69	0.5, 1.0	0.07

structure, family stress, current health status, and chronic health problems). The likelihood of a woman becoming depressed from one interview to the next was best predicted by stresses in her relationships with others, although being a woman with a hysterectomy also entered into this model. Depression at two interviews in succession, however, was best predicted by a woman being in poor health and by the number of her chronic health problems. (See reference 8 for a fuller discussion of these results.) An analysis of data from the Massachusetts study incorporating practically the same variables had practically the same results. As Avis and colleagues[9] comment, it would seem that 'health problems in general and stress are more predictive of depression in midlife women than menopausal transition'.

DISCUSSION

In summary, two studies which were broadly similar in design, based on samples roughly representative of menopausal women in two areas of North America, using the same measure of depression, came to very similar conclusions. I would predict that other researchers using the same methods, the same measures and similar populations would report approximately the same results. This does not mean, however, that I would predict the emergence of a new consensus on the relationship between menopause and depression. Researchers will continue to disagree for reasons which are partly methodological, partly theoretical and linguistic, and partly a reflection of differences in perspective and in the objectives of those asking the question.

The implications of a change in methodology can be illustrated using the Manitoba and Massachusetts studies and speculating on the implications for their results of a shift in any one of the following three parameters; the definition of menopausal status, the measurement of depression using the CES-D, the selection of women from the general population. Menopausal status is defined in both studies based on a woman's self-report of her current menstrual patterns. In another paper given at this Congress, Avis and colleagues[10] use depression data for a subset of the same women, but substituting for menopausal status an exact measure of estrogen levels and the date of a woman's last menstrual period. Using this definition, she would be able to link any increase in depression with a decline in estrogen. Had similar hormone data been available for all 2565 women in the Massachusetts study, then estrogen levels could have been substituted for the present definition of perimenopausal status and the association with depression re-examined, while at the same time controlling for health and social stress. The result may, or may not, have been the same, but would have been based on a more accurate measure of menopausal status.

Turning to the second parameter, the measurement of depression: in a previous analysis of the Manitoba data, a comparison was made between a woman's score on the CES-D and whether or not she reported two or more of the psychological symptoms from the Kupperman Index[11]. As might be expected, women identified as depressed on the basis of their CES-D scores also reported symptoms of nervous tension, depression and irritability on the general symptom checklist. When we reversed the direction of the comparison, however, and looked at how many women reporting these three symptoms also had scores of ≥ 16 on the CES-D, we found that between 28% and 43% of these women were not depressed as evaluated by this scale (the percentages varied from one interview to another). The implication, if one assumes that the CES-D is a more reliable and valid measure of depression, is that reliance on the symptoms of the Kupperman Index would lead to a correct identification of the woman who is depressed, but also to a gross overestimation of the prevalence of depression among women.

Interestingly, we found no association between these three symptoms and menopausal status; nevertheless, had we depended on the Kupperman Index alone, our perception of the prevalence of depression among women of menopausal age would have been quite different. It would also have been quite wrong as, judged by the standard methodological criteria, the CES-D is the more objective and scientific measure of depression. Describing the choice of this particular measure, McKinlay[6] wrote: "The

CES-D has been shown to be a valid, reliable and useful instrument for measuring depressive symptoms in the general community.... It also correlates well with clinical assessments of depression.... In addition to adequate reliability and validity (content, concurrent and discriminant), the CES-D has a similar factor structure within different subgroups of the population.... Moreover, because it measures states of general psychological malaise rather than specific diagnostic entities and symptoms which may occur at any period of life, the CES-D is considered especially appropriate for a study of menopause." In other words, our choice of the CES-D was based on sound methodological principles.

However, the choice of the CES-D reflected theoretical and conceptual priorities, as much as a concern for methodological niceties. We were interested in testing a model in which menopause was a causal factor in the onset of depression among women in midlife. If depression is thought of as lying at one end of a continuum extending to a total sense of well-being, then we wanted an instrument adequate for measuring mood at the depression end of this continuum. Other researchers may now be more interested in a model which posits an association between menopause and a decline in a woman's sense of well-being. Naturally, they will choose not the CES-D, but an instrument appropriate to the measurement of mood at a quite different point along the continuum from depression to well-being. The 'correctness' of a measure must always depend on its adequacy as a measure of the concept.

The problem is that there are many different concepts of psychological morbidity. As researchers explore other dimensions of the relationship between hormones and mood, we risk further confusion over the relationship between menopause and depression. Absence of a sense of well-being, for example, does not equate with the presence of depression. Precision in the use of language is unfortunately not a characteristic of menopause research.

The third parameter is the use of a sample of women broadly representative of midlife women. Earlier in this Congress, Malcolm Whitehead[12] discussed the differences in findings between studies looking at the relationship between menopause and depression when women are selected from the general as opposed to a clinical population. However, women who have undergone oophorectomy, or who are patients in menopause clinics, do not lie to researchers. When Barbara Sherwin[13], for example, reports on women who told her about their depression or their sexual dysfunction, we presume with her that they are speaking from their own experience. Using the results of general population surveys to tell such women that they are not depressed would be to invalidate this

166

experience. It would also be incorrect in scientific terms; the results of a general survey do not necessarily apply to a small, highly selective subgroup of women. It would, of course, be equally inappropriate to generalize from their experience to menopausal women as a whole.

While a psychologist rather than a clinical researcher, Barbara Sherwin is like many clinical researchers in being concerned primarily with the treatment and management of menopause as seen in a patient population. This patient-based, disease-based perspective results in the development of a model which focuses on the impact of declining estrogens on physical parameters – lipids, bone densities, or vaginal atrophy – and the benefits of replacing this estrogen through therapy. Clinical researchers assume also that their working model of what happens to a woman's body at menopause is universal, or, at least, that they have defined the normal parameters of the menopausal process. Given this assumption, large samples are unnecessary because the patient can represent the 'every-woman'.

Social scientists work from a very different perspective to the clinical researcher. Their model of menopause is more likely to be based on the presumption that the experience of becoming menopausal is not only diverse, but that it will vary based on a complex interplay between physiological, social and cultural factors. Menopause may vary with class, income or ethnicity, diet, whether a woman works, her type of work, whether she is married, has children, when these children were born and their number. In this model of menopause, a woman's response to the end of menses will have as much to do with social attitudes towards the menopausal woman as the impact of declining estrogens on sexual function. Indeed, the very expectation that postmenopausal women should be sexually active becomes a cultural artefact. Social scientists expect diversity among women, and are particularly concerned with the size and provenance of their samples.

In terms of the medical model, the objective when clinical researchers ask questions about the relationship between menopause and depression is to determine whether depression is a product of the same processes of estrogen decline as other symptoms associated with menopause. Evidence for the relationship is partly associational and based partly on a positive response to hormone replacement. The presence of depression is ascertained as simply as any other symptom; a woman is simply asked if she is depressed.

Social scientists have no commitment to treat, but rather aim to understand and explain. Their objective when asking questions about the relationship between menopause and depression is to evaluate the role of hormones relative to other factors which may trigger depression in women. In this model, evidence for the relationship has to hold under statistical tests in which the influence of menopause is parcelled out against the impact of other variables. Perhaps their most major contribution has been in terms of showing women that depression is not an inevitable concomitant of becoming menopausal.

REFERENCES

1. Holte, A. and Mikkelsen, A. (1982). Menstrual coping style, social background and climacteric symptoms. *Psychiat. Soc. Sci.*, **2**, 41–5
2. Hunter, M., Battersby, R. and Whitehead, M. (1986). Relationships between psychological symptoms, somatic complaints and menopausal status. *Maturitas*, **8**, 217–28
3. Dennerstein, L. (1993). Psychological wellbeing, midlife and the menopause. In Beg, G. and Hammar, M. *The Modern Management of the Menopause*, pp. 169–75. (Casterton: Parthenon Publishing)
4. McKinlay, S. (1993). Symptom patterns and health-care utilization among perimenopausal women in two North American populations. Presented at the *7th International Congress on the Menopause*, June, Stockholm
5. Kaufert, P. A., Gilbert, P. and Hassard, T. (1988). Researching the symptoms of menopause: an exercise in methodology. *Maturitas,* **10**, 117–31
6. McKinlay, J. B., McKinlay, S. M. and Brambilla, D. (1987). The relative contributions of endocrine changes and social circumstances to depression in mid-aged women. *J. Health Soc. Behav.*, **28**, 345–63
7. Radloff, L. S. (1977). The CES-D Scale: a self-report depression scale for research in the general population. *Appl. Psychol. Meas.*, **1**, 385–401
8. Kaufert, P. A., Gilbert, P. and Tate, R. (1992). The Manitoba project: a re-examination of the link between menopause and depression. *Maturitas,* **14**, 143–55
9. Avis, N. E., Brambilla, D., McKinlay, S. M. and Vass, K. (1993). A longitudinal analysis of the association between menopause and depression: results from the Massachusetts women's health study. In press
10. Avis, N., McKinlay, S., Vass, K., Brambilla, D. and Longcope, C. (1993). Hormone levels, symptoms, and the relation between menopause and depression. Presented at the *7th International Congress on the Menopause*, June, Stockholm
11. Blatt, M. G., Wiesbader, H. and Kupperman, H. S. (1953). Vitamin E and the climacteric syndrome. *Am. Med. Assoc. Arch. Intern. Med.*, **91**, 792–9
12. Whitehead, M. (1993). Psychosocial issues: the last two decades. Presented at the *7th International Congress on the Menopause;* Stockholm, June 1993
13. Sherwin, B. B. (1989). Clinical consequences of endocrine changes at the menopause. In van Hall, E. V. and Everaerd, W. (eds.) *The Free Woman – Women's Health in the 1990s,* pp. 680–7. (Carnforth: Parthenon Publishing)

19

Psychosocial factors and the menopause: results from the Norwegian Menopause Project

A. Holte, A. Mikkelsen, M. H. Moen, J. Skjœråsen, J. Jervell, K. T. Stokke and R. Wergelund

INTRODUCTION

Which health complaints are affected by the menopause? What is the prevalence of climacteric complaints? Which background factors increase the likelihood of reporting such complaints? How do women learn about the menopause, and what are their beliefs and attitudes to it? The answers to these questions have been rapidly changing through the years, not because the reality has changed, but because our knowledge stems largely from studies with methodological weaknesses[1]. Unfortunately, opinions about menopausal complaints are still based extensively on studies of self-selected clinical samples in which standard instruments of measurements have not been employed. Investigations of representative general population samples, and in particular prospective longitudinal research, are lacking.

This paper summarizes results of four studies by the Norwegian Menopause Project (NMP)[2], all of which used general population samples selected from the Community Registers in Norway by the Norwegian Central Bureau of Statistics. The 'Farmland study'[3] consisted of personal interviews exploring beliefs and attitudes about the menopause in a representative sample of women of different ages in a small Norwegian country settlement ($n = 61$). The 'Drammen survey'[4,5] consisted of a postal questionnaire about the 24 health complaints most frequently described in medical textbooks as associated with the menopause. A representative sample of 139 women, age 45–55, residing in the town of Drammen, were involved. The 'Oslo survey'[6-10] replicated this design, but was conducted in the city of Oslo ($n = 1886$). 'Prospect Oslo'[11-15] included a 5-year prospective longitudinal study of 177 healthy women who were selected randomly among those who had taken part in the Oslo survey and who were still menstruating regularly. In addition to measurements each year of the same health complaints as in our previous study, personality traits, psychological defence mechanisms, sex-role identification, marital adjustment, satisfaction with body appearance, quality of life and blood pressure were measured along with cytology and gynecological examination. Blood samples were collected at each examination and frozen for future analyses.

ATTITUDES AND BELIEFS

The Farmland study[3] yielded five important findings:

(1) Among the postmenopausal women 80% considered that their personal experiences with the 'change of life' had been better than that of *most* other women.

(2) Those who had not yet experienced the menopause had significantly more negative attitudes towards it than those who had experienced it.

(3) The women in the Farmland valley rarely talked to each other about the 'change of life'.

(4) Their knowledge about the menopause came only to a small extent from personal relationships with other women such as their mothers and female friends.

(5) Their main sources of information were women's magazines, books, radio and TV, reflecting a medical view based on experiences with patients.

The three latter findings were replicated in Drammen and Oslo. This may indicate that our culture contains a myth about how most women experience the change of life. The extent to which this affects the cultural forming of menopausal complaints is unknown, but may have important consequences as regards prevention.

PREVALENCE

Omitting 9% of women receiving hormone replacement therapy (HRT), 10% who were hysterectomized, and 5% who were bilaterally oophorectomized ($n = 200$), Table 1 shows the percentage of women, age 45–55, residing in Oslo, and reporting that they 'sometimes' or 'often' suffered from some of the 24 health complaints[6].

The highest prevalences of clinical relevance ('often') appeared 2–3 years after menopause. The figures are lower than those found in previous studies. However, few previous studies contained representative samples and they rarely differentiated between total and clinically relevant prevalence. This indicates that previously reported prevalences may have been overestimated as regards clinical relevance. The Oslo results were almost identical to those found previously in Drammen.

THE MENOPAUSAL SYNDROME

Factor analysis[9] showed that the complaints could be arranged into five independent clusters: vague somatic complaints, nervousness, mood swings, vasomotor complaints including vaginal dryness, and urogenital complaints. Again the analyses yielded remarkably similar results in Drammen and Oslo[5,9]. In both studies vasomotor complaints, including dryness of the vagina, were the only ones associated with menopausal status[4,6]. This indicates that the concept of the 'menopausal syndrome' should be restricted to include these complaints.

WHO HAS WHICH COMPLAINTS?

Multivariate analyses[4,8,10] showed that the reporting of usually having had similar complaints in connection with menstruation earlier in life was the best predictor of all clusters of complaints, except the vasomotor complaints. The relationships were specific: women with mood swings had suffered more frequently from mood complaints, women with vague somatic complaints from somatic complaints, etc. A simple explanation is most likely: at age 45–55 we tend to react in the same way as previously. Mood swings were also more frequent if the subject had poor social network; vague somatic complaints were more likely if the subject was gainfully employed or had low education or income. In general, psychological complaints were associated with a high number of negative life events during the past year. Variables that increased the likelihood of a 'menopausal syndrome' included menopausal status, age on reaching

Table 1 Complaints reported as being experienced 'sometimes' and 'often' according to menopausal status (percentage; n = 1686)

	Regular menstruation		Irregular menstruation		3yr postmenopause		> 5yr postmenopause	
	Sometimes	*Often*	*Sometimes*	*Often*	*Sometimes*	*Often*	*Sometimes*	*Often*
Hot flushes	35	8	48	28	44	45	47	32
Vaginal dryness	17	4	18	9	29	22	27	16
Nervousness	35	14	35	17	29	21	35	24
Pains	32	17	31	36	30	21	36	28
Sleeping problems	37	13	39	21	50	21	37	28
Feeling depressed	44	9	30	19	38	15	45	11
Irritability	57	10	49	17	46	14	51	10
Involuntary urination	10	2	10	–	11	–	7	–
Weight gain	28	15	26	18	24	25	30	18

(Modified from reference 6)

menopause, current cigarette smoking, the subject's mother having suffered from vasomotor complaints, chronological age, and having had negative expectations of the change of life.

CRITERIA AND AGE ON REACHING MENOPAUSE

From the longitudinal results[11-14] we learned that among non-treated subjects who had menstruated regularly until age 47, 97% did not menstruate again after 6 months of amenorrhea. The mean age on reaching the menopause among these women was 52.9 years (SD = 2.1). This may reflect the fact that HRT users and women with serious gynecological disorders more frequently suffer from conditions associated with early menopause. In addition they are probably smokers. Among healthy non-smokers (most women), the age on reaching menopause is significantly higher than in the general population. Our supposition, then, is that most women are wrongly informed about when to expect their menopause.

HEALTH COMPLAINTS AFFECTED BY THE MENOPAUSE

The longitudinal study made it necessary to change several truths[12]. Significant reductions after menopause were found in monthly headaches and tenderness in the breasts. Significant increases occurred not only in hot flushes, sweating and dryness of the vagina, but also in palpitations. Social dysfunction after the menopause also increased, but this was associated with increased hot flushes and sweating. There were no effects on measurements of anxiety, depression, personality traits and marital adjustment. A weak de-masculinization of sex-role identification was found among those who had low premenopausal scores. A new and intriguing finding was that feminine sex-role identification predisposes to vasomotor complaints, while masculinity protects against it. On the other hand, femininity seemed to protect against a decrease in the feeling of happiness and life-satisfaction after the menopause[14]. Preliminary analyses also indicate a significant reduction after the menopause in the frequency of sexual intercourse (59% of the sample), orgasms during intercourse (44%), sexual enjoyment (37%) and sexual interest (27%). Sexual difficulties (37%) increased significantly, but this was associated with increased dryness of the vagina and reports of the woman's partner lacking in sexual interest[12,13].

MENOPAUSE AND MOOD

In a final attempt to trace influences on mood, the menopause was found not to be accompanied by increased mood swings or by a deeper feeling of depression, but by a reduction in subjective well-being – a sense of happiness, life satisfaction, and regarding life as meaningful, worthwhile and rewarding. Fifty percent of women showed such a decrease, and this could not be attributed to increased vasomotor complaints or chronological age. Although our longitudinal approach has probably uncovered for the first time a direct influence of the menopausal development on mood, the mechanism behind it is still unknown.

REFERENCES

1. Holte, A. (1992). The search for a climacteric mood disorder: methodological problems and recent results. In Wijma, K. and von Schultz, B. (eds.) *Reproductive Life: Advances in Research in Psychosomatic Obstetrics and Gynaecology,* pp. 371–7. (Casterton: Parthenon)
2. Holte, A. (1992). The changing truths about how natural menopause affects health complaints: results from the Norwegian Menopause Projects. In Wijma, K. and von Schultz, B. (eds.) *Reproductive Life: Advances in Research in Psychosomatic Obstetrics and Gynaecology,* pp. 352–8. (Casterton: Parthenon)
3. Holte, A. and Mikkelsen, A. (1981). Cultural Myths and Climacteric Reaction: a Small Scale Norwegian Study. Paper presented at *Third International Congress on the Menopause,* Ostende
4. Holte, A. and Mikkelsen, A. (1982). Menstrual coping style, social background and climacteric symptoms. *Psychiatry Soc. Sci.,* **2**, 41–5
5. Mikkelsen, A. and Holte, A. (1982). A factor analytic study of climacteric symptoms. *Psychiatry Soc. Sci.,* **2**, 35–9
6. Holte, A. (1991). Prevalence of climacteric complaints in a representative sample of middle-aged women in Oslo, Norway. *J. Psychosom. Obstet. Gynaecol.,* **12**, 303–17
7. Holte, A. and Mikkelsen, A. (1990). Climacteric complaints as a major health problem in the ageing population year 2000: prognoses based on the distribution of climacteric complaints in a Scandinavian normal population. In Cortes de Prieto, J. (ed.) *Reproductive Medicine in the Human Society of the Year 2000,* pp. 233–43. (Alcala de Henares: University of Alcala de Henares Press)
8. Holte, A. and Mikkelsen, A. (1990). Psycho-social causes of climacteric complaints: the first results from a six-year prospective follow-up study of Norwegian women. In Cortes de Prieto, J. (ed.) *Reproductive Medicine in*

the Human Society of the Year 2000, pp. 245–53. (Alcala de Henares: University of Alcala de Henares Press)
9. Holte, A. and Mikkelsen, A. (1991). The menopausal syndrome: a factor analytic replication. *Maturitas,* **13,** 205–15
10. Holte, A. and Mikkelsen, A. (1991). Psycho-social determinants of menopausal complaints. *Maturitas,* **13,** 193–203
11. Holte, A. (1992). Influences of natural menopause on health complaints: a prospective study of healthy Norwegian women. *Maturitas,* **14,** 127–41
12. Holte, A. (1990). Influences of natural menopause on sexual behaviour and well-being: a prospective study of healthy Norwegian women. Paper presented at *Sixth International Congress on the Menopause,* Bangkok
13. Holte, A., Mikkelsen, A., Moen, M. H. and Skjaeråsen, J. (1992). Influences of natural menopause on sexual behaviour and well-being: a prospective study of healthy Norwegian women. Unpublished manuscript. Department of Behavioural Sciences in Medicine, University of Oslo, P.O. Box 1111, Blindern, N-0317 Oslo
14. Holte, A., Mikkelsen, A., Moen, M. H. and Skjaeråsen, J. (1992). Sex-role identification and menopause: A prospective study of healthy Norwegian women. Unpublished manuscript. Department of Behavioural Sciences in Medicine, University of Oslo, P.O. Box 1111, Blindern, N-0317 Oslo

20

The effects of estrogen therapy on mood and well-being

M. S. Hunter

This paper examines the nature of the relationship between estrogen and mood in menopausal women, and the effects of estrogen therapy upon mood and well-being. While the main focus is a review of the epidemiological and treatment studies, the scope is rather broader, placing this research in a socio-cultural context. The term depressed mood is used here to represent a continuum of self-reported depressive symptoms; where studies refer to clinical depression, or well-being specifically, this will be indicated.

In the 1970s Winokur[1], Weissman[2] and others concluded that women were not more likely to become depressed during the menopause transition than at other times. In 1980 the psychiatric diagnosis of involutional melancholia was deemed invalid and excluded from the 3rd edition of the *Diagnostic and Statistical Manual.* In the past 5 years or so there has, however, been an upsurge of interest in the possible psychoactive properties of estrogen. Claims have been made, first, that estrogen should be advocated as the treatment of choice for 'menopausal depression', and second, that estrogen might offer an additional bonus of lifting mood or increasing well-being in non-depressed, healthy women.

These two claims, or hypotheses, clearly refer to different subgroups of women and appear to be underpinned by different concerns. The first is no doubt motivated by a desire to alleviate depression – a problem which is common amongst menopause clinic attenders (approximately 50% would be considered clinical cases)[3]. However, this claim also assumes that depression is more prevalent for women during the menopause, and that depression experienced at the menopause has a hormonal basis. The second claim, if corroborated, could provide evidence with which to encourage women to use and adhere to hormone replacement therapy regimens. In this case estrogen has to be regarded as a pharmacological agent which lifts mood, rather than a replacement therapy.

Before discussing the evidence in relation to these claims, I want to look briefly at the possible mechanisms for the inferred action of estrogen. There is certainly support for a central nervous system activating effect of estrogen, from animal experiments and laboratory studies. It is proposed that estrogen has a monoamine oxidase inhibitory effect, leading to increased noradrenalin synthesis[4]. In addition, estrogen might influence tryptophan (the precursor of serotonin) release; a positive correlation has been reported between total plasma estrogen and free plasma tryptophan in postmenopausal women[5]. While there is some evidence in support of both possible mechanisms, a direct relationship between estrogen levels and depressed mood has not been generally supported.

EPIDEMIOLOGICAL AND CORRELATIONAL STUDIES

Are women more likely to be depressed or have psychological problems during the climacteric, or menopause transition? Studies comparing the experience of the menopause in different cultures tend to reveal a diversity of experience, suggesting that the meaning ascribed to it and women's reactions to it are in part culturally determined[6].

The results of cross-sectional studies of western populations have been inconclusive on the whole, some finding an increase in symptoms during the perimenopause, but the majority of studies finding no change. Attempts were made to overcome methodological problems, and, using prospective designs with standardized measures, several longitudinal studies of general population samples were carried out in North America and Europe in the 1980s[7-12]. In addition, two longitudinal studies are in progress in Australia and Sweden, with preliminary results being reported at this conference.

Few changes in emotional well-being or depressed mood were evident in these non-clinic samples. Dennerstein, reporting on the initial results of the Australian longitudinal study, found no significant differences in well-being between pre-, peri- and postmenopausal women. Overall, in these prospective studies considerable individual differences were found, but the majority of women did not regard the menopause as a major crisis. In my own study[10] there was a slight but significant increase in depressed mood, but menopausal status only accounted for 2% of the variation in depressed mood. Oldenhave (1991)[12] found an increase in psychological symptoms in perimenopausal women which was associated with reports of vasomotor symptoms. Avis, describing some new data from the Massachusetts study, which included hormonal measures, reported that while there was a slight increase in depressed mood at the time of the last menstrual period, again this was associated with reports of vasomotor symptoms, but not estrogen levels. Prospective studies that include concurrent hormonal measures, such as those from Massachusetts, Sweden and Australia should help to unravel these complex relationships further in the next few years.

For those who are depressed during the menopause transition, the main predictors appear to be past depression, socioeconomic status, stressful life events and chronic ill-health[13]. However, these variables are not specific to this time of life. Marital and employment status and social support also appear to moderate the development of depressed mood. Considering menopause-specific variables, women who have experienced surgical menopause, and those who hold negative beliefs about the menopause are more likely to become depressed when they reach the menopause. Psychosocial factors have been found to account for much more of the variation in psychological symptoms than stage of menopause[10].

If depression does occur at this time the following factors should be considered, and a hormonal cause not automatically assumed:

(1) The psychological significance of the menopause, including mixed feelings about fertility and aging.

(2) Reactions to social attitudes towards older women, feeling embarrassed or devalued.

(3) Anxiety and confusion about the process of the menopause transition, such as irregular periods, and not knowing how long it might last.

(4) Reactions to vasomotor symptoms, possibly affecting sleep.

(5) Coincidental life problems and role changes.

Epidemiological studies, therefore, do not support the claim that depressed mood or other psychological symptoms increase at the menopause, and certainly the cross-cultural variation in experience casts doubt upon the notion of an essentially biological cause of distress at this time. While it remains possible that hormonal changes might influence mood in some women, the effects of psychosocial factors are likely to be greater for the majority.

The next point to consider is the relationship between estrogen level and depressed mood. Most correlational studies find no significant association between depressed mood and estrogen levels[14,15,17,18]. Sherwin (1988), in one of a series of studies of surgically menopausal women, did find a positive correlation between ratings of confidence and elation and estrogen levels. However, this was true for treated but not untreated women, suggesting a possible pharmacological effect of estrogen[16]. It remains possible that withdrawal of estrogen might precipitate depressed mood: carefully designed research is needed to test this hypothesis.

HORMONE REPLACEMENT THERAPY STUDIES

Studies of the effects of estrogen therapy on depression or psychological symptoms are beset by methodological problems[19]. Samples are heterogeneous (some including depressed women, others exclude those with emotional problems; some use naturally, others surgically menopausal women), and different doses and types of estrogen regimens are used. The placebo effects are, in general, large, and few studies control for the effects of reduction in vasomotor symptoms upon well-being. It is also difficult to retain the blind status in studies when estrogen has such a marked effect on vasomotor symptoms. Some studies used standardized, others unstandardized measures. Finally, subjects' expectations and understandings of the treatments are very much influenced by the information they receive about the treatment trial – information which should be made explicit in research reports.

There is only space to provide a brief overview of some of the main studies, which are separated into those using general clinic samples, which include more women reporting depressive symptoms, and those selecting healthier, non-depressed subjects. It should be noted here that the results of treatment studies do not provide information about etiology.

General clinic samples

Klaiber's[4] original study of the benefits of high doses of estrogen for severely depressed psychiatric inpatients has not yet been replicated. Using menopause clinic samples, no significant improvements have been found with estrogen compared to placebo on standardized measures, such as the Beck Depression Scale[14,20], Hamilton Rating Scale[21], or General Health Questionnaire[20], despite improvements in vasomotor symptoms. Dennerstein and colleagues[22] did find an improvement on the Hamilton Rating Scale, after treating women who had undergone surgical menopause. Using vasomotor symptom reports as a covariate this improvement diminished, although it remained significant. Some studies find improvements in psychological symptoms using rating scales[20], while others do not[22]. A study by Montgomery and colleagues[23] is often quoted in support of the benefits of estrogen therapy for menopausal women. The effects of estrogen implants (50 mg) were compared with estrogen plus testosterone and a placebo. Despite an initial difference between estrogen and the placebo condition at 2 months post-implant for the perimenopausal women in the study, there were no overall significant differences between peri- or postmenopausal subgroups and the placebo group between 2 and 4 months post-implantation, nor for the postmenopausal women after 2 months.

Selected healthy samples

Sherwin[16], in one of a series of carefully conducted studies of surgically menopausal women, compared estrogen plus androgen or estrogen alone with a group who had been untreated (average time since operation being 3–4 years). Significant increases in ratings of confidence and feelings of elation, but no group differences on the MACL depression scale, were evident. Placebo effects and the effects of relief from vasomotor symptoms were not controlled for. However, in an earlier study, Sherwin and Gelfand did find positive effects of estrogen upon mood in a placebo controlled cross-over trial[24].

In another study, Myers and colleagues[25] included a placebo condition, and compared estrogen and estrogen with progestogen. Vasomotor symptoms reduced but no changes in mood were reported, as assessed by daily rating scales. In an attempt to overcome the confounding effects of vasomotor symptom relief, Ditkoff and co-workers[26] conducted a randomized double-blind study of 36 asymptomatic Hispanic American women, all of whom had undergone hysterectomy. Estrogen (0.625 mg), estrogen (1.25 mg) and a placebo condition were compared. There were small (2 scale points) but significant decreases in depressed mood, as assessed by the Beck Depression Scale, for both treated groups, but no dose response. However, all the women scored within the normal range in this study. Sherwin and Gelfand (1989)[27] compared the same doses as Ditkoff and co-workers and, while there was no placebo condition, those taking the 1.25 dose reported significantly more elation, better sleep and greater well-being than those taking the 0.625 dose. The estrogen levels produced by the 1.25 dose were considered by the authors to be in the supraphysiological range, suggesting that there may be a positive effect of estrogen upon well-being when higher doses are used.

CONCLUSIONS

Overall, women are not more likely to be depressed during the menopause transition than at other times of life. No clear correlation exists between estrogen levels and reports of depressive symptoms, and psychosocial factors are the most common cause of distress at this time of life.

There is no conclusive evidence that estrogen therapy improves depressed mood in clinic samples, over and above placebo effects. There is slightly more evidence of improvements in treated women who have previously undergone surgical menopause. There is some evidence – but again it is equivocal – of a slight improvement in well-being in selected healthy samples, and there may be a dose response. However, even if it were conclusively proved to be the case, the reasons for treating healthy women or encouraging them to use a pharmacological agent to 'feel better' should be obviously questioned – particularly when the majority of women do not feel more depressed during the menopause, and the major causal factors appear to be psychosocial in nature. It is also, after all, quite normal to feel low at times. For women who do feel depressed and want help there are psychological therapies, such as cognitive-behavior therapy that can be used to help people to find appropriate solutions to their problems.

I want to end by describing some unpublished data from a current study of a random sample of 100 45-year-old women drawn from general practice lists in South East England (Hunter and Liao). When asked about their future intentions about treatment at the menopause, 42% of these women expressed an intention to have hormone replacement therapy (HRT), 44% did not and 14% lacked sufficient information on which to base the decision. Those intending to take HRT were more likely to be depressed and had lower self-esteem than non-intenders. They gave non-specific reasons for their intention, such as 'it will make me feel better', 'I've heard it's a good thing'.

Such beliefs in HRT as a panacea should not be reinforced, nor should women be encouraged to attribute pre-existing, or concurrent, problems to the menopause, when they are more likely to have psychosocial causes. By advocating estrogen therapy as a treatment for psychological problems the belief that the menopause causes them is often, by implication, reinforced. This view of the menopause might, in turn, encourage the negative stereotypes which have been shown to be predictive of depressed mood at this time of life.

REFERENCES

1. Winokur, G. (1973). Depression and the menopause. *Am. J. Psychiatr.*, **130**, 92–3
2. Weissman, M. M. (1979). The myth of involutional melancholia. *J. Am. Med. Assoc.*, **242**, 742–4
3. Ballinger, S. (1985). Psychosocial stress and symptoms of the menopause: a comparative study of menopause clinic and non-patients. *Maturitas*, **7**, 315–27
4. Klaiber, E. L., Broverman, D. M., Vogel, W. and Kobayashi, Y. (1979). Estrogen replacement therapy for severe persistent depressions in women. *Arch. Gen. Psychiatr.*, **36**, 550–4
5. Aylward, M. (1976). Estrogens, plasma tryptophan levels in premenopausal patients. In Campbell, S. (ed.) *The Management of the Menopause and the Postmenopausal Years*, pp. 135–48. (Lancaster: MTP Press)
6. Avis, N. E., Kaufert, P. A., McKinlay, S. A. and Vass, K. (1993). The evolution of menopausal symptoms. In Burger, H. G. (ed.) *The Menopause*, pp. 17–32. (London: Bailliere Tindall)
7. McKinlay, S. M., Brambilla, D. J. and Posner, J. (1992). The normal menopause transition. *Maturitas*, **14**, 103–16
8. Kaufert, P. A., Gilbert, P. and Tate, R. (1992). The Manitoba Project; a re-examination of the relationship between menopause and depression. *Maturitas*, **14**, 143–56
9. Holte, A. (1992). Influences of natural menopause on health complaints; a prospective study of healthy Norwegian women. *Maturitas*, **14**, 127–41
10. Hunter, M. S. (1992). The S.E. England longitudinal study of the climacteric and postmenopause. *Maturitas*, **14**, 117–26
11. Matthews, K. A., Wing, R. R. and Kuller, L. H. (1990). Influences of natural menopause on psychological characteristics and symptoms of middle-aged healthy women. *J. Consult. Clin. Psychol.*, **58**, 345–63
12. Oldenhave, A. (1991). *Well-being and Sexuality in the Climacteric.* (Geneva: International Health Foundation)
13. Hunter, M. S. (1993). Predictors of menopausal symptoms: psychological aspects. In Burger, H. G. (ed.) *The Menopause*, pp. 36–46. (London: Bailliere Tindall)
14. Coope, J. (1981). Is oestrogen effective in the treatment of menopausal depression? *J. R. Coll. Gen. Pract.*, **31**, 134–40
15. Ballinger, C. B., Browning, M. C. K. and Smith, A. H. W. (1987). Hormone profiles and psychological symptoms in perimenopausal women. *Maturitas*, **9**, 235–51
16. Sherwin, B. B. (1988). Affective changes with estrogen and androgen replacement therapy in surgically menopausal women. *J. Affective Dis.*, **14**, 177–87
17. Alder, E. M., Bancroft, J. and Livingstone, J. (1992). Estradiol implants, hormone levels and reported symptoms. *J. Psychosom. Obstet. Gynaecol.*, **13**, 223–35
18. Owen, E. J., Siddle, N. C., McGarrigle, H. T. and Pugh, M. A. (1992). 25 mg

oestradiol implants – the dosage of first choice for subcutaneous oestrogen replacement therapy. *Br. J. Obstet. Gynaecol.,* **99**, 671–5

19. Kaufert, P. A. and Gilbert, P. (1988). Researching the symptoms of the menopause: and exercise in methodology. *Maturitas,* **10**, 117–31
20. Campbell, S. (1976). Double blind psychometric studies on the effects of natural oestrogens on postmenopausal women. In Campbell, S. (ed.) *Management of the Menopause and the Postmenopausal Years,* pp. 149–58. (Lancaster: MTP Press)
21. Thompson, J. and Oswald, I. (1977). Effect of oestrogen on the sleep, mood and anxiety of menopausal women. *Br. Med. J.,* **2**, 1317–19
22. Dennerstein, L., Burrows, G. D., Hyman, C. and Sharpe, K. (1979). Hormone therapy and affect. *Maturitas,* **1**, 247–59
23. Montgomery, J. C., Appelby, L., Brincat, M., Versi, E., Tapp, A., Fenwick, P. B. C. and Studd, J. W. W. (1987). Effect of oestrogen and testosterone implants on psychological disorders in the climacteric. *Lancet,* **7**, 297–9
24. Sherwin, B. B. and Gelfand, M. M. (1985). Sex steroids and affect in the surgical menopause: a double-blind cross-over study. *Psychoneuroendocrinology,* **10**, 325–35
25. Myers, L. S., Dixen, D., Morrissette, M., Carmichael, M. and Davidson, J. M. (1990). Effects of estrogen, androgen, and progestin on sexual psychophysiology and behaviour in postmenopausal women. *J. Clin. Endocrinol. Metab.,* **70**, 1124–31
26. Ditkoff, E. C., Crary, W. G., Cristo, M. and Lobo, R. A. (1991). Estrogen improves psychological function in asymptomatic postmenopausal women. *Obstet. Gynecol.,* **78**, 991–5
27. Sherwin, B. B. and Gelfand, M. M. (1989). A prospective one-year study of estrogen and progestin in postmenopausal women: effects on clinical symptoms and lipoprotein lipids. *Obstet. Gynecol.,* **73**, 759–66

Section 4

Urogenital symptoms around menopause

21

Estrogen deficiency and urinary incontinence

L. Cardozo and C. Kelleher

INTRODUCTION

The female genital and lower urinary tracts develop in close proximity, both arising from the embryological urogenital sinus. Human and animal studies have shown that the adult female urogenital tissues are estrogen sensitive, and estrogen receptors have been identified in the human vagina, urethra, bladder and pelvic floor[1-3]. It is therefore logical to expect changes in estrogen levels to influence the lower urinary tract and the genital tract in women.

Fluctuations in sex steroids, in particular estrogens, result in symptomatic, cytological and urodynamic changes. This has been demonstrated during the menstrual cycle, in pregnancy and following the menopause[4-7]. At the time of the menopause circulating estrogen levels fall, and the resulting urogenital atrophy causes symptoms of vaginal dryness, itching, burning, dyspareunia and discharge, as well as an increased incidence of urinary symptoms including dysuria, frequency, nocturia, urgency and incontinence.

EPIDEMIOLOGY

Improved life expectancy has resulted in a steady increase in the size of the postmenopausal population, to the extent that almost one-third of a woman's life will be spent in the estrogen-deficient postmenopausal state[8]. The true prevalence of postmenopausal urinary incontinence is unknown but it has been estimated at 16% in women over the age of 75 years[9]; 18% in women over the age of 70 years[10]; and 29% in women aged 61 years[2]. The role of estrogen deficiency in the pathogenesis of urinary incontinence compared to that of the aging process *per se* is still unclear.

In the large epidemiological study by Thomas and co-workers[9], the prevalence of incontinence was shown to increase with age but not specifically at the time of the menopause; in the study by Iosif and Bekassey[2], 70% of the incontinent elderly women related its onset to their last menstrual period. Both of these studies have deficiencies, but epidemiological data are undoubtedly difficult to collect. However, incontinence during the postmenopausal years is certainly very common. In a study of 228 women attending the Dulwich Menopause Clinic for hormone replacement therapy, 20% complained of severe urgency and nearly 50% complained of stress incontinence[11].

MECHANISM OF CONTINENCE

For continence to exist the urethral pressure must exceed the bladder pressure at all times except during micturition. This positive urethral closure pressure is produced by the four functional layers of the urethra; namely the epithelium, connective tissue, vascular tissue and muscle. All of these layers are affected by estrogen status[12].

Estrogens may aid continence by increasing urethral resistance, raising the sensory threshold of the bladder, increasing α-receptor sensitivity in the urethral smooth muscle[13,14], or possibly by a combination of all three. In addition, estrogen therapy has been shown to increase the number of intermediate and superficial cells in the vagina of postmenopausal women[15] and similar changes have been demonstrated in the urethra and bladder[16].

CAUSES OF POSTMENOPAUSAL URINARY INCONTINENCE

Incontinence in postmenopausal women may be due to a variety of causes (Table 1). To obtain a better understanding of the pathological processes of urinary incontinence and make an accurate diagnosis of the cause of incontinence urodynamic investigations are essential. Such investigations may be either simple or complex (Table 2): complex investigations are usually only available in specialist centers.

The treatment of urinary incontinence will depend on its cause, although simple measures should be implemented and will often lead to improvement for all diagnoses (Table 3). The treatment of detrusor instability and mild to moderate genuine stress incontinence is primarily

Table 1 Causes of urinary incontinence in women

Genuine stress incontinence (urethral sphincter incompetence)
Detrusor instability
Overflow incontinence (with chronic retention)
Fistulae
Congenital (e.g. epispadias, ectopic ureter)
Miscellaneous (e.g. urethral diverticulum)
Temporary (e.g. urinary tract infection, fecal impaction)
Functional

Table 2 Simple and complex urodynamic investigations

Simple	*Complex*
Mid-stream urine culture	Cystometry
Frequency/volume chart	Videocystourethrography
Pad test	Urethral pressure
Uroflowmetry	profilometry
'Eyeball urodynamics'	Ultrasound
	Ambulatory urodynamics
	Electromyography

Table 3 Simple measures in the management of urinary incontinence

Fluid restriction ($\leqslant 1.5\,l$/day)
Timing of intake
Timed/double voiding
Provision of a commode
Barrier cream
Treat chronic conditions (e.g. cough/constipation)
Monitor medication (e.g. diuretics)
Weight reduction?

conservative (Table 4). Surgery is appropriate for severe or refractory genuine stress incontinence (Table 5), and is seldom applicable for the treatment of detrusor instability unless all other measures have failed.

Genuine stress incontinence is most common among women in their reproductive years, whereas detrusor instability is seen more often in the elderly. Jolleys[17] found that the prevalence of stress incontinence reached a peak at the age of 50 years and declined thereafter.

Unfortunately, mixed urinary symptoms are common and the correlation between symptomatic and urodynamic diagnosis is known to be poor[18]. Jarvis and colleagues[19] found that urodynamic studies altered the manage-

Table 4 Conservative management of incontinence

Genuine stress incontinence
  pelvic floor exercises (with/without biofeedback)
  vaginal cones
  electrical stimulation
  devices (tampon/sponge/pessary)
  drugs (e.g. phenylpropanolamine, estrogen)
  pads/pants/catheters
  simple measures (see Table 3)

Detrusor instability
  bladder drill/biofeedback
  drugs (anticholinergic/smooth muscle relaxants)
  estrogen replacement
  electrical stimulation
  acupuncture/hypnotherapy/psychotherapy
  bed alarms/DDAVP (nocturnal enuresis)
  pads/pants/catheters
  simple measures (see Table 3)

Functional incontinence (e.g. immobility)
  commode/prompted or timed voiding
  incontinence aids (pads/pants/catheters)
  adequate laundry facilities
  fecal disimpaction

DDAVP, L-deamino-D-arginine vasopressin

Table 5 Surgical approach for the treatment of genuine stress incontinence

Anterior colporrhaphy (combined with Kelly or Pacey buttressing sutures)
Marshall–Marchetti–Krantz procedure
Colposuspension
Long needle bladder neck suspensions (Pereyra or Stamey)
Sling procedures
Periurethral injectables (e.g. GAX collagen)
Complex surgical procedures (e.g. artificial sphincter, neourethra)

GAX, glutaraldehyde cross-linked bovine collagen

ment of urinary incontinence in more than 30% of women after a clinical diagnosis had been made. It is therefore essential that adequate investigations are performed prior to treatment.

ESTROGENS IN UNDIAGNOSED INCONTINENCE

Early studies of the effect of estrogens on lower urinary tract dysfunction predated urodynamic studies and were largely subjective and uncontrolled.

The first report was from Salmon and co-workers[20] who treated 16 women with dysuria, frequency, urgency and incontinence for 4 weeks using intramuscular estrogen therapy. Twelve of them improved symptomatically. Thirty years later, Musiani[21] gave 110 stress incontinent women, Quinestradol, which is no longer available, and reported a cure rate of 33% and an improvement rate of 39%. Schleyer-Saunders[22] used estradiol implants to treat 100 postmenopausal women with undiagnosed urinary incontinence and found that 70% were significantly improved, reducing the need for surgery.

ESTROGEN THERAPY FOR URGE INCONTINENCE

Few controlled studies have been reported in the literature. Samsioe and co-workers[16] entered 34 women aged 75 years into a double-blind, placebo-controlled cross-over study of oral estriol 3 mg daily for 3 months. Despite the lack of objective assessment they found that urge incontinence and mixed incontinence were improved by estriol, but in women with stress incontinence there was no difference between estriol and placebo. Unfortunately we have not been able to reproduce their results.

We have recently reported the results of a double-blind placebo-controlled randomized multicenter study of oral estriol 3 mg/day in the treatment of 64 postmenopausal women with 'the urge syndrome'[23]. Women who entered the trial underwent urodynamic assessment and were divided into those with sensory urgency and those with detrusor instability. Treatment was for 3 months, after which patients were fully assessed both subjectively and objectively and side-effects were recorded. Patient compliance was confirmed by a significant improvement in the maturation index of vaginal wall smears with estriol when compared to placebo. Although estriol produced both subjective and objective improvement in lower urinary tract function it was not significantly better than placebo.

Estriol is a naturally occurring estrogen which binds to estrogen receptors but has a short nuclear retention time, so that long-term estrogenic effects are unlikely from a small once-daily dose. Estriol may effectively treat hot flushes and is useful in the management of vaginal atrophy, but it does not prevent osteoporosis. It is therefore a safe estrogen which should be effective in the treatment of postmenopausal 'urge syndrome'. However, our study failed to confirm any advantage of estriol over placebo in the treatment of this condition.

It is interesting to speculate whether this was because we used too low a dose, the wrong route of administration, or an inappropriate estrogen, and it is unclear whether low dose topical therapy, which improves genital atrophy without significant endometrial stimulation, is sufficient to treat urinary symptoms. Indeed it is possible that estrogen is actually no better than placebo for the management of postmenopausal women with this condition, although Fantl and co-workers[24] have suggested that estrogen supplementation raises the sensory threshold of the bladder.

In view of our disappointing results using estriol in the management of postmenopausal urinary urgency, we have recently assessed the efficacy of 17β-estradiol vaginal tablets (Vagifem) (C. J. Benness, B. G. Wise and L. D. Cardozo, unpublished data). These are well absorbed from the vagina and have been shown to cause maturation of the vaginal epithelium within 14 days[25].

One hundred and ten postmenopausal women suffering from urgency were randomized to receive either 25 μg 17β-estradiol or matching placebo each day for 6 months. All underwent urodynamic investigations and were divided into three groups: detrusor instability, sensory urgency and normal urodynamics. At the end of the treatment period the only significant difference between those receiving active or placebo therapy was the improvement in the symptom of urgency in those women with sensory urgency, which responded better to estradiol than placebo.

Eriksen and Rasmussen[26] showed in a 12-week double-blind, randomized, placebo-controlled trial that treatment with 25 μg 17β-estradiol tablets significantly improved lower urinary tract symptoms of frequency, urgency, and urge and stress incontinence compared to placebo. Unfortunately they did not select women on the basis of their urinary symptoms and the study lacked the benefit of objective urodynamic assessment.

ESTROGEN THERAPY FOR ATROPHIC VAGINITIS

Symptoms of genital atrophy may not arise until many years after the menopause, but they are thought to be very common. In a study of 61-year-old Swedish women, Iosif and Bekassy[2] reported one or more vaginal symptoms in over 50% of subjects, and the prevalence of these symptoms increased with age. Among a group of women aged 56–69 years, 22.3% reported local vaginal discomfort[27].

Although, in our study, vaginal estradiol had little effect on urinary symptoms, it has been shown to be useful in the management of atrophic vaginitis. In a placebo-controlled study of 164 women, 78.8% of those receiving Vagifem and 81.9% of the placebo group had moderate to severe vaginal atrophy prior to treatment. After 12 weeks' therapy only 10.7% of the Vagifem group but 29.9% of the placebo group had the same degree of atrophy[26].

Low-dose local therapy appears to be most beneficial in the management of symptoms due to vaginal atrophy; recently, a silicone vaginal ring releasing 5–10 μg estradiol/24 h for a minimum of 90 days was evaluated in 222 postmenopausal women with symptoms and signs of vaginal atrophy. Maturation of the vaginal epithelium, measured cytologically, significantly improved during treatment as well as symptoms of vaginal dryness, pruritus vulvae, dyspareunia and urinary urgency. Cure or improvement of atrophic vaginitis was recorded in more than 90% of subjects and most of the women found this form of treatment acceptable even during sexual intercourse[28].

ESTROGEN THERAPY FOR STRESS INCONTINENCE

The main parameter which has been used to assess the efficacy of estrogen therapy in the management of women with stress incontinence is urethral pressure profilometry. Caine and Raz[29] showed that 26 of 40 (65%) women with stress incontinence had increased maximum urethral pressures and symptomatic improvement whilst taking conjugated oral estrogen. Rud[30] treated 24 women with stress incontinence with high doses of oral estradiol and estriol in combination. He found a significant increase in transmission of intra-abdominal pressure to the urethra, as well as an increase in maximum urethral pressure. Seventy percent of the women were symptomatically improved; however, high doses of estrogen were employed over a short period of time and other studies have not all reported the same changes in urethral pressure profilometry.

Walter and co-workers[31] randomly allocated 29 incontinent, postmeno-pausal women with stable bladders to either estradiol and estriol or placebo (4 months' cyclical treatment). They found a significant improvement in urgency and urge incontinence (7 of 15 (47%) with estrogen therapy) but no improvement in stress incontinence. They were unable to demonstrate a change in urethral pressure profile parameters. Similarly, Wilson and colleagues[32] entered 36 women with urodynamically proven genuine stress incontinence into a double-blind, placebo-controlled study of cyclical oral estrone for 3 months and showed no difference in the subjective response, urethral pressure profile parameters or quantity of urine lost.

The only study to date which has shown a significant objective improvement in genuine stress incontinence using estrogen therapy was reported by Walter and co-workers[33]. In a randomized, placebo-controlled study of estriol 4 mg daily, they showed that nine of 12 (75%) women preferred estriol to placebo and that there was a significant objective decrease in urine loss with estriol compared to placebo. However, the numbers in this study were small.

ADVERSE EVENTS

Low-dose topical estrogen therapy, by avoiding the enterohepatic circulation and exerting a mainly local effect, is virtually free from side-effects. There have been occasional reports of vaginal bleeding in women with a uterus, but the endometrium usually remains atrophic despite prolonged treatment. Iosif[34] reported a series of 48 women receiving treatment with 0.5 mg estriol suppositories for 1–10 years. Vabra curettage showed the majority to have an inactive atrophic endometrium with only seven (15%) having a weakly proliferative endometrium after prolonged treatment. None of the women had evidence of hyperplasia or atypia. Mettler and Olsen[35] assessed the effect of long-term low-dose estradiol vaginal tablets (25 μg 17β-estradiol) on the endometrium. Fifty-one women received once or twice weekly treatment for up to 2 years. All nine women completing 2 years of treatment had an inactive atrophic endometrium and only three cases of weak endometrial proliferation were found after 1 year of treatment.

Reported side-effects and complications of systemic estrogen therapy in the management of postmenopausal urinary incontinence have also been few. Breast tenderness, heavy irregular withdrawal bleeding and palpitations have been reported, and there has been one case of myocardial infarction which was probably unrelated to therapy[32]. There have been no other documented problems despite the use of high doses of estrogen. However, the longest period of treatment reported in the literature was 4 months.

COMBINATION THERAPIES

It would appear that estrogens alone are helpful for the symptoms of urgency and urge incontinence, but not for stress incontinence. However, there have been reports of benefits from combination therapy using an estrogen and an α-adrenergic agonist. Beisland and colleagues[36] treated 24 menopausal women with genuine stress incontinence using phenylpropanolamine (50 mg twice daily orally) and estriol (1 mg/day vaginally), separately and in combination. They found that the combination cured eight women and improved a further nine, and was more effective than either drug alone. Further studies of this sort have been undertaken: Hilton and co-workers[37] recently reported the results of a double-blind, placebo-controlled study using estrogen (oral or vaginal) alone or with phenylpropanolamine, in 60 postmenopausal women with urodynamically proven genuine stress incontinence. They found that the symptoms of frequency and nocturia improved more with combined treatment than with estrogen alone, and that stress incontinence improved subjectively in all groups but objectively only in the combined group. It is likely that the effect of phenylpropanolamine on α-adrenergic receptors in the urethra is potentiated by the concomitant use of estrogen replacement therapy in postmenopausal women.

ESTROGENS IN THE TREATMENT OF RECURRENT URINARY TRACT INFECTION

A possible application for estrogen therapy in postmenopausal women with lower urinary tract dysfunction is in the treatment and prophylaxis of recurrent urinary tract infections. Estrogen therapy promotes recolonization of the vagina by lactobacilli, reducing both vaginal pH, and the proliferation of Gram negative fecal pathogens To date only small preliminary studies have been described in the literature.

Brandberg and co-workers[38] treated 41 elderly women with recurrent urinary tract infections with oral estriol and showed that their vaginal flora was restored to the premenopausal type, and that they required fewer antibiotics. In an uncontrolled study, Privette and colleagues[39] studied 12 women who experienced frequent urinary tract infections. They were all found to have atrophic vaginitis and had suffered a mean of four infections/patient/year. Treatment consisted of a combination of short-term douche and antibiotic for 1 week together with long-term estrogen therapy. During follow-up of 2–8 years there were only four infections in the entire group.

In a recent report Kjaergaard and co-workers[40] studied 23 postmenopausal women with recurrent urinary tract infections. The women were treated with vaginal estradiol or placebo for 5 months, following which there was improvement in vaginal cytology in the estradiol group only, but no difference in the number of urinary tract infections or patient satisfaction between the two groups. In the most recent study 40 elderly women with recurrent urinary tract infections were randomized to receive either oral estriol 3 mg daily for 4 weeks followed by 1 mg daily for 8 weeks, or matching placebo. There was no difference between estriol and placebo after the first treatment period but following the second treatment period, estriol was significantly more effective than placebo at reducing the incidence of urinary tract infections[41].

We have almost completed a large multicenter, double-blind placebo-controlled trial of oral estriol as a prophylactic agent against recurrent urinary tract infections in postmenopausal women. If it proves successful this type of weak estrogen therapy could be beneficial in the prevention of morbidity in both community-dwelling and institutionalized elderly women.

CONCLUSIONS

To date there have been few appropriate placebo-controlled studies using both subjective and objective parameters to assess the efficacy of estrogen therapy for the treatment of urinary incontinence. Further confusion arises from the heterogeneity of different investigations and consequently the best treatment in terms of dose, type of estrogen and route of administration is unknown.

It is possible that recurrent urinary tract infection may be treated or even prevented by estrogen therapy, but this is as yet unproven. Systemic estrogen replacement appears to alleviate the symptoms of urgency, urge incontinence, frequency, nocturia and dysuria, and low-dose topical estrogen is effective in the management of atrophic vaginitis. Although the latter appears to be free from side-effects, even following prolonged administration, it is unclear whether low-dose therapy is sufficient to treat urinary tract pathology.

There is no conclusive evidence that estrogen alone cures stress incontinence, although in combination with an α-adrenergic agonist there may be a place for estrogen therapy in the conservative management of genuine stress incontinence.

Estrogen supplementation definitely improves the quality of life of many postmenopausal women and makes them better able to cope with other disabilities. Perhaps the role of estrogen in the management of postmenopausal urinary disorders is as an adjunct to other methods of treatment such as surgery, physiotherapy or drugs. This is certainly a hypothesis which should be tested.

REFERENCES

1. Cardozo, L. D. (1990). Role of estrogens in the treatment of female urinary incontinence. *J. Am. Geriatric Soc.,* **38**, 326–8
2. Iosif, C. S. and Bekassy, Z. (1984). Prevalence of genito-urinary symptoms in

the later menopause. *Acta Obstet. Gynecol. Scand.,* **63**, 257–60

3. Batra, S. and Fosil, C. S. (1983). Female urethra, a target for estrogen action. *J. Urol.,* **129**, 418–20

4. Van Geelen, J. M., Doesburg, W. H., Thomas, C. M. G. and Martin, C. B. (1981). Urodynamic studies in the normal menstrual cycle: The relationship between hormonal changes in the menstrual cycle and urethral pressure profiles. *Am. J. Obstet. Gynecol.,* **141**, 384–92

5. Tapp, A. J. S. and Cardozo, L. D. (1986). The postmenopausal bladder. *Br. J. Hosp. Med.,* **35**, 20–3

6. McCallin, P. E., Stewart Taylor, E. and Whitehead, R. W. (1950). A study of the changes in cytology of the urinary sediment during the menstrual cycle and pregnancy. *Am. J. Obstet. Gynecol.,* **60**, 64–74

7. Solomon, C., Panagotopoulous, P. and Oppenheim, A. (1958). Urinary cytology studies as an aid to diagnosis. *Am. J. Obstet. Gynecol.,* **76**, 57–62

8. American National Institute of Health population figures. US Treasury Department. (MD, National Institutes of Health)

9. Thomas, T. M., Plymat, K. R., Blannin, J. and Meade, T. W. (1980). Prevalence of urinary incontinence. *Br. Med. J.,* **281**, 1243–5

10. Vetter, N. J., Jones, D. A. and Victor, C. R. (1981). Urinary incontinence in the elderly at home. *Lancet,* **2**, 1275–7

11. Cardozo, L. D., Tapp, A. and Versi, E. (1987). The lower urinary tract in peri and postmenopausal women. In Samsioe, E. and Bonne Eriksen, P. (eds.) *The Urogenital Oestrogen Deficiency Syndrome,* pp. 10–17.

12. Rud, T., Anderson, K. E., Asmussen, M., Hunting, A. and Ulmsten, U. (1980). Factors maintaining the urethral pressure in women. *Invest. Urol.,* **17**, 343–7

13. Versi, E. and Cardozo, L. D. (1988). Estrogens and lower urinary tract function. In Studd, J. W. W. and Whitehead, M. I. (eds.) *The Menopause,* pp. 76–84. (Oxford: Blackwell Scientific Publications)

14. Kinn, A. C. and Lindskog, M. (1988). Oestrogens and phenylpropanolamine in combination for stress urinary incontinence in postmenopausal women. *Urology,* **32**, 273–80

15. Smith, P. J. B. (1976). The effect of oestrogens on bladder function in the female. In Campbell, S. (ed.) *The Management of the Menopause and Postmenopausal Years,* pp. 291–8. (Lancaster: MTP)

16. Samsioe, G., Jansson, I., Mellstsrom,D. and Svandborg, A. (1985). Occurrence, nature and treatment of urinary incontinence in a 70 year old female population. *Maturitas,* **7**, 335–42

17. Jolleys, J. V. (1988). Reported prevalence of urinary incontinence in women in general practice. *Br. Med. J.,* **296**, 1300–2

18. Versi, E., Cardozo, L., Anand, D. and Cooper, D. (1991). Symptoms analysis for the diagnosis of genuine stress incontinence. *Br. J. Obstet. Gynaecol.,* **98**, 815–19

19. Jarvis, G. J., Hall, S., Stamp, S., Millar, D. R. and Johnson, A. (1980). An assessment of urodynamic examination in incontinent women. *Br. J. Obstet. Gynaecol.,* **87**, 893–6

20. Salmon, U. L., Walter, R. I. and Gast, S. H. (1941). The use of estrogens in the treatment of dysuria and incontinence in postmenopausal women. *Am. J. Obstet. Gynecol.,* **42**, 845–7

21. Musiani, U. (1972). A partially successful attempt at medical treatment of urinary stress incontinence in women. *Urol. Int.,* **27**, 405–10

22. Schleyer-Saunders, E. (1976). Hormone implants for urinary disorders in postmenopausal women. *J. Am. Geriatr. Soc.,* **24**, 337–9

23. Cardozo, L. D., Rekers, H., Tapp, A., Barnick, C., Shepherd, A., Schussler, B., Kerr-Wilson, R., Van Geelan, J., Barlebo, H. and Walter, S. (1993). Oestriol in the treatment of postmenopausal urgency – a multicentre study. *Maturitas* (in press)

24. Fantl, J. A., Wyman, J. F., Anderson, R. L., Matt, D. W. and Bump, R. C. (1988). Postmenopausal urinary incontinence: comparison between non-estrogen supplement and estrogen-supplemented women. *Obstet. Gynecol.,* **71**, 823–6

25. Nilsson, K. and Heimer, G. (1992). Low dose oestradiol in the treatment of urogenital oestrogen deficiency – a pharmacokinetic and pharmacodynamic study. *Maturitas,* **15**, 121–7

26. Eriksen, P. S. and Rasmussen, H. (1992). Low-dose 17-beta oestradiol vaginal tablets in the treatment of atrophic vaginitis: a double-blind placebo controlled study. *Eur. J. Obstet. Gynaecol. Reprod. Biol.,* **44**, 137–44

27. Hilton, P. and Stanton, S. L. (1983). The use of intravaginal oestrogen cream in genuine stress incontinence. *Br. J. Obstet. Gynaecol.,* **90**, 940–4

28. Smith, P., Heimer, G., Lindskog, M. and Ulsten, U. (1993). Oestradiol-releasing vaginal ring for treatment of post menopausal urogenital atrophy. *Maturitas,* **16**, 145–54

29. Caine, M. and Raz, S. (1973). The role of female hormones in stress incontinence. *Proceedings of the 16th Congress of the International Society of Urology,* Amsterdam

30. Rud, T. (1980). The effects of oestrogens and gestagens on the urethral pressure profile in urinary continent and stress incontinent women. *Acta Obstet. Gynecol. Scand.,* **59**, 265–70

31. Walter, S., Wolf, H., Barlebo, H. and Jansen, H. (1978). Urinary incontinence in postmenopausal women treated with oestrogens: a double-blind clinical trial. *Urol. Int.,* **33**, 135–43

32. Wilson, P. D., Faragher, B., Butler, B., Bu'lock, D., Robinson, E. L. and Brown, A. D. G. (1987). Treatment with oral piperazine oestrone sulphate for genuine stress incontinence in postmenopausal women. *Br. J. Obstet. Gynaecol.,* **94**, 568–74

33. Walter, S., Kjaergaard, B., Lose, G., Andersen, J. T., Heisterberg, L., Jakobsen, H., Klarskov, P., Moller-Hansen, K. and Lindskog, M. (1990). Stress urinary incontinence in postmenopausal women treated with oral estrogen (estriol) and alpha adrenoreceptor-stimulating agent (Phenylpropanolamine): a randomised double blind placebo controlled study. *Int. Urogynecol. J.,* **12**, 74–9

34. Iosif, C. S. (1992). Effects of protracted administration of estriol on the lower genitourinary tract in postmenopausal women. *Arch. Gynaecol. Obstet.,* **251**, 115–20

35. Mettler, L. and Olsen, P. G. (1991). Long term treatment of atrophic vaginitis with low dose oestradiol vaginal tablets. *Maturitas,* **14**, 23–31

36. Beisland, H. O., Fossberg, E., Moer, A. and Sander, S. (1984). Urethral sphincteric insufficiency in postmenopausal females: treatment with phenylpropanolamine and estriol separately and in combination. *Urol. Int.,* **39**, 211–16

37. Hilton, P., Tweddel, A. L. and Mayne, C. (1990). Oral and intravaginal estrogens alone and in combination with alpha adrenergic stimulation in genuine stress incontinence. *Int. Urogynaecol. J.,* **12**, 80–6
38. Brandberg, A., Mellstrom, D. and Samsioe, G. (1985). Peroral estriol treatment of older women with urogenital infections. *Lakartidningen,* **82**, 3399–401
39. Privette, M., Cade, R., Peterson, J. and Mars, D. (1988). Prevention of recurrent urinary tract infections in postmenopausal women. *Nephron,* **50**, 24–7
40. Kjaergaard, B., Walter, S., Knudsen, A., Johansen, B. and Barlebo, H. (1990). Treatment with low-dose vaginal estradiol in postmenopausal women. A double-blind controlled trial. *Ugeskrift For Laegar.,* **152**, 658–9
41. Kirkengen, A. L., Andersen, P., Gjersoe, E., Johannessen, G. A., Johnsen, N. and Bodd, E. (1992). Oestriol in the prophylactic treatment of recurrent urinary tract infections in postmenopausal women. *Scand. J. Primary Health Care,* **10**, 139–42

22

Endometrial changes during the perimenopausal years

S. K. Smith

INTRODUCTION

The mechanism of cyclical endometrial shedding evolved in higher primates in order to prepare the endometrium for implantation of an embryo. This development is regulated by ovarian steroids. The desire of women to maintain the beneficial systemic effects of ovarian steroids on the quality and longevity of their lives has exposed them to the inevitable problems of endometrial bleeding. This fascinating mechanism, at least viewed from the dispassionate perspective of a man, is poorly understood. In this section, the extent of the clinical problem will be considered and several new ideas concerning the regulation of endometrial bleeding considered.

THE CLINICAL PROBLEM

Natural cycles

It is the pattern of bleeding which defines the clinical problem. In natural, non-pregnant menstrual cycles bleeding may be regular but heavy, irregular, or may occur in the intermenstrual period in the presence of clearly defined menstrual episodes. The first type of bleeding occurs in ovulatory cycles[1] and is often associated with other symptoms including premenstrual syndrome and dysmenorrhea[2]. The second pattern arises from anovulatory cycles and is not usually associated with premenstrual syndrome or dysmenorrhea. The third type of bleeding may not be of endometrial origin but where it is it can arise from polyps or premenstrual endometrial breakdown.

MECHANISMS OF MENSTRUATION AND ENDOMETRIAL BLEEDING

Withdrawal bleeding

Natural menstruation arises from the withdrawal of estrogen and progesterone support from the endometrium. Initiation of bleeding arises with vasoconstriction of the spiral arterioles, followed by vasodilatation and extravasation of blood from the damaged vessels[3]. The volume of blood lost and the duration of bleeding reflects the complex interplay of vasoactive compounds, hemostasis, and the tissue remodelling that occurs at menstruation. It is assumed that the mechanism of bleeding arising from withdrawal of exogenous steroids is similar to that of the withdrawal of endogenous steroids but there is no evidence to substantiate this claim. Similarly, there is an assumption that the volume of the loss is less during hormone replacement therapy (HRT) withdrawal bleeding compared to natural bleeding, though this may not be the case (Rees, 1993, personal communication).

Markee's experiments define our understanding of menstruation[3]. Bleeding arises after intense vasoconstriction of the spiral arterioles. Various vasoconstrictive agents have been suggested to be involved in this process.

Prostaglandins

Vasoconstricting prostaglandins are synthesized by endometrium and are under hormonal control. Disturbances in the balance of constricting and dilating prostaglandins have been implicated in the etiology of heavy bleeding. While exogenous steroids regulate endometrial prostaglandin synthesis *in vivo*, in a pattern consistent with *in vitro* observations, the direct effects of HRT on endometrial prostaglandin synthesis and its effect on menstruation are poorly understood.

Endothelins

Endothelins 1, 2 and 3 are expressed in human endometrium[4], as are their α and β receptors[5]. Interestingly, there are marked cyclical changes in the expression of ligand and receptor, clearly suggesting steroidal regulation. Further work is needed to define their role in the initiation and regulation of endometrial bleeding and to determine the function of nitric oxide release in the control of uterine bleeding.

Regeneration

The role played by regeneration in controlling the volume and duration of bleeding remains unclear, though it is likely to be important as bleeding stops when the endometrium has re-established its epithelial lining and repaired its vasculature. Endometrium is a rich source of angiogenic growth factors which are able to promote the proliferation, migration and differentiation of endothelial cells, leading to new vessel formation.

Angiogenesis is a complex mechanism involving angiogenic growth factors, extracellular matrix (ECM) and proteases. Angiogenic growth factors, vascular endothelial growth factor (VEGF), acidic and basic fibroblast growth factor (FGF), endothelial growth factor (EGF) and transforming growth factor (TGF)-α are all expressed by human endometrium[6-8]. VEGF is expressed by glandular cells in the premenstrual phase of the cycle and is upregulated by hypoxia. Four splice variants are expressed, two of which are secreted products. In the early proliferative phase of the cycle, the stroma becomes infiltrated by VEGF-expressing cells. It is not yet clear what these cells are, but they are probably macrophages, as the other lymphocyte-derived cells, the large granular lymphocytes, do not express VEGF. In concert, the secreted VEGF from the desquamated epithelial cells and the invading macrophages probably provides a high concentration of VEGF. In addition, human endometrial epithelial cells express acidic and basic FGF. The problem is that FGF probably exists predominantly bound to heparan sulfate and heparin in the ECM, being released from dying cells. However, this would be the ideal circumstance in menstruating endometrium, where they could combine with VEGF and lymphocyte-derived TGF-α to promote angiogenesis.

This is a simplistic view of angiogenesis, which inevitably includes expression of metalloproteinases, tissue inhibitors of metalloproteinase and cell adhesion molecules. At present there is little information as to the *in vivo* or *in vitro* effects of HRT steroids on this mechanism.

HORMONAL REPLACEMENT THERAPY

Estrogen and cyclical progestagen therapy

Withdrawal bleeding occurs in about 85% of women using sequential HRT regimes[9]. While the dose and duration of progestagen therapy has been determined to prevent hyperplasia, only about 65% of the endometria demonstrate secretory change. Despite this, bleeding is cyclical and must arise in about 35% of cases from proliferative or atrophic endometrium. Bleeding occurs earlier in the progestagen regimen in these women than in those with secretory endometrium[10]. This bleeding arises before the end of medication and is thus not 'withdrawal bleeding'. It could reflect intermittent surging of endogenous estrogen synthesis or local steroid withdrawal, arising from depletion of steroid receptors induced by exogenous steroids. We have no objective data to explain this phenomenon. Even women in whom secretory change has occurred may bleed before the treatment is withdrawn. One approach has been to develop continuous combined therapies.

Continuous combined HRT

Continuous combined hormone therapy has a high incidence of irregular bleeding in the early months of treatment, ranging from 25 to 92% of women[11]. This declines with therapy to less than 5% after 1 year. However, this is influenced by the time from the last period[12] and the high incidence of women withdrawing from such studies[11,13]. Histological findings usually demonstrate atrophic changes, but detailed examination of the endometrial vasculature have, surprisingly, not been widely reported. Other studies investigating the atrophic effects of steroids on endometrium suggest a rounding-off of endothelial cells, resulting in gaps between the cells which permit red blood cells to pass into the stroma[14]. These changes appear focal on hysteroscopy. Loss of endothelial integrity might be expected to permit local release of proteolytic enzymes.

The endometrial changes induced by steroids which contribute to the loss of endothelial integrity are unknown, but angiogenic growth factors, cell adhesion molecules and the extracellular matrix are the key factors. As described, three angiogenic growth factors, VEGF, acidic and basic FGF are expressed in epithelial cells of endometrium throughout the normal menstrual cycle[6,7]. If this is the case, then the atrophic changes induced by continuous combined regimens would be expected to reduce VEGF synthesis per milligram of endometrium and inhibit the stroma which usually express the secreted growth factor. Both effects would reduce VEGF expression in endometrium, possibly leading to endothelial cell degradation. Endothelial cells express a wide range of growth factors and cytokines, not to mention specific adhesion molecules which are necessary for the maintenance of morphological integrity. Little is known of the effect of steroids on these mechanisms in women. Considering the clinical significance of endometrial bleeding it is surprising that so little research has been conducted in this area.

CONCLUSIONS

Hormone replacement therapy is not the elixir of youth but, if present assumptions concerning its beneficial effects on osteoporosis and cardiovascular disease are fully substantiated and if these benefits exceed the risks of therapy, it will relieve human suffering. There is an urgent need for directed basic molecular and cellular studies to determine the effects of steroids on the endometrial vasculature. Modest investment is likely, though not guaranteed, to lead to improved treatment regimens and even wholly new approaches to the problem of endometrial bleeding in older women.

REFERENCES

1. Haynes, P. J., Flint, A. P., Hodgson, H., Anderson, A. B. M. and Turnbull, A. C. (1980). Studies in menorrhagia (a) mefenamic acid, (b) endometrial prostaglandin concentration. *Int. J. Obstet. Gynaecol.*, **17**, 567–72
2. Bancroft, J., Williamson, L., Warner, P., Rennie, D. and Smith, S. K. (1993). Perimenstrual complaints in women complaining of PMS, menorrhagia, and dysmenorrhea: toward a dismantling of the premenstrual syndrome. *Psychosomatic Med.*, **55**, 133–45
3. Markee, J. E. (1940). Menstruation in intraocular endometrial transplants in the rhesus monkey. *Contrib. Embryol. Carnegie Inst.*, **28**, 219–308
4. Cameron, I. T., Davenport, A. P., van Papendorp, D., Baker, P. J., Huskisson, H. S., Gilmour, R. W., Brown, M. J. and Smith, S. K. (1992). Endothelin-like immunoreactivity in human endometrium. *J. Reprod. Fertil.*, **95**, 623–8
5. O'Reilly, G., Jones, D. S. C., Davenport, A. P., Cameron, I. T. and Smith, S. K. (1992). Presence of mRNA for endothelin-1, endothelin-2 and endothelin-3 in human endometrium, and a change in the ratio of ET_A and ET_B receptor subtype across the menstrual cycle. *J. Clin. Endocrinol. Metab.*, **75**, 1545–9
6. Charnock-Jones, D. S., Sharkey, A. M., Rajput-Williams, J., Burch, D., Schofield, J. P., Fountain, S. A., Boocock, C. A. and Smith, S. K. (1993). Identification and localization of alternatively spliced mRNAs for vascular endothelial growth factor in human uterus and estrogen regulation in endometrial carcinoma cell lines. *Biol. Reprod.*, **48**, 1120–8
7. Ferriani, R. A., Charnock-Jones, D. S., Prentice, A., Thomas, E. J. and Smith, S. K. (1993). Immunohistochemical localisation of acidic and basic fibroblast growth factors in normal human endometrium and endometriosis and the detection of their mRNA by PCR. *Hum. Reprod.*, **8**, 11–16
8. Haining, R. E. B., Schofield, J. P., Jones, D. S. C., Rajput-Williams, J. and Smith, S. K. (1991). The identification of mRNA for EGF and TGFα present in low copy number in human endometrium and decidua using RT-PCR. *J. Mol. Endocrinol.*, **6**, 207–14

9. Whitehead, M. I., Hillard, T. C. and Crook, D. (1990). The role and use of progestogens. *Obstet. Gynecol.,* **75**, 59–76S
10. Padwick, M. L., Pryse-Davies, J. and Whitehead, M. I. (1986). A simple method for determining the optimal dose of progestin in postmenopausal women receiving estrogens. *N. Engl. J. Med.,* **315**, 930–4
11. Archer, D. F. (1993). Hormone replacement therapy and uterine bleeding. *Menopausal Med.,* **1**, 1–3
12. Staland, B. (1981). Continuous treatment with natural oestrogen and progestogens. A method to avoid endometrial stimulation. *Maturitas,* **3**, 1145–56
13. Mattsson, L.-A., Cullberg, G. and Samsioe, G. (1982). Evaluation of a continuous oestrogen–progestogen regimen for climacteric complaints. *Maturitas,* **4**, 95–102
14. Johannisson, E. (1990). Endometrial morphology during the normal cycle and under the influence of contraceptive steroids. In: D'Arcangues, C., Fraser, I. S. and Newton, J. R. (eds.) *Contraception and Mechanisms of Endometrial Bleeding,* pp. 53–80. (Cambridge: Cambridge University Press)

23

Vaginosonography of the endometrium

J. H. J. M. Meuwissen and H. A. M. Brölmann

INTRODUCTION

Estrogen replacement therapy (HRT) offers the menopausal woman relief of menopausal symptoms and considerable protection against heart disease, stroke and osteoporosis. Despite these advantages, the widespread use of this therapy is limited by the risk of hyperstimulation of the endometrium and the problem of withdrawal bleeding after addition of progestogen.

The use of continuous and unopposed estrogen in the 1960s and 1970s led to an increase in hyperplasia and carcinoma[1,2]. Many epidemiologic case-control studies have shown a five-fold to 15-fold increased risk of endometrial carcinoma. This risk is considered both duration-dependent and dose-dependent. Studd and colleagues[4] stated that prolonged unopposed estrogen therapy may induce endometrial hyperplasia and, as a progression between cystic hyperplasia and adenomatous hyperplasia is possible in susceptible women, estrogen therapy must avoid hyperplastic change of the endometrium.

Hyperstimulation caused by estrogen use can be prevented by cyclic addition of progestogen for 13 days a month. This protective effect of progestogen is now generally accepted and the use of unopposed estrogen is considered to be forbidden for postmenopausal women with a uterus[3]. Addition of progestogen, however, is not without problems. Symptomatic side-effects may occur and there are unwanted metabolic changes and withdrawal bleeding. The acceptability of HRT is limited by these side-effects and withdrawal bleeding is one reason for poor compliance. Improving compliance and the uptake of HRT may be achieved by minimization of progestogen dosage and minimization of the frequency of progestogen addition. Research is necessary to determine whether this is possible without diminishing the safety of HRT.

NEW LOOK AT THE ENDOMETRIUM DURING HRT THROUGH VAGINOSONOGRAPHY

Since the report by Noyes in 1950[4], endometrial biopsy has been a routine examination in the evaluation of hormonal influences and diagnosis of endometrial pathology. Endometrial sampling is the mainstay for management of HRT in postmenopausal women. Although biopsy is an adequate means of obtaining histological evidence, this method is invasive and often painful and is therefore not suited for monitoring HRT.

Recent introduction of transvaginal ultrasound scanning (vaginosonography) permits the use of high frequency ultrasound close to the uterus. Vaginosonography allows the endometrial–myometrial interface to be seen clearly, and endometrial thickness can be measured. Vaginosonography is well tolerated by women.

Several recent studies have suggested that vaginosonography is a useful diagnostic technique for the detection of endometrial pathology. In postmenopausal women without estrogen therapy an 'endometrial width', properly speaking twice the thickness of the endometrium but in literature called 'endometrial thickness', of < 4 mm should indicate an atrophic state. In an endometrium with a thickness of ⩽ 8 mm pathology is unlikely. However, some case studies report otherwise. Endovaginal ultrasound evaluation of endometrial thickness is not sensitive enough to detect cancer of the endometrium and could not, therefore, replace histopathologic evaluation of endometrial tissue in women with postmenopausal bleeding. It may, however, give additional information about endometrial abnormalities[5-7].

What can vaginal ultrasound tell us about the endometrium during HRT?

Vaginal ultrasound can be used to monitor:

(1) The effects of estrogens on the endometrium;

(2) The effects of progestogens on the endometrium; and

(3) Endometrial thickness and histopathology.

Little is known about the growth of the endometrium during estrogen use in postmenopausal women and about the endometrial shedding potency of progestogens. In the menopausal clinic of the St. Joseph Hospital, Veldhoven, the endometrial thickness during HRT has been monitored by vaginosonography in an open trial since November 1989. The results of the study are presented devoid of interpretation and without conclusions. In view of the design of the study, only a few prudent indications for further research are given.

The design of the study: HRT with addition of progestogen 'on demand'

The study is an open prospective pilot study of postmenopausal women with no abnormal gynecological findings and free of clinical symptoms, who were treated with different kinds and dosages of estrogens.

The inclusion criteria were: amenorrhea for $\geqslant 3$ months, serum follicle stimulating hormone level > 25 U/l, estradiol level < 0.10 nmol/l and endometrial thickness $\leqslant 4$ mm. The latter demand was added because it has been demonstrated that endometrium with a thickness of $\leqslant 4$ mm is probably atrophic and without pathology. For this reason in our study baseline endometrial biopsies were not performed. Initially, we prescribed progestogens for 12 days as a routine before the start of estrogen treatment. Each woman participating in the study was provided with a chart on which the medication was clearly indicated. The women were asked to take the medication carefully and score possible bleeding by day on this chart.

Vaginosonograms were made with a 5.0 MHz probe (240 grade angle Combison 320). In this study, the distance between the echogenic intraluminar interfaces of the maximal endometrial thickness in the longitudinal plane (the endometrial width) is called endometrial thickness. If there is no intraluminal fluid or blood, this distance comprises two endometrial layers.

Timing of vaginosonography

Based on the inclusion criteria, the baseline endometrial thickness of the women who participated in this study was $\leqslant 4$ mm at the first vaginosonography. The second vaginosonography was performed 4–6 weeks after the start of estrogen use. When the endometrial thickness at the second vaginosonography was $\geqslant 8$ mm (the upper limit of normal) estrogen use was stopped and progestogen was administered for 12 days. If endometrial growth was moderate and the cut-off point of 8 mm had not been approached or reached, estrogen therapy was continued without progestogen addition. The next vaginosonography was then determined according to the increase of the endometrial thickness on linear interpretation: the interval was 4–6 weeks when there was a significant increase in endometrial thickness ($\geqslant 0.3$ mm/week) and 8–16 weeks when there was little or no endometrial growth.

Endometrial sampling, by use of a Pipelle sampler, was always carried out immediately after vaginosonography and also if the endometrial thickness was $\geqslant 8$ mm, if vaginal bleeding was observed during estrogen use, and if the duration of unopposed estrogen use was 6–12 months. In some women endometrial sampling was not possible because of narrowness of the cervical canal or other reasons. The pathologist who judged the histology was unaware of any information on duration/category of the patient.

In this research scheme, for safety reasons, the maximum treatment time was 2 years. After this period the woman was treated in the conventional way with progestogen addition each month or with estrogen/progestogen combinations.

Preliminary results

The effect of estrogens on the endometrium

Monitoring the endometrial thickness during unopposed continuous estrogen therapy showed that individual women differ in their sensitivity to estrogens. Some women seem to be very sensitive: the endometrial growth is $\geqslant 0.2$ mm/week, and in others the endometrial sensitivity for estrogens is very low: $\leqslant 0.04$ mm/week.

We treated 145 postmenopausal women with normal dose estrogen (estradiol valerate, 1 mg, premarin 0.625 mg, oral estradiol 2 mg daily, or transdermal estradiol 0.05 mg daily). Figure 1 shows the results of the first periods of continuous unopposed estrogen use. This shows the differences in response of the endometrium.

Some investigators have stated that endometrial growth during estrogen therapy is dose related. Because the study of HRT with progestogen on demand is an open study in which the needs of the participating women prevail above the demands of research, 48 changes of estrogen dose took place during the study. The endometrial growth during the different periods showed that endometrial growth is likely to be related to estrogen dose.

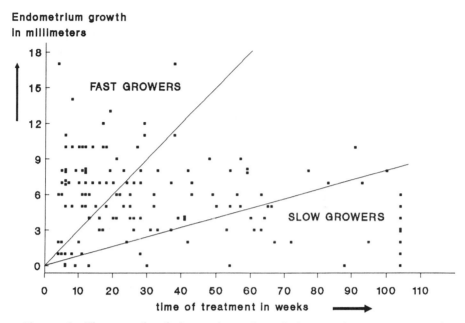

Figure 1 The growth of the endometrium during continuous unopposed estrogen replacement therapy in 145 postmenopausal women. ■, an endpoint for one woman. The endpoint is determined by the duration of the treatment or by passing the 8 mm limit of the endometrial thickness

The effect of progestogens on the endometrium

At present, there are two ways to assess the effect of progestogens on the endometrium. The first is to determine whether the progestogen causes a secretory transformation of the proliferative endometrium. The second method is based on the pattern of withdrawal bleeding and was developed by Padwick and colleagues[8]. They studied 96 postmenopausal women undergoing estrogen therapy who took also a progestogen for 12 days each month, and they correlated the day of onset of bleeding with the endometrial histology. Regardless of the preparation and dosage of the estrogen and progestogen used, proliferative endometrium was always associated with bleeding on or before day 10 of the addition of progestogen. Secretory endometrium or lack of endometrial tissue was associated with bleeding on day 11 or later.

Using vaginosonography of the endometrium before and 3 weeks after the start of progestogen therapy, it is possible to gain information on the endometrial shedding potency of progestogen and the relation of endometrial shedding and the pattern of withdrawal bleeding.

Vaginosonography was performed the day before the start of the progestogen treatment (initial endometrial thickness; day 1) and 1 week after the last tablet (final endometrial thickness; day 21). During this period no estrogens were used. In 81 postmenopausal women on HRT with progestogen addition, 159 progestogen challenge tests were performed. The onset of bleeding was expressed as the number of days counted from the day that the last progestogen tablet was used. A negative number corresponds to a withdrawal bleed that started before the last progestogen tablet was taken. The intensity was denoted on a four point scale as $-$, if there was no bleeding, $+$ if the bleeding was less than a normal menstruation, as $++$ if the bleeding was as a normal menstruation and as $+++$ if the bleeding was abundant. The duration of the withdrawal bleeding is expressed as the total number of days of the bleeding.

Initial endometrial thickness and endometrial shedding In the majority of women (145 out of 159) progestogen caused endometrial shedding. In seven tests there was no change and in another seven tests the endometrial thickness was increased after progestogen use. In most but not all cases, shedding of endometrium was accompanied by withdrawal bleeding. The thicker the endometrium at the moment progestogen therapy was started, the greater the probability of vaginal bleeding. If withdrawal bleeding occurred, the endometrial shedding was proportional to the initial endometrial thickness. However, about 20% of the postmeno-pausal women with 'no' endometrium (endometrial thickness $< 2\,mm$), who received progestogens before HRT was started, responded with withdrawal bleeding.

Withdrawal bleeding pattern and endometrial shedding Preliminary results indicated that:

(1) A more intense withdrawal bleeding corresponds to a larger initial thickness and more shedding of endometrium.

(2) The onset of withdrawal bleeding showed no significant correlation with endometrial shedding.

(3) The duration of withdrawal bleeding is positively correlated with endometrial shedding.

During our voyage of discovery we encountered several unexpected findings. The first curiosity was the possibility of endometrial shedding

Table 1 Histopathology and the thickness of the endometrium

Endometrial thickness (mm)	Histopathology					
	Adenomatous hyperplasia	Cystic hyperplasia	Proliferation	Slight proliferation	Atrophy	Indeterminable
≤ 4	0	0	11	18	20	16
5–6	4	2	21	16	20	4
7–8	1	2	20	15	1	5
9–10	2	2	34	16	1	4
11–12	2	2	31	14	0	5
13–14	2	3	22	4	0	0
15–16	—	1	14	2	1	0
17–18	0	0	4	1	0	0
≥ 18	0	2	7	2	1	1
Total	11	14	166	78	44	35

without withdrawal bleeding. As far as we know, this phenomenon, known in several animal species, was not known to exist in human. A point of interest in this respect is our impression that certain progestogens cause shedding of the endometrium without withdrawal bleeding more often than others. If this is so, then this could be of importance for compliance with HRT.

ENDOMETRIAL HISTOPATHOLOGY AND ULTRASOUND

In 1986 Gusberg[9] determined the cumulative risk of developing invasive carcinoma of the endometrium for patients with adenomatous hyperplasia. At the end of the seventh year, the percentage of cancer in the hyperplasia group was higher than in the control groups ($p = 0.01$). Patients with adenomatous hyperplasia are therefore at a higher risk for developing invasive carcinoma of the endometrium.

During our study, more than 300 biopsies were performed for indications described above. Comparison between endometrial thickness and histopathology is shown in Table 1. The correlation is not obvious.

Figure 2 presents the combined data of endometrial thickness, histopathology and duration of unopposed estrogen use in the period before the biopsy was performed. The data suggest that the development of endometrial hyperplasia is not correlated with the duration of unopposed estrogen use. Monitoring endometrial growth during HRT by vaginosonography cannot, therefore, prevent endometrial hyperplasia.

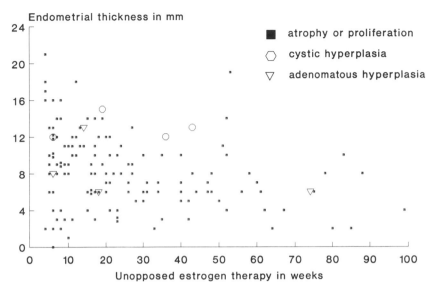

Figure 2 Endometrial thickness and histopathology combined with the duration of unopposed estrogen therapy in the previous period

REFERENCES

1. Ziel, H. K. and Finkle, W. D. (1975). Increased risk to endometrial carcinoma among users of conjugated estrogens. *N. Engl. J. Med.*, **293**, 1167–70
2. Smith, D. C., Pentice, R., Thompson, D. J. and Hermann, W. L. (1975). Association of exogenous estrogen and endometrial carcinoma. *N. Engl. J. Med.*, **293**, 1164–7
3. Leather, A. T. and Studd, J. W. W. (1990). Can the withdrawal bleed following oestrogen replacement therapy be avoided? *Br. J. Obstet. Gynaecol.*, **97**, 1071–9
4. Noyes, R. W., Hertig, A. T. and Rock, J. (1950). Dating the endometrial biopsy. *Fertil. Steril.*, **1**, 3–25
5. Osmers, R., Völksen, M. and Schauer, A. (1990). Vaginosonography for early detection of endometrial carcinoma? *Lancet*, **335**, 1569–75
6. Granberg, S., Wikland, M., Karlsson, B., Norström, A. and Friberg, A. G. (1991). Endometrial thickness as measured by endovaginal ultrasonography for identifying endometrial abnormality. *Am. J. Obstet. Gynecol.*, **164**, 47–52
7. Dorum, A., Kristensen, G. B., Langebrekke, A., Sornes, T. and Skaar, O. (1993). Evaluation of endometrial thickness measured by endovaginal ultrasound in women with postmenopausal bleeding. *Acta Obstet. Gynecol. Scand.*, 116–19
8. Padwick, M. L., Pryse-Davies, J. and Whitehead, M. I. (1986). A simple method for determining the optimal dosage of progestin in postmenopausal women receiving estrogens. *N. Engl. J. Med.*, **315**, 930–4
9. Gusberg, S. B. (1986). Current concepts in the control of carcinoma of the endometrium. *Cancer J. Clinicians*, **36**, 245–53

Section 5

Cardiovascular health and sex steroids

24

Vascular effects of sex steroids: where do we stand now?

O. Ylikorkala

Cardiovascular disorders will kill 50% of men and women now living in the Western world. Death from cardiovascular causes can be quite acceptable, at least for elderly people; it can be prompt and is thus devoid of long-term suffering and incapacity. However, a wide spectrum of cardiovascular complaints occurs in relatively young, active people. The true impact of these disorders on human health then becomes noticed. The prevention of cardiovascular disorders should be an essential step in every modern health care system.

DO ESTROGENS PROTECT AGAINST CARDIOVASCULAR DISORDERS?

There is a substantial evidence to suggest that female sex steroids protect against the development of occlusive vascular disorders. For example, it is well established that the risk of ischemic heart disease in fertile and premenopausal women is only approximately 20% that of men, but soon after the menopause, and in the presence of hypoestrogenism, the risk of cardiovascular disorders rises drastically, approaching that in men. That estrogens are of significance in this phenomenon gains further support from epidemiological surveys which strongly imply that estrogen therapy (HRT) protects against cardiovascular diseases (Table 1). It is noteworthy that addition of progestins to estrogen therapy does not negate the protective effect of estrogens on cardiovascular morbidity[10].

Table 1 Prospective studies of estrogen replacement therapy and coronary heart disease risk

Reference	Cohort size	Age of baseline (years)	End-points	Relative risk (ever-exposure)
1	32 317	30–55	Coronary heart disease	0.5*
2	1234	50+	Cardiovascular disease	1.9*
3	695	50–59	Coronary heart disease	0.3
4	2270	40–69	Fatal cardiovascular disease	0.4*
5	6093	18–54	Fatal cardiovascular disease	0.6
6	4544	45–54	Fatal coronary heart disease	0.5*
7	8841	40+	Fatal myocardial infarction	0.6*
8	1868	50–79	Fatal coronary heart disease	1.0
9	24 900	50–64	Myocardial infarction	0.8

*Significantly different from 1.0

Is epidemiological evidence sound?

The epidemiological data suggesting a beneficial effect of estrogen on cardiovascular health are prone to criticism. First, the long-term effects of HRT have never been tested in randomized, placebo-controlled prospective trials. Epidemiologists have claimed, therefore, that many benefits and risks of HRT found in observational studies may be caused by confounding factors or biases which are unavoidable in open clinical studies. For example, health conscious women who take notice of measures that may play a role in cardiovascular disorders may be more likely to start using HRT. The protection against cardiovascular disorders in these women may then be a result of non-medical measures rather than HRT. On the other hand, women belonging to families with an increased risk of cardiovascular disorders may be more likely to start using HRT. Any lack of protection afforded by HRT may then be a result of increased risk, rather than the lack of a protective effect. Another confounding factor is the subjectivity which is characteristic of risk judgement in HRT. Some women, for example, consider a small risk of cancer to be more significant than a large reduction in the risk of cardiovascular disorders, and this is

Table 2 The possible mechanisms by which the hormonal replacement therapy may protect against cardiovascular morbidity and mortality

Direct mechanisms
Endothelial cells
  prostacyclin
  endothelin-1
  nitric oxide
Vascular wall receptor stimulation
  flow changes

Indirect mechanisms
Lipids and lipoproteins
Insulin and carbohydrate metabolism
Vascular smooth muscle cells and connective tissue

also likely to bias patient selection.

We must therefore be ready to accept some criticism of the epidemiological studies on the benefits and risks of HRT. We have passed the time of well-controlled, randomized trials on the long-term effects of HRT, so the future will not bring epidemiologically sound clinical trials. Presently, women are well informed of the possible benefits and risks, and their recruitment into 'randomized' trials will not be possible.

Estrogens influence the vascular bed

Recent evidence of vascular effects of estrogens and progestins is more than welcome (Table 2). Estrogens may well protect blood vessels against atherosclerosis and other occlusive changes through their specific effect on vascular function. I shall start with the interplay between the vascular endothelium and platelets which is important in the development of occlusive vascular disorders[11]. Endothelial cells, which cover the luminal surface of all blood vessels, produce several vaso- and platelet-active agents, such as the anti-aggregatory and vasodilatory prostacyclin, vasoconstrictory endothelin-1 and vasodilatory 'endothelium-derived relaxing factor' which has been now identified as mainly nitric oxide. All these factors are of significance in vascular disorders. Platelets tend to adhere to and aggregate on damaged endothelium, and they can thereby trigger the formation of thrombi and other occlusive changes on vascular walls. One of the most characteristic phenomena during platelet aggregation is the release of pro-aggregatory and vasoconstrictive thromboxane A$_2$. The effects of estrogens and progestins on both prostacyclin and thromboxane A_2 should be considered.

Oral contraceptives and prostanoids

There are no data to suggest marked differences in prostacyclin and thromboxane A_2 production between women and men. Moreover, no clear cyclicity in prostacyclin production has been observed in healthy women of reproductive age[12]. However, the release of prostacyclin in a dissected vascular ring was shown to increase following the intake of oral contraceptive pills in women[13], and this agrees with a stimulation of between 20 and 40% in the urinary output of 2,3-dinor-6-keto-prostaglandin $F_{1\alpha}$ in women using combined pills, which are devoid of androgenic activity[14]; no change was seen in thromboxane A_2 output. These data do not provide uniform evidence that the vascular accidents reported to accompany the use of older types of oral pills could be due to changes in prostacyclin or thromboxane A_2; recent data from a case–control study suggest that the risk of cardiovascular disorders is not elevated in women using modern oral contraceptives[15].

Hormonal replacement therapy and prostanoids

In view of the risk of cardiovascular mortality following menopause it is pertinent to ask what happens to prostacyclin production at this time. Prostacyclin production may decrease by as much as 75%, as assessed by the release of 6-keto-prostaglandin $F_{1\alpha}$ (a metabolite of prostacyclin) in uterine arteries[16]. Although the *ex vivo* data from this study are very convincing, the urinary output of prostacyclin and thromboxane A_2 metabolites shows wide variation in postmenopausal women and no significant difference has been seen between pre- and postmenopausal women[17]. Nevertheless, 17β-estradiol stimulated prostacyclin production in a dose-dependent manner in a perfused umbilical artery preparation; this stimulation was reduced by addition of progesterone[18].

Clinical studies have been also undertaken to investigate the effects of HRT on prostacyclin and thromboxane A_2. In one study, 6 months' oral HRT did not significantly alter the urinary output of prostacyclin and thromboxane A_2 metabolites, but after the cessation of HRT, the urinary excretion of prostacyclin metabolites declined[19]. In another study, both oral and parenteral estrogens stimulated prostacyclin output by 27% and 9%, respectively, although the duration of therapy was only 3 months[19]. The data on HRT and prostanoids suggest, therefore, that HRT may eventually protect against cardiovascular disorders by changing the production of vasoactive prostanoids in the direction of prostacyclin dominance. However, more data are certainly needed on this relationship.

Other direct and indirect vascular effects of HRT

Besides its effects on prostanoids, there are several other mechanisms by which HRT may protect against vascular disorders (Table 2). Human blood vessels are known to contain specific receptors for estrogens, a further piece of evidence that blood vessels are a target for estrogen action. It is indeed known that HRT affects blood vessel performance in climacteric women, as assessed by Doppler ultrasound. There are also several studies on the changes in lipid and glucose metabolism in women using HRT, and these factors may be significant in the vasoprotection induced by HRT. In addition, there are very interesting vascular data on rabbits fed a cholesterol-rich diet together with estrogens. Considering all of the evidence, HRT can operate through different biological pathways to maintain the vascular health, and protect against cardiovascular morbidity and mortality. The epidemiological evidence on the vasoprotection induced by HRT (Table 1) may be sound.

REFERENCES

1. Stampfer, M. J., Willett, W. C., Colditz, G. A., Rosner, B., Speizer, F. E. and Hennekens, C. H. (1985). A prospective study of postmenopausal estrogen therapy and coronary heart disease. *N. Engl. J. Med.*, **313**, 1044–9
2. Wilson, P. W., Garrison, R. J. and Castelli, W. P. (1985). Postmenopausal estrogen use, cigarette smoking, and cardiovascular morbidity in women over 50: the Framingham Study. *N. Engl. J. Med.*, **313**, 1038–43
3. Eaker, E. D. and Castelli, W. P. (1987). Coronary heart disease and its risk factors among women in the Framingham Study. In Eaker, E. *et al.* (eds.) *Coronary Heart Disease in Women*, pp. 122–32. (New York: Haymarket Doyma)
4. Bush, T. L., Barrett-Connor, E., Cowan, L. D., Criqui, M. H., Wallace, R. B., Suchindran, C. M., Tyroler, M. A. and Rifkind, B. M. (1987). Cardiovascular mortality and non-contraceptive use of estrogen in women: results from the Lipid Research Clinics Program Follow-up Study. *Circulation*, **75**, 1102–9
5. Petitti, D. B., Perlman, J. A. and Sidney, S. (1987). Noncontraceptive estrogens and mortality: longterm follow-up of women in the Walnut Creek Study. *Obstet. Gynecol.*, **70**, 289–93
6. Hunt, K., Vessey, M., McPherson, K. and Coleman, M. (1987). Long-term surveillance of mortality and cancer incidence in women receiving hormone replacement therapy. *Br. J. Obstet. Gynaecol.*, **94**, 620–35
7. Henderson, B. E., Paganini-Hill, A. and Ross, R. K. (1988). Estrogen replacement

therapy and protection from acute myocardial infarction. *Am. J. Obstet. Gynecol.,* **159**, 312–17

8. Criqui, M. H., Suarez, L., Barrett-Connor, E., McPhillips, J., Wingard, D. L. and Garland, C. (1988). Postmenopausal estrogen use and mortality. *Am. J. Epidemiol.,* **128**, 606–14

9. Avila, M. H., Walker, A. M. and Jick, H. (1980). Use of replacement estrogens and the risk of myocardial infarction. *Epidemiology,* **1**, 128–33

10. Persson, I., Falkeborn, M., Lithell, H. and Adami, H. O. (1992). Hormone replacement therapy and cardiovascular diseases – with special emphasis on combined therapy. In Samsioe, G. (ed.) *Cardiovascular Diseases and HRT,* pp. 23–7. (New Jersey: Parthenon)

11. Ross, R. (1993). The pathogenesis of atherosclerosis: a perspective for the 1990s. *Nature (London),* **362**, 801–46

12. Tulppala, M., Viinikka, L. and Ylikorkala, O. (1992). Nonpregnant women with a history of habitual abortion have normal and luteal function independent production of prostacyclin and thromboxane A2. *Fertil. Steril.,* **57**, 1216–19

13. Sinzinger, H., Klein, K., Kaliman, J., Silbebauer, K. and Feigl, W. (1980). Enhanced prostacyclin formation in veins of women under chronic treatment with oral contraceptive drugs. *Pharmacol. Res. Commun.,* **12**, 515–21

14. Ylikorkala, O., Kuusi, T., Tikkanen, M. J. and Viinikka, L. (1987). Desogestrel- and levonorgestrel-containing oral contraceptives have different effects on urinary excretion of prostacyclin metabolites and serum high density lipoproteins. *J. Clin. Endocrinol. Metab.,* **65**, 1238–42

15. Thorogood, K. and Vessey, M. (1990). An epidemiological survey of cardiovascular disease in women taking oral contraceptives. *Am. J. Obstet. Gynecol.,* **163**, 274–81

16. Steinleitner, A., Stanczyk, F. Z., Lewin, J. H., d'Ablaing, G., Vijod, M. A., Shahbazian, V. L. and Lobo, R. A. (1989). Decreased *in vitro* production of 6-keto-prostaglandin F1a by uterine arteries from postmenopausal women. *Am. J. Obstet. Gynecol.,* **161**, 1677–81

17. Ylikorkala, O., Hirvonen, E., Saure, A. and Viinikka, L. (1990). Urinary excretion of prostacyclin and thromboxane metabolites in climacteric women: effect of estrogen-progestin replacement therapy. *Prostaglandins,* **39**, 33–7

18. Mäkilä, U. M., Wahlberg, L., Viinikka, L. and Ylikorkala, O. (1983). Regulation of prostacyclin and thromboxane production by human umbilical vessels: the effect of estradiol and progesterone in a superfusion model. *Prostaglandins Leukotrienes Med.,* **26**, 3–12

19. Foidart, J. M., Dombrowicz, N. and de Zignieres, B. (1991). Urinary excretion of prostacyclin and thromboxane metabolites in postmenopausal women treated with percutaneous estradiol (Oestrogel®) or conjugated oestrogens (Premarin®). In Dusitsin, N. and Notelovitz, M. (eds.) *Physiological Hormone Replacement Therapy,* pp. 99–107. (Carnforth: Parthenon)

25

Cardiovascular protection by estrogens with special emphasis on the arterial wall

J. Haarbo

INTRODUCTION

Cardiovascular diseases are very common among postmenopausal women, especially after the sixth decade. Efforts are therefore being made to identify possible risk factors and find therapies that could either prevent or alleviate these diseases. Several lines of evidence suggest that sex steroid hormones, especially estrogens, play a significant role in atherogenesis. The aim of the present paper is briefly to review the epidemiological and animal experimental evidence for a protective effect of hormone replacement therapy and then to discuss possible modes of action, especially regarding the arterial wall.

EPIDEMIOLOGICAL EVIDENCE

A large number of epidemiological studies have considered the protective effect of non-contraceptive estrogen use in postmenopausal women, as recently reviewed[1,2]. Until now there has only been one randomized, double-blind clinical trial of estrogen (cyclically combined with medroxy-progesterone acetate) replacement therapy in women[3]. That small but prospective study showed a reduction of about 70% in myocardial infarctions among estrogen users. However, this reduction was not statistically significant, probably because of the low sample size (84 pairs of women). The remaining about 30 observational (non-randomized) studies are either prospective (with[4] or without[5] internal controls) or case–control (community or hospital-based) studies. Three of the case–control studies may be particularly interesting because they showed significant beneficial effects of estrogen therapy using angiographically defined endpoints[6-8]. The consensus of all these studies is a reduction in cardiovascular risk of about 50% among estrogen users[1,2]. It is unlikely that this reduction is explained solely by confounding factors, especially selection bias. However, a randomized, prospective, placebo-controlled study with enough power to clearly determine the risk/benefit ratio of hormone replacement therapy is clearly needed. It is therefore with high expectations that we await the outcome of large ongoing studies in the United States[9].

ANIMAL STUDIES

The idea of using experimental animals to study the influence of estrogens on atherosclerosis is not new. Early studies with different formulations of estrogen indicated an anti-atherogenic action and suggested a possible mediating role of the lipid metabolism in plasma. Studies in different animal models have more recently investigated the effect of estradiol therapy alone, and combined with progestogen therapy[10-13]. We used ovariectomized, cholesterol-fed rabbits, which received orally 4 mg of 17β-estradiol, 1 mg of norethisterone acetate (NETA), 0.5 mg of levonorgestrel either as monotherapy or as continuously combined estrogen–progestogen regimens[10,11]. Both studies had an ovariectomized placebo group and a sham-operated group was included in the initial study[10]. The hormone doses given were selected to produce relevant serum hormone concentrations and a physiological effect on the endometrium as determined by the endometrial activities of estradiol dehydrogenase and isocitrate dehydrogenase. Both studies showed a large, statistically significant anti-atherogenic effect of estrogen monotherapy (Figures 1, 2). Furthermore, these progestogens, whether given alone or in conjunction with estrogen, had no impact on atherogenesis (Figures 1, 2). The beneficial influence of estrogen on the lipid metabolism contributed to the anti-atherogenic effect, but estradiol possessed, in addition, a significant anti-atherogenic effect, presumably exerted directly on the arterial wall (Figure 3). In keeping with these findings, a recent careful study of ovariectomized, cholesterol-fed monkeys showed that 17β-estradiol given alone and cyclically combined with progesterone had equal inhibitory effects on coronary artery atherosclerosis, which could not be explained by hormonal actions on plasma lipids or other known cardiovascular risk

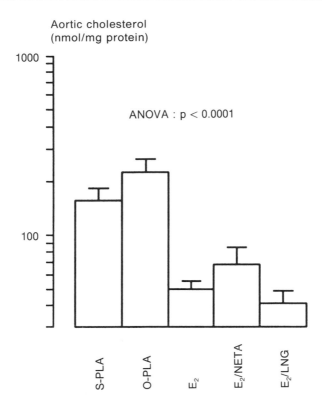

Aortic cholesterol
(nmol/mg protein)

Figure 1 Atherosclerosis in cholesterol-fed rabbits treated with sex hormones. S-PLA = sham-operated group; O-PLA = ovariectomized placebo group; E_2 = estradiol; NETA = norethisterone acetate; LNG = levonorgestrel. Data from ref. 10, with permission

factors[12]. Similar data have recently been obtained in the ovariectomized cholesterol-fed baboon[13].

In conclusion, estradiol has a significant anti-atherogenic effect in these species and the addition of a progestogen seems to have neutral effects. The beneficial effect of estrogen may be mediated in part by modulation of known cardiovascular risk factors and in part by a direct effect on the arterial wall.

MECHANISMS OF ACTION

It is beyond the scope of this paper to review in detail all the possible mechanisms by which estrogen may protect against atherothrombotic

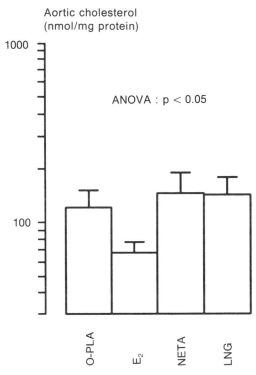

Aortic cholesterol
(nmol/mg protein)

ANOVA : p < 0.05

Figure 2 Atherosclerosis in hormone-treated ovariectomized rabbits with similar serum lipids and lipoproteins. O-PLA = ovariectomized placebo group; E_2 = estradiol; NETA = norethisterone acetate; LNG = levonorgestrel. Data from ref. 11, with permission

disease. However, the most established method of action, accounting for 25–50% of the reduction in cardiovascular disease risk, may be the beneficial effect on serum lipids and lipoproteins[14,15]. It has been shown repeatedly that estrogen decreases low density lipoprotein (LDL) cholesterol by approximately 10% and increases high density lipoprotein cholesterol correspondingly: the latter effect is counteracted by progestogen[16]. In addition, there may be significant beneficial effects of non-contraceptive estrogens on blood pressure, glucose tolerance, body fat distribution, hemostasis and the prostaglandin/thromboxane balance[17-20].

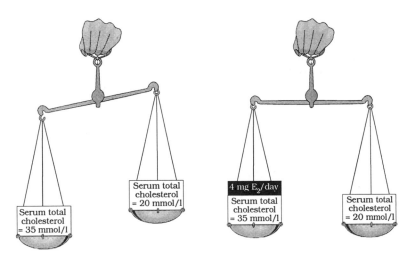

Figure 3 The left scale shows the increased degree of atherosclerosis associated with hypercholesterolemia, which can be neutralized by the addition of 4 mg 17β-estradiol (E$_2$)

Low density lipoprotein uptake and metabolism by the arterial wall

Some data suggest that the development of early atherosclerotic lesions is preceded by an increase in the concentration of undegraded LDL and in the rate of LDL degradation in the arterial wall[21]. Furthermore, it has recently been shown that aortic permeability (the amount of plasma cleared by the aortic wall; nl/h/cm^2) is a strong predictor for subsequent atherosclerosis[22].

Arterial uptake and degradation of LDL as well as arterial permeability to LDL can be measured *in vivo*, and this provides a possible approach to the study of the effects of estrogen on the arterial wall. It was demonstrated recently that estradiol (cyclically combined with progesterone) decreased the accumulation of LDL and its degradation products in cynomolgus monkey coronary arteries by >70%[21]. This hormonal effect was not explained by effects on plasma lipids or by cellular events in the arterial wall. These data therefore indicate a direct hormonal effect on the arterial wall. Using a different approach[22], we have studied the influence of 17β-estradiol on aortic permeability to LDL in ovariectomized rabbits fed a non-atherogenic diet in order to study early atherogenic processes. After 10 weeks, aortic permeability to LDL was measured 3 h after an intravenous injection of [^{125}I]LDL. The aortic permeability was calculated by the 'sink method', in which the aortic radioactivity is divided by the area under the curve for plasma radioactivity. Only the radioactivity in the aortic intima and inner media was used, because previous studies suggest that LDL may also enter the media from the adventitial side. Estradiol treatment reduced the plasma concentration of very low density lipoprotein cholesterol, whereas there were no differences with respect to LDL-cholesterol or high density lipoprotein cholesterol between the estradiol-treated and control animals. Aortic permeability to LDL and aortic cholesterol content were virtually identical in the two groups. The findings from these two studies therefore suggest that estradiol somehow changes the intra-arterial metabolism of LDL, perhaps by changing the intercellular matrix, leading to a shorter transit time of LDL in the arterial wall and therefore perhaps to less LDL oxidation.

REFERENCES

1. Bush, T. L. (1991). Extraskeletal effects of estrogen and the prevention of atherosclerosis. *Osteoporosis Int.,* 2, 5–11
2. Stampfer, M. J. and Colditz, G. A. (1991). Estrogen replacement therapy and coronary heart disease: a quantitative assessment of the epidemiologic evidence. *Prev. Med.,* 20, 47–63
3. Nachtigall, L. E., Nachtigall, R. H., Nachtigall, R. D. and Beckman, E. M. (1979). Estrogen replacement therapy I: a 10-year prospective study in the relationship to osteoporosis. *Obstet. Gynecol.,* 53, 277–81
4. Stampfer, M. J., Colditz, G. A., Willett, W. C., Manson, J. E., Rosner, B., Speizer, F. E. and Hennekens, C. H. (1991). Postmenopausal estrogen therapy and cardiovascular disease. *N. Engl. J. Med.,* 325, 756–62
5. Hunt, K., Vessey, M., McPherson, K. and Coleman, M. (1987). Long-term surveillance of mortality and cancer incidence in women receiving hormone replacement therapy. *Br. J. Obstet. Gynaecol.,* 94, 620–35
6. Gruchow, H. W., Anderson, A. J., Barboriak, J. J. and Sobocinski, K. A. (1988). Postmenopausal use of estrogen and occlusion of coronary arteries. *Am. Heart J.,* 115, 954–63
7. Sullivan, J. M., Zwaag, R. V., Lemp, G. F., Hughes, J. P., Maddock, V., Kroetz, F. W., Ramanathan, K. B. and Mirvis, D. M. (1988). Postmenopausal estrogen use and coronary atherosclerosis. *Ann. Intern. Med.,* 108, 358–63
8. McFarland, K. F., Boniface, M. E., Hornung, C. A., Earnhardt, W. and Humphries, J. O. (1989). Risk factors and noncontraceptive estrogen use in women with and without coronary disease. *Am. Heart J.,* 117, 1209–14
9. Healy, B. (1991). The Yentl syndrome. *N. Engl. J. Med.,* 325, 274–6
10. Haarbo, J., Leth-Espensen, P., Stender, S. and Christiansen, C. (1991). Estrogen monotherapy and combined estrogen-progestogen replacement therapy attenuate aortic accumulation of cholesterol in ovariectomized cholesterol-fed rabbits. *J. Clin. Invest.,* 87, 1274–9
11. Haarbo, J., Svendsen, O. L. and Christiansen, C. (1992). Progestogens do not affect aortic accumulation of cholesterol in ovariectomized cholesterol-fed rabbits. *Circ. Res.,* 70, 1198–1202

12. Adams, M. R., Kaplan, J. R., Manuck, S. B., Koritnik, D. R., Parks, J. S., Wolfe, M. S. and Clarkson, T. B. (1990). Inhibition of coronary artery atherosclerosis by 17-beta estradiol in ovariectomized monkeys. Lack of an effect of added progesterone. *Arteriosclerosis,* **10**, 1051–7

13. Kushwaha, R. S., Lewis, D. S., Carey, K. D. and McGill, H. C. (1991). Effects of estrogen and progesterone on plasma lipoproteins and experimental atherosclerosis in the baboon (*Papio* sp.). *Arteriosclerosis Thrombosis,* **11**, 23–31

14. Bush, T. L. and Miller, V. T. (1987). Effects of pharmacologic agents used during menopause: impact on lipids and lipoproteins. In Mishell, D. R. Jr (ed.) *Menopause, Physiology & Pharmacology,* pp. 187–208. (Chicago: Year Book Medical Publishers Inc.)

15. Bush, T. L., Barrett-Connor, E., Cowan, L. D., Criqui, M. H., Wallace, R. B., Suchindran, C. M., Tyroler, H. A. and Rifkind, B. M. (1987). Cardiovascular mortality and noncontraceptive use of estrogen in women: results from the lipid research clinics program follow-up study. *Circulation,* **75**, 1102–9

16. Haarbo, J., Hassager, C., Jensen, S. B., Riis, B. J. and Christiansen, C. (1991). Serum lipids, lipoproteins, and apolipoproteins during postmenopausal estrogen replacement therapy combined with either 19-nortestosterone derivatives or 17-hydroxy-progesterone derivatives. *Am. J. Med.,* **90**, 584–9

17. Bush, T. L. and Barrett-Connor, E. (1985). Noncontraceptive estrogen use and cardiovascular disease. *Epidemiol. Rev.,* **7**, 80–104

18. Barrett-Connor, E. and Laakso, M. (1990). Ischemic heart disease risk in postmenopausal women. Effects of estrogen use on glucose and insulin levels. *Arteriosclerosis,* **10**, 531–4

19. Haarbo, J., Marslew, U., Gotfredsen, A. and Christiansen, C. (1991). Postmenopausal hormone replacement therapy prevents central distribution of body fat after menopause. *Metabolism,* **40**, 1323–6

20. Lobo, R. A. (1990). Estrogen and cardiovascular disease. *Ann. N.Y. Acad. Sci.,* **592**, 286–94

21. Wagner, J. D., Clarkson, T. B., St. Clair, R. W., Schwenke, D. C., Shively, C. A. and Adams, M. R. (1991). Estrogen and progesterone replacement therapy reduces low density lipoprotein accumulation in the coronary arteries of surgically postmenopausal cynomolgus monkeys. *J. Clin. Invest.,* **88**, 1995–2002

22. Nielsen, L. B., Nordestgaard, B. G., Stender, S. and Kjeldsen, K. (1992). Aortic permeability to LDL as a predictor of aortic cholesterol accumulation in cholesterol-fed rabbits. *Arteriosclerosis Thrombosis,* **12**, 1402–9

26

Carbohydrate metabolism, cardiovascular disease and hormone replacement therapy

I. F. Godsland, C. Walton and J. C. Stevenson

INTRODUCTION

Our current understanding of the etiology of coronary heart disease (CHD) is based largely on the notion that chronic physiological disturbances, induced by genetic, environmental or lifestyle factors, cause pathological changes in the coronary artery wall, leading to atheroma, thrombosis and arterial occlusion. Cigarette smoking, raised blood pressure and hypercholesterolemia constitute the best-characterized risk factors for CHD, but together these may account for <50% of the actual incidence of the disease[1]. There is, therefore, considerable interest in other contributing factors; disturbances in carbohydrate metabolism, specifically as it relates to insulin metabolism, have recently achieved prominence in this respect.

CHD has hitherto been regarded as a health problem primarily of men, but there is increasing recognition that women may be equally affected, albeit at a later age[2]. The menopause may be of considerable importance in this respect. As described below, experimental studies suggest that the menopause might have significant effects on glucose and insulin metabolism, and that these effects might be reversed by hormone replacement therapy. However, the effects of the menopause and hormone replacement therapy on glucose and insulin metabolism remain relatively unexplored.

INSULIN AND GLUCOSE METABOLISM AND CARDIOVASCULAR DISEASE

An association between glucose and insulin metabolism and cardiovascular disease is suggested by the excess vascular disease mortality in diabetic men and women[3]. This possibility is strengthened by the observation that lesser degrees of glucose intolerance than those seen in diabetes are predictive of subsequent coronary heart disease[4-7]. While protein glycosylation provides a possible mechanism linking elevated glucose concentrations with coronary heart disease in diabetics[8,9], risk associated with lesser degrees of glucose intolerance is more likely to be mediated by insulin resistance and hyperinsulinemia.

Three prospective studies have found that plasma insulin concentrations are independent predictors for coronary heart disease[4,10,11]. Both men and women were included in the Busselton study[4], but the insulin response during an oral glucose tolerance test was an independent predictor of subsequent coronary heart disease only in men aged >60 years. A relatively low glucose load (50 g) was used in this study and glucose tolerance testing was not standardized according to time of day when the test was carried out, factors which may have limited the sensitivity of the study. The study of 986 Helsinki policemen, followed for 9.5 years[10], found plasma insulin concentration 2 h after an oral glucose load to be a strong independent predictor of coronary heart disease. Insulin was a stronger predictor than glucose. The 2-h plasma insulin concentration was also a significant predictor in the Paris prospective study of 6903 men followed for 15 years[11]. Studies of the prevalence of elevated insulin concentrations in patients with established coronary heart disease have been reviewed in detail by Stout[12]: 17 of 18 studies demonstrated significantly elevated insulin concentrations in individuals with established coronary disease. More recently, these associations have been demonstrated in a large group of women[13]. The elevated insulin concentrations described in these studies are likely to be due to insulin resistance, but insulin resistance *per se* does not appear to have been measured in patients with vascular disease.

Insulin diminishes plasma glucose concentrations by stimulating glucose elimination and suppressing hepatic glucose production. Pancreatic insulin secretion and the plasma glucose concentration are in a mutual feedback loop which appears to be set so that normoglycemia rather than normoinsulinemia is maintained. The sensitivity of insulin-dependent glucose regulation to insulin shows considerable variation between individuals[14] and appears to be the principal source of variation in plasma insulin levels in non-diabetic individuals. Non-diabetic individuals may thus exhibit a range of insulin sensitivities ranging from insulin sensitive to insulin resistant.

Associations between insulin concentrations and insulin resistance can be confounded by variation in insulin elimination rate[15], and it is necessary to obtain a true measure of insulin sensitivity if the importance of insulin resistance is to be evaluated accurately. We have recently compared insulin resistance, measured by mathematical modelling analysis of intravenous glucose tolerance test (IVGTT) glucose and insulin concentrations, in 40 healthy males and 39 males with angiographically proven coronary artery disease, and found insulin sensitivity to be reduced by 25.7% in the diseased group ($p < 0.05$, Ley and colleagues[16]). We have also compared insulin resistance in 38 healthy men and 14 men with cardiac syndrome X, a condition characterized by angina-like chest pain and an abnormal exercise electrocardiogram, in the absence of angiographic evidence of coronary artery disease. This condition may be associated with microvascular disease[17]. Insulin sensitivity in men with cardiac syndrome X was reduced by 31.1% ($p < 0.05$, Swan and co-workers[18] unpublished data). We have also compared IVGTT insulin concentrations in 23 healthy women and in 23 women with cardiac syndrome X, and found them to be elevated by 38.8% in the latter group ($p < 0.01$, Wynn Institute, unpublished data).

It has been proposed that hyperinsulinemia may increase risk of coronary heart disease by directly promoting atherogenesis[12] or by adversely affecting other cardiovascular disease risk factors. An association between hyperinsulinemia and hypertension has been found in a number of studies[19–21], and, in the few studies in which it has been measured, insulin resistance shows a positive relationship with blood pressure[22,23]. Insulin might affect blood pressure by enhancing renal sodium reabsorption[24] or sympathetic nervous system activity[25]. However, this possibility has been challenged, since neither insulin administration nor excessive endogenous insulin production are associated with elevated blood pressure[26–28]. There is, therefore, the possibility that elevated insulin concentrations and elevated blood pressure are linked through a common unknown intermediary. Significant relationships have also been found between elevated insulin concentrations and an adverse lipid and lipoprotein profile in large groups of healthy individuals, with high insulin concentrations being associated with high triglyceride and low high-density lipoprotein (HDL) or HDL_2-cholesterol concentrations[29–31].

The associations between elevated blood pressure, increased triglyceride concentrations, reduced HDL-cholesterol concentrations and hyperinsulinemia suggest that these disturbances, each of which has been shown to increase risk of coronary heart disease, constitute a distinct syndrome, with its origins in insulin resistance. This has been variously termed 'syndrome X'[32], 'the deadly quartet'[20] or 'familial combined dyslipidemic hypertension'[33]. 'Insulin resistance syndrome' would seem the most appropriate designation, however. Obesity has long been recognized as a frequent concomitant of these associated disturbances, and a central, or android, distribution of body fat appears to be the principal correlate[34]. Other components of the insulin resistance syndrome may include insulin-induced increases in levels of anti-fibrinolytic factor, plasminogen activator inhibitor-1 (PAI-1)[35], and increased proportions of the small, dense low-density lipoprotein (LDL) subfraction[36]. In support of the existence of a unique syndrome of insulin resistance, there is evidence for distinct clustering of these metabolic abnormalities[37–40], and an elevated insulin concentration may be predictive of subsequent development of elevated blood pressure and dyslipidemia[41]. Moreover, biochemical and physiological relationships can provide potential mechanisms for the observed associations. Insulin can affect lipoprotein metabolism by suppression of lipolysis[42], leading to reduced non-esterified fatty acid (NEFA) flux and reduced hepatic triglyceride synthesis[43]. NEFA concentrations may be increased in association with insulin resistance, suggesting resistance to the antilipolytic effects of insulin, and triglyceride concentrations may also be increased[44,45]. HDL concentrations are then reduced in association with the elevated triglyceride concentrations. Insulin stimulates synthesis of lipoprotein lipase and may also increase the activity of hepatic triglyceride lipase. Whether the activities of these enzymes are affected by insulin resistance is unclear, but it has been suggested that the elevated insulin concentrations associated with insulin resistance may promote release of hepatic triglyceride[32].

Increased insulin levels are typically associated with insulin resistance, but reduced uptake of newly secreted insulin by the liver may also be important. We have used mathematical modelling analysis of IVGTT insulin and C-peptide concentration profiles to provide measures of hepatic insulin uptake, and have found that this variable, rather than insulin sensitivity, correlates with HDL_2-cholesterol concentrations and systolic blood pressure in men, independently of body mass index, skinfold thickness ratio or serum triglyceride concentrations[46]. We have also observed reduced hepatic insulin uptake, as well as reduced insulin sensitivity and increased central fat deposition, in men with angina-like chest pain (Walton *et al.*, unpublished data). Furthermore, we have noted reduced insulin elimination in postmenopausal women[47], and we have evidence that hepatic insulin uptake is increased by hormone replacement therapy[48]. A possible underlying mechanism in some of these associations is provided by the observation that increased NEFA concentrations can reduce hepatic insulin uptake[49], and hepatic insulin uptake may prove to be of comparable importance to insulin sensitivity, with regard to metabolic correlates. This possibility may not have been raised hitherto due to the difficulty of estimating hepatic insulin uptake and peripheral insulin elimination.

INSULIN AND GLUCOSE METABOLISM AND THE MENOPAUSE

Some insight into whether or not the menopause affects insulin and glucose metabolism may be gained from experimental studies of the effects of estrogens and progesterone on isolated cell and tissue preparations. Early experimental investigations in animals consistently demonstrated increased pancreatic insulin secretion in response to glucose in animals treated with estrogens[50–52], and similar observations were subsequently made in islets isolated from estrogen-treated animals[53–55]. However, effects of estrogens are likely to be mediated secondarily through other substances, possibly glucocorticoids[56–59]. Progesterone also appears to augment the pancreatic insulin response to glucose, but by a direct action on the pancreas[53,60–63].

In addition to augmenting the pancreatic insulin response to glucose, experimental studies have indicated that estrogens may modify the sensitivity of insulin-dependent metabolic processes to insulin. Increased sensitivity of tissue glucose uptake and lipid synthesis have been demonstrated in estrogen-treated rats[64–66]. However, elevated plasma insulin concentrations, but with no improvement in glucose tolerance, have been observed in two experimental studies of the effects of progesterone[53,67]. Thus, while progesterone may augment pancreatic responsiveness it may also cause resistance to the glucoregulatory effects of insulin. Further studies have provided evidence for insulin resistance in tissues from progesterone-treated animals, with regard to both glucose and lipid metabolism[66,68–70]: this effect is very rapid, being detectable within 10 min of progesterone administration[70].

These studies suggest that the menopause is likely to have an appreciable effect on insulin and glucose metabolism. Estrogens and progesterone may augment the pancreatic insulin response to glucose, but the effects of the two hormones on insulin resistance appear to differ, with estradiol increasing, and progesterone decreasing, insulin sensitivity. Menopause might, therefore, be expected to result in some reduction in pancreatic insulin output and deterioration in glucose tolerance, but the effects on insulin sensitivity are likely to depend on the relative contributions of estradiol and progesterone to insulin sensitivity. It is conceivable that insulin sensitivity might increase with the reduction in progesterone concentrations at the menopause, but the overall effect may depend on the phase of the menstrual cycle during which insulin sensitivity is assessed in the premenopausal comparison group. There is some evidence that there is greater insulin resistance during the luteal phase when progesterone levels are high than during the follicular phase[71].

Discrimination of changes associated with the menopause from changes associated with aging is difficult. Changes observed in individual women followed through the menopause will be influenced by aging, and given the extended duration of the perimenopause, such studies are, in any case, extremely difficult to undertake. One alternative is to compare age-matched groups of pre- and postmenopausal women, but there is then uncertainty over uncharacterized differences that may determine time of onset of menopause, and it is extremely difficult to assemble age-matched groups of women who are unequivocally pre- and postmenopausal. Another possibility is to assemble groups of sufficient size and age range for effective characterization of age-related changes, which may then be corrected for statistically. A further consideration in studies of the menopause is the need to define menopausal status accurately. As mentioned above, if menopausal status is not evaluated, perimenopausal women may be included; measurement of plasma gonadotropin levels are necessary if this possibility is to be minimized.

We are aware of only three studies of the effects of the menopause on insulin and glucose metabolism. In the Framingham Study, fasting plasma glucose did not differ between pre- and postmenopausal women[72] and in the follow-up study[73] changes in fasting and glucose and insulin concentrations following an oral glucose tolerance test (OGTT) were of similar magnitude among women who became postmenopausal compared with those who remained premenopausal. We have recently completed a study in which the intravenous rather than the oral glucose tolerance test was used to compare glucose and insulin metabolism in pre- and postmenopausal women[47]. In addition to providing for an evaluation of glucose and insulin concentration differences, use of the IVGTT enables mathematical modelling analyses to be applied to the tolerance test glucose, insulin and C-peptide concentration profiles; these provide measures of some of the factors which underlie variation in glucose and insulin levels. The modelling analyses we have employed include a minimal model of glucose disappearance[74] and a combined pancreatic insulin secretion model[75,76]. In applying the minimal model of glucose disappearance, prediction of the glucose concentration profile from the insulin concentration profile provides a measure of insulin sensitivity. In applying the pancreatic insulin secretion model, both the insulin and C-peptide concentration profiles are simultaneously predicted to provide measures of true pancreatic insulin secretion, fractional insulin elimination rate and fractional hepatic insulin throughput. The latter measure provides an index of the proportion of newly secreted insulin which is released into the general circulation after passage through the liver. We studied 66 healthy, non-obese premenopausal women with regular menstrual cycles, and 92 postmenopausal women whose last menstrual period had been ⩾6 months previously and who had follicle stimulating levels >40 IU/ml. Multiple linear regression analyses and standardization were applied in each group to bring all metabolic measures to those that would obtain at a nominal common age at menopause. Comparison of the standardized data thus enabled the effect of the menopause to be distinguished. In accord with the two other reports of the effects of the menopause, we found no effect on glucose or insulin concentrations. However, the IVGTT C-peptide response was significantly lower in postmenopausal women and the model derived IVGTT pancreatic insulin secretion response was also reduced. The lack of any change in insulin concentrations was explained by reduced fractional insulin elimination. Insulin sensitivity was increased significantly by the menopause. This could relate to relatively low insulin sensitivity in our premenopausal women, who were tested during the luteal phase of the menstrual cycle. Mean insulin sensitivity (unstandardized) in postmenopausal women did not differ from that in luteal phase premenopausal women, and examination of the age-related changes in insulin sensitivity revealed that there was a marked, progressive decline with increasing age in postmenopausal women. In accord with this, we have previously reported a significant increase in IVGTT insulin response with increasing time since menopause[77]. A further divergence between the effects of the menopause and the metabolic characteristics of postmenopausal women was seen with the hepatic insulin throughput index. Mean hepatic insulin throughput was increased significantly in postmenopausal compared with premenopausal women, but standardization analysis suggested that menopause itself was associated with a slight reduction in hepatic insulin throughput. Again, examination of age-related variation in hepatic insulin throughput showed a rise with increasing age in postmenopausal women.

INSULIN AND GLUCOSE METABOLISM AND HORMONE REPLACEMENT THERAPY

If the insulin resistance syndrome does in fact develop in postmenopausal women, physiological reversal of the menopause by estrogen replacement should be associated with alleviation of these metabolic disturbances. The majority of studies of the effects of the native estrogen, 17β-estradiol, suggest an improvement in insulin sensitivity[78-81], whereas other have found no apparent effect, as demonstrated by unchanged OGTT glucose and insulin levels[82,83]. The non-native estrogens, conjugated equine estrogens, or the alkylated estrogens ethinylestradiol or mestranol, appear to have either no effect, or they raise insulin levels or impair glucose tolerance[82,84-88]. One study of conjugated equine estrogens found no effect on glucose tolerance, but lower insulin levels[89].

Hormone replacement therapy, administered to non-hysterectomized women, almost invariably employs a progestagen to minimize the possibility of endometrial hyperplasia, and the effects of such combination therapy are becoming an increasingly important consideration. A variety of synthetic progestagens are employed, including medroxyprogesterone acetate, dydrogesterone, levonorgestrel and norethisterone acetate. These may differ in their effects on glucose and insulin metabolism[15,90-93]. Luotola and co-workers[94] examined the effects of orally administered cyclical norethisterone acetate given with continuous 17β-estradiol in 30 postmenopausal women followed over 6 months. The combination had little effect, although in women who commenced the study with impaired glucose tolerance there was some improvement in glucose response. De-Cleyn and colleagues[95] studied 20 postmenopausal women before and 2 months after taking conjugated equine estrogens and then after 6 months of cyclically administered dydrogesterone (20 mg for 12 days) therapy. No significant changes in glucose tolerance test glucose and insulin concentrations were observed. We have recently followed 49 non-hysterectomized postmenopausal women, receiving 17β-estradiol (2 mg/day) and dydrogesterone (10 mg/day for 14 days). Mean oral glucose tolerance test incremental glucose and C-peptide responses did not change throughout the study, whereas the insulin response fell significantly after 12 cycles (unpublished data). The lack of change in glucose and C-peptide concentrations and reduction in insulin concentrations suggest that this sequential therapy improves insulin sensitivity and elimination in postmenopausal women. Elkind-Hirsch and colleagues[96] carried out IVGTT in six women with premature ovarian failure during the second cycle of a treatment comprising 25 days of estradiol (2 mg/day) and 10 days during which medroxyprogesterone acetate was given (5 mg/day, days 15–25)[96]. Insulin sensitivity did not differ between the hormone-free period and the period during which estradiol was given alone, but was reduced by the addition of medroxyprogeseterone acetate. The small sample size and the possibility of carry-over of steroid hormone effects from the preceding cycle render this study of doubtful value. We have also recently compared the effects of an oral therapy regimen, comprising conjugated equine estrogens (0.625 mg/day continuous) and levonorgestrel (75 μg/day for 12 days) with those of a transdermally administered regimen comprising patches delivering 17β-estradiol (50 μg/day for 14 days/cycle) followed by patches delivering both 17β-estradiol (50 μg/day) and norethisterone acetate (250 μg/day)[46]. Sixty women were randomized to receive either regimen and each woman underwent an IVGTT prior to treatment and at 3, 6 and 18 months of treatment. Tests at 3 months were carried out during both the estrogen-alone and estrogen plus progestagen phase of the treatment cycle. A further 29 women provided an untreated control group. Oral therapy caused a reduction in the initial plasma insulin response to the IVGTT. This resulted in a reduction in glucose elimination rate at the outset of the test and elevated glucose concentrations. These increased the stimulation of pancreatic insulin secretion and the overall insulin response. The transdermal treatment had no effect on glucose tolerance or insulin concentrations. Both treatments were associated with increased hepatic insulin uptake, but with the transdermal therapy this was compensated for by an increase in first-phase pancreatic insulin secretion. Neither treatment caused significant insulin resistance compared with baseline levels, but with the oral treatment, insulin resistance was significantly greater during the combined phase than the estrogen-only phase. Changes in glucose elimination rate, phase 2 IVGTT incremental insulin area, insulin resistance and the initial plasma insulin response induced by these two regimens after three and six cycles of treatment are illustrated in Figure 1. At 3 months, studies were carried out during both the estrogen-alone and combined phases of the treatment cycle: inclusion of the levonorgestrel progestagen in the oral therapy significantly increased the IVGTT insulin response and insulin resistance ($p < 0.01$ relative to the estrogen-alone phase).

Clearly, combined hormone replacement therapy regimens can differ substantially in their effects on insulin and glucose metabolism. Nevertheless there do appear to be combinations in which the improvements in glucose and insulin metabolism that may be seen with the native hormone are still apparent.

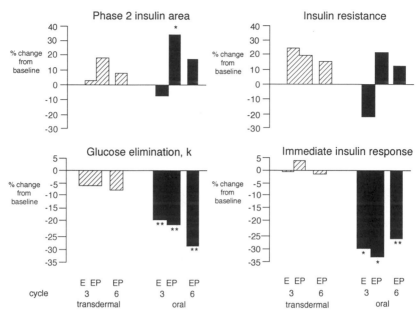

Figure 1 Changes in measures of glucose and insulin metabolism in 61 postmenopausal women receiving either transdermal estradiol/norethisterone acetate (▨) or oral conjugated equine estrogens/levonorgestrel (■) combined, cyclical hormone replacement therapy. During cycle 3, subjects were studied in both the estrogen alone phase (E) and the combined phase (EP) of the treatment cycle; during cycle 6, subjects were studied only during the combined phase (EP). (Adapted from reference 48). Significant changes relative to an untreated reference group: $^*p < 0.05$, $^{**}p < 0.01$, $^{***}p < 0.001$

CONCLUSIONS

Recent developments in our knowledge of the effects of hyperinsulinemia and insulin resistance possibly render disturbed insulin and glucose metabolism matters of greater importance in the assessment of cardio-vascular risk than in diabetes risk. Nevertheless, the effects of the menopause on insulin and glucose metabolism remain virtually unexplored. We have found evidence for reductions in pancreatic insulin secretion and insulin elimination associated with the menopause, but there appeared to be no adverse effect on insulin resistance, at least when luteal phase premenopausal women comprised the reference group. There was, however, evidence for progressive reductions in both insulin sensitivity and hepatic insulin elimination after the menopause, leading to increasing hyperinsulinemia with increasing menopausal age. The effects of administration of the native hormone, 17β-estradiol, are almost equally under-researched, although the weight of evidence favors improved insulin sensitivity and elimination in response to this hormone, thus strengthening the supposition that menopause might adversely affect insulin and glucose metabolism.

Given the known associations between insulin and other aspects of metabolism, it is relevant to consider what other effects the menopause has in these other areas. We have observed increased triglyceride concentrations and reduced HDL-cholesterol concentrations (specifically in the HDL_2 subfraction) in age-standardized comparisons between large groups of pre- and postmenopausal women ($n = 395$ and 147, respectively)[97]. We have also observed an increased proportion of android (central or abdominal) fat in postmenopausal compared with premenopausal women[98]. Others have observed similar effects on lipids and lipoproteins[72,73,99] and on fat distribution[100]. This combination of deteriorating insulin sensitivity and elimination, with increased triglyceride concentrations, reduced HDL-cholesterol concentrations and increased central fat is strongly reminiscent of the insulin resistance syndrome that is assuming such prominence in more general considerations of cardiovascular risk. The observation that estrogen therapy can alleviate some of these disturbances and can substantially reduce cardiovascular mortality must give weight to the hypothesis that it is coordinated metabolic disturbances, rather than a change in any one variable, that should be considered in modifying cardiovascular disease risk. The further observations that insulin action can stimulate blood flow, and that this effect is diminished in insulin resistant states[101], and that reduced blood flow can diminish insulin action[102] extends this hypothesis into areas of risk modification by estrogens that have hitherto been viewed in isolation from metabolic changes. The manifold metabolic and physiological inter-relationships that may be modified by the menopause are shown in Figure 2. There is experimental evidence for each of the connections shown, although their relative importance in postmenopausal women has yet to be investigated. Nevertheless, it is to be hoped that a growing awareness of these interdependencies may counter the somewhat parochial attitudes that seem to be developing around different factors underlying cardiovascular risk modification in postmenopausal women by estrogen replacement therapy.

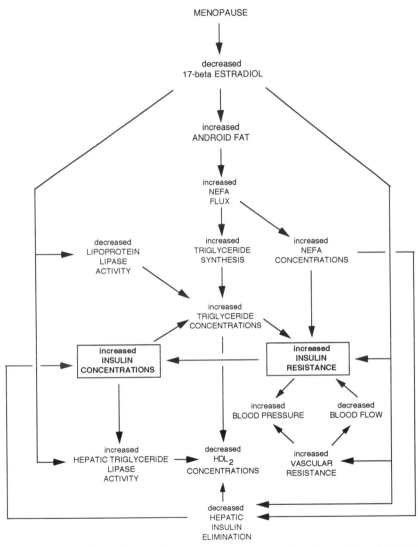

Figure 2 Possible effects of the menopause on interrelationships between glucose, insulin, lipid and lipoprotein metabolism and hemodynamics. Each illustrated connection is supported by published experimental findings (abbreviation: NEFA – non-esterified fatty acids)

REFERENCES

1. Wilson, P., Castelli, W. and Kannel, W. (1987). Coronary risk prediction in adults (The Framingham Heart Study). *Am. J. Cardiol.,* **59**, 91G–94G
2. Manolio, T. and Harlan, W. (1993). Research on coronary disease in women: political or scientific imperative? *Br. Heart J.,* **69**, 1–2
3. Jarrett, R. J. (1984). The epidemiology of coronary heart disease and related factors in the context of diabetes mellitus and impaired glucose tolerance. In Jarrett, R. J. (ed.) *Diabetes and Heart Disease,* pp. 1–24. (Amsterdam: Elsevier)
4. Welborn, T. and Wearne, K. (1979). Coronary heart disease incidence and cardiovascular mortality in Busselton with reference to glucose and insulin concentrations. *Diabetes Care,* **2**, 154–60
5. Jarrett, R., McCartney, P. and Keen, H. (1982). The Bedford Survey: ten year mortality rates in newly diagnosed diabetics, borderline diabetics and normoglycaemic controls and risk for coronary heart disease in borderline diabetics. *Diabetologia,* **22**, 79–84
6. Fuller, J., Shipley, M., Rose, G., Jarrett, R. and Keen, H. (1983). Mortality from coronary heart disease and stroke in relation to degree of glycaemia: the Whitehall Study. *Br. Med. J.,* **287**, 867–70
7. Donahue, R., Abbott, R., Reed, D. and Katsuhiko, Y. (1987). Post-challenge glucose concentration and coronary heart disease in men of Japanese ancestry. *Diabetes,* **36**, 689–92
8. Schleicher, E., Deufel, T. and Wieland, O. (1981). Non-enzymatic glycosylation of human serum lipoproteins: elevated εta-lysine glycosylated low density lipoprotein in diabetic patients. *FEBS Lett.,* **129**, 1–4
9. Steinbrecher, U. and Witztum, J. (1984). Glycosylation of low-density lipoproteins to an extent comparable to that seen in diabetes slows their catabolism. *Diabetes,* **33**, 30–4
10. Pyörälä, K., Savolainen, E., Kaukola, S. and Haapakoski, J. (1985). Plasma insulin as coronary heart disease risk factor: relationship to other risk factors and predictive value during $9\frac{1}{2}$ year follow-up of the Helsinki Policemen Study population. *Acta Med. Scand.,* **701** (Suppl.), 38–52
11. Fontbonne, A. and Eschwege, E. (1991). Insulin and cardiovascular disease: Paris Prospective Study. *Diabetes Care,* **14**, 461–9
12. Stout, R. (1990). Insulin and atheroma: 20-yr perspective. *Diabetes Care,* **13**, 631–54
13. Rönnemaa, T., Laakso, M., Pyörälä, K., Kallio, V. and Puukka, P. (1991). High fasting plasma insulin is an indicator of coronary heart disease in non-insulin-dependent diabetic patients and non-diabetic subjects. *Arteriosclerosis,* **11**, 80–90
14. Hollenbeck, C. and Reaven, G. (1987). Variations in insulin-stimulated glucose uptake in healthy individuals with normal glucose tolerance. *J. Clin. Endocrinol. Metab.,* **64**, 1169–73
15. Godsland, I., Walton, C., Felton, A., Proudler, A., Patel, A. and Wynn, V. (1992). Insulin resistance, secretion and metabolism in users of oral contraceptives. *J. Clin. Endocrinol. Metab.,* **74**, 64–70
16. Ley, C., Swan, J., Godsland, I., Walton, C., Crook, D. and Stevenson, J. C. (1993). Insulin resistance, lipids, body fat and coagulation factors in males with

suspected anginal and normal or abnormal coronary angiograms. *J. Am. Coll. Cardiol.,* in press

17. Dean, J., Jones, C., Hutchinson, S., Peters, J. and Henderson, A. (1991). Hyperinsulinaemia and microvascular angina ('syndrome X'). *Lancet,* **337,** 456–7

18. Swan, J. W., Walton, C., Godsland, I. F., Crook, D., Oliver, M. F. and Stevenson, J. C. (1993). Insulin resistance syndrome as a feature of cardiological syndrome X in non-obese men. *Br. Heart J.,* in press

19. Welborn, T., Breckenridge, A., Rubinstein, A., Dollery, C. and Fraser, T. (1966). Serum-insulin in essential hypertension and in peripheral vascular disease. *Lancet,* **1,** 1336–7

20. Modan, M., Halkin, H., Almog, S., Lusky, A., Eshkol, A., Shefi, M., Shitrit, A. and Fuchs, S. (1985). Hyperinsulinaemia: a link between hypertension, obesity and glucose intolerance. *J. Clin. Invest.,* **75,** 809–17

21. Manicardi, V., Camellini, L., Bellodi, G., Coscelli, C. and Ferrannini, E. (1986). Evidence for an association of high blood pressure and hyperinsulinaemia in obese man. *J. Clin. Endocrinol. Metab.,* **62,** 1302–4

22. Ferrannini, E., Buzziogli, G., Bonadonna, R., Glorico, M., Oleginni, M., Graziadel, L. and Pedrinelli, R. (1987). Insulin resistance in essential hypertension. *N. Engl. J. Med.,* **317,** 350–7

23. Shen, D.-C., Shieh, S.-M., Fuh, M.-T., Wu, D.-A., Chen, Y.-D. and Reaven, G. (1988). Resistance to insulin-stimulated-glucose uptake in patients with hypertension. *J. Clin. Endocrinol. Metab.,* **66,** 580–3

24. DeFronzo, R. (1981). The effect of insulin on renal sodium metabolism: a review with clinical implications. *Diabetologia,* **21,** 165–71

25. Landsberg, L. (1986). Diet, obesity and hypertension: an hypothesis involving insulin, the sympathetic nervous system and adaptive thermogenesis. *Q. J. Med.,* **61,** 1081–90

26. Mathias, C., da Costa, D., Fosbraey, P., Christensen, N. and Bannister, P. (1987). Hypotensive and sedative effects of insulin in autonomic failure. *Br. Med. J.,* **295,** 161–3

27. Sawicki, P., Heinemann, L., Starke, A. and Berger, M. (1992). Hyperinsulinaemia is not linked with blood pressure elevation in patients with insulinoma. *Diabetologia,* **35,** 649–52

28. Jarrett, R. (1992). In defence of insulin: a critique of syndrome X. *Lancet,* **340,** 469–71

29. Zavaroni, I., Dall'Aglio, E., Bruschi, A., Bonara, A., Pezzarosa, A. and Butturini, U. (1985). Evidence for an independent relationship between plasma insulin and concentrations of high density lipoprotein cholesterol and triglyceride. *Atherosclerosis,* **55,** 259–66

30. Wing, R., Bunker, C., Kuller, L. and Matthews, K. (1989). Insulin, body mass index and cardiovascular risk factors in premenopausal women. *Arteriosclerosis,* **9,** 479–84

31. Manolio, T., Savage, P., Burke, G., Liu, K., Wagenknecht, L., Sidney, S., Jacobs, D., Roseman, J. Jr, Donahue, R. and Oberman, A. (1990). Association of fasting insulin with blood pressure and lipids in young adults. The Cardia Study. *Arteriosclerosis,* **10,** 430–6

32. Reaven, G. (1988). Banting Lecture 1988: role of insulin resistance in human disease. *Diabetes,* **37,** 1595–607

33. Hunt, S., Wu, L., Hopkins, P., Stults, B., Kuida, H., Ramirez, M., Lalouel, J.-M.

and Williams, R. (1989). Apolipoprotein, low density lipoprotein subfraction, and insulin associations with familial combined hyperlipidemia: a study of Utah patients with familial dyslipidemic hypertension. *Arteriosclerosis, 9,* 335–44

34. Ostlund, R. Jr., Staten, M., Kohrt, W., Schultz, J. and Malley, M. (1990). The ratio of waist-to-hip circumference, plasma insulin level, and glucose intolerance as independent predictors of the HDL2 cholesterol level in older adults. *N. Engl. J. Med.,* **322,** 229–34

35. Juhan-Vague, I., Alessi, M., Joly, P., Thirion, X., Vague, P., Declerck, P., Serradimigni, A. and Collen, D. (1989). Plasma plasminogen activator inhibitor 1 in angina pectoris. Influence of plasma insulin and acute-phase response. *Arteriosclerosis,* **9,** 362–7

36. Krauss, R. (1991). The tangled web of coronary risk factors. *Am. J. Med.,* **90** (Suppl. 2A), 36–41

37. Zavaroni, I., Bonara, E., Pagliara, M., Dall'Aglio, E., Luchetti, L., Buananno, G., Bonati, P., Bergonzani, M., Gnudi, L., Passeri, M. and Reaven, G. (1989). Risk factors for coronary artery disease in healthy persons with hyper-insulinaemia and normal glucose tolerance. *N. Engl. J. Med.,* **320,** 702–6

38. Haffner, S., Fong, D., Hazuda, H., Pugh, H. and Patterson, J. (1988). Hyper-insulinaemia, upper body adiposity, and cardiovascular risk factors in non-diabetics. *Metabolism,* **37,** 338–45

39. Cambien, F., Warnet, J.-M., Eschwege, E., Jacqueson, A., Richard, J. and Rosselin, G. (1987). Body mass, blood pressure, glucose and lipids: does plasma insulin explain their relationships? *Arteriosclerosis,* **7,** 197–202

40. Ferranninni, E., Haffner, S., Mitchell, B. and Stern, M. (1991). Hyperinsulinaemia: the key feature of a cardiovascular and metabolic syndrome. *Diabetologia,* **34,** 416–22

41. Haffner, S. (1992). Prospective analysis of the insulin-resistance syndrome (Syndrome X). *Diabetes,* **41,** 715–22

42. Jones, D. and Arky, R. (1965). Effects of insulin on triglyceride and free fatty acid metabolism in man. *Metab. Clin. Exp.,* **14,** 1287–93

43. Ruderman, N., Richards, K., Valles de Bourges, V. and Jones, A. (1968). Regulation of production and release of lipoprotein by the perfused rat liver. *J. Lipid Res.,* **9,** 613–19

44. Howard, B. (1987). Lipoprotein metabolism in diabetes mellitus. *J. Lipid Res.,* **28,** 613–28

45. Reaven, G. and Chen, Y.-D. (1988). Role of insulin in regulation of lipoprotein metabolism in diabetes. *Diabetes/Metab. Rev.,* **4,** 639–52

46. Godsland, I., Crook, D., Walton, C., Wynn, V. and Oliver, M. (1992). Influence of insulin resistance, secretion, and clearance on serum cholesterol, triglycerides, lipoprotein cholesterol, and blood pressure in healthy men. *Arteriosclerosis Thrombosis,* **12,** 1030–5

47. Walton, C., Godsland, I., Proudler, A., Wynn, V. and Stevenson, J. (1993). The effects of the menopause on insulin sensitivity, secretion and elimination in nonobese, healthy women. *Eur. J. Clin. Invest.,* **23,** 466–73

48. Godsland, I., Gangar, K., Walton, C., Cust, M., Whitehead, M., Wynn, V. and Stevenson, J. (1993). Insulin resistance, secretion and elimination in postmenopausal women receiving oral or transdermal hormone replacement therapy. *Metabolism,* in press

49. Strömblad, G. and Björntorp, P. (1986). Reduced hepatic insulin clearance in rats with dietary-induced obesity. *Metabolism*, **35**, 323–7
50. Barnes, B., Regan, J. and Nelson, W. (1933). Improvement in experimental diabetes following the administration of amniotin. *J. Am. Med. Assoc.*, **101**, 926–7
51. Nelson, W. and Overholser, M. (1936). The effect of oestrogenic hormone on experimental pancreatic diabetes in the monkey. *Endocrinology*, **20**, 473–80
52. Griffiths, M. and Young, F. (1940). Does the hypophysis secrete a pancreotropic hormone? *Nature*, **146**, 266–7
53. Costrini, N. and Kalkhoff, R. (1971). Relative effects of pregnancy, estradiol and progesterone on plasma insulin and pancreatic islet insulin secretion. *J. Clin. Invest.*, **50**, 992–9
54. Howell, S., Tyhurst, M. and Green, I. (1977). Direct effects of progesterone on rat islets of Langerhans in vivo and in tissue culture. *Diabetologia*, **13**, 579–83
55. Faure, A. and Sutter-Dub, M.-T. (1979). Insulin secretion from isolated pancreatic islets in the female rat. Short and long term estradiol influence. *J. Physiol.*, **75**, 289–95
56. Kitay, J. (1963). Effects of estradiol on pituitary adrenal function in male and female rats. *Endocrinology*, **72**, 947–54
57. Kitay, J. (1963). Pituitary and adrenal function in the rat after gonadectomy and gonadal hormone replacement therapy. *Endocrinology*, **73**, 253–60
58. Rodriguez, R. (1965). Influence of oestrogens and androgens on the production and prevention of diabetes. In Leibel, B. and Wrenshall, G. (eds.) *On the Nature and Treatment of Diabetes*, pp. 288–307. (New York: Excerpta Medica)
59. Faure, A., Haourari, M. and Sutter, B.-C.-J. (1985). Insulin secretion and biosynthesis after oestradiol treatment. *Hormone Metab. Res.*, **17**, 378
60. Hager, D., Georg, J., Leitner, J. and Beck, P. (1972). Insulin secretion and content in isolated rat pancreatic islets following treatment with gestational hormones. *Endocrinology*, **91**, 977–81
61. Ashby, J., Shirling, D. and Baird, J. (1978). Effects of progesterone on insulin secretion in the rat. *J. Endocrinol.*, **76**, 479–86
62. Bailey, C. and Ahmed-Sorour, H. (1980). Role of ovarian hormones in the long-term control of glucose homeostasis. *Diabetologia*, **19**, 475–81
63. Neilsen, J. (1984). Direct effect of gonadal and contraceptive steroids on insulin release from mouse pancreatic islets in organ culture. *Acta Endocrinol.*, **105**, 245–50
64. McKerns, K., Coulomb, B., Kaleita, E. and DeRenzo, E. (1958). Some effects of *in vivo* administered oestrogens on glucose metabolism and adrenal cortical secretion *in vitro*. *Endocrinology*, **63**, 709–22
65. Gilmour, K. and McKerns, K. (1966). Insulin and estrogen regulation of lipid synthesis in adipose tissue. *Biochim. Biophys. Acta*, **116**, 220–8
66. Rushakoff, R. and Kalkhoff, R. (1981). Effects of pregnancy and sex steroid administration on skeletal muscle metabolism in the rat. *Diabetes*, **30**, 545–50
67. Beck, P. (1969). Progestin enhancement of the plasma insulin response to glucose in Rhesus monkeys. *Diabetes*, **18**, 146–52
68. Salans, L. (1971). Influence of progestin and estrogen on fat cell size, number,

glucose metabolism and insulin sensitivity. *Proceedings of the 53rd Meeting of the Endocrine Society,* Abstr. PA-59. (San Francisco, CA)

69. Sutter, B.-C.-J., Sutter-Dub, M., Leclerq, R. and Jacquot, R. (1973). Inhibition of insulin action by progesterone in the rat (abstract). *Diabetologia, 9,* 92

70. Sutter-Dub, M., Dazey, B., Hamdan, E. and Vergnaud, M. (1981). Progesterone and insulin-resistance: studies of progesterone action on glucose transport, lipogenesis and lipolysis in isolated fat cells of the female rat. *J. Endocrinol., 88,* 455–62

71. Valdes, C. and Elkind-Hirsch, K. (1991). Intravenous glucose tolerance test-derived insulin sensitivity changes during the menstrual cycle. *J. Clin. Endocrinol. Metab., 72,* 642–6

72. Kannel, W., Hjortland, M. and McNamara, P. (1976). Menopause and risk of cardiovascular disease: The Framingham Study. *Ann. Intern. Med., 85,* 447–52

73. Matthews, K., Meilahn, E., Kuller, L., Kelsey, S., Caggiula, A. and Wing, R. (1989). Menopause and risk factors for coronary heart disease. *N. Engl. J. Med., 321,* 641–6

74. Bergman, R., Ider, Y., Bowden, C. and Cobelli, C. (1979). Quantitative estimation of insulin sensitivity. *Am. J. Physiol., 236,* E667–77

75. Vølund, A., Polonsky, K. and Bergman, R. (1987). Calculated pattern of intraportal insulin appearance without independent assessment of C-peptide kinetics. *Diabetes, 36,* 1195–202

76. Watanabe, R., Vølund, A., Roy, S. and Bergman, R. (1989). Prehepatic beta-cell secretion during the intravenous glucose tolerance test in humans: application of a combined model of insulin and C-peptide kinetics. *J. Clin. Endocrinol Metab., 69,* 790–7

77. Proudler, A., Felton, C. and Stevenson, J. (1992). Ageing and the response of plasma insulin, glucose and C-peptide concentrations to intravenous glucose in postmenopausal women. *Clin. Sci., 83,* 489–94

78. Talaat, M., Habib, Y., Higazy, A., AbdelNaby, S., Malek, A. and Ibrahim, Z. (1965). Effect of sex hormones on the carbohydrate metabolism in normal and diabetic women. *Arch. Int. Pharmacodyn., 154,* 402–11

79. Silfverstolpe, G., Gustafson, A., Samsoie, G. and Svanborg, A. (1980). Lipid metabolic studies in oophorectomised women: effects induced by two different estrogens on serum lipids and lipoproteins. *Gynecol. Obstet. Invest., 11,* 161–9

80. Notelovitz, M., Johnston, M., Smith, S. and Kitchens, C. (1987). Metabolic and hormonal effects of 25 mg and 50 mg 17β estradiol implants in surgically menopausal women. *Obstet. Gynecol., 70,* 749–54

81. Cagnacci, A., Soldani, R., Carriero, P., Paoletti, A., Fioretti, P. and Melis, G. (1992). Effects of low doses of transdermal 17β-estradiol on carbohydrate metabolism in postmenopausal women. *J. Clin. Endocrinol. Metab., 74,* 1396–400

82. Larsson-Cohn, U. and Wallentin, L. (1977). Metabolic and hormonal effects of post-menopausal oestrogen replacement treatment. *Acta Endocrinol., 86,* 583–96

83. Crook, D., Montgomery, J., Godsland, I., Devenport, M., Marenah, C., Studd, J. and Wynn, V. (1991). Lipid and carbohydrate metabolism in premenopausal women given subdermal estradiol pellets. *Hormone Metab. Res., 23,* 174–7

84. Goldman, J. and Ovadia, J. (1969). The effect of estrogen on intravenous

glucose tolerance in women. *Am. J. Obstet. Gynecol.,* **103**, 172–8

85. Yen, S. and Vela, P. (1969). Carbohydrate metabolism and long term use of oral contraceptives. *J. Reprod. Med.,* **3**, 25–37

86. Thom, M., Chakravarti, S., Oram, D. and Studd, J. (1977). Effect of hormone replacement therapy on glucose tolerance in postmenopausal women. *Br. J. Obstet. Gynecol.,* **84**, 776–84

87. Spellacy, W., Buhi, W. and Birk, S. (1972). The effects of estrogens on carbohydrate metabolism: glucose, insulin and growth hormone studies on one hundred and seventy one women ingesting Premarin, mestranol and ethinyl estradiol for six months. *Am. J. Obstet. Gynecol.,* **114**, 378–92

88. Spellacy, W., Buhi, W. and Birk, S. (1982). The effects of two years of mestranol treatment on carbohydrate metabolism. *Metabolism,* **31**, 1006–8

89. Barrett-Connor, E. and Laakso, M. (1990). Ischaemic heart disease risk in postmenopausal women: effects of estrogen use on glucose and insulin levels. *Arteriosclerosis,* **10**, 531–4

90. Gershberg, H., Zorrilla, E., Hernandez, A. and Hulse, M. (1969). Effects of medroxyprogesterone acetate on serum insulin and growth hormone levels in diabetics and potential diabetics. *Obstet. Gynecol.,* **33**, 383–9

91. Beck, P., Zimmerman, D. and Eaton, R. (1976). Effects of gonadal steroids on arginine-stimulated glucagon and insulin secretion in women. Oral medroxy-progesterone acetate. In *Abstracts of the IXth Congress of the International Diabetes Foundation,* p. 34. (Amsterdam: Excerpta Medica)

92. Spellacy, W., Buhi, W. and Birk, S. (1974). Norgestrel and carbohydrate-lipid metabolism: glucose, insulin and triglyceride changes during 6 months time of use. *Contraception,* **9**, 615–25

93. Godsland, I., Crook, D., Simpson, R., Proudler, T., Felton, C., Lees, B., Anyaoku, V., Devenport, M. and Wynn, V. (1990). The effects of different formulations of oral contraceptive agents on lipid and carbohydrate metabolism. *N. Engl. J. Med.,* **323**, 1375–81

94. Luotola, H., Pyörälä, T. and Loikkanen, M. (1986). Effects of natural oestrogen-/progestogen substitution therapy on carbohydrate and lipid metabolism in post-menopausal women. *Maturitas,* **8**, 245–53

95. DeCleyn, K., Buytaert, P. and Coppens, M. (1989). Carbohydrate metabolism during hormonal substitution therapy. *Maturitas,* **11**, 235–42

96. Elkind-Hirsch, K., Sherman, L. and Malinak, R. (1993). Hormone replacement therapy alters insulin sensitivity in young women with premature ovarian failure. *J. Clin. Endocrinol. Metab.,* **76**, 472–5

97. Stevenson, J., Crook, D. and Godsland, I. (1993). Influence of age and menopause on serum lipids and lipoproteins in healthy women. *Atheroscler-osis,* **98**, 83–90

98. Ley, C., Lees, B. and Stevenson, J. (1992). Sex- and menopause-associated changes in body fat distribution. *Am. J. Clin. Nutr.,* **55**, 950–4

99. Jensen, J., Nilas, L. and Christiansen, C. (1990). Influence of menopause on serum lipids and lipoproteins. *Maturitas,* **12**, 321–31

100. Lapidus, L., Bengtson, C., Hällström, T. and Björntorp, P. (1989). Obesity, adipose distribution and health in women: results from a population study in Gothenburg, Sweden. *Appetite,* **12**, 25–35

101. Laakso, M., Edelman, S., Brechtel, G. and Baron, A. (1990). Decreased effect

of insulin to stimulate skeletal muscle blood flow in obese man. *J. Clin. Invest.*, **85**, 1844–52

102. Baron, A., Laakso, M., Brechtel, G. and Edelman, S. (1991). Mechanism of insulin resistance in insulin-dependent diabetes mellitus: a major role for reduced skeletal muscle blood flow. *J. Clin. Endocrinol. Metab.*, **73**, 637–43

27

Cardiac symptoms in middle-aged women

C. M. Oakley

The main concern in women is the steady increase in prevalence of coronary heart disease after the menopause. This change in prevalence is associated with changes in plasma lipids consonant with increased risk. Levels of low density lipoprotein (LDL) rise, with no change in total high density lipoprotein (HDL), although there is a fall in the major protective HDL_2 component of cholesterol. An earlier increase in coronary disease is seen in women after premature menopause as well as in those who have undergone oophorectomy. Administration of the natural estrogen, 17β-estradiol, brings about a rise in HDL_2 cholesterol; this enzyme is also a vasodilator which lowers blood pressure (possibly through a calcium antagonist effect) and is anti-thrombotic. In contrast to the protective effect of natural estrogen, synthetic estrogens, particularly when given in higher doses for oral contraception, increase cardiovascular risk, raising triglycerides, blood pressure and plasma insulin and adding to the thromboembolic risk through an increase in coagulation factors VIII, IX and X and a fall in anti-thrombin 3. The synthetic progestogens are androgenic and compound the risk.

The adverse effects of oral contraceptives containing synthetic estrogens and progestogens may be enhanced and the risks increased in women above the age of 35, particularly if they smoke, drink alcohol and are overweight.

A constellation of risk factors which include android adiposity with androgenic hormone profile, higher LDL:HDL ratio, increased insulin resistance and raised blood pressure is found commonly in the Asian community. This is probably genetic and helps to explain the increased prevalence of coronary disease in both sexes with the development of symptomatic coronary disease in Asians approximately 10 years earlier than in Europeans.

A number of trials of hormone replacement (HRT) have suggested that such treatment reduces cardiovascular risk, although there have been defects in the trials, mostly due to the use of unopposed estrogen without progestogen. The latter is now discouraged because of the increased risk of endometrial cancer in non-hysterectomized women treated with unopposed estrogen, and the tendency for longer term HRT. Sample sizes have often been small, the trials of short duration with respect to various different hormone products, observational, and mainly through questionnaires without case control or randomization. Notwithstanding these defects, however, a number of studies have suggested that HRT (including use at any time) reduces cardiovascular risk by about 50% and possibly more with continued use. However, the difficulties in analysis are shown from the Framingham Trial in which the relative risk from HRT was found to be increased to 1.7, though a re-analysis came up with a relative risk of only 0.5 in users similar to the other trials!

Angina-like pain with a positive exercise stress test but angiographically normal coronary arteries (syndrome X) is also more prevalent in women than in men and particularly in postmenopausal women. Many of the atypical symptoms in syndrome X are similar to those occurring in the mitral leaflet prolapse syndrome, a perplexing condition in which non-specific symptoms such as fatigue are associated with seeming cardiovascular symptoms including angina-like chest pains and shortness of breath, which are in no way explained by the mild hemodynamic fault. Although degenerative mitral valve changes with regurgitation become more frequent with increasing age, this syndrome is not confined to such patients but is found also in some younger patients with floppy valves and little or no regurgitation.

Syndrome X is usually associated with atypical chest pain symptoms in women who, although having positive stress tests, do not show ST-depression during pain on Holter monitoring. The literature is full of conflicting findings on the question of whether or not the pain is due to ischemia. Lactate production during pacing stress has been described, with an increase in coronary venous lactate compared with arterial blood lactate, but this is by no means a constant finding and has been present in only a minority of patients. Moreover, pacing stress is unphysiological and unlikely to stimulate maximal vasodilatation. Nevertheless, the concept of 'microvascular angina' has been introduced and a decreased coronary flow reserve shown. This might be caused by an abnormality in endothelium dependent vasodilatation. Some thallium stress studies have been said to show reversible defects, although it has not been explained why the defects should be focal in a disorder which presumably affects the entire coronary microvasculature. An intriguing recent concept has been developed by Collins and Poole-Wilson at Brompton National Heart Hospital. They postulate that estrogen deficiency may be responsible for decreased coronary vasodilator reserve because natural estrogen is a vasodilator. They have attempted to treat such patients with sublingual estrogens. A recent study at Hammersmith Hospital by Camici and Rosen using positron emission tomography and dipyridamole to induce maximum vasodilatation showed no difference between syndrome X patients and controls who were relatives of the patients. This was the first study to use controls and seems to be definitive at least in the particular patients studied. No doubt the condition is heterogeneous.

Dr. Schenck-Gustafsson described clinical symptoms and treatment in women, stressing again the frequent atypicality of symptoms, both in women with coronary artery disease and in women without (syndrome X). This atypicality of symptoms, the lower prevalence of coronary artery disease in women and the frequency of false positive exercise tests has been responsible for the high number of women found to have normal coronary arteries on angiography and perhaps for the conception of syndrome X. Because women develop coronary artery disease later than men, they are more likely than men of the same age to have single vessel coronary artery disease, and may even show normal coronary arteries after an infarct, suggesting that the infarct was caused by thrombotic occlusion induced by local vasoconstriction, perhaps at a point of minimal disease, followed by either auto or exogenous lysis. Patients with syndrome X may have real pain, and a low pain threshold, as has been shown by tests of somatic pain threshold which was also found to be low in these patients. It may be that some patients with syndrome X have a lowered threshold specifically to the perception of visceral pain.

Stress tests in women may be hard to interpret because of false-positive ST-segment depression, apparently not indicative of ischemia, and because some women fail to or are unable to complete the exercise test programme. Dr Astrom described the use of isotope techniques in the investigation of women with coronary artery disease, pointing out the increased predictive value of a positive thallium stress test compared with the unadorned ECG exercise test, although he admitted that false positives can occur due to take-up of thallium isotope in breast tissue.

Dr Juhlin-Dannfelt described the use of stress echocardiography in women with coronary artery disease, pointing out that it is inexpensive and involves no radiation. Moreover, a positive echo stress test has more specificity and hence prognostic value (though lower sensitivity) than a thallium stress test. Dobutamine stress rather than exercise tends to be preferred today in order to avoid movement. Digitized images before and after stress are superimposed in two planes on a quad screen to increase ease of recognition of the induced regional wall motion abnormality.

The increased incidence of atypical symptoms, false positive exercise and thallium stress tests, together with the lower prevalence of coronary artery disease at all ages up until the eighth or ninth decade, may be the reason why women tend not to be referred for surgery until they have more advanced disease than their male counterparts. This may contribute to the increased mortality of coronary bypass surgery in women, although other contributions to this include the smaller size of the arteries and higher incidence of diabetes in women.

Section 6

Hormones, mood and neurobiology

28

Hormones, mood and neurobiology – a summary

S. S. Smith

Alterations in circulating levels of the reproductive hormones estradiol and progesterone are not only associated with changes in reproductive capacity, but have also been shown to result in significant changes in mood and a variety of non-reproductive behaviors, from sensorimotor function to learning. Under pathological conditions, changes in seizure activity are also seen following elevations in steroid levels. Some of the diverse actions of these steroids may be mediated via classic genomic steroid receptor-mediated events. In addition to sites in the hypothalamus and midbrain where they facilitate reproductive function[1,2], classic receptors for estradiol and progesterone have also been localized to the amygdala[1,2], hippocampus[3] and locus coeruleus[4], where they may mediate some of the reported effects of these steroids on mood, learning and seizure activity. In addition, however, more recent findings have demonstrated that these steroids or their metabolites can act to modulate classic neurotransmitter receptors (Figure 1) for inhibitory and excitatory amino acids[5,6]. These findings suggest that steroids have the capacity to exert global actions throughout the brain, with important implications for their behavioral effects. Most recently, membrane receptors have been identified for the corticosteroids[7] and progesterone[8], suggesting an additional means of action[9] for steroid hormones.

In general, estradiol exerts excitatory actions and progestins exert inhibitory effects on the central nervous system (CNS). Elevated levels of estradiol are associated with 'activating' effects on mood and activity[10]. Mid-cycle peaks of this hormone can be associated with euphoria,

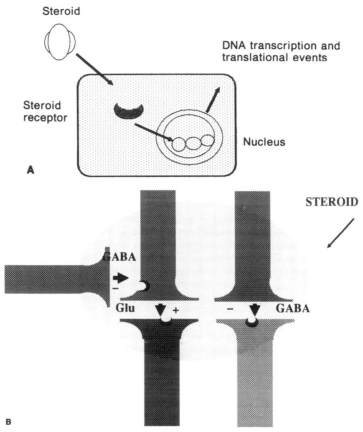

Figure 1 Classic actions of steroids (A) are exerted at cytosolic/nuclear receptors which, once bound to these lipophilic molecules, produce both transcriptional and translational events. In addition to these classic actions of these hormones, certain steroids exert actions on traditional neurotransmitter receptors (B), such as γ-aminobutyric acid (GABA) and the excitatory amino acids. In this case, steroids delivered by the vasculature or via the glial system would impact upon a neural circuit. The net effect of the steroid would be dependent upon the configuration of the particular circuit

irritability or high activity states[11], depending upon the susceptibility of the individual.

In addition, estradiol can act as an antidepressant[12]. Behavioral studies have suggested that the estrogen-dominant follicular phase is associated specifically with increases in repetitive, rapidly alternating tasks, such as walking, finger tapping frequency, word fluency and typing[13]. In general, these tasks involve alternating movements of the limbs or digits.

Increased levels of estradiol are also associated with activation of sensorimotor function. In both human and animal studies, increases in circulating estradiol are associated with increases in sensory perception for a number of modalities[14] including fine touch, two-point discrimination, hearing, olfaction and visual signal detection. Increases in locomotor activity[15,16], as well as improved limb coordination[17], are observed at this time. In addition, attentional mechanisms and short-term memory appear to be enhanced following cyclic elevations in estradiol[18,19].

In contrast to these 'activating' effects of estradiol, progestins are reportedly 'depressant' in terms of their effect on the CNS. At high doses, progesterone or its metabolites possess anesthetic properties[20-23]. Cyclic increases in this steroid have been associated with either tranquilizing, mood-stabilizing or depressant qualities[11,24]. In contrast to the facilitating effect of estradiol on rapidly performed, repetitive, alternating movements, the P-dominant luteal phase is associated with improved performance on perceptual restructuring tasks, such as mental subtraction, time estimation, maze performance and the embedded figures tasks[13]. What distinguishes these tasks from those enhanced during the estrogen-dominant phase is that they involve a response delay, rather than rapid movement.

The distinction between the activating, excitatory effects of estradiol and the depressant actions of the progestins is most clearly illustrated by their contrasting effects on convulsive activity. Elevations in estradiol across the hormone cycle have been associated with an increase in seizure activity[25,26]. This proconvulsant action of the steroid is dependent upon the type of seizure. Specifically, increases in generalized tonic-clonic seizures have been correlated with the estrogen-dominant follicular phase of the menstrual cycle[26]. That estradiol may directly facilitate seizure activity is suggested by the finding that local application of this steroid to the surface of the cat cerebral cortex induces focal seizures[27]. In contrast, cyclic increases in progesterone have been associated with decreases in seizure activity[28-30].

These contrasting actions of the two steroids on mood and behavior may be at least partially explained by their modulatory effect on amino acid receptor function. Estradiol has been shown in electrophysiological studies to amplify responses of neurons in the hippocampus[31], cortex (S. Smith, unpublished data) and cerebellum[32] to excitatory amino acids. In some cases, both quisqualate and N-methyl-D-aspartate (NMDA)-specific responses were augmented[31,32]. A recent report has provided evidence for an effect of this steroid on NMDA binding in the CA1 region of the hippocampus[33]. Chronic treatment with estradiol increased the binding

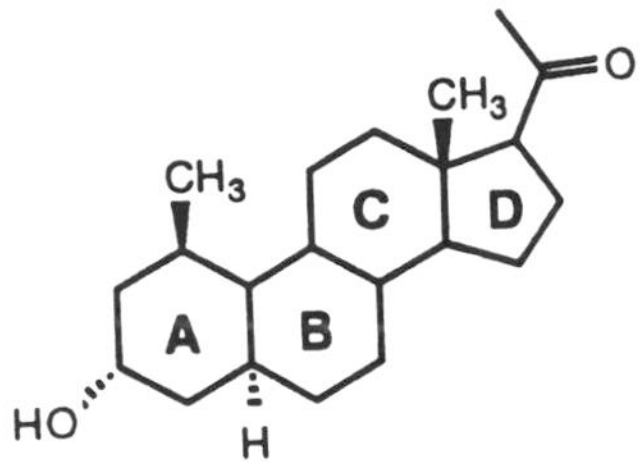

Figure 2 The structure of one of the most potent endogenous neuroactive steroids 3α,5α-THP

affinity of this excitatory amino acid. Further studies have confirmed that responses of neurons to afferent input[31,34] in these areas are also enhanced following increases in circulating levels of estradiol.

The depressant effects of progesterone are most likely due to its 3α-hydroxysteroid metabolite (Figure 2), 3α,5α-THP (3α-hydroxy-5α-pregnan-20-one or allopregnanolone)[35], which can be formed systemically or locally in widespread CNS sites from progesterone[36] and cholesterol[37]. Circulating and CNS levels of 3α,5α-THP correlated well with circulating levels of progesterone[38]. This metabolite was first shown to prolong the open time of Cl^- channels during γ-aminobutyric acid (GABA)-mediated increases in Cl^- conductance in cultured hippocampal and spinal cord neurons using the whole cell patch clamp technique[5]. Physiological levels of circulating progesterone also enhance GABA responses of cerebellar neurons, an effect due to the 3α,5α-THP metabolite[39]. In addition, alterations in benzodiazepine, muscimol and *t*-butyl-bicyclophosphorothionate (TBPS) binding have been noted following administration of 3α,5α-THP[4,40,41]. More recent studies suggest that this steroid binds to a novel site on the $GABA_A$ receptor[42,43] (Figure 3). Subtypes of the $GABA_A$ receptor exist[44] which have different affinities for the 3α-hydroxy C21 steroids[45,46]. Differential distribution of these subtypes throughout the CNS would then yield CNS areas with variable sensitivity to the GABA-enhancing actions of 3α,5α-THP[47], as has been demonstrated in frontal cortex and spinal cord[48], which implicate these CNS sites in particular as targets for the depressant effect of this steroid. In addition, neuronal sensitivity to the GABA-active 3α,5α-THP is inversely correlated with its circulating level, suggesting homologous steroidal modulation of $GABA_A$ receptor sensitivity[49].

The GABA-enhancing actions of 3α,5α-THP probably underlie the depressant effects of progesterone on mood, general activity, convulsant activity and anesthetized state, as was previously demonstrated for

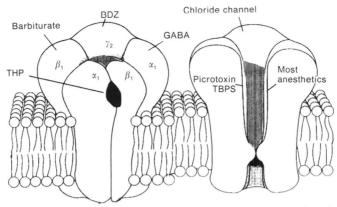

Figure 3 Theoretical binding site for the allopregnanolone (THP) class of compounds on the γ-aminobutyric acid-A (GABA$_A$) receptor. The GABA$_A$ receptor, composed of five subunits (each one a product of four membrane-spanning portions) contains binding sites for GABA, barbiturates, benzodiazepines (BDZ), picrotoxin, *t*-butyl-bicyclophosphorothionate (TBPS) and most anesthetic agents, in addition to a unique binding site for 3α,5α-THP (from reference 58 with permission)

a steroid anesthetic[50]. The anxiolytic properties associated with this compound are also probably due to the actions of this class of compounds at the GABA$_A$ receptor. Progesterone administration to subjects of either sex has been shown to produce effects similar to the benzodiazepines on such parameters as electrocardiogram (ECG), heart rate, blood pressure and respiratory rate[51]. Progesterone administration to female, estrogen-primed rats also exerts anxiolytic actions, as assessed using an animal model of anxiety, the conflict paradigm[52]. It is probably 3α,5α-THP rather than progesterone that exerts these anxiolytic actions. Both intraventricular and systemic administration of this metabolite have been shown to be anxiolytic in the rat[53,54]. In addition, systemic levels of progesterone which exert anxiolytic effects have been found to be well-correlated with elevated levels of 3α,5α-THP in the forebrain[55]. This latter finding provides strong evidence that the anxiolytic properties of progesterone may be due in fact to 3α,5α-THP.

As a corollary to these findings, a recent report suggests that progesterone exhibits withdrawal properties in a similar manner to other GABA-active agents such as benzodiazepines and barbiturates. Withdrawal from chronic exposure to physiological levels of progesterone is able to produce an anxiogenic action in estrogen-primed female rats[56]. It is probably withdrawal from 3α,5α-THP that produces this effect, as indomethacin, which blocks formation of the metabolite from progesterone, prevented the anxiogenic action of progesterone withdrawal. This finding may be relevant for studies examining anxiety related to the premenstrual syndrome[24,57] or dysphoria during the postpartum and postmenopausal periods. In these cases, changes in mood follow withdrawal from progesterone alone or in combination with estradiol.

Although estradiol appears to exert actions outside the hypothalamus which are primarily excitatory in nature, this hormone can also act to enhance GABA-ergic inhibition by two means: promoting conversion of progesterone to $3\alpha,5\alpha$-THP in some CNS sites[36], and increasing mRNA for glutamic acid decarboxylase (GAD), as has been demonstrated in the midbrain (M. McCarthy and S. Schwartz-Giblin, unpublished data). Both mechanisms would tend to enhance GABA inhibition and reinforce the effect of GABA-active progesterone metabolites. However, when both hormones are elevated during the cycle, synaptic responses to both excitatory and inhibitory input should be enhanced[58] simultaneously. This dual enhancement should tend to sharpen sensory perception to incoming stimuli, with improved performance the eventual outcome.

In addition to effects on inhibitory and excitatory amino acid receptor systems, reproductive hormones exert actions on the monoamine systems, long implicated in the pathogenesis of altered mood states. The locus coeruleus contains classic estradiol receptors[4], and thus has the potential for modulation by this steroid. In addition, it has long been known that estradiol can exert effects on the monoamine oxidase system[59], as well as on noradrenergic receptors[60], an effect dependent upon the dose, time course and CNS site. Catecholestrogens, which are formed locally in widespread CNS sites from estradiol[61], can act on the noradrenergic receptor and thus provide an additional avenue for steroid action. In addition to actions on the noradrenergic system, a number of studies have demonstrated significant effects of this steroid on the nigro-striatal dopamine system[62,63], which could have implications for effects on sensorimotor function as well as on affect. Changes in serotonin binding have also been noted across hormone state[64]. Thus, generalized changes in the monoamine system could underlie some of the mood changes associated with fluctuations in endogenous hormone levels.

The facilitating action of estradiol on learning and memory may result from more long-term effects of the steroid than are necessary to exert effects on neuronal responses. A recent study has demonstrated alterations in hippocampal dendritic spine density across the estrous cycle[65]. Increases in estradiol were shown to increase the number of dendritic spines in the CA1 region, an area known to contain classic receptors for

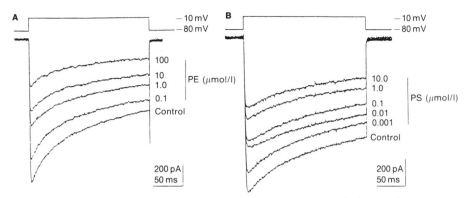

Figure 4 Concentration-dependent block by pregnenolone (PE), A, and pregnenolone sulfate (PS), B, on the voltage-gated Ca^{2+} current. Currents were evoked by a 200 ms voltage step to $-10\,mV$ from a holding potential of $-80\,mV$. A and B are two different hippocampal CA1 neurons. (Reprinted from reference 69 with permission from the author)

this steroid[3]. This neurotropic action of the steroid may result from classic genomic actions on oncogene proliferation[66] or, alternatively, could result from potentiation of excitatory amino acid receptor function.

A recent development in steroid research is the finding that steroid hormones (neurosteroids[67]) can be formed *de novo* in the brain from cholesterol, in addition to their systemic site of origin[68]. Of these, pregnenolone and pregnenolone sulfate have been found to exert a number of effects including suppression of voltage-gated calcium currents[69] (Figure 4) and potentiation of NMDA currents[70]. Behavioral studies suggest that this steroid may also play a role in learning[71], perhaps due to its ability to alter responses to NMDA. In addition, pregnenolone depresses the GABA-activated Cl^- current[72], an effect which may be anxiogenic. Thus, fluctuation in this steroid across the reproductive cycle or in response to other yet unidentified stimuli may significantly alter mood and behavior. A clearer understanding of the range of endogenous and synthetic neuroactive steroids which alter mood will prove useful for multiple clinical applications as these steroids possess anxiolytic, anticonvulsant, anesthetic and analgesic properties.

Alterations in circulating levels of estradiol, pregnenolone and progesterone or their metabolites are associated with diverse effects on mood, behavior and pathological states such as seizure activity (certainly many factors other than hormone level also contribute to these complex states). In general, estradiol exerts activating effects and progestins exert depressant actions on the CNS to bias in mood and behavior. In addition to classic genomic actions of the steroids, these hormones can also modulate classic neurotransmitter systems and may act at novel membrane steroid receptor sites. The discovery of the neurosteroids opens up additional possibilities for steroid action in the brain. The mechanisms by which steroids act to produce their diverse actions are only beginning to unfold.

ACKNOWLEDGEMENTS

The author is grateful to J. M. H. ffrench-Mullen for use of Figure 4. The author would also like to thank B. S. McEwen and K. W. Gee for helpful input.

REFERENCES

1. MacLuskey, N. J. and McEwen, B. S. (1980). Progestin receptors in rat brain, distribution and properties of cytoplasmic progestin-binding sites. *Endocrinology,* **106**, 192–202
2. Pfaff, D. and Keiner, D. (1973). Atlas of estradiol-concentrating cells in the central nervous system of the female rat. *J. Comp. Neurol.,* **151**, 121–58
3. Simerly, R. B., Chang, C., Muramatsu, M. and Swanson, L. W. (1990). Distribution of androgen and estrogen receptor mRNA-containing cells in the rat brain: an *in situ* hybridization study. *J. Comp. Neurol.,* **294**, 76–95
4. Heritage, A. S., Grant, L. D. and Stumpf, W. E. (1978). ^{3}H-Estradiol in catecholamine neurons of rat brainstem: combined localization by autoradiography and formaldehyde-induced fluorescence. *J. Comp. Neurol.,* **176**, 607–30
5. Majewska, M. D., Harrison, N. L., Schwartz, R. D., Barker, J. L. and Paul, S. M. (1986). Steroid hormone metabolites are barbiturate-like modulators of the GABA receptor. *Science,* **232**, 1004–7
6. Smith, S. S., Waterhouse, B. D. and Woodward, D. J. (1987). Sex steroid effects on extrahypothalamic CNS I: Estrogen augments neuronal responsiveness to ionophoretically applied glutamate in the cerebellum. *Brain Res.,* **422**, 40–51
7. Orichnik, M., Murray, T. F. and Moore, F. L. (1991). A corticosteroid receptor in neuronal membranes. *Science,* **252**, 1848–51
8. Tischkau, S. A. and Ramirez, V. D. (1993). A specific membrane binding protein for progesterone in rat brain: sex differences and induction by estrogen. *Proc. Natl. Acad. Sci. USA,* **90**, 1285–9
9. Schumacher, M., Coirini, H., Pfaff, D. W. and McEwen, B. S. (1990). Behavioral effects of progesterone associated with rapid modulation of exytocin receptors. *Science,* **250**, 691–4
10. Asso, D. and Braier, J. R. (1982). Changes with the menstrual cycle in psychophysiological and self-report measures of activation. *Biol. Psychol.,* **15**, 95–107
11. Friedman, R. C. (1982). *Behavior and the Menstrual Cycle.* (New York: Marcel Dekker)
12. Klaiber, E. L., Broverman, D. M., Vogel, W. L. and Kobayashi, Y. (1979). Estrogen

therapy for severe persistent depressions in women. *Arch. Gen. Psychiatry,* **36**, 550–4

13. Broverman, D. M., Klaiber, E. L., Kobayashi, Y. and Vogel, W. (1968). Roles of activation and inhibition in sex differences in cognitive abilities. *Psychol. Rev.,* **75**, 23–50

14. Zimmerman, E. and Parlee, M. B. (1973). Behavioral changes associated with the menstrual cycle: an experimental investigation. *J. Appl. Soc. Psychol.,* **3**, 335–44

15. Beatty, W. W. (1979). Gonadal hormones and sex differences in non-reproductive behaviors in rodents: organizational and activational influences. *Hormones Behav.,* **12**, 112–63

16. Morris, N. M. and Udry, J. R. (1970). Variations in pedometer activity during the menstrual cycle. *Obstet. Gynecol.,* **35**, 199–201

17. Hampson, E. and Kimura, D. (1988). Reciprocal effects of hormonal fluctuations on human motor and perceptual–spatial skills. *Behav. Neurosci.,* **102**, 456–9

18. Kopell, B., Lunde, D., Clayton, R., Moos, R. and Hamburg, D. (1969). Variations in some measures of arousal during the menstrual cycle. *J. Nerv. Mental Dis.,* **148**, 180–7

19. Patkai, P., Johannson, G. and Post, B. (1974). Mood, alertness and sympathetic-adrenal medullary activity during the menstrual cycle. *Psychosom. Med.,* **36**, 503–12

20. Selye, H. (1942). Correlations between the chemical structure and pharmacological actions of the steroids. *Endocrinology,* **30**, 437–53

21. Holzbauer, M. (1976). Physiological aspects of steroids with anesthetic properties. *Med. Biol.,* **54**, 227–42

22. Bixo, M. and Backstrom, T. (1990). Regional distribution of progesterone and 5α-pregnane-3,20-dione in rat brain during progesterone-induced 'anesthesia'. *Psychoneuroendocrinology,* **15**, 159–62

23. Carl, P., Hogskilde, S., Nielsen, J. W., Sorensen, M. B., Lindholm, M., Karlen, B. and Backstrom, T. (1990). Pregnanolone emulsion. A preliminary pharmacokinetic and pharmacodynamic study of a new intravenous anesthetic agent. *Anaesthesia,* **45**, 189–97

24. Backstrom, T. and Corstensen, H. (1974). Estrogen and progesterone in plasma in relation to premenstrual tension. *J. Steroid Biochem.,* **5**, 257–60

25. Logothetis, J., Harner, R., Morrell, F. and Torres, F. (1959). The role of oestrogen and catamenial exacerbations of epilepsy. *Neurology,* **9**, 352–60

26. Backstrom, T. (1976). Epileptic seizures in women related to plasma estrogen and progesterone during the menstrual cycle. *Acta Neurol. Scand.,* **54**, 321–47

27. Marcus, E. M., Watson, C. W. and Goldman, P. L. (1966). Effects of steroids on cerebral electrical activity; epileptogenic effects of conjugated estrogens and related compounds in the cat and rabbit. *Arch. Neurol.,* **15**, 521–32

28. Stitt, S. L. and Kinnard, W. J. (1968). The effect of certain progestins and estrogens on the threshold of electrically induced seizure patterns. *Neurology,* **18**, 213–16

29. Backstrom, T., Zetterlund, B., Blom, S. and Romano, M. (1984). Effects of intravenous progesterone infusions on the epileptic discharge frequency in women with partial epilepsy. *Arch Neurol. Scand.,* **69**, 240–8

30. Landgren, S., Aasly, J., Backstrom, T., Dubrovsky, B. and Danielsson, E. (1987).

61. Parvizi, N. and Ellendorf, F. (1983). Catecholestrogens in the brain: neuro-endocrine integration. *J. Steroid Biochem.*, **19**, 615–18

62. Becker, J. B. (1990). Estrogen rapidly potentiates amphetamine-induced striatal dopamine release and rotational behavior during microdialysis. *Neurosci. Lett.*, **118**, 169–71

63. Dluzen, D. E. and Ramirez, V. D. (1990). *In vitro* progesterone modulation of amphetamine-stimulated dopamine release from the corpus striatum of ovariectomized estrogen-treated female rats: response characteristics. *Brain Res.*, **517**, 117–22

64. Williams, J. and Uphouse, L. (1989). Serotonin binding sites during proestrus and following estradiol treatment. *Pharmacol Biochem Behav.*, **33**, 615–20

65. Wooley, C. S. and McEwen, B. S. (1992). Estradiol mediates fluctuation in hippocampal synapse density during the estrous cycle in the adult rat. *J. Neurosci.*, **12**, 2549–54

66. Murphy, L. J., Murphy, L. C. and Friesen, H. G. (1987). Estrogen induction of N-myc and c-myc protooncogene expression in the rat uterus. *Endocrinology*, **120**, 1882–8

67. Robel, P. and Baulieu, E. E. (1985). Neuro-steroids: 3β-hydroxy-delta-derivatives in the rodent brain. *Neurochem. Int.*, **7**, 953–8

68. McKay, S. A., Jenkin, G. and Thorburn, G. D. (1987). Peripheral plasma concentrations of pregnenolone sulphate, pregnenolone, progesterone and 20α-hydroxy-4-pregnen-3-one in ewes throughout the oestrus cycle. *J. Endocrinol.*, **113**, 231–7

69. Spence, K. T., Plata-Salaman, C. R. and ffrench-Mullen, J. M. H. (1991). The neurosteroids pregnenolone and pregnenolone-sulfate but not progesterone, block Ca^{++} currents in acutely isolated hippocampal CA1 neurons. *Life Sci.*, **49**, 235–9

70. Wu, F. S., Gibbs, T. T. and Farb, D. H. (1991). Pregnenolone sulfate: a positive allosteric modulator at the *N*-methyl-D-aspartate receptor. *Mol. Pharmacol.*, **40**, 333–6

71. Flood, J. F., Morley, J. F. and Roberts, E. (1992). Memory-enhancing effects in male mice of pregnenolone and steroids derived from it. *Proc. Natl. Acad. Sci. USA*, **89**, 1567–71

72. Mienville, J. M. and Vicini, S. (1989). Pregnenolone sulphate antagonizes $GABA_A$ receptor-mediated currents via a reduction of channel opening frequency. *Brain Res.*, **489**, 190–4

29

Ovarian steroids have diverse effects on brain structure and function

B. S. McEwen

INTRODUCTION

Ovarian steroids have numerous and profound effects on the central nervous system. These actions were first uncovered in relation to reproductive behaviors in lower animals[1], but more recently ovarian steroids have been found to affect such diverse non-reproductive processes as cognitive function, motor activity, seizure susceptibility and pain sensitivity, and pathological processes such as Parkinson's disease and Alzheimer's disease. At the same time, studies on animal brains have revealed a wide array of neurochemical and structural effects of ovarian steroids[1]. The purpose of this article is to provide a brief review of this information.

A BRIEF OVERVIEW OF MECHANISMS OF STEROID ACTION

Before proceeding to discuss ovarian steroid effects, it is important to point out that there are two types of mechanisms for steroid action. One involves well-characterized intracellular receptors which bind to DNA and regulate gene expression[2]; the other involves largely uncharacterized membrane sites for estrogen action that mediate rapid, non-genomic effects of estrogens[3] (see Chapter 39). Genomic and non-genomic effects of other steroids are recognized, and the most clear-cut example of a non-genomic effect is that of metabolites of progesterone and deoxy-corticosterone, which facilitate opening of the chloride channel of the

γ-aminobutyric acid (GABA$_A$) benzodiazepine receptor[3-5].

Intracellular, genomic receptors for estradiol are located primarily in the hypothalamus and preoptic area as well as in the anterior pituitary[6], but there are also estrogen sensitive neurons in other brain regions, including the hippocampal formation[6,7], which is an important brain structure for learning and memory[8]. Progesterone receptors are found in many of the same brain areas as estrogen receptors, where they are generally inducible by estrogens; however, there are also progestin receptors in the cerebral cortex that are not inducible by estrogens[9].

DIVERSE EFFECTS OF ESTROGENS ON NEUROCHEMISTRY

The actions of ovarian steroids on the adult brain have been elucidated in studies on experimental animals, mainly rats. They may be divided into two categories: effects on processes related to neurotransmission, and actions that affect neuronal structure and synaptic connectivity. Some examples of ovarian steroid effects on neurotransmitter systems in brain are given below.

Dopaminergic system

The effects of estrogen on the rodent brain include biphasic effects on dopaminergic activity which manifest themselves in spontaneous and drug-induced locomotor activity and stereotyped behaviors[10]. Direct action of estrogen in the caudate putamen is implicated in these effects[10], although there is no solid evidence for either membrane or intracellular estrogen receptors[11]. Estrogen effects on dopamine turnover and tyrosine hydroxylase levels in the incertohypothalamic and arcuate dopaminergic systems have also been described[12-15].

Neuropeptides

Various neuropeptide systems in neural tissue are regulated by estradiol. Estradiol induces receptors for oxytocin in the basal hypothalamus of the rat brain and this induction is linked to the activation of sexual behavior in the female rat[1]. Estrogen treatment also induces the mRNA for proenkephalin, an opiate peptide[1], while at the same time decreasing the mRNA for another opiate peptide, pro-opiomelanocortin[16,17]. Estradiol is also reported to induce the expression of at least two other neuropeptide systems: neurotensin[18] and galanin[19], in brain and/or pituitary tissue. There are undoubtedly many other estrogen effects on brain neuropeptide and

other neurotransmitter systems that remain to be discovered, and still others that there simply is not time to cover in this brief article.

GABA

Ovarian steroids also influence the expression of components of the inhibitory neurotransmitter, GABA. Estrogen treatment induces the mRNA for glutamic acid decarboxylase (GAD), the key enzyme in generating GABA from glutamate, in the CA1 region of the hippocampus, and sequential estradiol plus progesterone treatment reverses the effect of estradiol alone[20]. Estrogen treatment has also been reported to differentially regulate two forms of GAD mRNA (GAD 65 and GAD 67, reflecting two distinct genes) in different brain regions, increasing them in some brain regions and decreasing them in others[21].

In keeping with the complex regulation of GAD mRNA, $GABA_A$ receptor binding is also under complex regulation by ovarian steroids. $GABA_A$ receptor binding is decreased by estradiol treatment in midbrain and in basal hypothalamus, an effect reversed by sequential estradiol and progesterone treatment[22], whereas $GABA_A$ receptor binding is induced by estradiol in the CA1 region of hippocampus, an effect that is not changed by estradiol and progesterone replacement[23].

Cholinergic system

Estrogen treatment of ovariectomized adult female rats induces choline acetyltransferase (ChAT) activity in the basal forebrain and in several projection areas[24]. This induction occurs over a period of 24 h, and is expressed in a number of projection areas of the basal forebrain cholinergic system, namely, in the CA1 region of the hippocampus and frontal cortex, suggesting that ChAT is induced by estradiol in cholinergic cell bodies in the basal forebrain and then transported to nerve endings in hippocampus and cortex[24]. Acetylcholinesterase, the degradative enzyme for acetylcholine, is also induced by estradiol, suggesting that there is a general trophic effect of estradiol to enhance more than just the biosynthetic component of the basal forebrain cholinergic system[25]. Several laboratories have confirmed the inducibility of ChAT in the rat brain[26,27]. It is not known whether ChAT is induced in the human brain or in brains of infrahuman primates.

ESTROGENS, PROGESTINS AND SYNAPTIC TURNOVER

We have discovered that estradiol and progesterone regulate neuronal plasticity, particularly cyclic changes in the formation and break-down of synapses in the adult brain. These studies were stimulated, in part, by observations made in other laboratories that androgens and estrogens change neuronal morphology in the adult rat nervous system: estrogens were reported to increase synapse formation after neuronal damage, whereas castration and testosterone replacement were found to affect neuronal size and synaptic connectivity in the non-lesion adult male rat spinal cord[28,29]. In the CA1 region of hippocampus as well as in the ventromedial nucleus (VMN) of the hypothalamus, progestin receptors are induced by estrogen treatment[9]. We started our search for estrogen and progestin effects on brain morphology in the hypothalamus. Whereas the hippocampus is involved in learning and memory[8], the VMN is an important neural control site for sexual behavior in the female rat[6]. Estradiol and progesterone play an essential role in reproductive cycles by coordinating events in the reproductive tract with neural and neuro-endocrine processes[1,6]. In lower animals such as the rat, reproductive behavior is coordinated with these reproductive processes to increase likelihood of successful reproduction[6]. The coordination of sexual behavior with reproductive cycles is advantageous for the investigation of brain mechanisms which participate in and respond to circulating hormones[1,6].

In the adult female rat brain, we found that, during the 5-day estrous cycle, dendrites of neurons in the ventromedial hypothalamus sprout increased numbers of spines on dendrites and then lose them[30]. All of this happens rapidly during the estrous cycle, and the increase of spine density during the estrogen secretion phase of the cycle can be mimicked by giving estradiol for several days to ovariectomized female rats[30].

It was a much greater surprise, however, to discover that neurons of the CA1 region of hippocampus responded in a very similar way[31–33]. Increased spine numbers, as seen in the light microscope, are accompanied by increased numbers of synapses on spines, as shown in the electron microscope[31–33]. The fact that there is no change in synapses on dendritic shafts indicates that there is not a conversion of preexisting shaft synapses to spine synapses[33]. Thus it is highly likely that there is synaptogenesis under the influence of estrogen and then synaptic destruction during the later phase of the estrous cycle.

The loss of spines and spine synapses occurs during a 24-h period between the time of maximum sexual receptivity on the day of proestrus and the next day, the day of estrus. This loss is not due solely to the decline in estradiol: we found that simply removing estradiol results in a very slow rate of decrease of spine density. However, administration of progesterone accelerated the decline, and administering the antiprogestin, Ru486, during proestrus, was found to block the natural decline of synapse density[34].

CONCLUSIONS

In view of these diverse actions of ovarian steroids on brain function in animal studies, it is relevant to ask what are some of the clinical situations in which estrogens and progestins have been shown to have effects on neural processes. The following brief overview will indicate some of the studies on humans in which estrogens have been implicated.

Motor disturbances

Clinically, estrogens are recognized to exacerbate symptoms of Parkinson's disease[35]. Collectively, these effects imply antagonist actions of estradiol on the dopaminergic system, and animal experiments that were summarized above have supported such a role.

Epilepsy

Ovarian steroids are also implicated in epilepsy. Catamenial epilepsy varies according to the menstrual cycle, with the peak frequency of occurrence corresponding to the lowest ratio of progesterone to estradiol during the cycle[36,37]. Bearing in mind that there is some genetic and/or developmental predisposition to express seizures, there may be at least three types of hormone actions involved in the cyclic occurrence of epilepsy, or protection from seizures:

(1) Estrogen induction of excitatory synapses in hippocampus, leading to decreased seizure thresholds (see description above);

(2) Progesterone actions via the steroid metabolites which act via the $GABA_A$ receptor to decrease excitability[3]; and

(3) Hormone actions on the liver to increase clearance rates of antiseizure medication[37].

Premenstrual syndrome

Premenstrual tension is a cyclic mood disorder which in its most severe form is referred to as premenstrual syndrome (PMS). Its symptoms are eliminated by arresting the menstrual cycle[38], but specific hormonal causes are unknown[39]. Although there are indications that high estrogen and progesterone levels in the luteal phase may exacerbate symptoms of PMS, the administration of a gonadotropin releasing hormone agonist, along with low amounts of estradiol and progesterone in order to prevent ovarian hormone deficiency, has been reported to alleviate symptoms of PMS[38]. It remains to be determined whether PMS involves any of the specific morphological or neurochemical effects of ovarian steroids described above.

Pain

Recent studies in mice indicate that males and females use functionally distinct pain pathways, and that gonadal steroids, particularly estrogens, play a major role in regulating these pathways[40]. Thus basic research on pain mechanisms as well as clinical practice in treating pain must now take into consideration the sex differences in neural mechanisms mediating pain.

Depressive illness

One-month prevalence studies of mental disorders have revealed that males suffer more frequently from substance abuse and hostility/conduct disorders, whereas women are more prone to develop anxiety disorders and depressive illness[41]. Very few studies, however, provide any indication as to whether these disorders are related in any way to circulating gonadal hormones or to the actions of hormones during sexual differentiation. Unquestionably, early experience, social and cultural factors interact with the biological substrate to produce sex differences. Nevertheless, there is one report indicating that estrogen replacement in postmenopausal women produced a significant reduction in anxiety and depression[42]. Thus estrogen deficiency may contribute to depression and mood disorders in the postmenopausal state.

Cognitive function

Estrogens are also implicated in cognitive function in women. While, in humans, in contrast to the rat, sexual behavior is not tightly linked to the reproductive cycle, it is evident that there are effects of cyclic variations of estradiol on performance of spatial tasks and on fine motor skills[43], as well as paired-associate learning[44]. At present, it is not known whether the changes in human performance as a result of the presence or absence of estrogens has any connection to the hippocampus or to the formation and destruction of synapses. However, this possibility is very attractive and deserves further investigation.

Dementia

Following early reports that administration of estradiol, progesterone and testosterone to elderly women improved some measures of intellectual functioning[45], more recent work has demonstrated beneficial effects on verbal memory tests of estrogen replacement therapy in surgically menopausal women[46]. Moreover, two types of studies indicate a link to dementing illness in postmenopausal women: first, women with a history of cerebrovascular disease showed improved cognitive function on estrogen replacement therapy[47]; second, two other studies on elderly female Alzheimer's patients revealed improvements in tests of mental status over a period of 6 weeks of estrogen replacement therapy[48,49]. Furthermore, there are indications that women given estrogen replacement therapy are much less likely to develop dementing illness[50]. Taken together, these findings warrant further, more extensive investigations of the relationship between estrogens and both normal cognitive function as well as dementing illness.

CONCLUSION

There is ample evidence for a large number of effects of ovarian steroids on brain function from animal experiments and in clinical studies. Studies on experimental animals are beginning to reveal the specific neurochemical and structural consequences of estradiol and progesterone actions on the adult brain, and it is likely that much more will be learned in the near future. Clinical studies have begun to indicate the wide variety of actions exerted by estrogen on normal and pathological processes in the brain. It remains to be seen which of the mechanisms found in animal studies may explain the effects of ovarian hormones in humans, but it is likely that the structural changes produced by estradiol and the actions of estradiol on the dopaminergic, cholinergic, GABA and various neuropeptide systems will be found to be important in explaining changes in neurological, affective state and cognitive function which occur in some women after natural or surgical menopause.

ACKNOWLEDGEMENTS

Research in the author's laboratory described in this article is supported by NIH grant NS 07080. The author wishes to acknowledge his many laboratory colleagues who contributed to the work cited in this article.

REFERENCES

1. McEwen, B., Coirini, H., Danielsson, A., Frankfurt, M., Gould, E., Mendelson, M., Schumacher, A., Segarra, A. and Woolley, C. (1991). Steroid and thyroid hormones modulate a changing brain. *J. Steroid Biochem. Mol. Biol.*, **40**, 1–14
2. Yamamoto, K. (1985). Steroid receptor regulated transcription of specific genes and gene networks. *Annu. Rev. Genet.*, **19**, 209–52
3. McEwen, B. (1991). Steroids affect neural activity by acting on the membrane and the genome. *Trends Pharmacol. Sci.*, **12**, 141–7
4. Gee, K., Belelli, D. and Lan, N. (1990). Anticonvulsant steroids and the GABA/Benzodiazepine receptor-chloride ionophore complex. *Neurosci. Biobehav. Rev.*, **14**, 315–22
5. Paul, S. and Purdy, R. (1992). Neuroactive steroids. *FASEB J.*, **6**, 2311–22
6. Pfaff, D. W. (1980). *Estrogens and Brain Function.* (New York: Springer Verlag)
7. Loy, R., Gerlach, J. L. and McEwen, B. S. (1988). Autoradiographic localization of estradiol-binding neurons in the hippocampal formation and the enterohinal cortex. *Dev. Brain Res.*, **39**, 245–51
8. Eichenbaum, H. and Otto, T. (1992). The hippocampus – what does it do? *Behav. Neural Biol.*, **57**, 2–36
9. McEwen, B. S., Davis, P., Gerlach, J., Krey, L., MacLusky, N., McGinnis, M., Parsons, B. and Rainbow, T. (1983). In Bardin, C., Mauvais-Jarvis, P. and Milgrom, E. (eds.) *Progesterone and Progestin*, pp. 59–76. (New York: Raven Press)
10. van Hartesveldt, C. and Joyce, J. (1986). Effects of estrogen on the basal ganglia. *Neurosci. Biobehav. Rev.*, **10**, 1–14
11. Roy, E., Buyer, D. and Licari, V. (1990). Estradiol in the striatum: effects on behavior and dopamine receptors but no evidence for membrane steroid receptors. *Brain Res. Bull.*, **25**, 221–7
12. Lookingland, K. J. and Moore, K. E. (1984). Effects of estradiol and prolactin on incertohypothalamic dopaminergic neurons in the male rat. *Brain Res.*, **323**, 83–91
13. Blum, M., McEwen, B. S. and Roberts, J. (1987). Transcriptional analysis of tyrosine hydroxylase gene expression in the tuberoinfundibular dopaminergic neurons of the rat arcuate nucleus after estrogen treatment. *J. Biol. Chem.*, **262**, 817–21
14. Gunnett, J. W., Lookingland, K. J. and Moore, K. E. (1986). Comparison of the effects of castration and steroid replacement on incertohypothalamic dopaminergic neurons in male and female rats. *Neuroendocrinology*, **44**, 269–75
15. Sanghara, M. K., Grady, S., Smith, W., Woodward, D. J. and Porter, J. C. (1991). Incertohypothalamic A13 dopaminergic neurons: effect of gonadal steroids on tyrosine hydroxylase. *Neuroendocrinology*, **53**, 268–75

16. Wilcox, J. and Roberts, J. (1985). Estrogen decreases rat hypothalamic proopiomelanocortin messenger ribonucleic acid levels. *Endocrinology,* **117,** 2392–6

17. Treiser, S. and Wardlaw, S. (1992). Estradiol regulation of proopiomelanocortin gene expression and peptide content in the hypothalamus. *Neuroendocrinology,* **55,** 167–73

18. Alexander, M., Kiraly, Z. and Leeman, S. (1991). Sexually dimorphic distribution of neurotensin/neuromedin N mRNA in the rat preoptic area. *J. Comp. Neurol.,* **311,** 84–96

19. Kaplan, L., Gabriel, S., Koenig, J., Sundayk, M., Spindel, E., Martin, J. and Chin, W. (1988). Galanin is an estrogen-inducible, secretory product of the rat anterior pituitary. *Proc. Natl. Acad. Sci. USA,* **85,** 7408–12

20. Weiland, N. (1992). Glutamic acid decarboxylase messenger ribonucleic acid is regulated by estradiol and progesterone in the hippocampus. *Endocrinology,* **131,** 2697–702

21. McCarthy, M. M., Kaufman, L. C., Brooks, P. J., Pfaff, D. W. and Schwartz-Giblin, S. (1993). *Abstracts, Soc. Neurosci.,* **19,** 489

22. Schumacher, M., Coirini, H. and McEwen, B. S. (1989). Regulation of GABAa receptors in specific brain regions by ovarian hormones. *Neuroendocrinology,* **50,** 315–20

23. Schumacher, M., Coirini, H. and McEwen, B. (1989). Regulation of high-affinity GABAa receptors in the dorsal hippocampus by estradiol and progesterone. *Brain Res.,* **487,** 178–83

24. Luine, V. (1985). Estradiol increases choline acetyltransferase activity in specific basal forebrain nuclei and projection areas of female rats. *Exp. Neurol.,* **89,** 484–90

25. Luine, V. and McEwen, B. S. (1983). Sex differences in cholinergic enzymes of diagonal band nuclei in the rat preoptic area. *Neuroendocrinology,* **36,** 475–82

26. Kaufman, H., Vadasz, C. and Lajtha, A. (1988). Effects of estradiol and dexamethasone on choline acetyltransferase activity in various rat brain regions. *Brain Res.,* **453,** 389–92

27. Lapchak, P., Araujo, D., Quirion, R. and Beaudet, A. (1990). Chronic estradiol treatment alters central cholinergic function in the female rat: effect on choline acetyltransferase activity, acetylcholine content, and nicotinic auto-receptor function. *Brain Res.,* **525,** 249–55

28. Arnold, A. and Breedlove, M. (1985). Organizational and activational effects of sex steroids on brain and behavior: a reanalysis. *Horm. Behav.,* **19,** 469–98

29. Matsumoto, A. (1992). Sex steroid induction of synaptic reorganization in adult neuroendocrine brain. *Rev. Neurosci.,* **3,** 287–306

30. Frankfurt, M., Gould, E., Woolley, C. S. and McEwen, B. S. (1990). Gonadal steroids modify dendritic spine density in ventromedial hypothalamic neurons: a Golgi study in the adult rat. *Neuroendocrinology,* **51,** 530–5

31. Gould, E., Woolley, C., Frankfurt, M. and McEwen, B. S. (1990). Gonadal steroids regulate dendritic spine density in hippocampal pyramidal cells in adulthood. *J. Neurosci.,* **10,** 1286–91

32. Woolley, C., Gould, E., Frankfurt, M. and McEwen, B. (1990). Naturally occurring fluctuation in dendritic spine density on adult hippocampal pyramidal neurons. *J. Neurosci.,* **10,** 4035–9

33. Woolley, C. S. and McEwen, B. S. (1992). Estradiol mediates fluctuations in hippocampal synapse density during the estrous cycle in the adult rat. *J. Neurosci.*, **12**, 2549–54

34. Woolley, C. S. and McEwen, B. S. (1993). Roles of estradiol and progesterone in regulation of hippocampal dendritic spine density during the estrous cycle in the rat. *J. Comp. Neurol.*, **336**, 293–306

35. Bedard, P., Langelier, P. and Villeneuve, A. (1977). Oestrogens and extrapyramidal system. *Lancet,* 1367–8

36. Bonuccelli, U., Melis, G. B., Paoletti, A. M., Fioretti, P., Murri, L. and Muratoria, A. (1989). Unbalanced progesterone and estradiol secretion in catamenial epilepsy. *Epilepsy Res.,* **3**, 100–6

37. Herzog, A. G. (1991). Reproductive endocrine considerations and hormonal therapy for women with epilepsy. *Epilepsy,* **62** (Suppl. 6), S27–33

38. DeVane, G. W. (1991). Premenstrual syndrome. *J. Clin. Endocrinol. Metab.*, **72**, 250–1

39. Rubinow, D. R. (1992). The premenstrual syndrome: new views. *J. Am. Med. Assoc.*, **268**, 1908–12

40. Mogil, J., Sternberg, W., Kest, B., Marke, P. and Liebeskind, J. (1993). Sex differences in the antagonism of swim stress-induced analgesia: effects of gonadectomy and estrogen replacement. *Pain,* **17**, 53–8

41. Regier, D. A., Boyd, J. H., Burke, J. D., Rae, D. S., Myers, J. K., Kramer, M., Robbins, L. N., George, L. K., Karno, M. and Locke, B. Z. (1988). One-month prevalence of mental disorders in the United States. *Arch. Gen. Psychiatry,* **45**, 977–86

42. Best, N., Rees, M., Barlow, D. and Cowen, P. (1992). Effect of estradiol implant on noradrenergic function and mood in menopausal subjects. *Psychoneuroendocrinology,* **17**, 87–93

43. Hampson, E. (1990). Estrogen-related variations in human spatial and articulatory-motor skills. *Psychoneuroendocrinology,* **15**, 97–111

44. Phillips, S. and Sherwin, B. (1992). Variations in memory function and sex steroid hormones across the menstrual cycle. *Psychoneuroendocrinology,* **17**, 497–506

45. Caldwell, B. M. (1954). An evaluation of psychological effects of sex hormone administration in aged women. *J. Gerontol.,* **9**, 168–74

46. Phillips, S. and Sherwin, B. (1992). Effects of estrogen on memory function in surgically menopausal women. *Psychoneuroendocrinology,* **17**, 485–95

47. Funk, J., Mortel, K. and Meyer, J. (1991). Effects of estrogen replacement therapy on cerebral perfusion and cognition among postmenopausal women. *Dementia,* **2**, 268–72

48. Fillit, H., Weinreb, H., Cholst, I., Luine, V., McEwen, B. S., Amador, R. and Zabriskie, J. (1986). **11**, 337–345.q

49. Honjo, H., Ogino, Y., Naitoh, K., Urabe, M., Kitawaki, J., Yasuda, J., Yamamoto, T., Ishihara, S., Okada, H., Yonezawa, T., Hayashi, K. and Nambara, T. (1989). *In vivo* effects by estrone sulfate on the central nervous system-senile dementia (Alzheimer's type). *J. Steroid Biochem.,* **34**, 521–5

50. Birge, S. (1993). The role of estrogen deficiency in the aging central nervous system. In Lobo, R. (ed.) *Treatment of the Postmenopausal Woman,* (New York: Raven Press)

30

Activating effects of estradiol on brain activity

S. S. Smith

Numerous physiological and behavioral reports suggest that estradiol exerts activating effects on mood, behavior and brain excitability. Elevated levels of this hormone in the circulation are followed not only by events with reproductive significance[1], but are also associated with facilitation of an entire array of sensorimotor parameters. These include: increases in locomotor activity[2,3] and increases in sensory perception for a variety of modalities[4], including fine touch, hearing, olfaction and visual signal detection. In the rat, the receptive field size for whisker barrelfield[5] and pudendal nerve[6] are enhanced following chronic treatment with estradiol. Limb coordination is also improved. Rats in estrus perform more accurately in hurdle negotiation tasks, treadmill and balance beam walking and running in square wheels, measures of coordinated limb movement[7,8]. In man, rates of finger tapping are increased[9] and manual dexterity is enhanced[10] at the mid-cycle peak of this hormone.

A number of clinical studies suggest that increased levels of estradiol in the circulation are also correlated with 'activating' effects[11] on mood. Feelings of euphoria, elation or anxiety and increases in energy can reportedly occur at the time of the pre-ovulatory surge of estradiol[12,13]. Attentional mechanisms and short-term memory may also be enhanced following cyclic elevations in estradiol, as assessed by a reduced level of distractability[14-15]. Increased cortical levels of activation and increased alertness, as well as shorter reaction times are seen during the follicular (estrogen dominant) stage of the cycle[13,14]. In animal studies, results from two-stimulus and runway tests indicate that the ability to attend to a task is improved on the day of estrus, while distractability increases on diestrus (low estradiol)[15].

Further evidence for this activating action of estradiol is provided by reports of its proconvulsant action. Cyclic elevations in circulating estradiol can exacerbate ongoing convulsive activity, although this effect is dependent upon the seizure subtype[16,17]. Estradiol administration can also facilitate the acquisition of amygdala-kindled seizures in experimental animals[18]. This proconvulsant effect appears to be a direct action, as local application of estradiol to the surface of the cat cerebral cortex induces focal seizures characterized by 2–3 Hz spike and slow wave discharge[19]. However, the proconvulsant action of this steroid may depend upon the underlying central nervous system (CNS) mechanism which generates the seizure – for example, estradiol can exert anticonvulsant actions when administered to rats with picrotoxin-induced seizures[20].

A number of studies suggest that some of these activating effects may be due to the excitatory effect of estradiol on brain activity. Estradiol appears to activate neurons within multiple and widespread CNS sites. Within hours of systemic administration of this steroid, the metabolic activity of most CNS areas is markedly increased, as assessed by 2-deoxyglucose utilization studies[21]. A number of studies also suggest that estradiol is able to exert rapid, non-genomic actions on neuronal excitability. Results from the present laboratory have demonstrated that estradiol, applied locally by pressure ejection or systemically at physiological concentrations, can enhance excitatory responses of neurons within the cerebellum (Purkinje cells) to excitatory amino acid neurotransmitters within minutes[22,23] (Figure 1). This effect was specific for certain neurotransmitter receptor subtypes (quisqualate and NMDA)[24] (Figure 2), and was long-term, persisting for at least 6–8 h after exposure of the neuron to the steroid. More recent data suggest that these effects

Figure 1 (Opposite) Locally applied estradiol augments Purkinje cell responses to glutamate. Strip chart records (left) and corresponding peri-event histograms (right) indicate changes in Purkinje cell response to glutamate before (upper records), during (middle records) and after (lower records) continuous pressure ejection of estradiol (0.5 μmol/l in 0.01% propylene glycol–saline) at 1–2 P.S.I. Each histogram sums unit activity from 4–5 glutamate pulses (solid bar, 23 nA) of 10 s duration, occurring at 40 s intervals. Glutamate-induced excitation is indicated as a percent change in firing rate relative to spontaneous discharge (numbers next to bars). Purkinje cell responses to glutamate were significantly enhanced within seconds after the onset of estradiol application, and did not recover to control levels of response by 30 min after termination of steroid application. (Reprinted from reference 23 with permission)

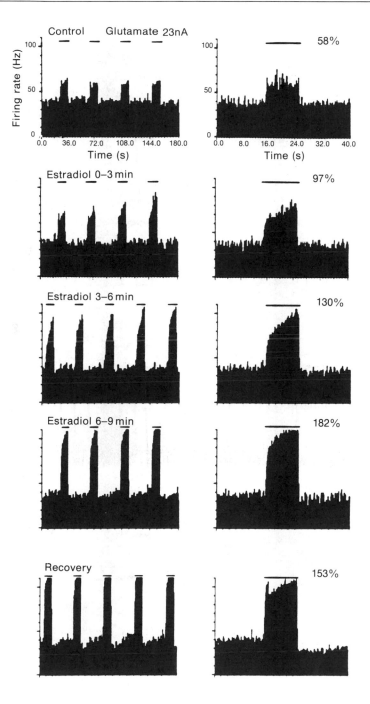

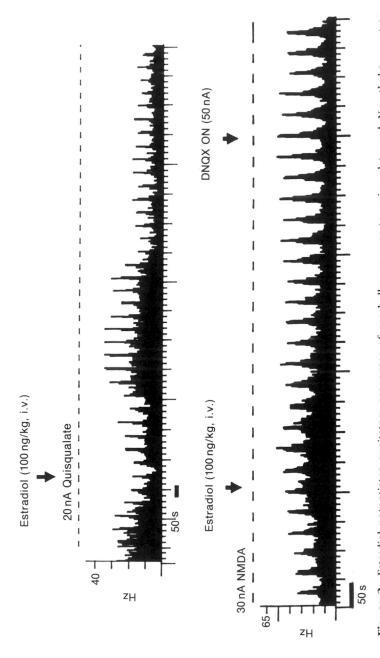

Figure 2 Estradiol potentiates excitatory responses of cerebellar neurons to quisqualate and *N*-methyl-D-aspartate (NMDA). Rate meter records demonstrate Purkinje cell responses to iontophoretic application of quisqualate or NMDA delivered as 20 s pulses (solid bars) at 50 s intervals over a period of 2 h. Responses of these neurons to NMDA are indirectly due to effects on the granule cell population. Each amino acid-induced excitation (numbers next to bars) is indicated as a percent increase in firing rate relative to spontaneous discharge and was evaluated before and for 5–6 min intervals after administration of estradiol (100 ng/kg, in 0.01% propylene glycol–saline) through a previously implanted jugular cannula in adult female Long-Evans rats (200–250 g), anesthetized with urethane (1.2 g/kg, intraperitoneally). Potentiation of quisqualate and NMDA-induced excitatory responses was achieved within 5–10 min after estradiol administration. (Reprinted from reference 24, with permission)

can occur in the cerebral cortex, and are observed in both male and female rats (S. Smith, unpublished data).

Potentiating effects of systemic estradiol on quisqualate[24] and glutamate[22] responses of Purkinje cells resulted in average increases of approximately 100% and 67–96%, respectively, by 15–30 min after injection of the steroid. In contrast, no effects on kainate responses of this system were observed. Local application of estradiol produced faster effects; glutamate responses more than doubled 3–5 min following the onset of continuous steroid application[23]. These effects were specific for the β isomer of estradiol, and were not dependent upon protein synthetic or classic steroid receptor-mediated mechanisms[22], suggesting a novel mechanism.

Initial studies of the neuromodulatory capacity of estradiol were performed in ovariectomized rats. More recent results suggest that the background steroid milieu can enhance the effectiveness of estradiol as a neuromodulatory agent. On estrus, following elevations of estradiol and progesterone in the circulation, estradiol produced a three-fold greater enhancement of quisqualate responses compared with results obtained on other days of the cycle[24]. Chronic exposure to estradiol may sensitize this system to the acute modulatory actions of the steroid. Although the cerebellar Purkinje cell does not appear to contain significant numbers of classic cytosolic/nuclear receptors for the steroid, the deep cerebellar nuclei have been shown to contain significant levels of mRNA for the estradiol receptor[25]. Thus, this hormone may be acting to up-regulate the binding capacity of its own receptor. Other long-lasting actions of estradiol on excitatory amino acid receptors or enzyme kinetics may also be involved.

Increases in neuronal sensitivity to excitatory amino acids following acute exposure to estradiol are not only observed in the cerebellum. A recent study has demonstrated that acute application of the β isomer of estradiol can also enhance responses of hippocampal CA1 pyramidal neurons to excitatory amino acid application[26], using the hippocampal slice preparation. This effect was specific for the non-N-methyl-D-aspartate (NMDA) receptor subtype, as responses to quisqualate, AMPA and kainate, but not NMDA, were enhanced by 1 min following application of 10 nmol/l estradiol to the slice.

This modulatory action of the steroid on potentiation of excitatory amino acid response appears to have a physiological outcome, as estradiol administration can also potentiate neuronal responses to stimulation, either electrically or behaviorally evoked[27]. Purkinje cell responses to forepaw stimulation were increased by an average of 30% 15 min following systemic injection of estradiol at a dose of 100 ng/kg (S. Smith, unpublished data; Figure 3). As glutamate is the excitatory neurotransmitter released at parallel fiber: Purkinje cell synapses, these results are consistent with previously published findings from this laboratory demonstrating estradiol-enhanced glutamate responsiveness of Purkinje cells. A peripheral effect of the steroid may also be involved in mediating this effect.

Estradiol has also been shown to enhance responses of hippocampal CA1 neurons to electrical stimulation of afferent pathways via increases in excitatory amino acid receptor sensitivity[26,28]. In the hippocampal slice preparation, 17β-estradiol (10 nmol/l) was able to produce a reversible depolarization and increased the amplitude of the Schaffer collateral-activated response (excitatory post-synaptic potential (EPSP)) less than 1 min after local application. The latter effect was blocked by the non-NMDA receptor antagonist 6-cyano-7-nitro-quinoxaline-2,3-dione (CNQX) but not by $\pm$-2-amino-phosphoropentanoic acid (AP5), suggesting that potentiation of non-NMDA receptors mediates this effect of the steroid (Figure 4).

In addition to these rapid effects of the steroid, estradiol was also demonstrated to exert long-term effects[26] on synaptic excitability using the hippocampal slice preparation, which may be due to more conventional genomic/receptor mechanisms. Chronic treatment with this steroid (10 μg, subcutaneously for 2 days) prolonged the EPSP and induced repetitive firing in response to Schaffer collateral stimulation to the CA1 region. An earlier report also suggested that estradiol was able to enhance responses of these neurons to electrical stimulation[29].

Other studies conducted in the hypothalamus also suggest that there are different short-term versus long-term effects of estradiol on neuronal excitability. In one study[30], chronic treatment with estradiol was shown to be excitatory, but not at excitatory amino acid receptors. Administration of estradiol (2 μg) for 1 week enhanced responses of neurons in the ventromedial nucleus of the hypothalamus to stimulation of afferent input and to application of acetylcholine[30]. In addition, inhibitory responses of these neurons to 5-hydroxytryptamine were also enhanced following chronic exposure to this steroid. The long-term nature of these changes may implicate genomic processes in the hypothalamus, a site rich in classic receptors for this steroid. Chronic estradiol administration (2 μg for 2 days) has also been shown to enhance responses of midbrain and pontine neurons to vaginal and somatosensory stimulation in the squirrel monkey[31].

Acute estradiol administration, although primarily excitatory outside the hypothalamus, can sometimes act in a depressant fashion. In particular,

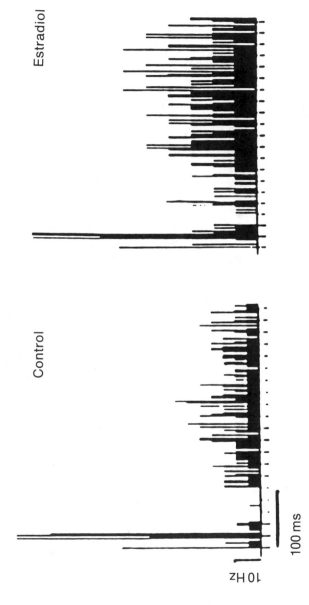

Figure 3 Purkinje cell responses to forepaw stimulation are enhanced after systemic administration of estradiol. Post-stimulus histograms indicate Purkinje cell responses to forepaw stimulation before (Control) and after systemic injection of estradiol (100 ng/kg, intravenously, in 0.01% propylene glycol–saline) to a urethane anesthetized rat in proestrus. Estradiol administration increased Purkinje cell responses by 35% above control responses

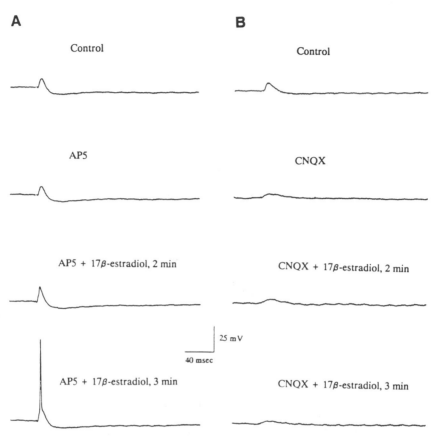

Figure 4 In CA1 hippocampus, synaptic potentiation by 17β-estradiol involves a non-N-methyl-D-aspartate (NMDA) component of the EPSP. The effect of AP5 and CNQX on synaptic responses of two different neurons that had exhibited synaptic potentiation by 17β-estradiol is shown. In control conditions, the Schaffer collaterals were stimulated with 0.1 ms, 50 μA pulses at a frequency of 0.1 Hz to elicit consistent subthreshold EPSPs. (A) In this neuron from an estrogen-primed animal, bath application of 50 μM AP5 had no significant effect on the Schaffer collateral-stimulated EPSP. In the presence of AP5, application of 17β-estradiol could still potentiate the EPSP. (B) In another neuron from an estrogen-primed animal, application of 10 μM 6-cyano-7-nitro-quinoxaline-2,3-dione (CNQX) significantly reduced the EPSP, leaving a small, presumably NMDA component. This residual component could not be potentiated by subsequent application of 17β-estradiol. (Reprinted from reference 26 with permission from the author)

neurons specialized for hypothalamic functions, such as reproduction and feeding behavior, are not activated by estradiol administration[32]. Acute

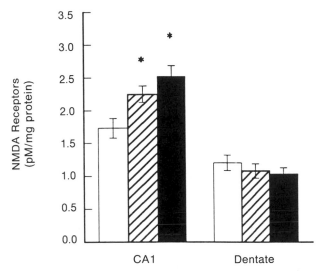

Figure 5 *N*-methyl-D-aspartate (NMDA) binding sites in the CA1 and dentate gyrus of the hippocampus. Treatment with estradiol (hatched bars) increased NMDA sites by 30% compared to ovariectomized rats (open bars) in the CA1 region. The level of NMDA binding after estradiol plus progesterone treatment (filled bars) was not significantly different from levels after treatment with estradiol alone. No steroid-induced changes in NMDA binding occurred in the dentate gyrus compared to ovariectomized animals (*$p < 0.05$). (Reprinted from reference 35 with permission from the author)

estradiol application hyperpolarizes neurons from the ventromedial hypothalamus involved in LHRH release[33], as well as glucose-sensitive neurons in feeding centers of the lateral hypothalamus[34]. In the latter case, this steroid has been shown to increase conductance of voltage-sensitive K^+ channels. The excitatory effects of the steroid, therefore, may be a more generalized effect. Earlier studies had reported variable effects of estradiol on neuronal activity in the hypothalamus.

There are several potential mechanisms by which estradiol may enhance excitatory amino acid responsiveness. First, chronic administration of physiological levels of estradiol has been shown to result in a 30% increase in NMDA receptor binding in the CA1 region of the hippocampus[35] (Figure 5). Thus, exposure to this steroid would amplify glutamate responses of neurons containing NMDA receptors, and could then enhance responses to afferent input. In addition, estradiol has been demonstrated to allosterically inhibit the activity of glutamate dehydrogenase, the enzyme which inhibits degradation of glutamate in the presence of high substrate availability[36]. Thus, glutamate actions would effectively be potentiated. Finally, estradiol can also increase release of glutamate from veratradine-stimulated hypothalamic synaptosomes[37]. Any one of these mechanisms could mediate the observed actions of estradiol on glutamate responses.

In addition to its direct actions on glutamate binding and degradation, estradiol exposure may also increase neuronal excitability by altering second messenger systems which have the capacity to potentiate excitatory amino acid responsiveness. As one example, estradiol (200 pmol/l) can amplify the level of phosphatidylinositol hydrolysis induced by activation of the Purkinje cell metabotropic receptor in estrogen-primed animals (S. Smith, unpublished data). Products of phosphatidylinositol hydrolysis, increased intracellular Ca^{2+} and protein kinase C, could then act to enhance glutamate responses due to activation of the NMDA receptor. In the hypothalamus, estradiol is also capable of depolarizing neuronal activity via a cAMP-dependent mechanism[34]. This effect, however, may be dependent upon classic receptor and genomic mechanisms. As some of the excitatory effects of this steroid occur in brain regions which do not concentrate estradiol, this mechanism may not be applicable.

In contrast to increasing excitatory amino acid function directly, activation of excitatory amino acid response may result from corresponding decreases in inhibitory amino acid response. Chronic exposure to estradiol results in a decrease in γ-aminobutyric acid (GABA)-A receptor density in many CNS sites[38]. In addition, estradiol treatment can suppress hyperpolarization induced by β-opioids and GABA-B receptor stimulation[39]. Thus, estradiol may also act via indirect mechanisms to increase neuronal excitability.

More recent studies have attempted to provide the link between the observed potentiating effects of estradiol on excitatory amino acid responses and the impact of this pharmacological effect on the activation of specific behaviors. This is accomplished by examining the actions of the steroids at the level of individual CNS circuits. The configuration of the circuit involved in a particular behavior will determine the outcome of estradiol effects on that behavior (i.e., due to presynaptic versus postsynaptic localization of amino acid receptors or the presence of inhibitory interneurons). This approach may help to explain the seeming incongruence between the proconvulsant and sometimes anticonvulsant actions of estradiol on different types of seizure activity.

Estradiol–circuit interactions have been evaluated most recently with regard to the facilitatory action of reproductive steroids on limb coordination. To this end, one relevant network to study is the olivo-cerebellar circuit, a necessary component of the motor system for achieving coordinated limb movement[40]. Within this circuit, inferior olivary neurons signal errors in limb position to cerebellar Purkinje cells[40]. As a result, Purkinje cell discharge is altered, thus resulting in a more appropriate limb position. One network strategy which could result in more accurate limb placement would target the strength of Purkinje cell responses to olivary (error signal) input, thereby increasing the sensitivity of the system to movement errors. (A heightened perception of 'error' in limb placement would allow for a more accurate correction in limb position.) Olivo-cerebellar synapses utilize glutamate primarily as their transmitter, and to a lesser extent aspartate, and contact quisqualate-selective excitatory amino acid receptor subtypes[41].

Again, based on pharmacological evidence, both local and systemic administration of estradiol specifically augments glutamate responses of Purkinje cells at AMPA- or quisqualate-sensitive receptor subtypes[23,24]. Therefore, one would expect increased response of the Purkinje cell to input from the inferior olive following increases in systemic estradiol. Cross-correlation analysis of olivo-cerebellar serial connections, recorded simultaneously, suggest that this is the case[42]. Responses of Purkinje cells to spontaneous olivary discharge are enhanced by an average of 30% on the night of estrus (Figure 6), following rises of estradiol concentrations in the circulation, compared with diestrus values. Thus, the Purkinje cell would exhibit enhanced perception of an error signal at this time, and the resultant change in discharge would produce a more accurate limb position. In this manner, increased responsiveness of the Purkinje cell to glutamate at quisqualate receptors could result in improved limb coordination, one behavioral change observed during cyclic elevation of the steroid.

A more recent finding suggests that estradiol-induced potentiation of NMDA receptor-mediated responses may also alter the behavior of populations of olivary neurons, recorded simultaneously with ensembles of microwires implanted chronically in the brain. An increase in the synchronization and oscillatory behavior of olivary neuron populations is a potential internal timing mechanism which may underlie hormone-associated improvements in rapid limb movements[43]. The observed effect of estradiol on facilitation of rapid limb movements[9,10] may be due to potentiation of this phenomenon. Administration of estradiol (30 ng, intraperitoneally) has been observed to increase the number of synchronized olivary neurons three-fold (S.S. Smith, unpublished data). The addition of progesterone enhanced this effect (Figure 7). These hormone-induced synchronized olivary oscillations could then be prevented by prior

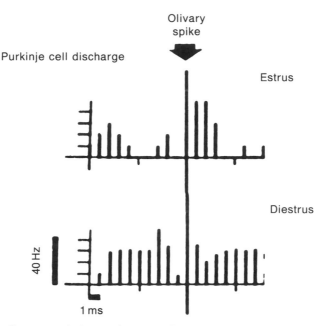

Figure 6 Cross-correlation analysis reveals a stronger olivo-cerebellar connectivity on estrus, following major elevations in the circulation of estradiol and progesterone, compared with similar values assessed on diestrus. In this figure, the firing of a cerebellar Purkinje cell is averaged around the spontaneous discharge of an olivary neuron (at arrow) recorded simultaneously across the estrous cycle of a rat. The Purkinje cell response (immediately following arrow) is greater on estrus than on diestrus. As this is a glutamatergic synapse contacting quisqualate receptors postsynaptically, these results suggest that estradiol enhances responses of Purkinje cells to spontaneously released glutamate at non-N-methyl-D-aspartate receptors. (Reprinted from reference 42 with permission)

administration of the NMDA antagonist MK-801 (100 mg, intraperitoneally). This finding suggests that estradiol enhances this network phenomenon via enhanced responses at NMDA receptors. Thus, studies at the network level confirm pharmacological findings, suggesting that potentiation of excitatory amino acid receptor function can lead to facilitation of activated states, such as seen during rapid and coordinated limb movement.

Estradiol as a reproductive hormone not only facilitates events which result in full reproductive capacity, but also enhances sensorimotor function, activates mood and can act in a proconvulsant fashion. Improvements in rapid, co-ordinated limb movements are observed when circulating levels of estradiol peak. In contrast, recent evidence also

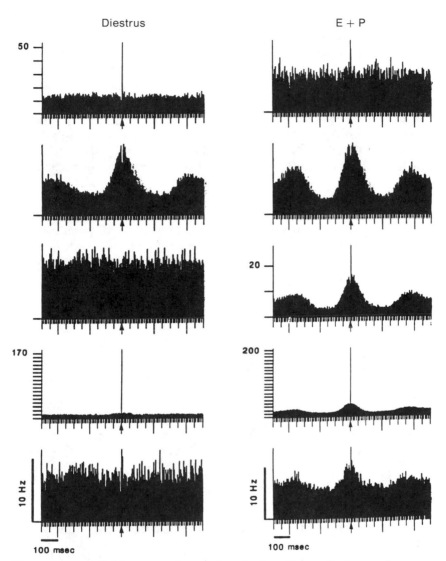

Figure 7 Estradiol increases the synchronized oscillatory discharge of a population of olivary neurons. Histograms of five olivary neurons recorded simultaneously are averaged around the spontaneous discharge of the neuron represented in the upper trace. The number of synchronized oscillating neurons is significantly increased after the administration of estradiol (E) (50 g, intraperitoneally) and progesterone (P) (50 ng, intraperitoneally), compared to those observed on diestrus. Administration of estradiol alone produced similar, but less extensive (by 50%) increases in synchronization

suggests that balance and co-ordination may be worsened when circulating levels of estradiol decline during the peri- and postmenopausal period (I. Persson, personal communication). Numerous reports suggest that estradiol can act to potentiate neuronal responses to excitatory amino acids in the cerebellum, cerebral cortex, hippocampus and hypothalamus. Other excitatory actions have been reported in the midbrain and pons. The impact of this pharmacological effect of this steroid on individual CNS circuits may serve to explain at least some of these effects of estradiol on mood and behavior. However, steroid level is only one of many factors which may have an impact on mood and performance in the human.

ACKNOWLEDGEMENTS

The author is grateful to R. L. Moss and N. G. Weiland for permission to reprint Figures 4 and 5. The author would also like to acknowledge J. K. Chapin for the development of computer software and neural network technology used to complete the steroid-circuit experiments.

REFERENCES

1. McEwen, B. S. (1988). Genomic regulation of sexual behavior. *J. Steroid Biochem.*, **30**, 179–83
2. Beatty, W. W. (1979). Gonadal hormones and sex differences in non-reproductive behaviors in rodents: organizational and activational influences. *Horm. Behav.*, **12**, 112–63
3. Morris, N. M. and Udry, J. R. (1970). Variations in pedometer activity during the menstrual cycle. *Obstet. Gynecol.*, **35**, 199–201
4. Zimmerman, E. and Parlee, M. B. (1973). Behavioral changes associated with the menstrual cycle: an experimental investigation. *J. Appl. Soc. Psychol.*, **3**, 335–44
5. Bereiter, D. A. and Barker, D. J. (1980). Hormone-induced enlargement of receptive fields in trigeminal mechanoreceptive neurons. I. Time course, hormones, sex and modality specificity. *Brain Res.*, **184**, 395–410
6. Kow, L.-M. and Pfaff, D. W. (1983). Effects of estrogen treatment on the size of receptive field and response threshold of pudendal nerve in the female rat. *Neuroendocrinology*, **13**, 299–313
7. Becker, J. B., Snyder, P. J., Miller, M. M., Westgate, S. A. and Jenuwine, M. J. (1987). The influence of estrous cycle and intrastriatal estradiol on sensorimotor performance in the female rat. *Pharmacol. Biochem. Behav.*, **27**, 53–9
8. Smith, S. S. (1991). Network properties of the olivo-cerebellar circuitry during spontaneous alterations in limb coordination. In *Proc. Soc. Neurosci.*, 551.7
9. Becker, D., Creutzfeldt, O. D., Schwibbe, M. and Wuttke, W. (1982). Changes in psychological, EEG and psychological parameters in women during the spontaneous menstrual cycle and following oral contraceptives. *Psychoneuroendocrinology*, **7**, 75–90

10. Hampson, E. and Kimura, E. (1988). Reciprocal effects of hormonal fluctuations on human motor and perceptual-spatial skills. *Behav. Neurosci.*, **102**, 456–9

11. Asso, D. and Braier, J. R. (1982). Changes with the menstrual cycle in psychophysiological and self-report measures of activation. *Biol. Psychol.*, **15**, 95–7

12. Friedman, R. C. (1982). *Behavior and the Menstrual Cycle*. (New York: Marcel Dekker)

13. Backstrom, T., Sanders, D., Leask, R., Davidson, D., Warner, P. and Bancroft, J. (1983). Mood, sexuality, hormones and the menstrual cycle. II. Hormone levels and their relationship to the premenstrual syndrome. *Psychosomatic Med.*, **45**, 503–7

14. Patkai, P., Johannson, G. and Post, B. (1974). Mood, alertness and sympathetic-adrenal medullary activity during the menstrual cycle. *Psychosom. Med.*, **36**, 503–12

15. Birke, L. I., Andrew, R. J. and Best, S. M. (1979). Distractibility changes during the estrous cycle of the rat. *Anim. Behav.*, **18**, 95–8

16. Logothetis, J., Harner, R., Morrell, F. and Torres, F. (1959). The role of oestrogen and catamenial exacerbations of epilepsy. *Neurology*, **9**, 352–60

17. Backstrom, T. (1976). Epileptic seizures in women related to plasma estrogen and progesterone during the menstrual cycle. *Acta Neurol. Scand.*, **54**, 321–47

18. Buterbaugh, G. G. (1987). Postictal events in mygdala-kindled female rats with and without estradiol replacement. *Exp. Neurol.*, **95**, 697–713

19. Marcus, E. M., Watson, C. W. and Goldman, P. L. (1966). Effects of steroid on cerebral electrical activity: epileptogenic effects of conjugated estrogens and related compounds in the cat and rabbit. *Arch. Neurol.*, **15**, 521–32

20. Schwartz-Giblin, S., Korotzer, A. and Pfaff, D. W. (1989). Steroid hormone effects on picrotoxin-induced seizures in female and male rats. *Brain Res.*, **476**, 240–7

21. Namba, H. and Sokoloff, L. (1984). Acute administration of high doses of estrogen increases glucose utilization throughout brain. *Brain Res.*, **291**, 391–4

22. Smith, S. S., Waterhouse, B. D. and Woodward, D. J. (1987). Sex steroid effects on extrahypothalamic CNS I: Estrogen augments neuronal responsiveness to ionophoretically applied glutamate in the cerebellum. *Brain Res.*, **422**, 40–51

23. Smith, S. S., Waterhouse, B. D. and Woodward, D. J. (1988). Locally applied estrogens potentiate glutamate-evoked excitation of cerebellar Purkinje cells. *Brain Res.*, **475**, 272–82

24. Smith, S. S. (1989). Estrogen produces long-term increases in excitatory neuronal responses to NMDA and quisqualate. *Brain Res.*, **503**, 354–7

25. Simerly, R. B., Chang, C., Muramatsu, M. and Swanson, L. W. (1990). Distribution of androgen and estrogen receptor mRNA-containing cells in the rat brain: an *in situ* hybridization study. *J. Comp. Neurol.*, **2**, 76–95

26. Wong, M. and Moss, R. L. (1992). Long-term and short-term electrophysiological effects of estrogen on the synaptic properties of hippocampal CA1 neurons. *J. Neurosci.*, **12**, 3217–25

27. Smith, S. S., Woodward, D. J. and Chapin, J. K. (1989). Sex steroids modulate motor-correlated increases in cerebellar discharge. *Brain Res.*, **476**, 307–16

28. Wong, M. and Moss, R. L. (1991). Electrophysiological evidence for a rapid

membrane action of the gonadal steroid, 17β-estradiol, on CA1 pyramidal neurons of the rat hippocampus. *Brain Res.*, **543**, 148–52

29. Teyler, T. J., Vardaris, R. M., Lewis, D. and Rawitch, A. B. (1980). Gonadal steroids: effects on excitability of hippocampal pyramidal cells. *Science*, **209**, 1017–18

30. Kow, L.-M. and Pfaff, D. W. (1985). Estrogen effects on neuronal responsiveness to electrical and neurotransmitter stimulation: an *in vitro* study on the ventromedial nucleus of the hypothalamus. *Brain Res.*, **347**, 1–10

31. Rose, J. D. and Michael, R. P. (1978). Facilitation by estradiol of midbrain and pontine unit responses to vaginal and somatosensory stimulation in the squirrel monkey. *Exp. Neurol.*, **58**, 46–58

32. Bueno, J. and Pfaff, D. W. (1976). Single unit recording in hypothalamus and preoptic area of estrogen-treated and untreated ovariectomized female rats. *Brain Res.*, **101**, 67–78

33. Kelly, M. J., Kuhnt, U. and Wuttke, W. (1980). Hyperpolarization of hypothalamic parvocellular neurons by 17β-estradiol and their identification through intracellular staining with procion yellow. *Exp. Brain Res.*, **40**, 440–7

34. Minami, T., Oomura, Y., Nabekura, J. and Fukuda, A. (1990). 17β-estradiol depolarization of hypothalamic neurons is mediated by cyclic AMP. *Brain Res.*, **519**, 301–7

35. Weiland, N. G. (1992). Estradiol selectively regulates agonist binding sites on the *N*-methyl-D-aspartate receptor complex in the CA1 region of the hippocampus. *Endocrinology*, **131**, 662–8

36. Pons, M., Michel, F., Descomps, B. and Crastes de Paulet, A. (1978). Structural requirements for maximal inhibitory allosteric effect of estrogens and estrogen analogues on glutamate dehydrogenase. *Eur. J. Biochem.*, **84**, 257–66

37. Fleischmann, A., Makman, M. H. and Etgen, A. M. (1990). Ovarian steroids increase veratridine-induced release of amino acid neurotransmitters in preoptic area synaptosomes. *Brain Res.*, **507**, 161–3

38. Schumacher, M., Corini, H. and McEwen, B. S. (1989). Regulation of high-affinity GABA$_A$ receptors in specific brain regions by ovarian hormones. *Neuroendocrinology*, **50**, 315–20

39. Kelly, M. J., Loose, M. D. and Ronnekleiv, O. K. (1992). Estrogen suppresses μ-opioid- and GABA$_B$-mediated hyperpolarization of hypothalamic arcuate neurons. *J. Neurosci.*, **12**, 2745–50

40. Houk, J. C. and Gibson, A. R. (1987). Sensorimotor processing in the cerebellum. In *New Concepts in Cerebellar Neurobiology*, pp. 387–416. (New York: Alan R. Liss)

41. Monaghan, D. T. and Cotman, C. W. (1986). Distribution of *N*-methyl-D-aspartate-sensitive L-[^{3}H]glutamate binding sites in rat brain. *J. Neurosci.*, **5**, 2909–19

42. Smith, S. S. (1993). Female sex steroid hormones: from receptors to networks to performance – actions on the sensorimotor system. *Prog. Neurobiol.*, in press

43. Ebner, T. J. and Bloedel, J. R. (1987). *New Concepts in Cerebellar Neurobiology*, pp. 371–86. (New York: Springer-Verlag)

31

Effects of natural and synthetic gestagens on mood and brain excitability

T. Bäckström

The effects of progesterone and progestagens on mood are generally considered to be negative. A number of reports concern the negative effects of oral contraceptives on mood, and mood changes related to the menstrual cycle in the premenstrual syndrome (PMS) are also well-known. Recent reports have also described negative mood changes during hormone replacement therapy with the addition of progestagens.

MOOD CHANGES DURING THE MENSTRUAL CYCLE AND THE PREMENSTRUAL SYNDROME

The menstrual cycle is characterized by cyclic changes of sex hormones produced by the ovary. Many chronic illnesses are influenced by these hormones, and since several organ systems have receptors for the hormones, an influence on their function is understandable. The function of the central nervous system is also affected: cyclic changes in epileptic seizures can be seen in many fertile women with epilepsy[1]. A variety of symptoms has been described as showing a cyclical pattern[2], most commonly, mental symptoms with depression, irritability, lack of energy and tension, and somatic symptoms of bloatedness, breast tenderness and changes in appetite[3,4].

The etiology of PMS is still unknown. A temporal relationship to the luteal phase of the menstrual cycle is, however, clear and many facts suggest that one or several provoking factors are produced by the corpus luteum. Symptoms start to develop in parallel with the initial development of the corpus luteum, and they disappear when estradiol and progesterone reach follicular phase levels at the end of the luteal phase[5]. During the preovulatory estradiol peak there are very few negative symptoms, but rather a period of well-being[5].

In anovulatory cycles the corpus luteum does not develop and there is no production of progesterone or its metabolites in the end of the cycle. Anovulatory cycles, whether spontaneous or induced by treatment with gonadotropin releasing hormone analogs, show diminished cyclical mood changes compared to ovulatory cycles[6-8]. High-dose estradiol implants, which cause anovulation, are reported to be effective in abolishing cyclical mood changes[9]. Danazol also inhibits ovulation and is reported to be effective[10], but it also has side-effects.

PMS patients were studied during two menstrual cycles with daily prospective ratings and daily blood samples for estradiol and progesterone measurements. The cycle with higher luteal phase concentrations of both estradiol and progesterone was associated with more severe premenstrual symptoms than the cycle with lower concentrations[11]. The results suggest that the severity of the symptoms is related to higher plasma levels during the luteal phase.

EFFECTS OF EXOGENOUS PROGESTAGENS ON MOOD

There are indications that only certain women are sensitive to production of negative mood changes by progestagens. Cullberg[12] noted that only women who had previously suffered from PMS reacted badly when taking oral contraceptives. This suggests that women with PMS are more sensitive to hormonal provocation than are women without. We also have some endocrine indications that the hypothalamo–pituitary unit is more sensitive to ovarian hormones in women with PMS than in controls[13]. This is important as it suggests that it would be possible to predict which patients would experience negative mood changes during hormone replacement therapy (HRT) – those who in their fertile life suffered from PMS.

In women taking combined oral contraceptives, a triphasic oral contraceptive pill is more likely to provoke symptoms than is a monophasic pill[14]. Qualitative differences also seem to exist between the progestagenic compounds. In one study desorgestrel was found to be less likely to provoke symptoms than was levonorgestrel[15].

POSTMENOPAUSAL HORMONE REPLACEMENT THERAPY

The estrogen/gestagen sequential replacement therapy given to post-menopausal women produces the same hormonal variations as during an ovulatory menstrual cycle; the estrogen-only treatment is similar to an anovulatory cycle. Women taking gestagen in the last part of the treatment period show a significant cyclicity in their mood and physical signs, whereas those receiving only estrogen show no deterioration of mood at the end of the treatment cycle[16]. The results suggest that progestagens, alone or in combination with estrogen, are involved in the provocation of the mood changes. A higher dose of a progestagen gives more severe symptoms than a lower dose[17].

POSSIBLE MEDIATORS OF PROGESTAGEN EFFECTS ON MOOD

Increasing numbers of reports indicate direct effects of ovarian steroids on the central nervous system. Many regions of the brain fulfil all criteria for being target organs for the steroids[18]. There are several possible mediators of the steroid hormone effects on mood within the central nervous system. One of the most interesting is the γ-aminobutyric acid-A (GABA-A) receptor, where both agonistic and perhaps antagonistic actions of steroids exist[19]. However, the exact chain of events between the action of a steroid and a particular mood in women is not yet established. Today we only know of agonists to the GABA-A receptor which have sedative effects. GABA-receptor antagonists, or so called 'inverse-agonists', which are anxiogenic substances, might also exist, however. The inverse-agonists are known to exist among benzodiazepines active at the GABA-A receptor but this has not yet clearly been shown for the steroids[20]. Some of the GABA-A receptor agonistic progesterone metabolites are very potent depressants of central nervous system function. This is particularly true for those steroids with a 3α-hydroxy-5 reduced molecule[21,22]. In an anesthesia model we have noticed that 5α-pregnane-3α-ol,20-one (3α-OH-DHP) is about eight times more potent than the most potent barbiturate known today, methohexital[23]. In an epilepsy model, 3α-OH-DHP is more potent than clonazepam, a benzodiazepine used in epilepsy treatment[24]. 3α-OH-DHP has also been tested clinically as an anesthetic[25].

Both anxiolytic and anxiogenic steroids might be produced by the corpus luteum in women with PMS or may be metabolites of exogenous progestagens in HRT and oral contraceptives. 5-Reduced steroids are produced by the corpus luteum and liver[26]. Progesterone, and probably also progestagens, can also be metabolized to 5-reduced steroids within the brain[27]. In studies of rat brain, all investigated areas had increased estradiol and progesterone concentrations at the time of high ovarian production[28].

ACKNOWLEDGEMENTS

This work was supported by CoCensys Ltd., Irvine CA, USA, Swedish Medical Research Council, Samverkansnämden i Norrland.

REFERENCES

1. Bäckström, T. (1976). Epileptic seizures in women in relation to variations of plasma estrogen and progesterone during the menstrual cycle. *Acta Neurol. Scand.*, **54**, 321–47
2. Dalton, K. (1984). *The Premenstrual Syndrome and Progesterone Therapy.* (London: William Heineman (1985))
3. Moos, R. H. (1969). Typology of menstrual cycle symptoms. *Am. J. Obstet. Gynecol.*, **103**, 390–402
4. Bancroft, J. and Bäckström, T. (1985). Premenstrual syndrome. *Clin. Endocrinol.*, **22**, 313–36
5. Bäckström, T., Sanders, D., Leask, R., Davidson, D., Warner, P. and Bancroft, J. (1983). Mood, sexuality, hormones and the menstrual cycle II. Hormone levels and their relationship to the premenstrual syndrome. *Psychosom. Med.*, **45**, 503–7
6. Hammarbäck, S., Ekholm, U.-B. and Bäckström, T. (1991). Spontaneous anovulation causing disappearance of symptom cyclicity in women with premenstrual syndrome. *Acta Endocrinol.*, **125**, 132–7
7. Muse, K. N., Cetel, N. S., Futterman, L. A. and Yen, S. S. C. (1984). The premenstrual syndrome, effects of 'medical ovariectomy'. *N. Engl. J. Med.*, **311**, 1345–9
8. Hammarbäck, S. and Bäckström, T. (1988). Induced anovulation as treatment of premenstrual tension syndrome – a double-blind crossover study with GnRH-agonist versus placebo. *Acta. Obstet. Gynaecol. Scand.*, **67**, 159–66
9. Magos, A. L., Brincat, M. and Studd, J. W. (1986). Treatment of the premenstrual syndrome by subcutaneous estradiol implants and cyclical oral norethisterone: placebo controlled study. *Br. Med. J.*, **292**, 1629–33
10. Watts, J. F., Edwards, R. L. and Butt, W. R. (1985). Treatment of premenstrual syndrome using danazol: preliminary report of a placebo-controlled, double-blind, dose ranging study. *J. Int. Med. Res.*, **13**, 127–8
11. Hammarbäck, S., Damber, J.-E. and Bäckström, T. (1989). Relationship between symptom severity and hormone changes in patients with premenstrual syndrome. *J. Clin. Endocrinol. Metab.*, **68**, 125–30
12. Cullberg, J. (1972). Mood changes and menstrual symptoms with different gestagen/estrogen combinations. A double blind comparison with placebo. *Acta Psychiatr. Scand.*, **236**(Suppl.), 1–46
13. Bäckström, T., Smith, S., Lothian, H. and Baird, D. T. (1985). Prolonged follicular

phase and depressed gonadotrophins following hysterectomy and corpus luteectomy in women with premenstrual tension syndrome. *Clin. Endocrinol., 22,* 723–32

14. Bancroft, J., Sanders, D., Warner, P. and Loudon, N. (1987). The effects of oral contraceptives on mood and sexuality: comparison of triphasic and combined preparations. *J. Psychosom. Obstet. Gynaecol., 7,* 1–8

15. Bäckström, T., Lindhe, B.-Å., Cavalli-Björkman, B., Nordenström, S. and Hansson, Y. (1992). Effects of oral contraceptives on mood: a randomized comparison of three phasic and monophasic preparations. *Contraception, 46,* 253–68

16. Hammarbäck, S., Bäckström, T., Holst, J., von Schoultz, B. and Lyrenäs, S. (1985). Cyclical mood changes as in the premenstrual tension syndrome during sequential estrogen-progestagen postmenopausal replacement therapy. *Acta Obstet. Gynecol. Scand., 64,* 515–18

17. Magos, A. L., Brewster, E., Sing, R., O'Dowd, T. M. and Studd, J. W. W. (1986). The effect of norethisterone in postmenopausal women on oestrogen therapy: a model for the premenstrual syndrome. *Br. J. Obstet. Gynaecol., 93,* 1290–6

18. Pfaff, D. W. and McEwen, B. (1983). Action of estrogens and progestins on nerve cells. *Science, 219,* 808–14

19. Majewska, M. D., Harrison, N., Shwartz, R., Barker, J. and Paul, S. (1986). Steroid hormone metabolites are barbiturate-like modulators of the GABA receptor. *Science, 232,* 1004–7

20. Braestrup, C., Schmiechen, R., Neef, G., Nielsen, M. and Petersen, E. N. (1982). Interaction of convulsive ligands with benzodiazepine receptors. *Science, 216,* 1241–3

21. Gyermelz, L., Iriarte, J. and Crabbe, P. (1986). Structure–activity relationship of some steroidal hypnotic agents. *J. Med. Chem., 11,* 117–25

22. Gee, K. (1988). Steroid modulation of the GABA/benzodiazepine receptor-linked chloride ionophore. *Mol. Neurobiol., 2,* 291–317

23. Norberg, L., Wahlström, G. and Bäckström, T. (1987). The anaesthetic potency of 3α-hydroxy-5α-pregnan-20-one and 3α-hydroxy-5β-pregnan-20-one determined with an intravenous EEG-threshold method in male rats. *Acta Pharmacol. Toxicol. Scand., 61,* 42–7

24. Landgren, S., Aasly, J., Bäckström, T., Dubrowsky, B. and Danielsson, E. (1987). The effect of progesterone and its metabolites on the interictal epileptiform discharge in the cat's cortex. *Acta Physiol. Scand., 131,* 33–42

25. Carl, P., Hogskilde, S., Nielsen, J. W., Sorensen, M. B., Lindholm, M., Karlen, B. and Bäckström, T. (1990). Pregnanolone emulsion. A preliminary pharmacokinetic and pharmacodynamic study of a new intravenous anaesthetic agent. *Anesthesia, 45,* 189–97

26. Bäckström, T., Andersson, A., Baird, D. T. and Selstam, G. (1986). 5-alpha-pregnan-3,20-dione in peripheral and ovarian vein blood of women of different stages of the menstrual cycle. *Acta Endocrinol., 111,* 116–21

27. Karavolas, H. J., Bertics, P. J., Hodges, D. and Rudie, N. (1984). Progesterone processing by neuroendocrine structures. In Celotti, F. (ed.) *Metabolism of Hormonal Steroids in the Neuroendocrine Structures,* pp. 149–83. (New York: Raven Press)

28. Bixo, M., Bäckström, T. and Winblad, B. (1984). Regional progesterone accumulation in the brain of the PMSG-treated female rat. *Acta Physiol. Scand., 122,* 355–9

32

The significance of steroid action at the GABA$_A$ receptor complex

D. A. Finn and K. W. Gee

INTRODUCTION

The γ-aminobutyric acid$_A$ (GABA$_A$) receptor complex (GRC) is a member of the ligand-gated family of receptors and contains several distinct, but interacting, modulatory sites which participate in the regulation of GABA-gated chloride ion conductance. Ultimately, ligands interacting with these modulatory sites adjust the gain of membrane chloride ion conductance and thereby influence the state of central nervous system (CNS) excitability. For example, benzodiazepine receptor agonists, barbiturates and GABA-positive steroids potentiate GABA-gated chloride ion conductance, while benzodiazepine receptor inverse agonists and GABA-negative steroids attenuate the actions of GABA. The identification of the steroid metabolites in the brain which interact with the GRC, termed neuroactive steroids, emphasizes the importance of these endogenous steroids as neuromodulators and provides an exciting new avenue for pharmacologic intervention in the treatment of neuropsychiatric disorders responsive to treatment via the GRC.

It was only within the last 10 years that the reported rapid (within seconds) onset of action of steroids was found to be mediated via an interaction with the GRC. The initial *in vitro* evidence was provided by electrophysiological studies demonstrating enhancement of GABA-stimulated chloride conductance by the synthetic steroid anesthetic alphaxalone (3α-hydroxy-5α-pregnan-11,20-dione) in rat brain[1]. These findings were soon extended to both the 5α- and 5β-reduced, 3α-

hydroxylated metabolites of progesterone and deoxycorticosterone. Subsequent studies identified the progesterone metabolite, 3α-hydroxy-5α-pregnan-20-one (3α,5α-P) and the deoxycorticosterone metabolite, 3α,21-dihydroxy-5α-pregnan-20-one (5α-THDOC) as the most potent GABA agonist steroid modulators at the GRC.

MECHANISM OF ACTION

Electrophysiological studies determined that 3α,5α-P and 5α-THDOC potentiate GABA-induced chloride conductance by increasing both the frequency (i.e. a benzodiazepine-like effect) and duration (i.e. a barbiturate-like effect) of channel opening in various cell preparations and in cells containing recombinantly expressed receptors[2-4]. The threshold concentration for enhancement of GABA-gated currents was 10–30 nM. At higher concentrations, the pregnane steroids directly activated the GABA$_A$ receptor. Intracellularly applied alphaxalone and 3α-hydroxy-5β-pregnan-20-one (3α,5β-P) had no discernible effects on the GABA$_A$ receptor, suggesting that the steroid binding site can only be accessed extracellularly[5]. In contrast to pentobarbital, which potentiated GABA-gated currents over a range of concentrations that also depressed currents mediated by glutamate receptor subtypes, alphaxalone and several endogenous steroids greatly enhanced GABA-gated currents, but had no direct effect on glutamate receptors[5]. In addition, progesterone administration *in vivo* enhanced GABAergic responses of cerebellar Purkinje neurons with a time lag consistent with the conversion of progesterone into an active metabolite[6]. *In vitro* studies demonstrated that both the 5α- and 5β-reduced 3α-hydroxylated metabolites of progesterone and deoxycorticosterone enhanced the binding of [^{3}H]flunitrazepam and [^{3}H]muscimol to the benzodiazepine and GABA$_A$ receptors, respectively, and allosterically inhibited the binding of [^{35}S]*t*-butylbicyclophosphorothionate ([^{35}S]TBPS) to the channel component of the GRC in a non-competitive manner[7]. Both 3α,5α-P and 5α-THDOC were also found to enhance GABA-stimulated chloride uptake in rat brain synaptoneurosomes at nanomolar concentrations[8]. The rapid effects and remarkable potency of these steroids on GABA-stimulated chloride conductance and uptake, combined with their heterotropic cooperativity at known sites on the GRC, suggested an independent site of action at the GRC.

Stringent structure–activity requirements were also observed for an action of the neuroactive steroids at the GRC, as determined by binding, chloride uptake and electrophysiological studies[7]. The stereoselectivity provided additional evidence for a specific site of action at the GRC. The two key features necessary for activity are a 5α- or 5β-reduced steroid A-ring and a 3α-OH group. Among all the endogenously occurring steroids examined, 3α,5α-P is the most potent, followed by its 5β-stereoisomer (3α,5β-P) and 5α-THDOC. The 3β-analogs (3β-hydroxy, 5α- or 5β-reduced pregnanes) are devoid of activity. Similarly, progesterone, estradiol, corticosterone, 5α-dihydroxytestosterone and cholesterol are inactive. An interesting modification is the reduction of the C-20 ketone to the hydroxyl, resulting in 5α-pregnanediol. This steroid has efficacy only in the presence of GABA, unlike 3α,5α-P and 5α-THDOC which can potentiate and directly activate GABA-gated currents. In addition, 5α-pregnanediol has limited efficacy in modulating [^{35}S]TBPS binding[9], in potentiating GABA-stimulated chloride uptake[10] and in the magnitude of GABA-evoked whole-cell currents (Callachan and Lambert, unpublished work), compared to 3α,5α-P.

Definitive evidence for an independent and specific site of action on the GRC for neuroactive steroids was provided by the observation of a steroid recognition site on recombinantly expressed GRCs derived from human cDNAs[4,11]. The binding and electrophysiology results obtained in recombinantly expressed receptors are consistent with similar studies using cell preparations and brain homogenates. The predicted heterotropic cooperative interactions between sites on the GRC and the stereoselectivity of steroid action are identical. Expression of various GABA$_A$ receptor subunits in human embryonic kidney 293 cells, which lack GABA$_A$ receptors or GABA, therefore provides an additional mechanism for understanding steroid action in the brain. Studies in brain regions or homogenates are complicated by the heterogeneity of GABA$_A$ receptor subtypes: the exact stoichiometry of subunits conferring functional GABA$_A$ receptors in specific brain regions is unknown.

Although the evidence is not as compelling as that for the GABA-agonist neuroactive steroids, steroids with GABA-negative actions have also been reported (e.g. pregnenolone sulfate and dehydroepiandrosterone sulfate (DHEAS)). Micromolar concentrations of pregnenolone sulfate and DHEAS antagonize GABA-gated chloride uptake in synaptoneurosomes and conductance in cultured neurons[12,13] in a non-competitive manner. Pregnenolone sulfate decreases channel opening frequency without affecting channel burst duration[14]. Recent work in recombinant GABA$_A$ receptors indicated that pregnenolone sulfate potentiated GABA-gated current at 0.1 and 1 nM concentrations in 50% of oocytes, but inhibited GABA-gated currents in 100% of oocytes at higher concentrations[15]. In addition, co-application of pregnenolone sulfate and 3α,5α-P implies that the inhibition by pregnenolone sulfate is exerted through a mechanism independent of the potentiation by $3\alpha,5\alpha$-P. Pregnenolone sulfate has also been shown to markedly reduce glycine-activated chloride currents[16] and to specifically enhance N-methyl-D-aspartate (NMDA)-gated currents[17] and NMDA-mediated elevations in intracellular calcium[18]. The excitatory actions of pregnenolone sulfate therefore appear to be due to an interaction with a number of neurotransmitter systems, rather than to a specific interaction with the GRC.

PHYSIOLOGICAL SIGNIFICANCE

An understanding of the physiological role of neuroactive steroids is extremely important. It is apparent that these endogenously occurring steroids can reach levels that are capable of modulating the GRC. Levels of $3\alpha,5\alpha$-P and 5α-THDOC in brain and plasma have been shown to fluctuate in response to stress and during the estrus and menstrual cycles of rats and humans, respectively[19,20]. Brain and plasma levels of $3\alpha,5\alpha$-P temporally follow those of progesterone: peak brain levels are observed in estrus in the rat and dramatically increase during pregnancy[21]. Both $3\alpha,5\alpha$-P and 5α-THDOC are detected in male rat brain, but the levels are low under most circumstances. Exposure of male rats to swim stress resulted in a rapid 4 to 20-fold increase in $3\alpha,5\alpha$-P and 5α-THDOC[20]. The brain levels of these 3α-hydroxysteroids measured after swim stress in males (approximately $3–10\,ng/g$ or $10–30\,nmol/l$) and during the estrus cycle (approximately $4–12\,ng/g$) and pregnancy ($\geq 30\,ng/ml$ or $100\,nmol/l$) in females[20,21] are, therefore, within the range of concentrations previously shown to potentiate the *in vitro* action of GABA at the GRC.

It is not yet established whether the endogenous neuroactive steroids found in the brain originate from peripheral sources (e.g. adrenals or gonads) or from *de novo* synthesis in the brain, although indirect evidence suggests that *de novo* synthesis of neurosteroids occurs. The enzymes responsible for the reduction of progesterone and deoxycorticosterone to their GRC-active metabolites, 5α-reductase and 3α-hydroxysteroid oxidoreductase, are present in the brain and localized primarily in the white matter or glia[22–24]. Estrus cycle-related changes in the brain levels of these enzymes have also been detected[22]. After castration and adrenalectomy, pregnenolone and dehydroepiandrosterone persist in the brain despite several weeks of peripheral steroid hormone deficit[25], suggesting independence with respect to peripheral sources. The most important evidence comes from studies conducted in brain-derived mitochondria and cell culture models which demonstrate that steroidogenesis occurs. The conversion of cholesterol to pregnenolone has been shown in rat brain-derived mitochondria[26]. Several cell culture models, comprised of glial cells or neurons and glia, have demonstrated the biosynthesis of cholesterol, pregnenolone, progesterone and 3α,5α-P following incubation with mevalonolactone[27–30]. It is unclear whether 5α-THDOC is actually synthesized *de novo*.

Nonetheless, it is important to consider that there are two potential sources of neuroactive steroids in the brain. One pool consists of steroids derived from peripheral sources and the second consists of steroids synthesized in the brain (neurosteroids). Therefore, brain levels of a neuroactive steroid may come from two different sources. The ultimate physiological significance of the different sources will depend on the steroid concentration achieved and the brain region affected. This is particularly important since there can be a big difference between steroids which reach the brain from distant sources and are in relatively low concentrations in the blood and brain extracellular fluid and steroids that are made locally in the CNS and can provide a high local concentration to adjacent brain cells.

Behavioral and biochemical studies

Behaviorally, the GABA-agonist neuroactive steroids possess anesthetic, hypnotic, anticonvulsant and anxiolytic properties. Both 3α,5α-P and 5α-THDOC are potent anxiolytics in several animal models of anxiety. The light/dark transition test is based on the natural tendency of rodents to explore novel environments, but avoid open, brightly lit areas, which are aversive to the rodent[31]. A variety of clinically established anxiolytics, including benzodiazepines and barbiturates, increase the number of transitions between the light and dark boxes. 5α-THDOC, injected intraperitoneally, significantly increased the number of light/dark transitions at doses of 7.5–15 mg/kg in male Swiss-Webster mice[32]. There was no decrease in generalized locomotion, although a trend for sedation was found following a dose of 30 mg/kg. Subsequent studies in male Swiss-Webster mice found that intraperitoneal administration of 5α-THDOC, 3α,5α-P and diazepam produced a dose-dependent anxiolytic activity in the light/dark transition test[33]. The doses producing significant increases in the number of light/dark transitions were as follows: 5α-THDOC (20 and 40 mg/kg), 3α,5α-P (10, 20 and 40 mg/kg) and diazepam (1, 5, 10 and 20 mg/kg). The 3β-stereoisomer of 3α,5α-P had no anxiolytic activity. In addition, the specific benzodiazepine antagonist CGS-8216 was unable to block the anxiolytic action of 3α,5α-P. In the open-field test, which measures the antagonism between the tendency to explore a novel environment and the tendency to remain still in an aversive (brightly lit) environment, 5α-THDOC (20 mg/kg), 3α,5α-P (20 mg/kg) and diazepam (10 mg/kg) significantly increased open-field activity compared to vehicle control[33]. An increase in open-field activity is characteristic of anxiolytics. Consistent with the results for light/dark transition, 3β,5α-P did not increase open-field activity over that of vehicle. In a lick suppression conflict paradigm[34] conducted in Sprague-Dawley rats, intraperitoneal administration of 5α-THDOC (10, 15 and 20 mg/kg) significantly increased punished responding[32]. There was no effect of 5α-THDOC on non-punished licking, although a trend toward sedation was found following the 20 mg/kg dose. Likewise, intraperitoneal administration of 3α,5α-P (20 mg/kg) disinhibited punished induced suppression of drinking[33]. 3α,5α-P produced a significant increase (237%) in the number of shocks received, whereas intraperitoneal chlordiazepoxide (10 mg/kg) produced a 197% increase in punished responding. Intracerebroventricular administration of 3α,5α-P (1.25, 5 and 10 μg) and 3α,5β-P (2.5, 5 and 10 μg) resulted in anxiolytic effects on the elevated plus maze[35]. Both steroids significantly increased the proportion of open-arm entries at all three doses and significantly increased the proportion of time spent on the open arms at the two highest doses tested. Administration of 10 μg of 3α,5α-P also caused sedation, measured by a decrease in locomotor activity. The anxiolytic action of 3α,5β-P was blocked by intraperitoneal administration of picrotoxin (0.75 mg/kg). This dose of picrotoxin did not significantly affect behavior on the plus maze. There was no effect of the 3β-stereoisomer of 3α,5α-P on either elevated plus maze behavior or locomotor activity.

In addition to the anxiolytic actions of some neuroactive steroids discussed above, 5α-THDOC also had inhibitory influences on aggression and defeat-induced analgesia in mice[36]. Administration of 3α,5α-P, but not 3β,5α-P, produced a potent analgesic response in mice[37]. 5α-THDOC also possessed potent sleep-inducing properties in rats[38]. In contrast, pregnenolone sulfate decreased pentobarbital-induced sleep time by approximately 30%[39]. These behavioral responses closely follow the anticipated patterns based on *in vitro* evidence, indicating that GABAergic steroids modify the functioning of central $GABA_A$ receptors *in vivo*, and may therefore participate in the physiological control of CNS excitability.

Due to the fluctuating progesterone and 3α,5α-P levels during the estrus and menstrual cycle, it is not surprising that behavioral and biochemical experiments have demonstrated estrus cycle-related differences in anxiety levels and seizure susceptibility and in sensitivity to benzodiazepines and barbiturates. Behavioral experiments indicated that female rats in metestrus were more anxious than proestrus females, as measured by burying behavior[40]. Females in proestrus were also more sensitive to the anxiolytic action of diazepam than were ovarectomized females[41] or females in metestrus[40]. Ovarectomized females trained to discriminate pentobarbital from saline were also observed to generalize test doses of progesterone to pentobarbital[42]. Although animal models and human studies suggest that anxiety levels vary during the estrus/menstrual cycle, it has been difficult to correlate emotional symptoms of premenstrual syndrome (PMS) with endogenous levels of 3α,5α-P, even though 3α,5α-P is anxiolytic[33,35]. Functional measurements of GRC sensitivity using a cuneate slice preparation indicated that the potentiating effect of pentobarbital was increased during estrus, whereas the potentiating effect of flurazepam was unchanged during the estrus cycle[43]. Chloride uptake studies indicated that ovarectomized females exhibited a reduced efficacy of GABA-stimulated chloride ion transport and lack of effect of diazepam to potentiate GABA-stimulated uptake, when compared to proestrus females[41]. One study indicated that there were no estrus cycle-related differences in the K_d or B_{max} for [^{3}H]flunitrazepam or [^{3}H]muscimol in cortex, striatum or hippocampus[44].

The variation in results presented above may result from measuring estrus cycle-related changes in GRC sensitivity to the effects of modulators other than neurosteroids (i.e. GABA, benzodiazepines or barbiturates). Recent work in our laboratory evaluated GRC sensitivity during the estrus cycle by measuring sensitivity to neurosteroids directly[45]. Allosteric modulation of [^{35}S]TBPS binding to the chloride ionophore was used as the measure of GRC sensitivity[46,47]. The results in washed tissue and in washed tissue plus 3 μM (+)bicuculline (to minimize the influence of endogenous GABA levels) indicate that 3α,5α-P is more potent in diestrus 1 than in estrus. The increased potency of 3α,5α-P during diestrus 1 (when endogenous levels of 3α,5α-P are low) and decreased potency of 3α,5α-P during estrus (when endogenous levels of 3α,5α-P are high) suggest that sensitivity of the GRC may change (via *de novo* synthesis of new receptor subtypes or post-translational modifications) to maintain homeostatic regulation of brain excitability.

Seizure susceptibility

The anticonvulsant action of progesterone and its metabolite are well documented. Over 50 years ago, Seyle first reported that progesterone protected rodents against pentylenetetrazol (metrazol)-induced seizures[48]. The prolonged latency of progesterone's anticonvulsant effect relative to that of its metabolites implied that progesterone was metabolized for activity. Subsequent studies demonstrated that $3\alpha,5\alpha$-P protected against metrazol-, (+)bicuculline- and picrotoxin-induced seizures, with maximum potency against (+)bicuculline-induce seizures[49]. The high potency of $3\alpha,5\alpha$-P against (+)bicuculline-induced seizures is consistent with its GABA-agonist action at the GRC. There was no protection by $3\alpha,5\alpha$-P against electric shock- and strychnine-induced seizures[49].

Recent animal studies investigating estrus cycle-related and sex differences in seizure susceptibility found a small but significant sex difference in metrazol seizure threshold[50]. Although there was considerable overlap between the scattergrams, the threshold dose for onset to seizures was lower in males than in females. In female rats a positive correlation between progesterone levels and (+)bicuculline seizure threshold was observed, although there was no significant difference between estrus cycle days or between males and females[51]. Recent work in our laboratory found estrus cycle-related and male/female differences in seizure susceptibility only for convulsant drugs specific for the GRC (i.e. methyl-6,7-dimethoxy-4-ethyl-β-carboline-3-carboxylate (DMCM)) and (+)bicuculline)[52]. (+)Bicuculline seizure threshold for onset to first myoclonic jerk was significantly lower in females in estrus than in females in diestrus 1 or males. The threshold for onset to generalized convulsions or tonic extension was significantly higher in males than in females in estrus or diestrus 1. DMCM seizure threshold for onset to all three seizure types was lowest in males and significantly lower in females in estrus than in females in diestrus 1. The higher seizure threshold in females in diestrus 1 versus estrus is consistent with recent *in vitro* data indicating that $3\alpha,5\alpha$-P is more potent in diestrus 1[45]. In addition, there were no estrus cycle-related or male/female differences in seizure susceptibility to picrotoxin, metrazol or strychnine[52]. Administration of $3\alpha,5\alpha$-P prior to infusion with metrazol significantly increased the threshold dose for onset to seizures and provided equal protection against generalized and tonic convulsions. Interestingly, the threshold dose for onset to first myoclonic jerk was significantly higher in females in diestrus 1 than females in estrus or in males[53]. These results suggest that there is a selective interaction between convulsant drugs specific for the GRC and estrus cycle-related changes in neuroactive steroid levels and potency.

Several clinical studies on the association between seizures and menses in female epileptics led to the hypothesis that cyclical variations in seizure susceptibility (i.e. catamenial epilepsy) may be correlated with changes in ovarian steroid levels[54-56]. Although some reports contained conflicting results regarding whether high levels of progesterone or estrogen increased the incidence of seizures, a recent clinical study indicates that seizure susceptibility in women with catamenial epilepsy is better correlated with levels of the GRC-active progesterone metabolite 5α-pregnanediol than estrogen[57]. One study in female epileptics found that infusion of progesterone to achieve plasma levels observed during the luteal phase of the menstrual cycle significantly reduced electroencephalographic spike frequency in four of the seven patients[58]. Another prospective study found that in a subset of women with epilepsy, changes in seizure frequency were observed in relation to hormonal variations during the menstrual cycle[59]. In the luteal phase when progesterone levels were high, the number of generalized seizures was low. These results suggest that progesterone and its metabolites may play a role in epileptic seizures.

CONCLUSIONS

It is now apparent that the neuroactive steroids, whether via peripheral sources or *de novo* synthesis in the brain, can alter brain excitability, and ultimately behavior, through an interaction at a specific steroid site on the GRC. In addition, selective enhancement of GABA-gated inhibition in particular brain regions may occur, based on recent evidence demonstrating brain regional differences in neuroactive steroid potency and in the coupling of steroid recognition sites to the GRC. This suggests that subtypes of the steroid recognition site may exist, and provides the potential for additional specificity of neuroactive steroid action. The physiological significance of neuroactive steroids in modulating brain excitability is further complicated by recent results indicating an inverse relationship between neuroactive steroid levels and potency at the GRC during the estrus cycle. Therefore, the increased potency of 3α,5α-P during diestrus 1 (when endogenous levels of 3α,5α-P are low) and decreased potency of 3α,5α-P during estrus (when endogenous levels of 3α,5α-P are high) suggest that sensitivity of the GRC may change (via *de novo* synthesis of new receptor subtypes or post-translational modifications) to maintain homeostatic regulation of brain excitability. It may be then, that behavioral changes due to endogenous GRC-active neurosteroid levels (e.g. anxiety or seizure susceptibility) would be observed only in disease states, when metabolism is altered or when the affinity of the receptor for neurosteroids does not change, so that the normal brain homeostasis is upset. This could explain the difficulty in correlating emotional symptoms of PMS with endogenous levels of 3α,5α-P. Further support for this notion is provided by the report that up to 75% of all women of fertile age notice some kind of cyclical mood changes, but only 5–10% of these women actually suffer from PMS[60]. Nonetheless, the neuromodulation of brain excitability by steroids via an interaction at the GRC provides insight into another mechanism by which the endocrine system may influence brain function and behavior.

REFERENCES

1. Harrison, N. L. and Simmonds, M. A. (1984). Modulation of the GABA receptor complex by a steroid anesthetic. *Brain Res.*, **323**, 287–92
2. Majewska, M. D., Harrison, N. L., Schwartz, R. D., Barker, J. L. and Paul, S. M. (1986). Steroid metabolites are barbiturate-like modulators of the GABA receptor. *Science*, **232**, 1004–7
3. Peters, J. A., Kirkness, E. F., Callachan, H., Lambert, J. J. and Turner, A. J. (1988). Modulation of the $GABA_A$ receptor by depressant barbiturates and pregnane steroids. *Br. J. Pharmacol.*, **94**, 1257–69
4. Puia, G., Santi, M. R., Vicini, S., Pritchett, D. B., Purdy, R. H., Paul, S. M., Seeburg, P. H. and Costa, E. (1990). Neurosteroids act on recombinant human $GABA_A$ receptors. *Neuron*, **4**, 759–65
5. Lambert, J. J., Peters, J. A., Sturgess, N. C. and Hales, T. G. (1990). Steroid modulation of the $GABA_A$ receptor complex: electrophysiological studies. In *Steroids and Neuronal Activity*, (Ciba Foundation Symposium 153), pp. 56–82. (Chichester: John Wiley & Sons)
6. Smith, S. S., Waterhouse, B. D. and Woodward, D. J. (1987). Sex steroid effects on extrahypothalamic CNS. II. Progesterone, alone and in combination with estrogen, modulates cerebellar responses to amino acid neurotransmitters. *Brain Res.*, **422**, 52–62
7. Belelli, D., Lan, N. C. and Gee, K. W. (1990). Anticonvulsant steroids and the GABA/benzodiazepine receptor-chloride ionophore complex. *Neurosci. Biobehav. Rev.*, **14**, 315–22
8. Morrow, A. L., Suzdak, P. D. and Paul, S. M. (1987). Steroid hormone metabolites potentiate GABA receptor-mediated chloride ion flux with nanomolar potency. *Eur. J. Pharmacol.*, **142**, 483–5
9. Gee, K. W., Bolger, M. B., Brinton, R. E., Coirini, H. and McEwen, B. S. (1988). Steroid modulation of the chloride ionophore in rat brain: structure activity requirements, regional dependence and mechanism of action. *J. Pharmacol. Exp. Ther.*, **246**, 803–12
10. Belelli, D. and Gee, K. W. (1989). 5α-Pregnan-3α,20α-diol behaves like a partial agonist in the modulation of GABA-stimulated chloride ion uptake by synaptoneurosomes. *Eur. J. Pharmacol.*, **167**, 173–6
11. Lan, N. C., Chen, J. S., Belelli, D., Pritchett, D., Seeburg, P. H. and Gee, K. W. (1990). A steroid recognition site is functionally coupled to an expressed $GABA_A$-benzodiazepine receptor. *Eur. J. Pharmacol. Mol. Pharmacol. Sec.*, **188**, 403–6
12. Majewska, M. D. and Schwartz, R. D. (1987). Pregnenolone sulphate: an endogenous antagonist of the γ-aminobutyric acid receptor complex in brain? *Brain Res.*, **404**, 355–60

13. Majewska, M. D., Demirgoren, S., Spivak, C. E. and London, E. D. (1990). The neurosteroid dehydroepiandrosterone sulphate is an allosteric antagonist of the GABA$_A$ receptor. *Brain Res.*, **526**, 143–6

14. Mienville, J. M. and Vicini, S. (1989). Pregnenolone sulphate antagonizes GABA$_A$-receptor-mediated currents via a reduction of channel opening frequency. *Brain Res.*, **489**, 190–4

15. Zaman, S. H., Shingai, R., Harvey, R. J., Darlison, M. G. and Barnard, E. A. (1992). Effects of subunit types of the recombinant GABA$_A$ receptor on the response to a neurosteroid. *Eur. J. Pharmacol. Mol. Pharmacol. Sec.*, **225**, 321–30

16. Wu, F. S., Gibbs, T. T. and Farb, D. H. (1990). Inverse modulation of γ-aminobutyric acid- and glycine-induced currents by progesterone. *Mol. Pharmacol.*, **37**, 597–602

17. Wu, F. S., Gibbs, T. T. and Farb, D. H. (1991). Pregnenolone sulphate: a positive allosteric modulator at the *N*-methyl-D-aspartate receptor. *Mol. Pharmacol.*, **40**, 333–6

18. Irwin, R. P., Maragakis, N. J., Rogawski, M. A., Purdy, R. H., Farb, D. H. and Paul, S. M. (1992). Pregnenolone sulfate augments NMDA receptor mediated increases in intracellular Ca^{2+} in cultured rat hippocampal neurons. *Neurosci. Lett.*, **141**, 30–4

19. Holzbauer, M., Birmingham, M. K., DeNicola, A. F. and Oliver, J. T. (1985). *In vivo* secretion of 3α-hydroxy-5α-pregnan-20-one, a potent anaesthetic steroid, by the adrenal gland of the rat. *J. Steroid Biochem.*, **22**, 97–102

20. Purdy, R. H., Morrow, A. L., Moore Jr., P. H. and Paul, S. M. (1991). Stress-induced elevations of γ-aminobutyric acid type A receptor-active steroids in the rat brain. *Proc. Natl. Acad. Sci. USA*, **88**, 4553–7

21. Paul, S. M. and Purdy, R. H. (1992). Neuroactive steroids. *FASEB J.*, **6**, 2311–22

22. Karavolas, H. J., Bertics, P. J., Hidges, D. and Rudie, N. (1984). Progesterone processing by neuroendocrine structures. In Celotti, F., Naftolin, F. and Martini, L. (eds.) *Metabolism of Hormonal Steroids in the Neuroendocrine Structures*, pp. 149–70. (New York: Raven Press)

23. Krieger, N. R. and Scott, R. G. (1989). Nonneuronal localization for steroid converting enzyme: 3α-hydroxysteroid oxidoreductase in olfactory tubercle of rat brain. *J. Neurochem.*, **52**, 1866–70

24. Celotti, F., Melcangi, R. C., Negri-Cesi, P., Ballabio, M. and Martini, L. (1987). Differential distribution of the 5α-reductase in the central nervous system of the rat and the mouse: are the white matter structures of the brain target tissue for testosterone action? *J. Steroid Biochem.*, **26**, 125–9

25. Baulieu, E. E. and Robel, P. (1990). Neurosteroids: a new brain function? *J. Steroid Biochem. Mol. Biol.*, **37**, 395–403

26. McCauley, L. D., Lan, N. C., Tomich, J. M., Shively, J. E. and Gee, K. W. (1993). Benzodiazepines and peptides stimulate pregnenolone synthesis in brain mitochondria. *J. Neurochem.*, in press

27. Hu, Z. Y., Bourreau, E., Jung-Testas, I., Robel, P. and Baulieu, E. E. (1987). Neurosteroids: oligodendrocyte mitochondria convert cholesterol to pregnenolone. *Proc. Natl. Acad. Sci. USA*, **84**, 8215–19

28. Jung-Testas, I., Hu, Z. Y., Baulieu, E. E. and Robel, P. (1989). Steroid synthesis in rat brain cell cultures. *J. Steroid Biochem.*, **34**, 511–19

29. Jung-Testas, I., Hu, Z. Y., Baulieu, E. E. and Robel, P. (1989). Neurosteroids:

biosynthesis of pregnenolone and progesterone in primary cultures of rat glial cells. *Endocrinology*, **125**, 2082–91

30. Barnea, A., Hajibeigi, A., Trant, J. M. and Mason, J. I. (1990). Expression of steroid metabolizing enzymes by aggregating fetal brain cells in culture: a model for developmental regulation of the progesterone 5α-reductase pathway. *Endocrinology*, **127**, 500–4

31. File, S. E. (1980). The use of social interaction as a method of detecting anxiolytic activity of chlordiazepoxide-like drugs. *J. Neurosci. Methods*, **2**, 219–38

32. Crawley, J. N., Glowa, J. R., Majewska, M. D. and Paul, S. M. (1986). Anxiolytic ctivity of an endogenous adrenal steroid. *Brain Res.*, **398**, 382–5

33. Weiland, S., Lan, N. C., Mirasedeghi, S. and Gee, K. W. (1991). Anxiolytic activity of the progesterone metabolite 5α-pregnan-3α-ol-20-one. *Brain Res.*, **565**, 263–8

34. Vogel, J., Beer, B. and Clody, D. (1971). A simple reliable conflict procedure for testing antianxiety agents. *Psychopharmacology*, **21**, 1–7

35. Bitran, D., Hilvers, R. J. and Kellogg, C. K. (1991). Anxiolytic effects of 3α-hydroxy-5α[β]-pregnan-20-one: endogenous metabolites of progesterone that are active at the GABA$_A$ receptor. *Brain Res.*, **561**, 157–61

36. Kavaliers, M. (1988). Inhibitory influences of the adrenal steroid, 3α,5α-tetrahydrocorticosterone on aggression and defeat-induced analgesia in mice. *Psychopharmacology*, **95**, 488–92

37. Kavaliers, M. and Wiebe, J. P. (1987). Analgesic effects of the progesterone metabolite, 3α-hydroxy-5α-pregnan-20-one, and possible modes of action in mice. *Brain Res.*, **415**, 393–8

38. Mendelson, W. B., Martin, J. V., Perlis, M., Wagner, R., Majewska, M. D. and Paul, S. M. (1987). Sleep induction by an adrenal steroid in the rat. *Psychopharmacology*, **93**, 226–9

39. Majewska, M. D., Bluet-Pajot, M. T., Robel, P. and Baulieu, E. E. (1989). Pregnenolone sulfate antagonizes barbiturate-induced sleep. *Pharmacol. Biochem. Behav.*, **33**, 701–3

40. Fernandez-Guasti, A. and Picazo, O. (1990). The actions of diazepam and serotonergic anxiolytics vary according to the gender and the estrous cycle phase. *Pharmacol. Biochem. Behav.*, **37**, 77–81

41. Bitran, D., Hilvers, R. J. and Kellogg, C. K. (1991). Ovarian endocrine status modulates the anxiolytic potency of diazepam and the efficacy of γ-aminobutyric acid-benzodiazepine receptor-mediated chloride ion transport. *Behav. Neurosci.*, **105**, 651–60

42. Heinsbroek, R. P. W., van Haaren, F., Zantvoord, F. and van de Poll, N. E. (1987). Discriminative stimulus properties of pentobarbital and progesterone in male and female rats. *Pharmacol. Biochem. Behav.*, **28**, 371–4

43. Westerling, P., Lindgren, S. and Meyerson, B. (1991). Functional changes in GABA$_A$ receptor stimulation during the oestrous cycle of the rat. *Br. J. Pharmacol.*, **103**, 1580–4

44. Hamon, M., Goetz, C., Euvrard, C., Pasqualini, C., Le Dafniet, M., Kerdelhue, B., Cesselin, F. and Peillon, F. (1983). Biochemical and functional alterations of central GABA receptors during chronic estradiol treatment. *Brain Res.*, **279**, 141–52

45. Finn, D. A. and Gee, K. W. (1993). The influence of estrus cycle on neurosteroid

potency at the GABA$_A$ receptor complex. *J. Pharmacol. Exp. Ther.*, **205**, 1374–9

46. Squires, R. F., Casida, J. E., Richardson, M. and Saederup, E. (1983). [^{35}S]*t*-Butylbicyclophosphorothionate binds with high affinity to brain-specific sites coupled to gamma-aminobutyric acid-A and ion recognition sites. *Mol. Pharmacol.*, **23**, 326–36

47. Gee, K. W., Lawrence, L. J. and Yamamura, H. I. (1986). Modulation of the chloride ionophore by benzodiazepine receptor ligands: influence of γ-aminobutyric acid and ligand efficacy. *Mol. Pharmacol.*, **30**, 218–25

48. Seyle, H. (1942). The antagonism between anesthetic steroid hormones and pentamethylenetetrazol (metrazol). *J. Lab. Clin. Med.*, **27**, 1051–3

49. Belelli, D., Bolger, M. B. and Gee, K. W. (1989). Anticonvulsant profile of the progesterone metabolite 5α-pregnan-3α-ol-20-one. *Eur. J. Pharmacol.*, **166**, 325–9

50. Kokka, N., Sapp, D. W., Witte, U. and Olsen, R. W. (1992). Sex differences in sensitivity to pentylenetetrazol but not in GABA$_A$ receptor binding. *Pharmacol. Biochem. Behav.*, **43**, 441–7

51. Wilson, M. A. (1992). Influences of gender, gonadectomy, and estrous cycle on GABA/BZ receptors and benzodiazepine responses in rats. *Brain Res. Bull.*, **29**, 165–72

52. Finn, D. A., Ostrom, R. and Gee, K. W. (1993). The influence of estrus cycle on neurosteroid potency and seizure susceptibility. *Proc. West. Pharmacol. Soc.*, in press

53. Finn, D. A., Ostrom, R. and Gee, K. W. (1993). Estrus cycle and sensitivity to convulsants and the anticonvulsant effect of 3α-hydroxy-5α-pregnan-20-one (3α,5α-P). *Soc. Neurosci. Abst.*, **19**, 1539

54. Laidlaw, J. (1956). Catamenial epilepsy. *Lancet*, **2**, 1235–7

55. Newmark, M. E. and Penry, J. K. (1980). Catamenial epilepsy: a review. *Epilepsia*, **21**, 281–300

56. Schechter, D., Labar, D. R., Pedley, T. A., Ottman, R. and Endicott, J. (1989). Influence of the menstrual cycle on seizures. *Epilepsia*, **30**, 704

57. Rosciszewska, D., Buntner, B., Guz, I. and Zawisza, L. (1986). Ovarian hormones, anticonvulsant drugs and seizures during the menstrual cycle in women with epilepsy. *J. Neurol. Neurosurg. Psychiatry*, **49**, 47–51

58. Backstrom, T., Zetterlund, B., Blom, S. and Romano, M. (1984). Effects of continuous progesterone infusion on the epileptic discharge frequency in women with partial epilepsy. *Acta Neurol. Scand.*, **69**, 240–8

59. Backstrom, T. (1976). Epileptic seizures in women in relation to variations of plasma estrogen and progesterone during the menstrual cycle. *Acta Neurol. Scand.*, **54**, 321–47

60. Andersch, B., Wendestam, C., Hahn, L. and Ohman, R. (1986). Premenstrual complaints. I. Prevalence of premenstrual symptoms in a Swedish urban population. *J. Psychosom. Obstet. Gynaecol.*, **5**, 39–49

33

An open trial of estrogen therapy for dementia of the Alzheimer type in women

T. Ohkura, K. Isse, K. Akazawa, M. Hamamoto, Y. Yaoi and N. Hagino

INTRODUCTION

Disturbance of the cholinergic neurotransmitter system is the most significant change of all neurochemical pathologies of dementia of the Alzheimer type (DAT)[1-3]. Acetylcholine is presently considered the most important neurotransmitter in memory and cognitive function[4,5]. Many investigators have reported a marked reduction in the activity of choline acetyltransferase (ChAT), an enzyme involved in the synthesis of acetylcholine in the cerebral cortex, striatum, and hippocampus of the brains of DAT patients[2]. Recently, the decrease of nicotinic acetylcholine receptors (n-Ach-R) in the cerebral cortex of DAT brains has also been reported[6-8]. In contrast, estrogen administration has been associated with increases in both the synthesis and activity of ChAT[9-11], and increases in the binding sites of hypothalamic n-Ach-R in rats[12]. The effects of estrogen in rats, however, show sex differences: estradiol administration increased the activity of ChAT in the nucleus of the diagonal band in oophorectomized females, but caused decreases or had no effect in castrated males[13].

In postmenopausal women, estrogen administration has been associated with a positive effect on attention span, concentration and libido[14,15]. Improvements in memory function have been noted in both pre- and postmenopausal estrogen-deficient women[14,16] and in surgically menopausal women[17] during estrogen replacement therapy (ERT). Serum levels

Table 1 Clinical summary of patients

Patient	Age (years)	Duration of illness (years)	Severity of dementia	Sulpiride (mg/day)	Mianserin (mg/day)
Group A					
KK	87	6	severe	50	—
ME	57	7	severe	30	10
KM	85	7	mild	—	—
MN	77	5	severe	—	—
OY	80	17	severe	—	—
Group B					
HM	76	7	moderate	50	10
KA	74	2	moderate	30	10
NR	70	3	mild	50	—
SY	70	4	moderate	30	20
WS	68	4	moderate	50	—
MY	78	5	mild	50	10

of estrone sulfate are lower in women with DAT than in senile women without DAT[18]. In the aging rat, the cessation of cyclic changes in circulating estrogen has been associated with suppression of hippocampal function; supplemental estradiol has been shown to restore this function[19]. Based on these observations, we speculate that the decline or cessation of cyclic changes in circulating estrogen in menopausal and postmenopausal women may be a contributing factor in the etiology of DAT.

These observations also suggest the utility of ERT in postmenopausal patients with DAT. In fact, Fillit and colleagues[20] and Honjo and co-workers[18] both reported improvements in psychometric assessments of estrogen-treated DAT patients in two separate studies. Their evaluations of therapeutic efficacy of estrogen in DAT patients included only psychometric assessment. This study reports psychometric assessment, regional cerebral blood flow (rCBF) and electroencephalogram (EEG) activity in DAT patients treated with ERT. No previous study has assessed the effects of estrogen in DAT patients using rCBF and EEG measurements.

SUBJECTS AND METHODS

Subjects

This protocol was approved by the Ethical Committee of Tokyo Metropolitan Institute of Gerontology. Informed consent was obtained from all participants and their spouses or guardians. Eleven female patients with DAT were identified and enrolled in the study (Table 1). Group A included five in-patients of the Tokyo Metropolitan Tama Geriatric Hospital (mean age ($\pm$ SE) 77.2 $\pm$ 5.4 years) whose dementia was diagnosed as severe (4) or mild (1). Group B included six out-patients of the same hospital (mean age 72.7 $\pm$ 1.6 years) whose dementia was diagnosed as moderate (4) or mild (2). The mean duration of illness ($\pm$ SE) in groups A and B was 8.4 $\pm$ 2.2 years and 4.2 $\pm$ 0.7 years, respectively. Patients in group B with moderate dementia had a shorter duration of illness and less severe symptoms than patients with moderate dementia in group A, and thus were treated as out-patients. Diagnostic Statistics Manual of Mental Disorders, third edition (revised) (DSM III-R)[21] criteria were used to establish DAT diagnosis and dementia severity. Multiple infarct dementia was excluded by the Hachinski ischemic score[22]. No patient had a Hachinski score >4. To supplement the DAT diagnosis, all patients were also evaluated by rCBF measurement with single photon emission computed tomography (SPECT) using *N*-isopropyl-*p*[^{123}I]iodoamphetamine ([^{123}I]IMP), computerized tomography (CT) and EEG.

The minimal required psychotropic drug dosages for sulpiride (30–50 mg/day) (common doses: 150–300 mg/day) and mianserin hydrochloride (10–20 mg/day) (common doses: 30–60 mg/day) were administered to eight patients before and during the studies, but the types and the doses of those drugs before, during and after ERT were fixed (Table 1). All patients underwent a pretreatment gynecologic examination including vaginal, cervical and endometrial Papanicolaou's smears. Gynecologic follow-up examinations were also performed during and after ERT to evaluate side-effects.

Estrogen administration protocol

ERT consisted of 0.625 mg of conjugated estrogens (Premarin) administered orally twice a day, continually for 6 weeks. Premarin comprises at least 10 estrogens; the estrogens present in the greatest amount are the sodium salts of estrone sulfate, equilin sulfate and 17α-dihydroequilin sulfate.

Psychometric assessment

Patient assessment before, during and after ERT consisted of the Mini-Mental State Examination (MMS)[23], Hasegawa Dementia Scale (HDS)[24], Hamilton Depression Rating Scale (HRS)[25] and the GBS-Scale (GBS)[26]. The scores for the MMS and HDS evaluations are inversely related to the degree of dementia (the higher the score the lower the degree of dementia). The scores for the HRS and GBS tests are directly related to the degree of symptoms of depression (HRS) and the degree of clinical symptoms of dementia (GBS).

Psychometric assessments were performed once in group A and three times in group B before ERT was initiated. The mean value of the three assessments in group B was regarded as the 'before treatment' value. During ERT, the assessment was performed twice (3 weeks and 6 weeks after the initial administration) in both groups and the mean value was regarded as the 'treatment' value. The last assessment was performed once 3 weeks after the termination of ERT. The HRS and GBS in both groups were performed once during each of three periods: 2–3 weeks before ERT, during weeks 4–6 of ERT, and 3 weeks after termination of ERT. All of the psychometric assessments were performed on all patients.

Regional cerebral blood flow (rCBF) measurement

SPECT was performed 15 min after intravenous injection of 6 mCi [^{123}I]IMP, using a rolling gamma camera GE400-AC. Box regions of interest (ROI) $12 \times 12 \, mm^2$ were set in 8 mm-thick horizontal slices parallel to the orbitomeatal line (OM-line) to count ROI activity in each cortex and basal nucleus. According to Johnson and colleagues[27], relative [^{123}I]IMP uptake was calculated as the ratio of each cortical ROI activity to the mean (right and left) cerebellar ROI counts (cortico-cerebellar ratio: CCR). The measurement was performed in 13 regions in each hemisphere at the levels of OM-20 (20 mm above OM-line), OM-50 (approximately 50 mm above OM-line) and OM-70 (approximately 70 mm above OM-line). SPECT was performed once within 1 month of initiation of ERT. Repeat SPECT was performed on all patients during weeks 4–6 of ERT.

Quantitative EEG

EEG activity from 21 channels (10–20 International Electrode System) was simultaneously recorded on paper and magnetic tape. Artifact-free resting records from Fp_1, Fp_2, F_3, F_4, C_3, C_4, P_3, P_4, O_1 and O_2 (ipsilateral ear reference) were quantified using fast Fourier transformation (FFT) analysis. EEG epochs (1024 points, sampling interval 5 ms) were average-accumulated ten times using a Signal Processor (San-Ei, 7T 18). The mean absolute power values for six frequency bands (Table 2) of each subject were calculated before and during ERT.

EEG was performed once within 1 month of initiation of estrogen administration and performed again during weeks 4–6 of ERT. Two EEGs

Table 2 Frequency bands of electroencephalography

δ	2.0–3.8 Hz
$\theta 1$	4.0–5.8 Hz
$\theta 2$	6.0–7.8 Hz
$\alpha 1$	8.0–9.8 Hz
$\alpha 2$	10.0–13.8 Hz
β	14.0–20.0 Hz

(patients MN and SY) were excluded from the statistical analysis because of interruption by artifacts.

Determination of serum levels of steroids and pituitary hormones

Blood samples were taken from all patients in group B before and 3 weeks after the initiation of ERT to determine serum levels of estradiol, estriol, testosterone, androstenedione, dehydroepiandrosterone sulfate (DHEA-S), luteinizing hormone (LH), follicle stimulating hormone (FSH) and prolactin. The samples were measured by radioimmunoassay (RIA) at Mitsubishi Yuka BioClinical Laboratories, Inc. (MBC). Using the MBC assay kit (DIRIA-ESTRK, Sorin Biomedica, Italy), the sensitivity of RIA for serum estradiol was 10 pg/ml and the mean ($\pm$SE) value of serum estradiol during the mid-follicular phase (days 6–9) of 15 women with the normal menstrual cycle in Koshigaya Hospital was 38.1 ± 3.9 pg/ml, which was lower than that measured by the other kits.

Statistical analysis

All statistical analyses were performed by the paired t-test.

RESULTS

Psychometric assessment

MMS

During ERT, one of the five patients in group A showed an increased MMS score from 4 to 7. In group B, five of the six patients showed an increase of 1.5–4.5 points in MMS scores: the mean ($\pm$SE) value of the six patients increased significantly from 15.3 ± 3.1 to 17.6 ± 2.9 ($p < 0.02$). The MMS score decreased after the termination of ERT in

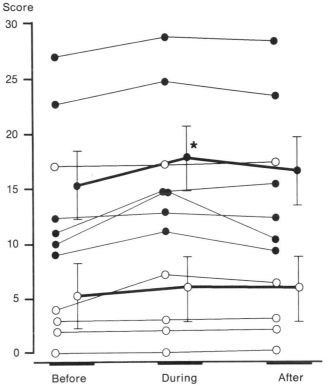

Figure 1 Changes in Mini-Mental State Examination (MMS) scores before, during and after estrogen therapy in out-patients with mild to moderate dementia of the Alzheimer type (DAT) (●) and in in-patients with mild to severe DAT (○). Vertical bars indicate the range of standard error. The full score for MMS is 30 points. $^*p < 0.02$ vs. before

group B to 16.2 ± 3.1, but was not significantly different from the pre-treatment score (Figure 1).

HDS

During ERT, the HDS scores of two patients in group A increased by 2 and 2.5 points, respectively, but no change in score was seen in the other three patients. In group B, HDS scores during ERT increased by 1–7.6 points and the mean ($\pm$ SE) value of the six patients increased significantly from 11.5 ± 4.2 to 14.9 ± 4.9 ($p < 0.05$). The HDS score decreased after

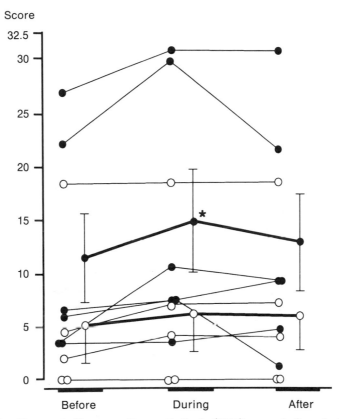

Figure 2 Changes in Hasegawa Dementia Scale (HDS) scores before, during and after estrogen therapy for out-patients with mild to moderate dementia of the Alzheimer type (DAT) (●) and in-patients with mild to severe DAT (○). Vertical bars indicate the range of standard error. The full score for HDS is 32.5 points. $^{*}p < 0.05$ vs. before

the termination of ERT to 12.8 ± 4.5, which was not significantly different from the pretreatment score (Figure 2).

HRS

In three patients in group A, HRS scores during ERT decreased from 10 to 9, 4 to 1, and 3 to 0. In the other two patients, the HRS scores before ERT were 0 and did not change. The mean value of the five patients in group A was not significantly different before, during and after ERT. The

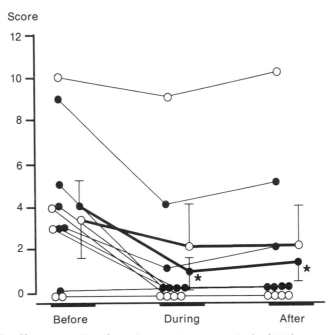

Figure 3 Changes in Hamilton Depression Rating Scale (HRS) scores before, during and after estrogen therapy in out-patients with mild to moderate dementia of the Alzheimer type (DAT) (●) and in-patients with mild to severe DAT (○). Vertical bars indicate the range of standard error. *$p < 0.02$ vs. before

mean HRS ($\pm$ SE) score in group B decreased significantly from 4 ± 1.2 to 0.8 ± 0.7 ($p < 0.02$). The HRS score in group B after the termination of ERT was 1.2 ± 0.8, still significantly lower ($p < 0.02$) than the pretreatment score (Figure 3).

GBS

The GBS scores of the two patients in group A decreased during ERT from 104 to 96 and 69 to 64. No changes in the GBS scores were seen in the other three patients. In group B, the GBS score of each patient decreased during ERT; the mean ($\pm$ SE) GBS score of the group showed a significant decrease from 35.2 ± 7.8 to 22.7 ± 6.9 ($p < 0.01$). The mean GBS score increased to 34.7 ± 7.8 after the termination of ERT, which

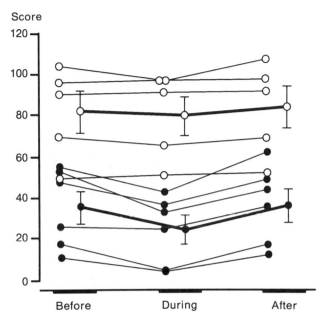

Figure 4 Changes in the GBS-Scale (GBS) scores before, during and after estrogen therapy in out-patients with mild to moderate dementia of the Alzheimer type (DAT) (●) and in-patients with mild to severe DAT (○). Vertical bars indicate the range of standard error

was not significantly different from the pretreatment score and was significantly higher than during ERT ($p < 0.001$) (Figure 4).

Regional cerebral blood flow (rCBF)

The mean rCBF during ERT increased significantly for the total study population, 23.0% in the right lower frontal region at OM-20 ($p < 0.02$) and 7.1% in the right primary motor area at OM-70 ($p < 0.01$) (Figure 5). In the other regions, no significant changes in the rCBF were observed during ERT.

Electroencephalogram

The mean absolute power values of δ band in both Fp_1 and Fp_2 decreased significantly during ERT ($p < 0.02$ and $p < 0.05$, respectively) in the nine patients of groups A and B. The mean power values of $\theta 2$

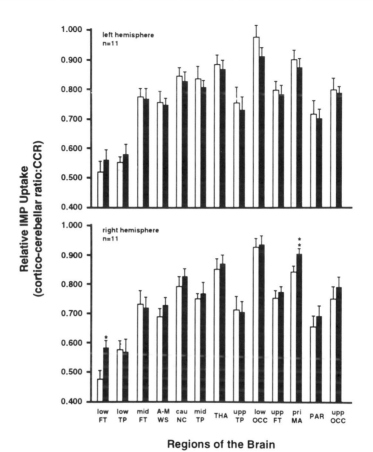

Figure 5 Changes in regional cerebral blood flow (rCBF) before and during estrogen therapy. The rCBF is represented by the cortico-cerebellar ratio. Open and closed columns indicate before and during estrogen therapy, respectively. $^*p < 0.02$ vs. before, $^{**}p < 0.01$ vs. before. Low FT = lower frontal region; low TP = lower temporal region; mid FT = middle frontal region; A-M WS = watershed area; cau NC = caudate nucleus; mid TP = middle temporal region; THA = thalamus; upp TP = upper temporal region; low OCC = lower occipital region; upp FT = upper frontal region; priMA = primary motor area; PAR = parietal region; upp OCC = upper occipital region

band in both O_1 and O_2 also decreased significantly during the treatment ($p < 0.05$ and $p < 0.02$, respectively, Figure 6).

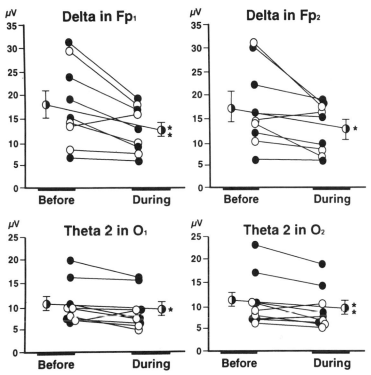

Figure 6 Significant changes in absolute power values in quantitative electroencephalogram before and during estrogen therapy. ●, out-patients with mild to moderate DAT; ○, in-patients with mild to severe DAT. Vertical bars indicate the range of standard error (groups A and B, $n = 9$). No significant changes were observed in any regions and bands other than those illustrated here. $^*p < 0.05$ vs. before, $^{**}p < 0.02$ vs. before

Serum levels of steroids and pituitary hormones

During ERT, the mean serum estradiol levels significantly increased from 10.2 ± 0.2 pg/ml to 29.7 ± 7.2 pg/ml ($p < 0.05$) in group B (estradiol levels < 10 pg/ml ($n = 5$) before ERT were calculated as 10 pg/ml). The mean serum estriol levels increased from 2.2 ± 0.2 pg/ml to 5.3 ± 1.4 pg/ml, but this was not statistically significant (estriol levels < 2 pg/ml ($n = 4$) before ERT were calculated as 2 pg/ml). The serum levels of other steroid hormones (testosterone, androstenedione and DHEA-S) showed no significant changes. ERT significantly suppressed serum levels of LH and FSH ($p < 0.01$ and $p < 0.001$, respectively) and significantly increased prolactin levels ($p < 0.05$). The mean prolactin

Table 3 Serum hormone levels before and during estrogen administration

	Before	*During*
Estradiol (pg/ml)	10.2 ± 0.2	29.7 ± 7.2*
Estriol (pg/ml)	2.2 ± 0.2	5.3 ± 1.4
Testosterone (ng/ml)	0.55 ± 0.07	0.60 ± 0.04
Androstenedione (ng/ml)	0.47 ± 0.06	0.41 ± 0.16
Dehydroepiandrosterone sulfate (ng/ml)	347 ± 93	356 ± 92
Luteinizing hormone (mIU/ml)	20.2 ± 2.9	1.9 ± 0.6**
Follicle stimulating hormone (mIU/ml)	85.4 ± 10.8	6.4 ± 2.3+
Prolactin (ng/ml)	24.6 ± 7.9	54.7 ± 11.1*

Data are presented as mean ± SE
*$p < 0.05$ vs. before; **$p < 0.01$ vs. before; +$p < 0.001$ vs. before

level before ERT exceeded the normal prolactin level (normal range < 14.6 ng/ml). Table 3 presents a summary of serum levels of hormones before and during estrogen administration.

Gynecological changes and side-effects

The maturation index (MI) of vaginal smears of all patients changed from 'shift to the left' before ERT to 'shift to the right' or 'a peak in the middle' during ERT. Senile vaginitis, observed in four of the 11 patients at baseline, was not observed during and after estrogen administration.

In Papanicolaou's smears, one patient's diagnosis changed from a baseline class II (primarily vaginal and cervical) to class IIIa (vaginal, cervical and endometrial), but returned to class II (vaginal, cervical and endometrial) on a repeat smear following withdrawal bleeding caused by the termination of estrogen administration; a follow-up endometrial biopsy showed no abnormal changes. In the other ten patients, no abnormality in Pap smears before, during and after ERT was observed. Withdrawal bleeding occurred in ten of the 11 patients. Transient breast tenderness or redness of the papilla mammae was observed in most cases.

DISCUSSION

No pharmacologic treatment has yet been proven effective in DAT except tacrine, a cholinesterase inhibitor[28]. Treatment with acetylcholine precursors such as phosphatidylcholine or lecithin[29] or anticholinesterase drugs such as physostigmine[30] or tetrahydroaminoacridine[31] is based on the observed reduction of activity of the ChAT enzyme – synthesis of acetylcholine from choline and acetyl-CoA is catalyzed intraneuronally by

ChAT – in the cerebral cortex, striatum and hippocampus of DAT patients[2]. These cholinergic precursors have not been shown effective in improving cognitive function, although some evidence suggests that they may slow the rate of cognitive decline. In comparison to the cholinergic precursors, the anticholinesterase drugs in DAT patients are more encouraging[28,31].

As an alternative approach to modifying the central cholinergic deficit, Fillit and colleagues[20] gave 2 mg/day of micronized estradiol to 7 female patients with DAT for 6 weeks. Only three patients showed significant improvements in attention, orientation, mood and social interaction as measured by psychometric assessment such as MMS, HRS, and Randt Memory Test[32]. Response to estradiol therapy in three patients appeared to be correlated with higher baselines of HRS and cognitive status (MMS and Randt Memory Test). Three years later, Honjo and colleagues[18] reported that five of seven female DAT patients treated with a dose of 1.25 mg/day conjugated estrogens (Premarin) over 6 weeks showed significant improvements in HDS, and six of seven showed improvements in a new screening test for dementia developed by the Japanese National Mental Health. They noted special improvements in memory, orientation and calculation.

In our study, improvements in psychometric assessment were observed in only two group A patients. However, apparent improvements in clinical symptoms in these two patients were observed not only by the authors but also by the nurses and the patients' families, whose observations were reflected in the changes in the GBS scores. This low response rate in the group A patients may be related to their degree of dementia at baseline, except for one patient whose MMS and HDS scores at baseline were 17 and 18.5, respectively. The MMS, HDS and HRS scores were very low in four of the five group A patients at baseline, suggesting that the depressive condition was a negligible clinical feature in this group. Patients in group B showed statistically significant improvements in all psychometric tests. The improvements, however, disappeared and the scores returned to the baseline levels after the termination of ERT, suggesting the value of ERT in these patients. All the families of the group B patients described improvements in patients' deeds in daily life. These families, including those of the group A patients KK and ME, requested continuation of ERT long-term. Improvements were noted in recent and/or distant memory (in attention, orientation, changes in personality related to mood, and vegetative symptoms (such as feeding and sleeping), as previously observed by Fillit and colleagues[20]).

Antidepressant effects of conjugated estrogens have been suggested by others[33,34]. These antidepressant effects may, however, be related to the levels of depression at baseline. Fillit and co-workers[20] indicated that the higher the HRS scores (increased degree of depressive symptoms), the higher the antidepressant effect of estrogen. They observed a median baseline HRS score of 21 for estrogen responders, compared to the median baseline HRS score of 9 for non-responders. The median HRS score in our study was much lower at baseline: 4 in group A and 3.5 in group B. The low HRS score was due partly to the chronic administration of low doses of sulpiride and mianserin, except in three patients of group A.

Even though our patients demonstrated low HRS scores, they responded well and demonstrated improved cognitive function during ERT. The effect of ERT on DAT was therefore not considered to be secondary to the improvement in depressive symptoms. However, although HRS scores were low at baseline, they decreased further, and so a link between cognitive function and depressive symptoms could not be dismissed.

Improvement in memory function in association with ERT has been observed in postmenopausal women by Furuhjelm and Fedor-Freybergh[14] and Hackman and Galbraith[16], and in surgically menopausal women by Sherwin[17]. Ditkoff and colleagues[35] observed an overall improvement in mood and quality of life in postmenopausal women on ERT. Hagino[19] demonstrated that early aging female rats exhibited a decrease in hippocampal function that was restored during ERT.

The mechanism by which estrogen may affect cognitive and emotional function in DAT is not known. Some studies have suggested links between estrogen and increases in the synthesis and activity of ChAT[9-11]. Other studies have demonstrated that estrogens have effects on neural cells[36]. Estradiol has been described as a trophic factor during neuronal development[37] and also appears to play a role in the reparative neuronal response to injury[38]. Arimatsu and Hatanaka[39] showed that estrogen enhanced survival of cultured amygdala neurons. Many links between ERT and improved cognitive and emotional function have been hypothesized and continue to be studied.

Nuwayhid and co-workers[40] reported that intravenous administration of Premarin or 17β-estradiol produced a marked decrease in uterine vascular resistance and an increase in uterine blood flow, but did not affect other regional blood flows in ewes. However, Goldman and colleagues[41] noted an effect of intravenous estradiol on cerebral circulation in rats; within 10 min of estradiol injection, blood flow increased significantly in the frontal cortex (47%), hippocampus (36%), basal ganglia (33%) and cerebellum (27%); females were more affected than males.

The rCBF studies have suggested that [^{123}I]IMP uptake measured by SPECT in DAT patients reflects severity of dementia[27,42]. Hamamoto and colleagues[42] compared mild and moderate dementia, and observed a reduction in circulation to the temporal and parietal regions in the right hemisphere, but not in the left hemisphere. We have also observed an increase of rCBF in the right lower frontal region in association with ERT. This suggests that the increased [^{123}I]IMP uptake observed in our study may be related to the increased activity of cholinergic neurons, and that ERT may improve, in part at least, cerebral cortical function of DAT patients.

Quantitative EEG can be used to detect minor changes in brain function. It is non-invasive, provides a direct sample of brain activity in a numerical form, and is not influenced by motivational factors and practice effect as is neuropsychological examination. Quantitative EEG studies by Penttila and co-workers[43], Soininen and Parianen[44] and Uchiyama and colleagues[45], revealed that θ power values increase in mild DAT; as the level of DAT increases to moderate, α power values decrease; when the level of DAT becomes severe, δ power values increase in addition. In our study, during ERT we noted a decrease in absolute power values of δ and $\theta2$ bands, an observation that goes against the normal EEG evidence of the progression of DAT. However, the observed improvement in EEG did not always correspond to the degree of improvement in clinical symptoms. Continued study is necessary to understand EEG findings during ERT.

In our study, ERT increased the mean serum estradiol level up to the values of mid-follicular phase of the normal menstrual cycles in healthy women. Furthermore, ERT suppressed serum levels of LH and FSH, but did not affect serum levels of testosterone, androstenedione or DHEA-S. Prolactin levels, which were elevated prior to estrogen administration, perhaps due to the administration of small doses of sulpiride, increased further during ERT. Increases in prolactin levels are considered to be one of the causes for slight breast tension.

The patient whose Pap smear diagnosis changed from class II to class IIIa during ERT may be the result of improved surveillance. All subjects underwent vaginal, cervical and endometrial smear tests, but endometrial smears were often difficult to obtain in the elderly, whose uterine orifice was tightly closed. In this patient, after the initiation of ERT, the uterine orifice enlarged enough to allow a better endometrial smear sample to be obtained. Therefore, the possibility exists that class IIIa tissue was present but undiagnosed before ERT. Adequate observation of the endometrium is necessary when estrogen is used long-term.

ACKNOWLEDGEMENTS

The authors wish to express their gratitude to Ms Akiko Yamaguchi and Ms Yukari Ogino for preparation of the manuscript. The authors also wish to express their gratitude to Mr Kevin D. Pawley for his editorial assistance. The study was supported by Grants-in-Aid for Scientific Research, The Ministry of Health and Welfare and The Ministry of Education, Science, and Culture, in Japan.

REFERENCES

1. Whitehouse, P. J., Price, D. L., Struble, R. G., Clark, A. W., Coyle, J. T. and DeLong, M. R. (1982). Alzheimer's disease and senile dementia: loss of neurons in the basal forebrain. *Science*, **215**, 1237–9
2. Bartus, R. T., Dean, R. L. III, Beer, B. and Lippa, A. S. (1982). The cholinergic hypothesis of geriatric memory dysfunction. *Science*, **217**, 408–17
3. Coyle, J. T., Price, D. L. and DeLong, M. R. (1983). Alzheimer's disease: a disorder of cortical cholinergic innervation. *Science*, **219**, 1184–90
4. Drachman, D. A. and Leavitt, J. (1974). Human memory and the cholinergic system. A relationship to aging? *Arch. Neurol.*, **30**, 113–21
5. Perry, E. (1988). Acetylcholine and Alzheimer's disease. *Br. J. Psychiatry*, **152**, 737–40
6. Nordberg, A. and Winblad, B. (1986). Reduced number of [^{3}H]nicotine and [^{3}H]acetylcholine binding sites in the frontal cortex of Alzheimer brains. *Neurosci. Lett.*, **72**, 115–19
7. Kellar, K. J., Whitehouse, P. J., Martino-Barrows, A. M., Marcus, K. and Price, D. L. (1987). Muscarinic and nicotinic cholinergic binding sites in Alzheimer's disease cerebral cortex. *Brain Res.*, **436**, 62–8
8. Whitehouse, P. J., Martino, A. M., Marcus, K. A., Zweig, R. M., Singer, H. S., Price, D. L. and Kellar, K. J. (1988). Reductions in acetylcholine and nicotine binding in several degenerative diseases. *Arch. Neurol.*, **45**, 722–4
9. Luine, V., Park, D., Joh, T., Reis, D. and McEwen, B. (1980). Immunochemical demonstration of increased choline acetyltransferase concentration in rat preoptic area after estradiol administration. *Brain Res.*, **191**, 273–7
10. Luine, V. N. (1985). Estradiol increases choline acetyltransferase activity in specific basal forebrain nuclei and projection areas of female rats. *Exp. Neurol.*, **89**, 484–90
11. Kaufman, H., Vadasz, C. and Lajtha, A. (1988). Effects of estradiol and dexamethasone on choline acetyltransferase activity in various rat brain regions. *Brain Res.*, **453**, 389–92
12. Morley, B. J., Rodriguez-Sierra, J. F. and Clough, R. W. (1983). Increase in hypothalamic nicotinic acetylcholine receptors in prepubertal female rats administered estrogen. *Brain Res.*, **278**, 262–5
13. Luine, V. N. and McEwen, B. S. (1983). Sex differences in cholinergic enzymes of diagonal band nuclei in the rat preoptic area. *Neuroendocrinology*, **36**, 475–82
14. Furuhjelm, M. and Fedor-Freybergh, P. (1976). The influence of estrogens on

the psyche in climacteric and post-menopausal women. In Van Keep, P. A., Greenblatt, R. B. and Albeaux-Fernet, M. M. (eds.) *Consensus on Menopause Research*, pp. 84–93. (Baltimore: University Park Press)

15. Vanhulle, G. and Demol, R. (1976). A double-blind study into the influence of estriol on a number of psychological tests in post-menopausal women. In Van Keep, P. A., Greenblatt, R. B. and Albeaux-Fernet, M. M. (eds.) *Consensus on Menopause Research*, pp. 94–9. (Baltimore: University Park Press)

16. Hackman, B. W. and Galbraith, D. (1976). Replacement therapy with piperazine oestrone sulphate ('Harmogen') and its effect on memory. *Curr. Med. Res. Opin.*, 4, 303–6

17. Sherwin, B. B. (1988). Estrogen and/or androgen replacement therapy and cognitive functioning in surgically menopausal women. *Psychoneuroendocrinology*, 13, 345–57

18. Honjo, H., Ogino, Y., Naitoh, K., Urabe, M., Kitawaki, J., Yasuda, J., Yamamoto, T., Ishihara, S., Okada, H., Yonezawa, T., Hayashi, K. and Nambara, T. (1989). *In vivo* effects by estrone sulfate on the central nervous system – senile dementia (Alzheimer's type). *J. Steroid Biochem.*, 34, 521–5

19. Hagino, N. (1981). Aged limbic system. Interactions of estrogen with catecholaminergic and peptidergic synpatic transmissions. *Biomed. Res.*, 2, 85–108

20. Fillit, H., Weinreb, H., Cholst, I., Luine, V., McEwen, B., Amador, R. and Zabriskie, J. (1986). Observations in a preliminary open trial of estradiol therapy for senile dementia-Alzheimer's type. *Psychoneuroendocrinology*, 11, 337–45

21. American Psychiatric Association (1987). *Diagnostic and Statistical Manual of Mental Disorders*, 3rd edn. revised. (Washington, DC: American Psychiatric Association)

22. Hachinski, V. C., Iliff, L. D., Zilhka, E., Du Boulay, G. H., McAllister, V. L., Marshall, J., Russell, R. W. R. and Simon, L. (1975). Cerebral blood flow in dementia. *Arch. Neurol.*, 32, 632–7

23. Folstein, M. F., Folstein, S. E. and McHugh, P. R. (1975). Mini-Mental State: a practical method for grading the cognitive state of patients for the clinician. *J. Psychiatr. Res.*, 12, 189–98

24. Hasegawa, K. (1983). The clinical assessment of dementia in the aged: a dementia screening scale for psychogeriatric patients. In Bergener, M. (ed.) *Aging in the Eighties and Beyond, Highlights of the Twelfth International Congress on Gerontology*, pp. 207–18. (New York: Springer Publishing)

25. Hamilton, M. (1976). Development of a rating scale for primary depressive illness. *Br. J. Soc. Clin. Psychol.*, 6, 278–96

26. Gottfries, C. G., Brane, G., Gullberg, B. and Steen, G. (1982). A new rating scale for dementia syndromes. *Arch. Gerontol. Geriatr.*, 1, 311–30

27. Johnson, K. A., Holman, B. L., Mueller, S. P., Rosen, T. J., English, R., Nagel, J. S. and Growdon, J. H. (1988). Single photon emission computed tomography in Alzheimer's disease. Abnormal Iofetamine I 123 uptake reflects dementia severity. *Arch. Neurol.*, 45, 392–6

28. Farlow, M., Gracon, S. I., Hershey, L. A., Lewis, K. W., Sadowsky, C. H. and Doran-Ureno, J. (1992). A controlled trial of tacrine in Alzheimer's disease. *J. Am. Med. Assoc.*, 268, 2523–9

29. Little, A., Levy, R., Chuaqui-Kidd, P. and Hand, D. (1985). A double-blind, placebo controlled trial of high-dose lecithin in Alzheimer's disease. *J. Neurol. Neurosurg. Psychiatry*, 48, 736–42

30. Blackwood, D. H. R. and Christie, J. E. (1986). The effects of physostigmine on memory and auditory P 300 in Alzheimer-type dementia. *Biol. Psychiatry*, **21**, 557–60

31. Summers, W. K., Majovski, L. V., Marsh, G. M., Tachiki, K. and Kling, A. (1986). Oral tetrahydroaminoacridine in long-term treatment of senile dementia, Alzheimer type. *N. Engl. J. Med.*, **315**, 1241–5

32. Brown, E. R., Randt, C. T. and Osborne, D. P. Jr. (1983). Assessment of memory disturbance in aging. In Agnoli, A., Crepaldi, G., Spano, P. F. and Trabucci, M. (eds.) *Aging Brain and Ergot Alkaloids*, pp. 131–7. (New York: Raven Press)

33. Klaiber, E. L., Broberman, D. M., Vogel, W. and Kobayashi, Y. (1979). Estrogen therapy for severe persistent depressions in women. *Arch. Gen. Psychiatry*, **36**, 550–4

34. Gerdes, L. C., Sonnendecker, E. W. W. and Polakow, E. S. (1982). Psychological changes effected by estrogen–progestogen and clonidine treatment in climacteric women. *Am. J. Obstet. Gynecol.*, **142**, 98–104

35. Ditkoff, E. C., Crary, W. G., Cristo, M. and Lobo, R. A. (1991). Estrogen improves psychological function in asymptomatic postmenopausal women. *Obstet. Gynecol.*, **78**, 991–5

36. McEwen, B. S., Biegon, A., Fischette, C. T., Luine, V. N., Parsons, B. and Rainbow, T. C. (1984). Toward a neurochemical basis of steroid hormone action. In Martini, L. and Ganong, W. E. (eds.) *Frontiers in Neuroendocrinology*, Vol. VIII, pp. 153–76. (New York: Raven Press)

37. Toran-Allerand, C. D. (1981). Cellular aspects of sexual differentiation of the brain. In Jagiello, G. and Vogel, H. J. (eds.) *Bioregulation of Reproduction*, pp. 43–57. (New York: Academic Press)

38. Jones, K. J. (1988). Steroid hormones and neurotrophism: relationship to nerve injury. *Metab. Brain Dis.*, **3**, 1–18

39. Arimatsu, Y. and Hatanaka, H. (1986). Estrogen treatment enhances survival of cultured amygdala neurons in a defined medium. *Dev. Brain Res.*, **26**, 151–9

40. Nuwayhid, B., Brinkman, C. R. 3rd, Wood, J. R. Jr., Martinek, H. and Assali, N. S. (1975). Effects of estrogen on systemic and regional circulations in normal and renal hypertensive sheep. *Am. J. Obstet. Gynecol.*, **123**, 495–504

41. Goldman, H., Skelley, E. B., Sandman, C. A., Kastin, A. J. and Murphy, S. (1976). Hormones and regional brain blood flow. *Pharmacol. Biochem. Behav.*, **5** (Suppl. 1), 165–9

42. Hamamoto, M., Yamazaki, M., Igarashi, H., Miyazaki, T., Isse, K., Uchiyama, M., Tanaka, K., Chiba, K. and Terashi, A. (1990). Single photon emission computed tomography in Alzheimer-type dementia. In Nagatsu, T., Fisher, A. and Yoshida, M. (eds.) *Basic, Clinical, and Therapeutic Aspects of Alzheimer's and Parkinson's Diseases*, Vol. II, pp. 59–62. (New York: Plenum Press)

43. Penttila, M., Parianen, J. V., Soininen, H. and Riekkinen, P. J. (1985). Quantitative analysis of occipital EEG in different stages of Alzheimer's disease. *Electroenceph. Clin. Neurophysiol.*, **60**, 1–6

44. Soininen, H. and Parianen, J. V. (1988). Quantitative EEG in the diagnosis and follow-up of Alzheimer's disease. In Giannitrapani, D. and Murri, L. (eds.) *The EEG of Mental Activities*, pp. 42–9. (Basel: Karger)

45. Uchiyama, M., Isse, K., Tanaka, K., Kuroda, A., Komazaki, H., Hamamoto, M., Igarashi, H. and Miyazaki, T. (1990). A clinical EEG study of Alzheimer-type

dementia. In Nagatsu, T., Fisher, A. and Yoshida, M. (eds.) *Basic, Clinical, and Therapeutic Aspects of Alzheimer's and Parkinson's Diseases*, Vol. II, pp. 159–62. (New York: Plenum Press)

Section 7

Estrogen effects on extragenital target tissues

34

Hormone replacement therapy – standardized or individually adapted doses? – effect on bone mass

C. Christiansen

INTRODUCTION

Osteoporosis is a major public health problem occurring primarily among the postmenopausal population. Its relationship to loss of ovarian function was originally described in an elegant clinical study of the disease by Albright and colleagues more than 50 years ago[1]. However, there are still questions about the use of sex steroids in the prevention and treatment of the disease, that clinicians face on a regular basis.

This review evaluates the role of sex steroids, paying particular attention to the routes of administration, dose and the requisites for patient monitoring given that patients respond differently to the same dose of estrogen.

EFFICACY

There are a large number of studies that have evaluated the effect of estrogen administration upon bone mass in postmenopausal women[2]. In general, all studies have drawn similar conclusions. Estrogen intervention reduces bone remodelling to premenopausal levels and thus reduces the rate of loss of skeletal tissue. The effects persist for as long as therapy is provided (at least 15 years) and are lost when estrogens are discontinued. All estrogens appear capable of inhibiting bone loss, provided adequate doses are administered and adequate serum levels are obtained.

Considerable epidemiological data support the concept that estrogens will reduce the risk of osteoporotic fracture among the aging female population[2]. Several studies have demonstrated reduction in the risk of both hip and distal radius fractures. Fewer data are available for vertebral fractures, but one epidemiological study and one prospective clinical trial have both shown dramatic reductions in crush fractures with estrogen use[3,4].

Estrogens have similar effects when used in the treatment of osteoporosis. Clear reductions in bone turnover are seen and further bone loss is prevented[5]. Small but significant increments in bone mass are seen, especially in those who present with increased bone remodelling. Again the route of administration does not appear to influence the outcome.

ORAL VERSUS PERORAL THERAPY

Although oral steroid administration is convenient in clinical practice, its rapid absorption produces marked fluctuations in serum concentrations. Also, during the drug's first pass through the liver, hepatic cells are exposed to very high hormone concentrations, with estrogen levels in the portal vein exceeding those in the general circulation by four- or fivefold[6]. The clinical effects of this phenomenon are not clear, but it may be associated with several metabolic side-effects. Parenteral estrogen administration does not affect hepatic protein synthesis in the same way as does oral estrogen[7,8].

It is now clear that all routes of administration have similar effects upon the skeleton. Thus, estrogens can be administered across the skin, (percutaneously, subcutaneously, or transdermally) as well as orally[9]. The important factor for the skeleton appears to be the dose administered rather than its route.

Most commonly, estrogens are given by the oral, percutaneous, or transdermal routes. The intravaginal route should not be used for skeletal (or other systemic) effects since absorption is variable. In some countries pellets are implanted subcutaneously allowing estrogen administration on a 3- or 6-month schedule[10]. The difficulty in removing the pellet should this be necessary makes this perhaps a less desired method, although it clearly has some advantages for some individuals.

DOSE AND DURATION

As noted above, the critical factor for estrogen effects on the skeleton appears to be dose and the serum level that is obtained. Original dose–

338

response studies performed using micronized estradiol and conjugated equine estrogens indicated that 2 mg/day and 0.625 mg/day, respectively, was sufficient to reduce bone loss in postmenopausal women[7].

An early study of 3 mg percutaneous estradiol demonstrated it to be highly effective in preventing bone loss in all parts of the skeleton[11]. Over a 2-year period, placebo-treated and calcium-treated postmenopausal women showed a significant reduction of 5–7% in bone mineral content of the distal forearm, the spine and the total skeleton. Values remained constant or showed a slight increase on all bone compartments in postmenopausal women receiving cyclic percutaneous estradiol. In another study[12] two comparable groups of postmenopausal women were treated with either 1.5 mg or 3 mg of percutaneous estradiol. Both groups responded well to treatment and were not losing bone during the study. This suggests that in the majority of postmenopausal women 1.5 mg of percutaneous estradiol is sufficient to provide optimum protection against bone loss.

For transdermal estrogen a dose of 50 μg/day appears to reduce both spinal and femoral neck bone loss[13].

There is inadequate information about the dose of estrogen administered by the subcutaneous route.

The duration of therapy required is not clear, but appears to be at least 5 years[14], and may be 10 years or lifelong. In practice, those patients who remain on treatment for 1 year will want to continue on treatment. For patients who present after fracture it is probable that lifetime therapy is required. In all patients a system of regular patient monitoring must be initiated.

INDIVIDUAL RESPONSE AND PATIENT MONITORING

Not all women will develop symptomatic osteoporosis – even without preventive intervention. Some may be protected by the development of a high peak bone mass during their premenopausal years. A significant proportion of postmenopausal women will only lose bone at a slow rate over the first postmenopausal decade when bone loss is accelerated. These women will probably never lose enough bone to become osteoporotic.

The decision to prescribe estrogen for a particular patient is often based on issues other than the risk of osteoporosis. However, when sex steroids are to be used primarily for the purpose of prevention of osteoporosis it is useful to obtain an estimate of bone mass or density. These tests, which are becoming increasingly available to the clinician, allow an estimate of the risk of the disease. Thus, they are similar to

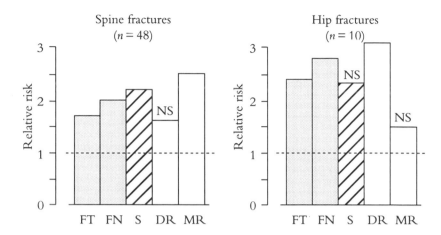

Figure 1 Long-term fracture risk prediction with bone mineral measurements made at various sites. Data adapted from Melton, L. J. *et al.* (1991)[18]: FT = femoral trochanter, FN = femoral neck, S = spine, DR = distal radius, MR = mid-radius, NS = not significant. Data are taken from 304 women (age 30–94 years) followed for a mean of 7.8 years (range 0.1–10.2 years)

measurement of cholesterol or blood pressure. In the case of bone density, the lower the value, the greater the risk of fracture[15]. All methods of measurement and skeletal sites appear to be able to give an indication of the overall risk of fracture (Figure 1). There may be some site specificity, as might be expected. Thus, measurement of the hip is more able to predict the risk of hip fracture than results from other sites in the skeleton[16]. However, the difference is not particularly great, and in practice the importance is in the decision that the measurement is required. With increasing availability of biochemical indicators of bone remodelling, these biochemical tests have been suggested as indicators of remodelling rate and thereby markers for increased rates of bone loss[17].

If the treatment is provided primarily to prevent osteoporosis it may be important to monitor the effect of treatment to ensure that the administered dose is optimal. Bone mass measurement after 1 year helps determine if the treatment is effective and can improve compliance. The biochemical markers that are affected dramatically by estrogen therapy may also be shown to be very efficient tools by which to monitor the effects of therapy.

REFERENCES

1. Albright, F., Smith, P. H. and Richardson, A. M. (1941). *J. Am. Med. Assoc.*, **116**, 2465–70
2. Lindsay, R. (1988). Sex steroids in the pathogenesis and prevention of osteoporosis. In Riggs, B. L. (ed.) *Osteoporosis: Etiology, Diagnosis and Management*, pp. 333–45. (New York: Raven Press)
3. Ettinger, B., Genant, H. K. and Cann, C. E. (1987). *Ann. Int. Med.*, **106**, 40–6
4. Lindsay, R., Hart, D. M., Forrest, C. and Baird, C. (1980). *Lancet*, **2**, 1151–3
5. Seibel, M. J., Cosman, F., Shen, V. *et al.* (1993). *J. Bone Min. Res.*, **8**, 881–90
6. Ottoson, U.-B. (1984). *Acta Obstet. Gynecol. Scand.*, **m127**, 5–37
7. Jensen, J., Riis, B. J., Strom, V. *et al.* (1987). *Am. J. Obstet. Gynecol.*, **156**, 66–71
8. Hassager, C., Riis, B. J., Strom, V. *et al.* (1987). *Circulation*, **76**, 753–8
9. Christiansen, C. and Lindsay, R. (1991). *Osteoporosis Int.*, **1**, 7–15
10. Studd, J., Savvas, M., Waston, N. *et al.* (1990). *Am. J. Obstet. Gynecol.*, **163**, 1474–7
11. Riis, B. J., Thomsen, K., Strom, V. *et al.* (1987). *Am. J. Obstet. Gynecol.*, **156**, 61–5
12. Wimalawansa, S. (1990). In Christiansen, C. and Overgaard, K. (eds.) *Osteoporosis*, vol. 3, pp. 1917–22
13. Stevenson, J. C., Cust, M. P., Gangar, K. F. *et al.* (1990). *Lancet*, **336**, 265–9
14. Consensus Report (1991). Consensus Development Conference: prophylaxis and treatment of osteoporosis. *Am. J. Med.*, **90**, 107–10
15. Johnston, C. C. Jr., Melton, L. J. III, Lindsay, R. and Eddy, D. M. (1989). *J. Bone Min. Res.*, **4**, 1–7
16. Cummings, S. R., Black, D. M., Nevitt, M. C. *et al.* (1993). *Lancet*, **341**, 72–4
17. Christiansen, C., Riis, B. J. and Rodbro, P. (1987). *Lancet*, **1**, 1105–7
18. Melton, L. J. *et al.* (1991). Abstract no. 213, Annual Meeting of the American Society for Bone and Mineral Research, 1991. *J. Bone Min. Res.*, **6** (suppl. 1)

35

Comparison of the effects of estrogen and the progestins progesterone, dydrogesterone and 20α-dihydroxydydrogesterone on proliferation and differentiation of normal adult human osteoblast-like cells

H. J. J. Verhaar, C. A. Damen, S. A. Duursma and B. A. A. Scheven

INTRODUCTION

It has been established that estrogen/gestagen replacement therapy prevents bone loss in postmenopausal women[1,2]. It has also been reported that substitution therapy with these hormones is able to increase bone mineral content for at least 3 years in early postmenopausal women and for at least 1 year in 70-year-old women[3,4]. The mode of action by which these sex steroids exert their anabolic effects on bone has not yet been completely unraveled. The demonstration of active estrogen and (inducible) progesterone receptors in the nuclei of normal human osteoblast-like (HOB) cells has suggested possible direct effects of these hormones on osteoblast function[5,6]. Recently, we have reported that both 17β-estradiol and progesterone were able to stimulate growth of HOB cells *in vitro*. In general, progesterone showed a stronger proliferation-inducing effect, whereas estradiol was more potent in stimulating HOB cell differentiation[7]. In the present study we have extended these observations by investigating the effects of the progestationally-active retrosteroid dydrogesterone and 20α-dihydroxydydrogesterone on HOB cells[8]. When administered to women, dydrogesterone is completely metabolized, 20α-dihydroxydydrogesterone being the main metabolite[8]. The biological activity of this metabolite is unknown. The effects of the three mentioned progestins, alone or in combination with estradiol, on proliferation and differentiation of HOB cells have been evaluated in this study.

MATERIALS AND METHODS

Reagents

17β-Estradiol and progesterone were purchased from Sigma. Both dydrogesterone and 20α-dihydroxydydrogesterone were obtained from Solvay Duphar BV (Weesp, The Netherlands).

Human osteoblast (HOB) cultures

Adult human trabecular bone explants were dissected from femoral heads obtained during orthopedic surgery. Osteoblast-like cell cultures were subsequently established from these bone particles as described previously[7,9,10]. Culture was performed in 10% fetal bovine serum (FBS) in minimal essential medium (MEM) supplemented with 2 mM glutamine, 0.1 mg/ml streptomycin, 100 U/ml penicillin and 2.5 mg/ml fungizone in 5% CO_2/air at 37°C. These bone-derived cells displayed specific osteoblast features[7,9-11]. HOB from bone samples derived from different patients were harvested using 0.05% trypsin/0.02% EDTA treatment, and subsequently pooled before subculture in 96-well culture plates (5000 cells/well). After 3–5 days preculture in MEM/FBS, the medium was replaced with serum-free, phenol red-free MEM containing 1 mg/ml bovine serum albumin (BSA) and the supplements as above. After 4 h, medium was replaced with either control medium or medium containing estradiol, progesterone, dydrogesterone or 20α-dihydroxydydrogesterone. The following assays were carried out in the 96-well plates after incubation of the cultures for 1 day in serum-free medium.

BrdU-incorporation

DNA synthesis was studied by immunochemical determination of the amount of 5-bromo-2'-deoxy-uridine (BrdU), a thymidine analog, incorporated into cellular DNA[12]. The cultures were labelled with 10 μmol/l BrdU (Amersham) for 24 h, fixed in 70% ethanol for 30 min at 4°C, followed by a 15 min treatment with 4 N HCl. After subsequent washing in 0.1 mol/l borate solution (pH 8.5) and twice in PBS, the cells were overlayered with a specific mouse anti-BrdU monoclonal antibody (0.5 μg/ml; Boehringer-Mannheim) for 60 min at room temperature. After reaction with goat anti-mouse IgG conjugated with peroxidase for 60 min, antibody labelling was detected using ABTS as substrate (Boehringer-Mannheim). The absorbance of the reaction was quantified with a microtiter plate reader at 414 nm. The results were expressed as a percentage of control values.

Total cell number assay

Total cell numbers were determined using methylene blue staining of fixed adherent cells as described previously[7,13,14]. Cultures were fixed with neutral buffered formalin for 30 min at room temperature, stained with 0.1% methylene blue in 0.01 mol/l borate buffer (pH 8.6) for 30 min, followed by a rinse procedure with borate buffer. Then the dye was eluted in a 1:1 ethanol (v/v 99.8%) and 0.1 mol/l HCl solution, and the absorbance at 595 nm was measured using an automatic microtiter plate reader. Results were calculated relative to control absorbance values.

Analysis of alkaline phosphatase (AP) activity

Histochemical staining of the cells for AP activity was carried out using a Sigma kit (No. 84) with α-naphthol phosphate as substrate and Fast Blue BB as coupler. The number of positive cells was counted using an inverted microscope.

Statistics

Results from the experiments (using different pooled cell populations) were subjected to an overall statistical evaluation using the Student–Newman–Keul's one-way analysis of variance.

RESULTS

The progestin dydrogesterone and its metabolite 20α-dihydroxydydrogesterone, at concentrations of 10^{-12} mol/l and 10^{-10} mol/l, stimulated total HOB cell numbers to the same extent (Figure 1). Maximum stimulation was reached with the concentration of 10^{-10} mol/l for both

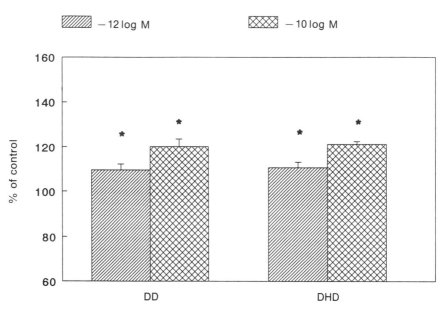

Figure 1 Effect of dydrogesterone (DD) and 20α-dihydroxydydrogesterone (DHD) on total human osteoblast-like cell numbers using the methylene blue assay. Means ± SEM are expressed relative to control values ($n = 6$). $^*p < 0.05$ vs. controls

of these compounds (Figure 1), as was also the case for progesterone itself[7]. Figure 2 depicts the results obtained from HOB cultures incubated with estradiol, progesterone, dydrogesterone and 20α-dihydroxydydrogesterone at concentrations of 10^{-10} mol/l in serum-free and phenol red-free medium for 1 day. All three progestins manifested an equal stimulatory effect on total cell numbers; this was significantly greater than that exerted by estradiol (Figure 2). Combining estradiol with each of the progesterone compounds did not result in a further enhancement of total HOB cell numbers (Figure 2).

Progesterone, dydrogesterone and 20α-dihydroxydydrogesterone at doses of 10^{-10} mol/l stimulated DNA synthesis to the same extent and were each significantly more potent enhancers of DNA replication than was estradiol (Figure 3). The combination of estradiol with progesterone, dydrogesterone or 20α-dihydroxydydrogesterone resulted in a consistently greater increase of DNA synthesis, although this was not statistically different from that induced by the different progestins alone (Figure 3).

The effect of estradiol, progestin, dydrogesterone and 20α-dihydroxydydrogesterone on osteoblast differentiation was studied using alkaline

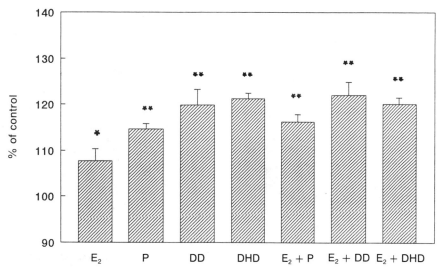

Figure 2 Comparison of the effect of 17β-estradiol (E$_2$), progesterone (P), dydrogesterone (DD) and 20α-dihydroxydydrogesterone (DHD) at a concentration of 10^{-10} mol/l on total human osteoblast-like cell numbers using the methylene blue (total cell number) assay. Means $\pm$ SEM are expressed relative to control values ($n = 6$). $^*p < 0.05$ vs. controls; $^{**}p < 0.05$ vs. controls and cultures treated with estradiol alone

phosphatase (AP) as a marker for mature osteoblast phenotype. Histochemical analysis of HOB cultures incubated with 10^{-10} mol/l of these steroids revealed a significant increase in AP activity (Figure 4). The number of AP-positive cells in the estradiol-treated cultures was significantly greater than that in cultures incubated with progestins (Figure 4). The progestins all affected HOB differentiation to the same extent. Combining estradiol with different progestins did not further increase AP activity over that seen with estradiol treatment alone.

DISCUSSION

In this study, we have confirmed the stimulatory effects of estradiol and progesterone and have shown for the first time the anabolic effects of dydrogesterone and 20α-dihydroxydydrogesterone on mitogenesis and differentiation of human osteoblast-like cells derived from explants dissected from femoral heads obtained from women undergoing orthopedic surgery. The three progestins tested enhanced proliferation of the human-derived osteoblasts to a greater extent than estradiol. The

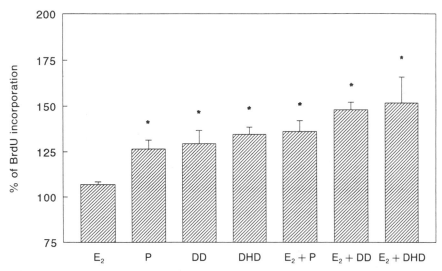

Figure 3 Comparison of the effect of 17β-estradiol (E₂), progesterone (P), dydrogesterone (DD) and 20α-dihydroxydydrogesterone (DHD) on bromodeoxy-uridine (BrdU) incorporation (measure of DNA synthesis) into human osteoblast-like cells, derived from female trabecular bone samples. The cells were treated with 10^{-10} mol/l of the mentioned hormones for 1 day in serum-free medium. Results ± SEM are expressed as relative to control absorbance values. *Significantly different compared to controls and cultures treated with estradiol alone ($p < 0.05$)

progestins were equally potent in stimulating HOB proliferation. Although not statistically significant, an increased stimulation of DNA replication in HOB cells was obtained by combining estradiol with either progesterone, the retrosteroid dydrogesterone or 20α-dihydroxydydrogesterone, compared with the progestins alone. Coinciding with their effects on osteoblast replication, the steroids stimulated differentiation in human osteoblasts. Compared to the progestins, estradiol demonstrated a more distinct stimulatory effect on alkaline phosphatase activity in HOB cells. The progestins had equal effects on HOB differentiation.

The fact that the progestationally active compounds were equally potent in stimulating HOB mitogenesis suggests an equal affinity for the specific progesterone receptor. The maximal effects of the progestins at different doses might be due to a rapid saturation of the low numbers of progesterone receptors on HOB cells[5]. The action of estradiol is likely to occur via active estrogen receptors in the nucleus of HOB cells[5]. Estrogen and the progestins may regulate transcription and expression of proto-oncogenes, which may play a role in the regulation of cell growth and

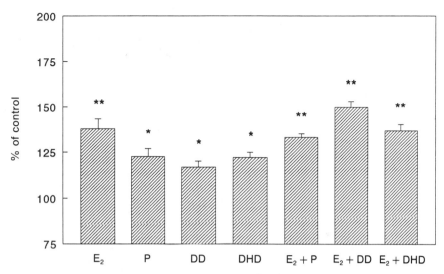

Figure 4 Comparison of the effects of 17β-estradiol (E$_2$), progesterone (P), dydrogesterone (DD) and 20α-dihydroxydydrogesterone (DHD) at a concentration of 10^{-10} mol/l, on the number of cells showing alkaline phosphatase activity as visualized by cytochemical staining of the human osteoblast like cultures Mean $\pm$ SEM relative to control values ($n = 6$). $^*p < 0.05$ vs. controls; $^{**}p < 0.05$ vs. controls and cultures treated with progesterone, dydrogesterone or dihydroxydydrogesterone

differentiation in our short-term 1-day cultures[15,16]. Estradiol has been reported to enhance c-*jun* mRNA levels (within 30 min) in a dose-dependent manner, suggesting a possible role for c-*jun* as an early regulatory gene of the action of the steroid[17].

Mediation of the hormone's actions by local factors cannot be excluded. It is known that estradiol and progesterone are capable of inducing insulin-like growth factors (IGF-I/-II) and their binding proteins in osteoblast-like cultures[18–22]. These growth factors exert direct effects on osteoblast proliferation and differentiation and may mediate the stimulatory effects of estradiol and the different progestins in our cultures[13,23–27]. Recent data from the literature demonstrated that progesterone increased IGF-II levels in the conditioned medium of HOB cultures, while no effective concentrations of IGF-I could be demonstrated: this may indicate additional anabolic effects of progesterone on bone-forming cells via IGF-II[28]. Recently, it was suggested that human osteoblast-like cells are capable of synthesizing estrogen, which also could be an important mechanism in the local regulation of bone volume[29].

Our present results lead us to formulate the hypothesis that direct effects of estrogen and progestins on osteoblasts may be one mechanism by which these steroids exert their anabolic effects on bone *in vivo*[3,4].

ACKNOWLEDGEMENT

This work was financially supported by Solvay Duphar BV (Weesp, The Netherlands), to whom the authors express their gratitude.

REFERENCES

1. Riis, B. J., Jensen, J. and Christiansen, C. (1987). Cyproterone acetate, an alternative gestagen in postmenopausal oestrogen/gestagen therapy. *Clin. Endocrinol. (Oxf.)*, **26**, 327–34
2. Riis, B. J., Thomsen, K., Strøm, V. and Christiansen, C. (1987). The effect of percutaneous estradiol and natural progesterone on postmenopausal bone loss. *Am. J. Obstet. Gynaecol.*, **156**, 61–5
3. Christiansen, C., Christensen, M. S. and Transbøl, I. (1981). Bone mass in postmenopausal women after withdrawal of oestrogen/gestagen replacement therapy. *Lancet*, **1**, 459–61
4. Jensen, G. F., Christiansen, C. and Transbøl, I. (1982). Treatment of postmenopausal osteoporosis. A controlled therapeutic trial comparing oestrogen/gestagen, 1,25-dihydroxyvitamin D_3 and calcium. *Clin. Endocrinol. (Oxf.)*, **16**, 515–24
5. Eriksen, E. F., Colvard, D. S., Berg, N. J., Graham, M. L., Mann, K. G., Spelsberg, T. C. and Riggs, B. L. (1988). Evidence of estrogen receptors in normal human osteoblast-like cells. *Science*, **241**, 84–6
6. Komm, B. S., Terpening, C. M., Benz, D. J., Graeme, K. A., Gallegos, A., Korc, M., Greene, G. L., O'Malley, B. W. and Haussler, M. R. (1988). Estrogen binding, receptor mRNA, and biologic response in osteoblast-like osteosarcoma cells. *Science*, **241**, 81–4
7. Scheven, B. A. A., Damen, C. A., Hamilton, N. J., Verhaar, H. J. J. and Duursma, S. A. (1992). Stimulatory effects of estrogen and progesterone on proliferation and differentiation of normal human osteoblast-like cells *in vitro*. *Biochem. Biophys. Res. Commun.*, **186**, 54–60
8. Van Amsterdam, P. H., Overmars, H., Scherpenisse, P. M., de Bree, H. and Post, L. C. (1980). Dydrogesterone: metabolism in man. *Eur. J. Drug Metab. Pharmacokin.*, **5**, 173–84
9. Beresford, J. N., Gallager, J. A., Poser, J. W. and Russell, R. G. G. (1984). Production of osteocalcin by human bone *in vitro*. Effects of 1,25-$(OH)_2D_3$, parathyroid hormone and glucocorticoids. *Metab. Bone Rel. Res.*, **5**, 229–34
10. Auf'mkolk, B. and Schwartz, E. (1985). Biochemical characterizations of human osteoblasts in culture. In *Normal and Abnormal Bone Growth: Basic and Clinical Research*, pp. 201–14. (Alan R. Liss Inc.)
11. Chavassieux, P. M., Chenu, C., Valentin-Opran, A., Merle, B., Delmas, D., Hartmann, D. J., Saez, S. and Meunier, P. J. (1990). Influence of experimental

conditions on osteoblast activity in human primary bone cell cultures. *J. Bone Min. Res.,* **5**, 337–43

12. Gratzner, H. G. (1982). Monoclonal antibody to 5-bromo- and 5-iodo-deoxyuridine: a new reagent for detection of DNA replication. *Science,* **218**, 474–5

13. Oliver, M. H., Harisson, N. K., Bishop, J. E., Cole, P. J. and Laurent, G. J. (1989). A rapid and convenient assay for counting cells cultured in microwell plates. *J. Cell Sci.,* **92**, 513–18

14. Scheven, B. A. A., Hamilton, N. J., Fakkeldij, T. M. V. and Duursma, S. A. (1991). Effects of recombinant human insulin-like growth factor I and II (IGF-I/-II) and growth hormone (GH) on the growth of normal adult human osteoblast-like cells and human osteogenic sarcoma cells. *Growth Reg.,* **1**, 160–7

15. Beato, M. (1989). Gene regulation by steroid hormones. *Cell,* **56**, 335–44

16. Clarke, C. L. and Sutherland, R. L. (1990). Progestin regulation of cellular proliferation. *Endocrine Rev.,* **11**, 266–301

17. Subramaniam, M., Rasmussen, K., Riggs, B. L. and Spelsberg, T. C. (1991). Estrogen induces rapid expression of c-*jun* mRNA levels in normal human osteoblast-like cells. *J. Bone Min. Res.,* **6** (suppl. 1), abstract no. 25, 589

18. Ernst, M., Heath, J. K. and Rodan, G. A. (1989). Estradiol effects on proliferation mRNA for collagen and insulin-like growth factor-I, and PTH-stimulated adenyl cyclase activity in osteoblastic cells from calvariae and long bone. *Endocrinology,* **125**, 825–33

19. Gray, T. K., Mohan, S., Linkhart, T. A. and Baylink, D. J. (1989). Estradiol stimulates *in vitro* the secretion of insulin-like growth factors by the clonal osteoblastic cell line, UMR 106. *Biochem. Biophys. Res. Commun.,* **158**, 407–12

20. Schmid, C., Ernst, M., Zapf, J. and Froesch, E. R. (1989). Release of insulin-like growth factor carrier proteins by osteoblasts: stimulation by estradiol and growth hormone. *Biochem. Biophys. Res. Commun.,* **160**, 788–94

21. Lempert, U. G., Strong, D. D., Mohan, S., Demarest, K. and Baylink, D. J. (1992). Effect of progesterone on the mRNA levels of insulin-like growth factors (IGFs), IGF-binding proteins (IGFBPs) and type-1 and type-2 IGF-receptors in human osteoblastic cells. *Bone Min.,* **17** (suppl. 1), abstract no. 60, 86

22. Gray, T. K. (1989). Estrogens and the skeleton: cellular and molecular mechanisms. *J. Steroid Biochem.,* **34**, 285–7

23. Kasperk, C. H., Wergedal, J. E., Mohan, S., Long, D. L., Lau, K. H. and Baylink, D. J. (1990). Interactions of growth factors present in bone matrix with bone cells: effects on DNA synthesis and alkaline phosphatase. *Growth Factors,* **3**, 147–58

24. Slootweg, M. C., Hoogerbrugge, C. M., De Poorter, T. L., Duursma, S. A. and Van Buul-Offers, S. C. (1990). The presence of classical insulin-like growth factor (IGF) type-I and -II receptors on mouse osteoblasts: autocrine/paracrine growth effect of IGFs? *J. Endocrinol.,* **125**, 271–7

25. Centrella, M., McCarthy, T. L. and Canalis, E. (1990). Receptors for insulin-like growth factors-I and -II in osteoblast-enriched cultures from fetal rat bone. *Endocrinology,* **126**, 39–44

26. Wergedal, W. E., Mohan, S., Lundy, M. and Baylink, D. J. (1990). Skeletal growth factor and other growth factors known to be present in bone matrix stimulate proliferation and protein synthesis in human bone cells. *J. Bone Min. Res.,* **5**, 179–86

27. Merriman, H. L., La Tour, D., Linkhart, T. A., Mohan, S., Baylink, D. J. and Strong, D. D. (1990). Insulin-like growth factor-I and insulin-like growth factor-II induce c-*fos* in mouse osteoblastic cells. *Calcif. Tissue Int.*, **46**, 258–60
28. Tremollieres, F. A., Strong, D. D., Baylink, D. J. and Mohan, S. (1992). Progesterone and promegestone stimulate human bone cell proliferation and insulin-like growth factor-2 production. *Acta Endocrinol. (Copenh.)*, **126**, 329–37
29. Purohit, A., Flanagan, A. M. and Reed, M. J. (1992). Estrogen synthesis by osteoblast cell lines. *Endocrinology*, **131**, 2027–9

36

Ovarian failure and the musculoskeletal system

G. Heytmanek

The menopause does not consist of hot flushes alone, but comprises an intricate and complex picture, including osteoporosis, atherosclerosis and psychiatric manifestations. It is also important not to neglect the many individual symptoms that at first sight do not seem to bear any relation to the menopause, such as arthralgia[1] or dryness of the eyes[2].

Investigations of the menopause usually deal mainly with epidemiology, osteoporosis or atherosclerosis; only a very small number of studies are based on anthropometric aspects. However, muscle mass, adipose tissue content and their effects on the hormonal system must not be neglected.

Hagen[3] was one of the first to suggest that a certain minimum body weight or minimum level of subcutaneous fatty tissue, respectively, is necessary for the onset of menarche and the occurrence of regular menstrual cycles. This was confirmed by numerous studies[4]. There is thus sufficient proof for the existence in principle of a direct correlation between the duration of the ovarian function on the one hand and individual anthropometric parameters on the other. It is still unclear whether this connection is genetically determined or whether it is determined by an endocrine function of muscle and adipose tissue.

It is well known that the peripheral adipose tissue aromatizes C-19 steroids, produced by both the adrenals and postmenopausally in the ovary, into C-18 steroid compounds. Thus the peripheral estrogen level also depends on the amount of tissue capable of such aromatization. A study by Matsumine[5] suggests that peripheral aromatization is the major source of circulating estrogens in men and postmenopausal women. The conversion was almost the same as that reported from human adipose tissue, suggesting that the contributions of muscle and fat to extraglandular production of estrogen in these subjects might be similar. This was the first direct confirmation of muscle aromatase activity and indicates the possible importance of muscle as an extragenital source of estrogen in both men and postmenopausal women.

In the same year Brodie and colleagues[6] found that estrogen biosynthesis occurs not only in reproductive tissue of the female but also in such diverse sites as testis, adipose tissue and muscle. Their rationale for the clinical use of aromatase inhibitors is that compounds interacting with aromatase in all tissues could provide both selective and effective inhibition of estrogen production (4-hydroxyandrostene-3,17-dione). This compound causes rapid competitive inhibition in estrogen synthesis in women with breast cancer, reducing mean serum levels to 36% of those before treatment. There was no effect on gonadotropin levels, indicating that reduction in estrogen levels was due to inhibition of peripheral aromatization. In spite of the fact that all patients had relapsed following previous therapy, complete or partial tumor regression occurred in 30%.

These two studies suggest the importance of the muscular system, not only as supporting structure but also as hormonally active tissue.

Cauley[7] compared grip strength in the menopause, physical activity, estrogen use and anthropometric factors in women with or without hormone replacement therapy. Multiple regression analysis revealed that only height, age and physical activity were independent determinants of grip strength, and height was the major determinant of upper body strength in older women. The reduction in physical activity with advancing age may contribute to a decline in strength, and modest increases in physical activity may retard the loss of strength that accompanies aging; the loss of ovarian estrogen may also be related to the loss of strength in postmenopausal women.

Similar studies, such as that by Notelovitz[8], have also concluded that hormone replacement therapy after ovarian insufficiency can only be advantageous. Jensen[9] suggests that high-dose postmenopausal hormone therapy changes body composition by increasing muscle mass and that since the body weight remains unchanged, a proportionate decrease in the fat mass seems to occur.

In a cross-sectional population study, Kyllonen[10] compared muscle strength and bone mineral density in healthy postmenopausal women and found that height, isometric muscle strength and endurance of muscles were not significant predictors of bone mineral density. Weight and age were the most significant predictors of isometric muscle strength. Mobility of the spine, body fat content and aerobic threshold had no correlation with bone mineral density. The authors of the NHANES I epidemiologic follow-up study[11] concluded that their findings are the first evidence from a prospective study that anthropometric indicators other than body mass index may be independently related to risk of hip fracture.

Aloia[12] studied cross-sectional and longitudinal changes in body composition with age in white women, to determine the relationship between body cell mass and menopause, and between body fat and bone mass. There was statistical evidence for a curvilinear component to loss of total body potassium, with negligible rates of loss before menopause. Longitudinal measurements also indicated a relationship between proximity to menopause and the rate of loss of potassium. Total body potassium was significantly related to total body calcium and bone density of the spine radius and femoral neck. Total body fat was not related to any of these measurements. There was no evidence to suggest that adiposity plays a major role in protecting against bone loss.

Serum sex hormone levels may be related to the risk of several diseases in postmenopausal women. Cauley[13] measured serum concentrations of estrone, estradiol, testosterone and androstenedione. Neither age nor time since menopause was a significant predictor of sex hormone level. The degree of obesity was a major determinant of estrone and estradiol: estrone levels of obese women were about 40% higher than those in non-obese women. There was a weak relationship between obesity and androgens. Physical activity was an independent predictor of serum estrone. More active women had lower estrogen levels. There was a positive relationship between muscle strength and estrogen levels.

The association between body mass and fat distribution and sex hormone concentrations in postmenopausal women was also studied by Kaye[14]. After adjustment for body mass index and other related factors, waist to hip circumference ratio was significantly and negatively associated with levels of sex hormone binding globulin, luteinizing hormone and follicle stimulating hormone, and demonstrated a significant curvilinear relationship with free testosterone. These data suggest that abdominal adiposity in menopausal women is associated with a relatively more androgenic hormone profile.

Reid[15] concluded that total body fat is the most significant predictor of bone mineral density throughout the skeleton, and this relationship is not explicable in terms of either estrone production in fat tissue or the dependence of skeletal load-bearing of fat mass. The mechanism underlying this relationship is an important question to be addressed in bone biology.

In another study, Reid[16] studied the relationship between upper-arm anthropometry and soft-tissue composition in postmenopausal women. Multiple regression analysis showed that the anthropometric indices were more closely correlated with fat than with lean mass. It is concluded that all of these indices are useful measures of fat mass but that none, including arm muscle area, is a specific index of lean mass in normal postmenopausal women.

Another study of the authors' department found that in both fertile and postmenopausal women there are phase-significant correlations between sex hormone concentrations and body form. There is plenty of evidence for this from the relationship between body form and hormonally controlled events. Hagen and colleagues[3] postulated the necessity of a certain minimum weight or minimum subcutaneous fat content, respectively, for the beginning of menarche as well as for the development of regular menstrual cycles. However, the relationship between body form and menopausal age has not yet been examined. Only the body measurement index (body weight/body height) has been correlated with age, and an increase in age at menopause. In 110 healthy, central European postmenopausal women (not hysterectomized nor ovariectomized), age 38–61 years (mean 50.8 years), body measurements were taken according to Kussmann[17]. Only factor 1 (postcephalic breadth–circumference) showed a significant positive correlation with menopausal age, while factor 2 (postcephalic length–height) showed a significant negative correlation. In all women, increases in all breadth and circumferential measurements correlated with increasing menopausal age. Decreasing length and height measurements also correlated with increasing menopausal age. Women with a later menopause were therefore smaller and more obese than women with an earlier menopause. This shows that there is a direct correlation between the duration of ovarian function, on the one hand, and the size of individual anthropometric parameters, on the other. It is, however, unclear whether this connection is genetically determined or whether the endocrine competence of muscle and adipose tissue is responsible. Although, as with the Sherman study, no statistically significant correlation between individual menopausal age and body weight could be ascertained, most length–height measurements correlated negatively and most breadth–circumference measures correlated positively with menopausal age. The positive correlation between shoulder/chest index and menopausal age suggests that women with gynoidal fat distribution have a later menopause than women with androidal build.

ACKNOWLEDGEMENT

B. Hartmann for his support of our study at the 1st Department of Gynecology and Obstetrics, University of Vienna, Austria.

REFERENCES

1. Metka, M., Heytmanek, G., Enzelsberger, H., Schurz, B. and Kurz, Ch. (1988). Der Gelenkschmerz in der Prä- und Postmenopause, Arthropathia Climacterica. *Geburtsh. Frauenheilk.,* **48**, 232–4
2. Metka, M., Enzelsberger, H., Knogler, W., Schurz, B. and Aichmaier, R. (1991). Ophthalmic complaints as a climacteric symptom. *Maturitas,* **14**, 3–8
3. Hagen, Ch., Christiansen, C. and Chrisstiansen, M. S. (1982). Climacteric symptoms, fat mass and plasma concentrations of LH, FSH, PRL, estradiol 17-beta and androstenedione in the early postmenopausal period. *Acta Endocrinol.,* **101**, 87–92
4. Lauritzen, Ch. (1982). *Das Klimakterium der Frau.* (Verlag Schering)
5. Matsumine, H., Hirato, K., Yanaihara, T., Tamada, T. and Yoshida, M. (1986). Aromatization by skeletal muscle. *J. Clin. Endocrinol. Metab.,* **63**, 717–20
6. Brodie, A. M., Wing, L. Y., Goss, P., Dowsett, M. and Coombs, R. C. (1986). Aromatase inhibitors and their potential clinical significance. *J. Steroid Biochem.,* **9**, 859–61
7. Cauley, J. A., Pertini, A. M., LaPorte, R. E., Sandler, R. B., Baylers, C. M., Robertson, R. J. and Selemenda, C. W. (1987). The decline of grip strength in the menopause: relationship to physical activity, estrogen use and anthropometric factors. *J. Chronic Dis.,* **40**, 115–20
8. Notelovitz, M., Martin, D., Tesar, R., Khan, F. Y., Probart, C., Fields, C. and McKenzie, L. (1991). Estrogen therapy and variable resistance weight training increase bone mineral in surgically menopause women. *J. Bone Min. Res.,* **6**, 583–90
9. Jensen, J., Christiansen, C. and Rodbro, P. (1986). Estrogen–progesterone replacement therapy changes body composition in early postmenopausal women. *Maturitas,* **8**, 209–16
10. Kyllonen, E. S., Vaananen, H. K., Heikkinen, J. E., Kurttila-Matero, E., Martikkala, V. and Vanharanta, J. H. (1991). Comparison of muscle strength and bone mineral density in healthy postmenopausal women: a cross-sectional population study. *Scand. J. Rehab. Med.,* **23**, 153–7
11. Farmer, M. E., Harris, T., Madans, J. H., Wallace, R. B., Coroni-Huntley, J. and White, L. R. (1989). Anthropometric indicators and hip fracture. The NHANES I epidemiologic follow-up study. *J. Am. Geriatr. Soc.,* **37**, 9–16
12. Aloia, J. F., McGowan, D. M., Vaswani, A. N., Ross, P. and Cohn, S. H. (1991). Relationship of menopause to skeletal and muscle mass. *Am. J. Clin. Nutr.,* **53**, 1378–83
13. Cauley, J. A., Gutai, J. P., Kuller, L. H., LeDonne, D. and Powell, J. G. (1989). The epidemiology of serum sex hormones in postmenopausal women. *Am. J. Epidemiol.,* **129**, 1120–31
14. Kaye, S. A., Folsom, A. R., Soler, J. T., Prineas, R. J. and Potter, J. D. (1991).

Association of body mass and fat distribution with sex hormone concentrations in postmenopausal women. *Int. J. Epidemiol.,* **20**, 151–6

15. Reid, I. R., Ames, R., Evans, M. C., Sharpe, S., Gamble, G., France, J. T., Lim, T. M. and Cundy, T. F. (1992). Determinant of total body and regional bone mineral density in normal postmenopausal women — a key role for fat mass. *J. Clin. Endocrinol. Metab.,* **75**, 45–51

16. Reid, I. R., Evans, M. C. and Ames, R. (1992). Relationships between upper-arm anthropometry and soft-tissue composition in postmenopausal women. *Am. J. Clin. Nutr.,* **56**, 463–6

17. Knussmann, R. (1988). Sumatometry. In Knussmann, R. (ed.) *Anthropology.* (Stuttgart: Fischer Verlag)

37

Ovarian failure and joints

G. Holzer

INTRODUCTION

Both osteoporosis and osteoarthritis are widespread obstructive conditions, which become more frequent with age, especially in women after the menopause. Based on this fact, it is necessary to consider whether tissues of the musculoskeletal system should be regarded as target organs of sex hormones. While the therapeutic use of sex hormones is widely accepted for the prophylaxis of osteoporosis, its use in the prophylaxis and therapy of osteoarthrosis is still an experiment.

HISTORICAL REVIEW

The role of the endocrinological environment (especially with regard to sex hormones) in the pathogenesis of joint disorders has been considered since the beginnings of medicine. These considerations were consolidated by the clinical experience, according to which joint disorders can arise contemporaneously with the menopause, or how the course of these disorders may be influenced under these circumstances.

In the book *On Female Diseases*, Hippocrates said that with 'light menses the pain goes into the limbs of arms and legs and into the small of the back'. 'The woman will have pain in the region around the neck, in the spine and in the lumbar region'. The pain is not always localized in the same place, but 'now and then there'. The symptoms arise 'especially in women who are not married'[1].

Celsus[2] wrote that 'ailments of the joints of hands and feet are long-lasting and arise often'. Eunuchs or 'other women than those whose menses is suppressed' are only rarely concerned.

The French neurologist Charcot[3] showed in some of his works the connection between polyarthritis on the one side and menopause, pregnancy, birth and lactation on the other. Fox[4] was one of the first to describe the clinical picture in detail and first used the expression 'climacteric arthritis'. It arises in women at the time of the menopause and is characterized by intermittent joint disorders and by swelling of the fingers with shining skin. According to Fox the prognosis is good. Pineles[5] pointed out that the hormonal environment at the time of the menopause is a cause of the Heberden–Rosenbach knot, which was described first by Heberden in 1802.

Umber[6] described the affliction, especially of the small finger joints, which concerns practically only women, as 'endocrine chronic peri-arthritis (destruens)'. It progresses slowly over years and decades without fever and is directly connected with functional anomalies of the sexual glands (menarche, menopause and sterilization). His[7] explained that the menopausal arthritides with swellings and pain arise before, during and after the menopause, progress for 1 or 2 years and remain constant afterwards, often accompanied by relief of pain.

Menge[8] caused a stir with his publication in 1924. He saw the clinical picture of 'arthropathia ovaripriva' in women castrated by means of X-rays and, less often, in postmenopausal women, who developed symptoms in the knees (usually bilateral) and sometimes in the shoulders and joints of the fingers. The subjective complaints differed from light to so severe that the patient could not walk or move the shoulders. Objectively he only found severe crepitations. The symptoms sometimes disappeared spontaneously, but could also persist for years. At this time other studies by Cecil and Archer[9], Hall[10] and Weil[11] were also published.

According to Wagenhäuser[12] the frequent occurrence of arthrosis of the fingers in postmenopausal women etiologically points to disturbances in the endocrine balance. But 'in this case the estrogen deficiency itself does not seem to be a direct reason, but the secondary stimulation of the hypophysis caused by the insufficient hormone production by the gonads'. From 1941 on Silberberg and Silberberg[13] were the first to make a number of experimental studies, followed later on by Rosner[14].

CLIMACTERIC ARTHRALGIAS

Synonyms for this condition include climacteric arthritis (Fox), arthritis of the menopause (Cecil/Archer), arthropathia ovaripriva (Menge), menopause arthralgia (Hall) and arthropathia climacterica (Metka). All of these mean joint disorders, which arise in connection with menopause (pre-, peri- or postmenopausal). Clinically these disorders are characterized by pains and swellings of one or usually more symmetrically affected joints, especially the proximal (PIP) and the distal interphalangeal joints (DIP) of the fingers. The joints of the feet and large joints such as the shoulders, knees or hips can also be affected. Involvement of the PIP joints can be judged the leading symptom. These disorders usually have a good prognosis, although permanent lesions can occur.

Differential diagnosis

The diagnosis of climacteric arthralgia is an exclusion diagnosis. As well as arthritis urtica, inflammatory changes of the joints such as rheumatoid arthritis and mono- and polyarthritis of other origin, such as Reiter's syndrome and psoriatic arthritis, have to be excluded. If the hands are concerned, neurological disorders such as the cervical syndrome should be taken into consideration.

Epidemiology

The rheumatic disorders, including degenerative joint disorders, account for a high proportion of the total morbidity of the population in epidemiologic studies[15,16]. While the morbidity of osteoarthrosis is equal between the two sexes[15,16], review data show differences between the sexes regarding age, severity of the disorder and other parameters. In the age group >50 years, women are affected more frequently and more severely than men: that is, more joints are involved[15,17]. The severity of rheumatic disorders correlates directly with the severity of climacteric symptoms[18]. Recently an extremely high rate of preceding hysterectomies and other gynecologic surgery was reported in patients with osteoarthrosis[19]. Among women attending an out-patient department because of climacteric symptoms, about 70% complain, when asked, about pain in the joints, especially the proximal and distal joints of the fingers (Metka, Holzer and Chlud, manuscript in preparation).

Pathogenesis of osteoarthrosis

The models of the etiology of osteoarthrosis which are valid today assume two pathways for the cause of the initial lesion of the cartilage, which is the key event: on one side the biomechanic path with definable pre-arthrosis (deformations or dysfunctions) and localized overexertion of the cartilage, and on the other the biochemical path with reduced resistance of the cartilage, caused by endogenous enzymatic degradation (hypothetically). The discrepancy between the possibility of strain and the effective strain causes the endogenous or exogenous damage of cartilage with following (primary or secondary) osteoarthrosis[20].

Biochemically, early damage is associated with pathological hydration of the cartilage, presumably caused by the injured network of collagen fibres. The network loses its tight linkage, and water is absorbed. This causes a functional deterioration of the matrix and a loss of proteoglycans. Repeated mechanical strain results in additional deformation, reduced elasticity and increased pressure on the subchondral bone[21]. All these lesions cause fissures on the surface of the cartilage.

The connections between the chondrocytes, the metabolic center of the cartilage and of the extracellular matrix, are discontinued, which causes metabolic reactions in the chondrocytes. In spite of the increased proliferative rate in the initial phase an inferior matrix develops.

Effects of steroid hormones at joints

Sex hormones exert their effects by a variety of complex mechanisms. These mechanisms are triggered by the binding of the free steroid molecule to specific receptors, especially in the nucleus. There an interaction with the genetic material of the target cell occurs. In this way the hormone–receptor complex induces or stops biological reactions of the hormone in the target cells[22].

Steroid hormones stimulate collagen, protein and prostaglandin synthesis. In the immune system they regulate both the formation of antibodies and the proliferation and differentiation of stem cells.

In the past, the uterus, vagina, breasts, brain and hypophysis have been described as typical target organs for female sex hormones. Recent studies have shown receptors for steroid hormones in other tissues, including larynx, gingiva, spleen, in the cardiovascular and central nervous systems, and in chondrocytes[23,24]. It has to be kept in mind that the effects of steroid hormones do not need specific receptors, but can also take place directly[25].

EXPERIMENTAL STUDIES

The effect of circulating sex hormones on the development of degenerative osteoarthrosis was studied by Silberberg and Silberberg[13,26]. They found that mice of a particular breed had a predisposition for the development of osteoarthrosis of a certain pattern: female mice fell ill more rarely, and in male animals orchiectomy influenced the course of the disease favorably. While androgens worsened the pathogenesis, therapy with estrogens ameliorated the result. However, Sokoloff and Jay[27] could not support the results of Silberberg and Silberberg regarding the benefit of estrogens.

In the late 1970s, Rosner and colleagues[28] studied estrogens. Their model for the experimental development of osteoarthrosis was partial menisectomy in immature female New Zealand white rabbits. A single administration of estrogen every 14 days resulted in no amelioration of the clinical condition. With lower doses, femoral fissures of the cartilage and ulcerations occurred.

To be able to control the endogenous production of estrogen, this group continued their studies in female rabbits after oophorectomy. The drugs were given more often than before, but with the same cumulative dosage, in order to keep a permanent circulating level. The results were compared with the results of treatment with placebo and with tamoxifen, a non-steroidal antagonist. Animals treated with estrogen showed increased erosive changes of the cartilage compared to control animals, while animals which had received tamoxifen showed a statistically significant reduction in arthrotic lesions of the cartilage[14].

LABORATORY TESTS

In 1962 Priest and colleagues[29] reported that estrogen has a suppressive effect on the synthesis of proteoglycans in cartilage. The studies of Silberberg and Silberberg[13,26,30] showed increased condensation and fibrillation of cartilage matrix and a reduced proliferative rate of the chondrocytes caused by estrogens. Biochemically, this means that estrogens cause a transient inhibition of proteoglycan synthesis and an increase (active or passive) in collagen synthesis[31]. The inhibitory effect of estrogens is connected therefore with dehydration, increased deposition of cytoplasmatic glycogen and an apparent increase in collagen content.

Further *in vitro* studies showed that estrogens stimulate prostaglandin synthesis by acting directly on the chondrocyte[32]. High exogenous concentrations of prostaglandin also inhibit proteoglycan synthesis. Presumably this effect of estrogens is mediated by receptors, since cytoplasmatic and nuclear estrogen receptors were later found in the chondrocyte of the cartilage[23,24].

Discussion is centering on whether inflammatory and immunologic reactions have an influence on the pathogenesis of osteoarthrosis, and whether they are of etiologic importance. These processes can be influenced by estrogens[33] and this is currently being studied.

CLINICAL STUDIES

During the last decade treatments and drugs for a number of joint disorders have been developed which fit a causal therapy (gout and rheumatic fever). The drug treatment of degenerative joint disorders such as osteoarthrosis is currently possible on a small scale, although epidemiologic data show clearly the importance of these disorders[34]. The literature contains numerous contradictory statements regarding the therapy of climacteric arthralgias with 'ovarial substances'. Curschmann stated in 1932 that the older products were more likely to have had a very uncertain efficacy[35]. The tendency for spontaneous healing, which occurs with many joint symptoms in connection with the menopause[7], was not always considered sufficiently.

In a small trial of therapy with estrogens Kellgren[36] found no subjective improvement of the pain, but slight deterioration. No positive effect on the development of arthrotic processes could be found.

Prill[37] reported good results after estrogen therapy. Although Dequeker showed initial disappearance of symptoms when estrogen was given[18], he had to revise the effect of a long-term estrogen therapy for the small joints of the fingers[17].

Our team followed up 152 patients who initially complained of severe arthralgias: 23% reported complete disappearance and 48% a significant improvement[38]. In a recent study the proportion experiencing significant improvement was even slightly higher[20].

A follow-up study using X-rays of the knee-joints[39] showed that therapy with hormones (for prophylaxis of osteoporosis) caused a lower incidence of osteoarthrosis rather than an increased risk.

SEX HORMONES AND RHEUMATOID ARTHRITIS

Far more epidemiologic and etiologic studies of joint disorders and sex hormones deal with the significance of these hormones in rheumatoid arthritis[40,41]. Not only pregnancy[43–45], but also the phase of the menstrual cycle[42] has effects on the activity of rheumatoid arthritis.

SEX HORMONES AND JAW JOINTS

There are reports of osteoarthrosis of the jaw joint (art. temporomandibu-laris) associated with hormonal disorders. According to Ganshorn[46] there is a prevalence of women with this condition and a temporal connection between the onset of the arthralgia and estrogen production in puberty. Other authors report a second peak of disorders of the jaw joints in postmenopausal women[47,48].

According to Loewit[49] about two-thirds of patients with this condition are female. The authors found only six (about 25%) patients with normal hormone levels. They considered endocrine influences to be important indirect causes for the development of osteoarthrosis of the jaw joints.

THE FUTURE

After coordination of the present epidemiologic references with the partly contradictory experimental and clinical studies, an etiologic connection between osteoarthrosis and sex hormones might be possible. In order to verify this hypothesis further studies are necessary. Clinical efficacy of hormone replacement has to be tested in prospective studies, and the effect of steroid hormones on different joints has to be studied in animals.

REFERENCES

1. Hippokrates. (1982). Über Faruenkrankheiten. In Grensemann, H. (ed.) *Hippokratische Gynäkologie*, p. 131. (Wiesbaden: Steiner Verlag)
2. Celsus. (1935). Buch IV Kap. 31. In *Celsus De Medicina* (Trans. Spencer, W.G.) Vol I, p. 455. (Heinemann – London, Harvard University Press – Cambridge)
3. Charcot, J. M. (1889). *Maladies des Viellards. Oevres Completes*, Vol. 7
4. Fox, R. F. (1895). The varieties of rheumatoid arthritis. *Lancet*, **ii**, 79–84
5. Pineles, F. (1908). Zur Pathogenese der Heberdenschen Knoten. *Wr. Klin. Wschr.*, **21**, 902–4
6. Umber, F. (1924). Zur Nosologie der Gelenkerkrankungen. *Münch. Med. Wschr.*, **71**, 4
7. His, W. (1927). Die Gelenkerkrankungen während der Klimax. *Monatschr. Geburtsch. Gynäkol.*, **75**, 26–31
8. Menge, C. (1924). Über Arthropathia ovaripriva. *Z. Gynäkol.*, **48**, 1617
9. Cecil, R. L. and Archer, B. H. (1925). Arthritis of the menopause. *J. Am. Med. Assoc.*, **84**, 75
10. Hall, F. C. (1938). Menopause arthralgia. *N. Engl. J. Med.*, **219**, 1015–26
11. Weil, M. P. (1929). Rheumatismus der Menopause. *Med. Welt*, 1425–7
12. Wagenhäuser, F. (1970). Die Arthrosen der kleinen Gelenke. In Schoen, R., Böni, A. and Miehlke, K. (eds.) *Klinik der Rheumatischen Erkrankungen*, pp. (Berlin: Springer-Verlag)
13. Silberberg, M. and Silberberg, R. (1963). Modifying action of estrogen on the evolution of osteo-arthritis in mice of different ages. *J. Endocrinol.*, **72**, 449–51
14. Rosner, I. A., Malemud, C. J., Goldberg, V. M., Getzky, L. and Moskowitz, R.

(1982). Pathologic and metabolic responses of experimental osteoarthritis to estradiol and an estradiol antagonist. *Clin. Orthop.,* **171**, 280–6

15. Peyron, J. G. (1986). Osteoarthritis. *Clin. Orthop.,* **213**, 13–19
16. Wagenhäuser, F. J. (1977). *Die Rheumamorbidität.* (Bern: Huber)
17. Dequeker, J. and de Profit, G. (1978). The effect of long-term oestrogen treatment on the development of osteoarthrosis at the small hand joints. *Maturitas,* **1**, 27
18. Dequeker, J. and Ferrin, J. (1972). Effect of long-term estrogen therapy on bone remodeling with women with natural menopause. In Van Keep, P. A., Greenblatt, R. B. and Albeaux-Fernet, M. (eds.) *Consensus on Menopause Research,* p. 124–8. (Lancaster: MTP)
19. Spector, T. D., Brown, G. C. and Silman, A. J. (1988). Increased rates of previous hysterectomy and gynecological operations in women with osteoarthritis. *Br. Med. J.,* **297**, 899–900
20. Hackenbroch, M. (1986). Periphere Arthrosen. In Jäger, M. and Wirth, C. J. (eds.). *Praxis der Orthopädie,* p. 638. (Stuttgart: Thieme)
21. Radin, E. L. and Paub, I. L. (1972). Role of mechanical factors in pathogenesis of primary osteoarthritis. *Lancet,* **i**, 1370
22. Baulieu, E. E., Atgar, M., Best-Belpomme, M., Corvol, P., Courvalin, J. C., Mester, J., Milgrom, E., Robel, P., Rochefort, H. and de Catalogne, D. (1975). Steroid hormone receptors. *Vitamins Hormones,* **33**, 649–736
23. Rosner, I. A., Manni, A., Malemud, C. J., Boja, B. A. and Moskowitz, R. W. (1982). Estradiol receptors in articular chondrocytes. *Biochem. Biophys. Res. Commun.,* **106**, 1379
24. Young, C. N. and Stack, N. T. (1982). Estrogen and glucocorticoid receptors in adult canine articular cartilage. *Arthritis Rheum.,* **25**, 568
25. Mackintosh, D. and Mason, R. M. (1988). Pharmacological actions of 17-beta-oestradiol on articular cartilage chrondrocytes and chondrosarcoma chondrocytes in the absence of oestrogen receptors. *Biochem. Biophys. Acta,* **964**, 295–302
26. Silberberg, M. and Silberberg, R. (1941). Changes in bones and joints in various strains of mice. *Am. J. Anat.,* **68**, 69
27. Sokoloff, L. and Jay, G. E. Jr (1961). Failure of orchiectomy to affect degenerative joint disease in STR/IN mice. *Proc. Soc. Exp. Biol. Med.,* **108**, 792
28. Rosner, I. A., Goldberg, V. M., Getzky, L. and Moskowitz, R. W. (1979). Effects of estrogen on cartilage and experimentally induced osteoarthritis. *Arthritis Rheum.,* **22**, 52–8
29. Priest, R. E. and Complitz, R. N. (1952). Inhibition of synthesis of sulphated mucopolysaccharides by estradiol. *J. Exp. Med.,* **116**, 565
30. Silberberg, M. and Silberberg, R. (1970). Linked modification of the affect of estrogen on joints and cortical bone of female mice. *J. Gerontol.,* **16**, 201
31. Silberberg, R. and Halser, M. (1971). Stimulation of articular cartilage of young adult mice by hormones. *Pathol. Microbiol.,* **37**, 23–36
32. Rosner, I. A., Malemud, C. J., Hassid, A. I., Goldberg, V. M., Boja, B. A. and Moskowitz, R. W. (1983). Estradiol and tamoxifen stimulation of lapine articular chondrocytes prostaglandin synthesis. *Prostaglandins,* **26**, 123–38
33. Goldberg, V. M., Moskowitz, R. W., Rosner, I. A. and Malemud, C. J. (1981). The role of estrogen and oophorectomy in immune synovitis. *Semin. Arthritis Rheum.,* **11** (Suppl.), 134–9

34. Kalbhen, D. A. (1982). *Arthrosis Deformans*, p. 9. (Basel: Eular Verlag)
35. Curschmann, H. (1932). Zur Therapie endokrin bedingter Gelenkerkrankungen. *Fortschr. Ther.*, **8**, 33–7
36. Kellgren, J. H. and Moore, R. (1952). Generalized osteoarthritis and Heberden's nodes. *Br. Med. J.*, **1**, 181
37. Prill, H. J. and Lauritzen, C. (1970). Das Klimakterium. In Schwalm, H., Döderlein, G. *Klinik der Frauenheilkunde und Geburtshilfe*, pp. 374–5. (Berlin, München, Wien)
38. Metka, M., Heytmanek, G., Enzelsberger, H., Schurz, B. and Kurz, Ch. (1988). Der Gelenksschmerz in der Prä- und Postmenopause. *Geburtsh. Frauenheilkunde*, **48**, 232–4
39. Hannan, M. T., Felson, D. T., Anderson, J. J., Naimark, A. and Kannel, W. B. (1990). Estrogen use and radiographic osteoarthritis of the knee in women. *Arthritis Rheum.*, **33**, 525–32
40. Da Silva, J. A. and Hall, G. M. (1992). The effects of gender and sex hormones on outcome in rheumatoid arthritis. *Clin. Rheumatol.*, **6**, 196–219
41. Lahita, R. G. (1985). Sex steroids and rheumatoid arthritis. *Arthritis Rheum.*, **28**, 121–6
42. Latman, N. S. (1983). Relation of menstrual cycle phase to symptoms of rheumatoid arthritis. *Am. J. Med.*, **73**, 947–50
43. Linos, A., Worthington, J. W., O'Fallow, W. M. and Kusland, L. T. (1983). Case-controlled study of rheumatoid arthritis and prior use of oral contraceptives. *Lancet*, 1299–300
44. Silman, A. J. (1986). Is pregnancy a risk factor in the causation of rheumatoid arthritis? *Ann. Rheum. Dis.*, **45**, 1031–4
45. Pritchard, M. H. (1992). An examination of the role of female hormones and pregnancy as risk factors for rheumatoid arthritis. *Br. J. Rheumatol.*, **31**, 395–9
46. Ganshorn, M. and Gärtner, F. (1975). Untersuchungen über mögliche Zusammenhänge zwischen Kiefergelenkserkrankungen und weiblichen Sexualhormonen. *ZWR*, **84**, 726–8
47. Arnaudow, M. (1966). Zur Ätiologie der Arthrosis deformans der Kiefergelenke. *Dtsche. Zahnärztl. Zeitschr.*, **21**, 127–30
48. Hupfauf, L. (1963). Symptomatik und Genese chronischer Kiefergelenkserkrankungen. *Dtsche. Zahnärztl. Zeitschr.*, **18**, 225–35
49. Loewit, K., Wense, Th. and Wunderer, H. (1973). Hormonelle Störungen und Arthropathien der Kiefergelenke. *Österr. Z. Stomatol.*, **70**, 122–5

38

The use of estrogen replacement as an adjunct therapy in rheumatoid arthritis

G. Hall and T. Spector

INTRODUCTION

The possible effect of sex hormones on rheumatic disorders has attracted considerable attention for several years. Much of this interest is based on the epidemiological studies that point toward a higher incidence of several arthritides in women that exhibit a peak age of onset during the perimenopausal period. Gynecologists will recognize the high prevalence of joint pains that accompanies other climacteric symptoms and we found that as many as 67% of new patients attending a menopause clinic suffered troublesome rheumatic symptoms, many of these being readily definable conditions such as osteoarthritis and carpal tunnel syndrome[1]. The prevalence of rheumatoid arthritis in the UK is approximately 1–2% and females are three times as likely as men to acquire the condition. Other observations pointing towards an effect of sex hormones in the etiopathogenesis of rheumatoid arthritis include the frequent remission of disease during pregnancy, the relapse following parturition, a possible protective effect of the oral contraceptive pill and the less favorable outcome seen in women with rheumatoid arthritis compared with their male counterparts, particularly after the menopause[2–4].

Early studies of estrogen extracts in the 1930s and 60s in rheumatoid arthritis were encouraging but side-effects were common[5,6]. More recent studies have shown an amelioration of carpal tunnel syndrome and fibromyalgia with estrogen replacement therapy (ERT)[1] but a small Dutch study of ERT in rheumatoid arthritis was negative[7]. This is a large prospective randomized study of ERT in postmenopausal rheumatoid arthritis designed to assess its effects on bone metabolism over 2 years and disease activity over 6 months[8].

PATIENTS AND METHODS

Patients

A total of 346 clinic attenders with rheumatoid arthritis were invited to participate in a 2-year study of osteoporosis in rheumatoid arthritis, and were not informed of any possible beneficial effect on their rheumatoid disease activity. The first 200 patients to reply and satisfy the inclusion criteria were included (> 3 years since the last monthly period or follicle stimulating hormone > 15 μg/l). Patients continued with their routine anti-rheumatic medication as prescribed by their respective rheumatologist and this could be altered at his discretion, not the investigators'. Sixty six percent of patients were receiving stable doses of a concurrent slow-acting antirheumatic drug, such as penicillamine or methotrexate, and 21% were receiving low-dose corticosteroids.

Treatment

Patients were randomly allocated to receive either transdermal estradiol 50 μg daily with oral norethisterone 1 mg daily for 12 days per month (Estrapak 50® or Estraderm 50® if hysterectomized) or a placebo tablet (calcium supplement).

Assessments

Patients were assessed by the same observer, blinded to treatment, at entry, 3 and 6 months. Two objective and two subjective parameters of disease activity were measured: a Ritchie articular index (AI, which scores 28 groups of joints for tenderness to pressure; 0 = no discomfort, 3 = extreme tenderness; maximum score = 84); the erythrocyte sedimentation rate (ESR); early morning stiffness and a visual analog pain score (VPS, 10 cm, 0 = no pain, 10 = extreme pain). Functional disability was assessed at baseline using a standardized Health Assessment Questionnaire. Serum estradiol levels were measured at entry, 3 and 6 months using radioimmunoassay to give an indication of compliance.

Table 1 Characteristics of estrogen replacement therapy (ERT) and placebo groups. Values are means and standard deviation (unless otherwise indicated)

| | ERT | | | Placebo | |
	All		*Compliers*		*Placebo*
Number (mean, SD)	77		42		91
Age (years)	56.2	(5.4)	56.8	(5.3)	56.0 (4.6)
Menopausal years	7.7	(5.7)	8.5	(6.5)	8.1 (5.9)
Disease duration	11.6	(10.5)	10.2	(8.4)	12.2 (9.2)
Estradiol (pmol/l)	73.0	(148.1)	74.9	(133.0)	60.8 (136.2)
ESR (mm/h)	33.7	(24.0)	38.3	(25.7)	34.8 (23.9)
AI (0–84)	10.5	(8.2)	12.2	(8.5)	11.7 (9.3)
VPS (cm)	4.2	(2.6)	4.6	(2.6)	4.4 (2.7)
EMS (min)	33.2	(36.4)	40.4	(39.6)	49.7 (49.9)
HAQ (0–3)	1.54 (0.9)		1.43 (0.92)		1.52 (1.05)
Steroid users	19	(21%)	9	(21%)	16 (21%)

AI, Ritchie articular index; VPS, visual analog pain score; EMS, early morning stiffness; ESR, erythrocyte sedimentation rate; HAQ, Health assessment questionnaire (0 = no disability, 3 = severe disability); 0–84 is the score range, as above

RESULTS

There were 91 and 77 patients completing placebo and ERT, respectively, after 6 months and patient details are given in Table 1. Patient groups were similar in all baseline characteristics including age, menopausal status, rheumatoid arthritis disease duration and activity, except early morning stiffness which was higher in the placebo group. Patients allocated to placebo were significantly heavier ($p = 0.01$) but baseline estradiol levels were similar. There was no overall effect of ERT on disease activity compared with placebo.

However, two pharmacokinetic studies have shown that, using this transdermal estradiol dose, one should observe a mean steady concentration of serum estradiol of between 122 (SE, 27) and 138 (SE, 10) pmol/l[9,10]. Retrospective analysis of this cohort showed that 35 (42%) patients allocated to ERT failed to achieve estradiol levels > 100 pmol/l at either 3 or 6 months and this subgroup (termed 'poor compliers') were excluded from further analysis. Mean estradiol levels in the remaining 42 (58%) patients ('compliers') were 224 and 194 pmol/l after 3 and 6 months treatment, respectively, compared with 40 and 45 pmol/l, respectively, in the 'poor compliers'.

When comparing the 'compliers' with placebo there were significant improvements after 6 months in AI and VPS. The net effects of ERT compared with placebo after 6 months were; AI–29% ($p < 0.001$),

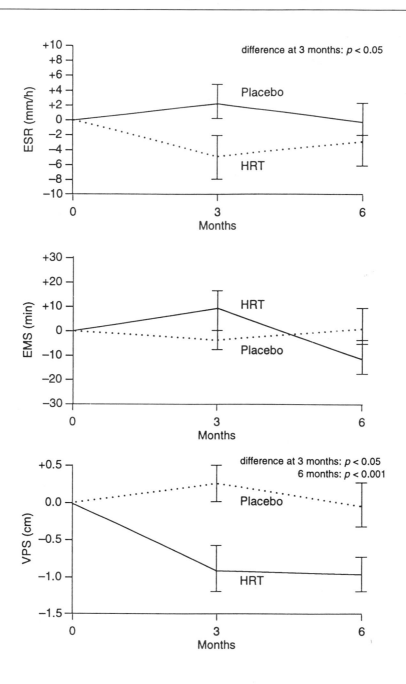

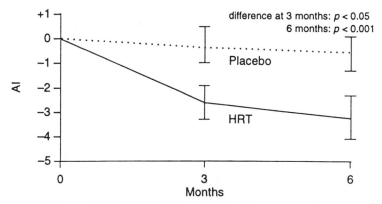

Figure 1 Changes in disease activity variables. Hormone replacement therapy compliers vs. placebo (mean values with standard error). ESR, erythrocyte sedimentation rate; HRT, hormone replacement therapy; EMS, early morning stiffness; VPS, visual analog pain score; AI, Ritchie articular index

ESR−9% (NS), early morning stiffness−25% (NS) and VPS−22% ($p < 0.05$) (Figure 1). Comparing 'compliers' with 'poor compliers' confirmed significant improvements in AI, early morning stiffness ($p < 0.001$) and VPS ($p < 0.05$) after 6 months in the compliers group. There were no notable differences in response to therapy in patients temporally closer to the menopause or in hysterectomized patients.

DISCUSSION

This is the largest randomized study to date of ERT in rheumatoid arthritis and shows that it has no overall effect on disease activity when used as an adjunct therapy with concomitant antirheumatic medications. However, a subgroup of patients were identified who failed to achieve expected serum estradiol levels. Following exclusion of this group, there were significant improvements in some parameters of disease activity, notably the articular index and pain score. Although the placebo effects of ERT are well documented, improvements in the objective measures of disease activity suggest that there may be a genuine effect of estrogen in rheumatoid arthritis. Any effect may also have been partly disguised by the use of other antirheumatic therapies.

We have assumed that inadequate compliance is the principal reason for the suboptimal estradiol levels in the 'poor compliers' based on the studies that suggest that as many as 40% of patients stop taking ERT after

6 months[11]. Clearly other possible reasons include poor drug absorption and drug interactions. Compliance was understandably poor in this group of urban patients, some with considerable disability, many receiving at least three other drugs and most unaware of any potential benefit of ERT.

Why should estrogen have any effect on disease activity? Certainly our findings corroborate the animal studies of Holmdahl and colleagues[12] who found that castration of female mice with a type II collagen model of arthritis led to an exacerbation of their disease which was subsequently reversed with estrogen therapy. They later found that the postparturition flare that occurs in the same model could be prevented with estrogen[13]. There are several potential mechanisms by which estrogen may have an anti-inflammatory action. Estrogen receptors have been isolated on human CD8 T cells[14] and in the thymus[15] and Cutulo and associates recently isolated receptors in the synovium[16]. The effects of estrogens on cytokines are also interesting. Pacifici and co-workers have shown that monocyte secretion of the proinflammatory cytokine, interleukin-1, is elevated following the menopause and these levels can be suppressed within 1 month of ERT[17].

Our previous findings have suggested that ERT is helpful for the treatment of climacteric rheumatological conditions such as carpal tunnel syndrome and fibromyalgia, albeit probably through different mechanisms[1]. This study suggests that there may be an ameliorating effect of ERT in rheumatoid arthritis when used as an adjunct therapy and providing adequate estradiol levels are gained. Importantly, this study also shows that ERT can be prescribed for bone loss in rheumatoid arthritis, itself associated with a two-fold increased risk of osteoporotic fracture[18], without fear of a disease flare. Further studies are planned that ensure satisfactory compliance and using higher doses of estrogens in patients who are not receiving concomitant antirheumatic therapies.

ACKNOWLEDGEMENT

This study was partly funded by Ciba Pharmaceuticals, UK.

REFERENCES

1. Hall, G. M., Spector, T. D. and Studd, J. W. W. (1992). Carpal tunnel syndrome and hormone replacement therapy. *Br. Med. J.*, **304**, 382
2. Pope, R. M., Yoshinoya, S., Rutstein, J. and Persillin, R. H. (1983). Effects of pregnancy on the prognosis and serology of rheumatoid arthritis. *Am. J. Med.*, **74**, 973–9
3. Spector, T. D. and Hochberg, M. C. (1990). The protective effect of the oral

contraceptive pill on rheumatoid arthritis. *J. Clin. Epidemiol.*, **43**, 1221–30
4. da Silva, J. A. P. and Hall, G. M. (1992). Effects of gender and sex hormones on outcome in rheumatoid arthritis. *Baillières' Clin. Rheumatol.*, **6**, 193–219
5. Cohen, A., Dubbs, A. W. and Myers, A. (1940). The treatment of atrophic arthritis with estrogenic substance. *N. Engl. J. Med.*, **222**, 140–2
6. Gilbert, M., Rotstein, J., Cunningham, C., Estrin, I., Davidson, A. and Pincus, G. (1964). Norethynodrel with mestranol in treatment of rheumatoid arthritis. *J. Am. Med. Assoc.*, **190**, 235
7. van den Brink, H. R., van Everdingen, A., van Wijk, M. J. G., Jacobs, J. W. G. and Bijlsma, J. W. J. (1992). Adjuvant estrogen therapy has no effect on disease activity in postmenopausal women with rheumatoid arthritis. *Arthritis Rheum.*, **35**, S202
8. Hall, G. M., Daniels, M., Huskisson, E. C. and Spector, T. D. (1994). A randomized controlled trial of hormone replacement therapy in postmenopausal rheumatoid arthritis. *Ann. Rheum. Dis.*, in press
9. Selby, P. L. and Peacock, M. (1986). Dose dependent response of symptoms, pituitary and bone to transdermal oestrogen in postmenopausal women. *Br. Med. J.*, **293**, 1337–9
10. Powers, M. S., Schenkel, L., Darley, P. E., Good, W. R. and Balestra, J. C. (1985). Pharmacokinetics and pharmacodynamics of transdermal dosage forms of 17B-estradiol: comparison with conventional oral estrogens used for hormone replacement therapy. *Am. J. Obstet. Gynecol.*, **152**, 1099–106
11. Ryan, P. J., Harrison, R., Blake, G. M. and Fogelman, I. (1992). Compliance with hormone replacement therapy (HRT) after screening for osteoporosis. *Br. J. Obstet. Gynaecol.*, **99**, 325–8
12. Holmdahl, R., Carlsten, H., Jansson, L. and Larsson, P. (1989). Oestrogen is a potent immunomodulator of murine experimental rheumatoid disease. *Br. J. Rheumatol.*, **28**, 54–8
13. Mattson, R., Mattson, A., Holmdahl, R., Whyte, A. and Rook, G. A. (1991). Maintained pregnancy levels of oestrogen afford complete protection from post partum exacerbation of collagen induced arthritis. *Clin. Exp. Immunol.*, **85**, 41–7
14. Stimson, W. H. (1988). Oestrogen and human T-lymphocytes. Presence of specific receptors in the T-suppressor/cytotoxic subset. *Scand. J. Immunol.*, **28**, 345–50
15. Luster, M. I., Hayes, H. T., Korach, K., Tucker, A. N., Dean, J. H., Greenlee, W. F. and Boorman, G. A. (1984). Estrogen immunosuppresion is regulated through estrogenic responses in the thymus. *J. Immunol.*, **133**, 110–16
16. Cutulo, M., Accardo, S., Villaggi, B., Clerico, P., Bagnesco, M., Coviello, D. A., Carruba, G., Casto, M. L. and Castagnetta, L. (1993). Presence of estrogen-binding sites on macrophage-like synoviocytes and CD8+, CD29+, CD45RO T lymphocytes in normal and rheumatoid synovitis. *Arthritis Rheum.*, **36**, 1087–97
17. Pacifici, R., Rifas, L., McCracken, R., Vered, I., McMurty, C., Avioli, L. and Peck, W. A. (1989). Ovarian steroid treatment blocks a postmenopausal increase in blood monocyte interleukin-1 release. *Proc. Natl. Acad. Sci.*, **86**, 2398–2402
18. Spector, T. D., Hall, G. M., McCloskey, E. V. and Kanis, J. (1993). The prevalence of vertebral fractures in postmenopausal rheumatoid arthritis. *Br. Med. J.*, **306**, 558

39

Effects of sex hormones on connective tissue

J. Huber

From an embryological standpoint, the epidermis and subcutaneous connective tissue develop from different germ layers. The epidermal part of the skin grows up from the ectoderm, the corium and the subcutis from the mesenchyma. Both are endocrine working 'units' of the mammalian organism, converting different steroids from one form to another. An important biological function which occurs in the subcutaneous fat is the aromatization of C19 steroids to C18 steroids, and the reduction of testosterone and progesterone. Subcutaneous fat tissue is of increasing importance in the diagnosis and treatment of endocrinological problems and of climacteric symptoms.

ULTRASOUND OF THE SKIN AS A SCREENING TOOL FOR THE MANAGEMENT OF OSTEOPOROSIS

The results of lumbar densitometry and skin ultrasound investigation on the upper side of the left arm were compared in 144 patients. In 25 of these patients, a bone density below 80% was diagnosed, and of these, 23 patients were found to have a skin thickness of < 1 mm. However, in the group as a whole, a low skin thickness was found in a total of 54 women.

In conclusion, ultrasound of the skin has a high sensitivity but a low specificity when used as a screening tool for low bone density.

Other indications for the use of ultrasound of the skin

In the subcutis, the vasoactivity of ovarian steroids is clinically important. 17β-Estradiol acts as a vasodilator, causing the release of nitric oxide by the endothelial cells. The 'key' in this biological procedure is nitric oxide synthetase, which is enhanced by 17β-estradiol.

The vasoconstrictor effect of progesterone is well documented by Doppler-derived parameters. Estrogen dependency of subcutaneous venectasies, especially observed under the pill and during hormone replacement therapy, is being studied presently by the author. It is postulated that topical use of progesterone can be efficacious in cases of venectasis; the same treatment protocol is well used in the treatment of mastalgia.

Skin ultrasound examination is applied also for another indication – that of the documentation of subcutaneous water retention, induced by estrogen.

The diuretic effect of progesterone can also be observed and was also investigated biochemically by the author. A dose regimen of $400\,\mu$g progesterone, intravaginally, elevated the serum aldosterone level by blocking aldosterone receptors. On the other hand, the sodium level declined. Progesterone also antagonizes the estradiol-induced water retention effect in the subcutis, and this is clinically very significant.

SUPPRESSION OF 5α-REDUCTASE ENZYME ACTIVITY

In the subcutaneous layer of the skin, testosterone is converted to the biologically active dihydrotestosterone which is responsible for the hirsutism disorder.

In a prospective randomized behavioral study, the possible suppression of 5α-reductase activity in order to improve the hirsute condition was investigated. Finasteride® dissolved in benzol was used topically. In 18 hirsute patients, Finasteride was compared to 12 placebo controls. The preliminary results of Finasteride application to the same region twice daily, after a treatment period of 6 weeks, were encouraging; in 14 cases, the patient herself reported an improvement.

SUBCUTANEOUS ANATOMY

Fifteen years ago, Nurnberger, a dermatologist, and Muller, a pathologist, published a paper in the *Journal of Dermatology* concerning the gender specificity in the anatomical situation of the subcutis. They demonstrated accurately the so-called 'standing fat divisions' only in the female subcutis. In the male, they are polygonal and connected.

Nurnberger concluded that a relationship between the anatomical situation and sex steroids existed, and these conclusions were verified in further studies. Two observations substantiate this association:

(1) The 'standing fat divisions' occur normally in females only (this was well-known hundreds of years ago, as can be seen in the famous picture, the 'Pelzchen', from Rubens.)

(2) If males are orchidectomized or treated with cyproteronacetate they change in the female subcutaneous feature.

In conclusion, a topical androgen deficiency is thought to be involved in this gender-specific skin architecture. This fact formed the basis for another prospective behavioral study, undertaken to investigate the biological effect of the topically applied androgen, Andractim®.

The preliminary results show an improvement of the condition of the skin in more than 50% of patients treated. However, the standardization and fair comparison of the results have proven to be a problem in this trial.

It is likely that a number of other main biological reactions occur in the subcutaneous fat – those involving cytokines, paracrinological procedures and free radical reactions.

In summary, it appears that the subcutis is set to become an increasingly interesting organ from an endocrinological point of view.

40

Ovarian failure and the skin

H. Kuhl

It is well established that skeletal mass decreases gradually in women after reaching a maximum between the ages of 20 and 30 years. After the menopause the rate of bone loss may be accelerated due to estrogen deficiency. The bone consists not only of minerals: up to one-third comprises an organic matrix which is more than 90% collagen. Therefore, changes in the synthesis and/or degradation of collagen may play an important role in the development of postmenopausal osteoporosis. As 50–75% of total protein in the skin is collagen, aging and loss of ovarian activity may affect the skin in a similar way. In fact, a concomitant fall in skin collagen content and bone density occurs during the first 15 years after the menopause: this can be prevented effectively by estrogen replacement therapy[1]. Using X-ray measurement, Brincat and colleagues[2] found a close correlation between skin thickness and metacarpal index. Similar observations have been made by Loch and Pech, using ultrasonic measurement of skin thickness[3]. As early as 1963, McConkey and co-workers[4] noticed an association between thin transparent skin and osteoporosis, and in 1970, Black and colleagues[5] reported decreased skin collagen content in women with osteoporosis. The results indicate that dermal and bone collagen are controlled by the same endocrine factors, and that the decline in skin and bone collagen after the menopause has a common etiology: estrogen deficiency.

The female skin is characterized by the typical distribution and appearance of subcutaneous fat and of body hair which are under the control of estrogens and androgens. Human skin fibroblasts and hair follicles contain estrogen and androgen receptors and show a high metabolic activity[6-11]. Therefore, the loss of estrogen after the menopause while androgen levels remain unaltered, may cause a change in the activity of hair follicles and sebaceous glands, even though the skin shows a high local capacity for aromatization of androgens to estrogens[12,13]. Moreover, estrogen deficiency may lead to a reduction in mitotic and metabolic activity of epidermal and dermal cells and consequently to dehydration and a decrease in collagen content of the dermis, and may cause a reduction in dermal blood flow. These changes can superimpose and enhance the age-dependent thinning and decrease of turgor, tension and resilience of the skin. Finally, the wrinkling of skin has been attributed to the deleterious influence of UV-irradiation on elastic fibres and collagen. There are numerous animal experiments and *in vitro* investigations on the action of sex steroids on skin. Several clinical studies have been carried out in order to distinguish between the effects of aging, solar irradiation and estrogen deficiency.

EFFECT OF AGING ON SKIN

The study of Shuster and colleagues[14] on forearm skin collagen, dermal thickness and collagen density revealed an age-dependent linear decrease in skin collagen by 1% per year throughout adult life of both women and men. Initial skin collagen content was considerably less in females than in men. This difference reflects approximately 15 years of age and may explain the earlier aging of the skin of women as compared to men. While in men there was also a gradual decline in skin thickness, in women it remained nearly constant until the fifth decade, after which a significant thinning occurred[14]. There was also a highly significant relationship between thickness and collagen content of skin in older but not in younger women. Collagen density (ratio collagen/thickness) was lower in women than in men and decreased with age, indicating that skin collagen decreases more rapidly than skin thickness. During aging, the collagen fibers degenerate and become coarsened. Possibly the packing of fibrils in the collagen bundles is looser or ground substance between collagen bundles decreases more slowly than collagen. The data obtained from the forearm skin hold true for all skin sites of the body, whether sun-exposed or protected[14]. The findings of a considerably higher skin collagen content and collagen density in women with hirsutism suggest an influence of androgens, whereas skin thickness was not significantly increased[15]. In postmenopausal women, synthesis of type III collagen, a constituent of both skin and bone collagen, can be stimulated by treatment with anabolic steroids to a higher degree than with estrogen and progestogen[16].

The turgor and appearance of the skin is dependent on an intact network of elastic fibers in the dermis which ascend into the dermal papillae and reach the basal lamina of the dermal–epidermal junction. Ultrastructural investigations demonstrated that chronological aging of the skin begins at the age of 30 years[17]. Between 30 and 70 years a minority, and after the age of 70 years the majority, of fibers exhibit progressive disintegration. In men and women over 45 years, the papillary dermal elastic fibers are thickened and focally clumped. There are large interindividual variations with a marked decrease in elastic fibers in some elderly individuals, but also focal decreases or increases in others. Until the age of 70 years, the elastin and elastic microfibrils are synthesized[17].

Aging of skin is associated with a marked decline in the hyaluronic acid content and a simultaneous rise in other acid mucopolysaccharides (e.g. chondroitin sulfate B)[18]. The loss of hyaluronic acid leads to dehydration of the skin. In old skin, vascular sclerosis of differing degree may be observed. As the activity of the basal layers of the epidermis is dependent on nutrition by the dermal capillary circulation, an impaired vascularization and blood flow may decrease the activity of dermal cells.

EFFECT OF SUN EXPOSURE OF THE SKIN

Symptoms such as pruritus, flushing, bruising, thinning and dryness can be observed more frequently in sun-exposed skin of postmenopausal women than in protected skin[19]. Most of the wrinkling of aging skin is assumed to be the cumulative result of chronic injury from solar irradiation, which causes degeneration into a porous structure of elastic fibers in the upper dermis[17,20]. Chronic ultraviolet exposure of the skin may also cause the production of abnormal elastin, which is incorporated into the elastic microfibrils[17].

In sun-exposed skin, the vascular walls of postcapillary venules and of arterial and venous capillaries are thickened by the development of a layer of basement membrane-like material[21]. The premature death of epidermal cells of aging skin is more pronounced in sun-exposed skin[22]. Lipid peroxidation may be involved in the process of aging of epidermal cells. Lipid peroxidation, which is induced by superoxide radicals, is strongly enhanced by small amounts of melanin[22].

EFFECT OF ESTROGEN DEFICIENCY ON SKIN

Epidermis

Gradual atrophy of the epidermis begins after the age of 30 years and is

Table 1 Effect of bilateral ovarectomy on epidermal thickness (planimetric measurements) and on epidermal [³H]thymidine labelling (labelling index) (after reference 24)

	Before ovarectomy	1 month after ovarectomy	4 months after ovarectomy	7 months after ovarectomy
Epidermal thickness (cm²)	49.3 ± 8.5	48.9 ± 6.3	44.6 ± 6.3**	42.0 ± 5.1**
[³H]thymidine labelling index	25.7 ± 8.8	13.1 ± 12.6*	14.3 ± 9.8**	18.6 ± 10.5

*$p < 0.05$; **$p < 0.01$

intensified between 40 and 50 years. The boundary between epidermis and dermis becomes almost straight, perhaps secondary to atrophy of the dermal papillae, and the rate of epidermal cell proliferation decreases. The atrophy progresses in older age and the epidermis becomes transparent.

Castration leads to thinning of the epidermis, which can be prevented by estrogen treatment. In pharmacologically high doses, however, estrogens can depress epidermal DNA and protein synthesis *in vitro* and, therefore, may inhibit proliferation[20]. Investigations with cultured epidermal samples indicate that estradiol does not directly control proliferation of human epidermis[23]. In all probability, the influence of estrogens on the epidermis is mediated by other hormones and growth factors. On the other hand, the mitotic activity in the epidermis is limited to the basal cell layers, and the epidermal activity is dependent on the dermal capillary circulation. The epidermal atrophy corresponds to the atrophy of the vessels. Estrogen treatment increases the number of capillaries and causes dilation of arterioles and venules, resulting in an improved nutrition of the basal layer of the epidermis. In contrast to estradiol, progesterone-stimulated cell proliferation shortens the cornification rate of epidermal cells and increases epidermal thickness, while testosterone enhances keratinization of the epidermic cells[23].

The comprehensive study of Rauramo and Punnonen[24,25] on the effect of abrupt estrogen deprivation revealed a significant decrease of epidermal thickness. During the 1st month after bilateral ovarectomy, some women showed an alteration, but thereafter, epidermis became thinner with increasing time after castration. After 4 months, thickness was significantly decreased by 9% and after 7 months by 14% (Table 1). There was no correlation between epidermal thickness and the labelling indices, as within 1 month after ovarectomy a rapid fall in DNA synthesis by

Table 2 Decrease in skin collagen content after the menopause (after reference 2)

n	Time after menopause	Skin collagen content ($\mu g/mm^2$)
19	0–3 months	189.6 ± 55.2
14	6–7 months	193.4 ± 55.6
19	1 year	161.1 ± 44.8
16	1.5–2 years	191.7 ± 73.5
14	3 years	192.4 ± 66.9
15	4–5 years	146.6 ± 54.0
13	6–7 years	147.1 ± 57.7
15	8–9 years	154.5 ± 81.3
12	10–15 years	130.6 ± 30.6
11	≥ 16 years	108.6 ± 23.3

50% was observed, which thereafter remained in this range (Table 1). Obviously, the decline in mitosis rate precedes the thinning of epidermis.

Dermis

The most important constituents of connective tissue in the dermis are collagen and elastin fibers, fibroblasts, and ground substance containing mucopolysaccharides, non-collagenous protein and water[18]. Collagen (largely type I, but also type III) and elastin are produced by fibroblasts in a low-molecular weight, soluble form; these are polymerized to insoluble cross-linked collagen peptide chains. These fibrils are aggregated to fibers. The majority of amino acids contained in collagen are glycine, proline and hydroxyproline. Hydroxyproline is uniquely found in collagen and may serve as a marker for collagen degradation. Animal experiments have shown that estrogens enhance polymerization of soluble collagen to the insoluble form, retard degradation and prolong the half-life of collagen by more than 100%[26]. This suggests that estrogen deprivation may cause an accelerated degradation of collagen.

Clinical investigations in postmenopausal women have revealed a continuous decline of skin collagen content during the first 15 years after menopause, after which it stabilized (Table 2)[1,2]. The average loss of dermal collagen was 2.1%/postmenopausal year[2]. There was also a linear decline in skin thickness which was less pronounced than that of collagen content (Table 3); the average decrease in skin thickness during the first 19 years after the menopause was 1.13%[2]. There was a highly significant correlation between skin thickness and collagen content, and both

Table 3 Decrease in skin thickness (X-ray measurements) after the menopause (after reference 2)

n	Time after menopause	Skin thickness (mm)
12	0–3 months	0.88 ± 0.14
10	6–9 months	0.77 ± 0.15
20	1 year	0.75 ± 0.16
17	1.5–2 years	0.81 ± 0.13
9	3 years	0.80 ± 0.14
15	4–5 years	0.77 ± 0.14
14	6 years	0.73 ± 0.12
12	7–10 years	0.81 ± 0.12
12	11–19 years	0.69 ± 0.14
12	⩾20 years	0.64 ± 0.12

were independent of chronological age of the women, but correlated significantly with menopausal age[1,2]. Treatment with estradiol and testosterone implants prevented effectively the fall in collagen content and thickness of skin[1]. In postmenopausal women, skin collagen content can be significantly increased by estradiol therapy, the effect being the more pronounced the lower the collagen content was before[27]. There appears to be an optimum skin collagen content which cannot be exceeded by higher doses of estrogen.

In young women, premature estrogen deprivation appears to cause accelerated degeneration of dermal elastic fibers. Ultrastructural examination of skin biopsies of three women (30–37 years) with a history of premature ovarian failure revealed degenerative changes in 6–10% of the elastic fibers (formation of lacunae, peripheral fragmentation, granular degeneration, splitting of fibers into strands) which are normally seen in women aged 50–70 years[19]. These findings indicate a relationship between estrogen deprivation and premature aging of dermal elements.

The ground substance which has a gel-like consistency, fills the space between fibrous and cellular elements of the dermis. It contains acid and neutral mucopolysaccharides, non-collagenous protein, water, and compounds derived from blood plasma. It represents a depot which binds water and electrolytes in a three-dimensional structure of acid mucopolysaccharides and their protein complexes[18,28]. The predominant acid mucopolysaccharide in young skin is hyaluronic acid, which is a polymer of alternating N-acetylglucosamine and glucuronic acid units. Hyaluronic acid is produced in a low-molecular weight form which is subsequently polymerized and complexed with proteins. There is a close correlation between the content of high-molecular weight hyaluronic acid and of water, and 25% of tissue water is bound to hyaluronic acid[28,29].

It has been demonstrated that treatment of mice with estrogens increases the content of hyaluronic acid in skin four- to five-fold and increases the ratio of hyaluronic acid/protein 3.5-fold, while the water content doubles[28,29]. This suggests that estrogen deprivation results in a decline of hyaluronic acid and a loss of water storage, i.e. a dehydration of tissue.

Sweat glands, hair follicles and sebaceous glands

In all probability, estrogens have no influence on sweat glands. Androgens stimulate sebaceous mitoses and increase sebum production, while estrogens do not affect mitosis rate in the sebaceous gland but decrease sebum production[9]. The change from vellus hair to terminal hair is under androgenic control; estrogens may play a role, as they are taken up by the hair follicles. The deprivation of estrogens leads to a predominance of androgenic influence and may change the appearance of facial and body hair. Sebaceous glands and hair follicles are very active in metabolizing sex steroids[11].

REGULATION OF MITOTIC AND METABOLIC ACTIVITY OF THE SKIN

The mechanism of action of sex steroids on the skin is still unclear. There is no doubt that various hormones and growth factors are involved in the regulation of fibroblast activity. Human fibroblasts contain not only estrogen and androgen receptors[6,7], but also receptors for growth hormone (hGH) and insulin-like growth factor (IGF-I, somatomedin-C)[30,31]. Growth of cultured human fibroblasts can be stimulated by hGH, but the effect is at least partly mediated by IGF-I which is produced locally by the fibroblasts[32]. IGF-I production by cultured human fibroblasts is also increased by platelet-derived growth factor (PDGF), fibroblast growth factor (FGF), epidermal growth factor (EGF) and macrophage growth factor[33]. Moreover, thyroid hormones, glucocorticoids and insulin may also influence fibroblast IGF-I synthesis, but only in the presence of cytokines such as PDGF. The findings indicate a complex regulation of fibroblast activity by endocrine and autocrine factors.

The main source of IGF-I is the liver, and hepatic production of IGF-I is stimulated by hGH. In postmenopausal women the serum levels of hGH and IGF-I are 50% lower than in premenopausal women, while hGH-binding protein is unchanged[34]. hGH treatment of men and women older than 60 years resulted in a strong increase in the IGF-I levels[35]. Pituitary secretion of hGH is dependent on sex and age, whereby estradiol levels play an important role[36]. Transdermal estradiol therapy increased significantly IGF-I, but not hGH levels, while oral treatment with ethinyl-estradiol increased hGH and decreased IGF-I levels[34,37]. The hepatic production of hGH-binding protein was also stimulated, but free hGH remained elevated. It may be assumed that some of the effects of estrogens on the skin are mediated and modulated by IGF-I and other factors. It has been demonstrated that treatment of rats with hGH increased collagen content and mechanical strength of the skin[38]. As a consequence, the acceleration of the age-dependent skin collagen loss and the decrease in epidermal DNA synthesis in women with estrogen deficiency may be caused at least partly by the fall in hGH and IGF-I levels or a decrease in local IGF-I production. Changes in the local concentration or activity of other hormones and cytokines may also play a role.

CONCLUSION

Estrogens are directly and indirectly involved in the regulation of the activity of epidermal cells and fibroblasts. Therefore, estrogen deprivation may accelerate the age-dependent degenerative changes in the skin. Estrogen deficiency is associated with a decrease in the rate of mitosis of epidermal cells, resulting in epidermal atrophy. It decreases dermal vascularization and blood flow, which is important for nutrition of the basal layers of epidermis. Estrogen deprivation leads to a reduction in polymerization of low molecular weight collagen and to enhanced collagen degradation, and possibly reduces collagen synthesis. This results in a degeneration of collagen fibers. It also causes an accelerated degeneration of elastin fibers. It decreases synthesis and polymerization of hyaluronic acid and consequently reduces water storage in the network of acid mucopolysaccharides. Therefore, estrogen deficiency enhances the age-dependent decrease in skin thickness.

REFERENCES

1. Brincat, M., Moniz, C. F., Kabalan, S., Versi, E., O'Dowd, T., Magos, A. L., Montgomery, J. and Studd, J. W. W. (1987). Decline in skin collagen content and metacarpal index after the menopause and its prevention with sex hormone replacement. *Br. J. Obstet. Gynaecol.*, **94**, 126–9

2. Brincat, M., Kabalan, S., Studd, J. W. W., Moniz, C. F., de Trafford, J. and Montgomery, J. (1987). A study of the decrease of skin collagen content, skin thickness, and bone mass in the postmenopausal woman. *Obstet. Gynecol.*, **70**, 840–5

3. Loch, E. G. and Pech, A. (1991). Osteoporosis screening using ultrasonic measurement of skin thickness. XII World Congress of Gynaecology and Obstetrics (FIGO), Abstract 0754

4. McConkey, B., Fraser, G. M., Bligh, A. S. and Whitely, H. (1963). Transparent skin and osteoporosis. *Lancet*, **I**, 693–5

5. Black, M. M., Shuster, S. and Bottoms, E. (1970). Osteoporosis, skin collagen, and androgen. *Br. Med. J.*, **II**, 773–4

6. Hasselquist, M. B., Goldberg, N., Schroeter, A. and Spelsberg, T. C. (1980). Isolation and characterization of the estrogen receptor in human skin. *J. Clin. Endocrinol. Metab.*, **50**, 76–82

7. Keenan, B. S., Meyer, W. J. III, Hadjian, A. J. and Migeon, C. J. (1975). Androgen receptor in human skin fibroblasts – characterization of a specific 17β-hydroxy-5α-androstan-3-one-protein complex in cell sonicates and nuclei. *Steroids*, **25**, 535–52

8. Mowszowicz, I., Riahi, M., Wright, F., Bouchard, P., Kuttenn, F. and Mauvais-Jarvis, P. (1981). Androgen receptor in human skin cytosol. *J. Clin. Endocrinol. Metab.*, **52**, 338–44

9. Ebling, F. J. (1973). The effects of cyproterone acetate and oestradiol upon testosterone stimulated sebaceous activity in the rat. *Acta Endocrinol.*, **72**, 361–5

10. Rampini, E., Davis, B. P., Moretti, G. and Hsia, S. L. (1971). Cyclic changes in the metabolism of estradiol by rat skin during the hair cycle. *J. Invest. Dermatol.*, **57**, 75–80

11. Sansone-Bazzano, G., Seeler, A. K., Cummings, B. and Reisner, R. M. (1979). Steroid hormone metabolism in skin and isolated sebaceous glands: preliminary observations on the effect of age. *J. Invest. Dermatol.*, **73**, 118–22

12. Schweikert, H. U., Milewich, L. and Wilson, J. D. (1976). Aromatization of androstenedione by cultured human fibroblasts. *J. Clin. Endocrinol. Metab.*, **43**, 785–95

13. Berkovitz, G. D., Fujimoto, M., Brown, T. R., Brodie, A. and Migeon, C. J. (1984). Aromatase activity in cultured human genital skin fibroblasts. *J. Clin. Endocrinol. Metab.*, **59**, 665–71

14. Shuster, S., Black, M. M. and McVitie, E. (1975). The influence of age and sex on skin thickness, skin collagen and density. *Br. J. Dermatol.*, **93**, 639–43

15. Shuster, S., Black, M. M. and Bottoms, E. (1970). Skin collagen and thickness in women with hirsuties. *Br. Med. J.*, **II**, 772

16. Hassager, C., Jensen, L. T., Podenphant, J., Riis, B. J. and Christiansen, C. (1990). Collagen synthesis in postmenopausal women during therapy with anabolic steroids or female sex hormones. *Metabolism*, **39**, 1167–9

17. Braverman, I. M. and Fonferko, E. (1982). Studies in cutaneous aging: I. The elastic fiber network. *J. Invest. Dermatol.*, **78**, 434–43

18. Danforth, D. N. and Buckingham, J. C. (1964). Connective tissue mechanisms and their relation to pregnancy. *Obstet. Gynecol. Surv.*, **19**, 715–32

19. Bolognia, J. L., Braverman, I. M., Rousseau, M. E. and Sarrel, P. M. (1989). Skin changes in menopause. *Maturitas*, **11**, 295–304

20. Sharad, P. and Marks, R. (1977). A pharmacological effect of oestrone on human epidermis. *Br. J. Dermatol.,* **97**, 383–6
21. Braverman, I. M. and Fonferko, E. (1982). Studies in cutaneous aging: II. The microvasculature. *J. Invest. Dermatol.,* **78**, 444–8
22. Serri, F., Bartoli, G. M., Seccia, A., Borrello, S. and Galeotti, T. (1979). Age-related mitochondrial lipoperoxidation in human skin. *J. Invest. Dermatol.,* **73**, 123–5
23. Tammi, R. (1982). Effects of sex steroids on human skin in organ culture. *Acta Dermatovenereol.,* **62**, 107–12
24. Punnonen, R. (1972). Effect of castration and peroral estrogen therapy on the skin. *Acta Obstet. Gynecol. Scand.,* Suppl. **21**, 1–44
25. Rauramo, L. (1976). Effect of castration and peroral estradiol valerate and estriol succinate therapy on the epidermis. In Campbell, S. (ed.) *The Management of the Menopause and Postmenopausal Years,* pp. 253–62. (Lancaster: MTP Press)
26. Skosey, J. L. and Damgaard, E. (1973). Effect of estradiol benzoate on the degradation of insoluble collagen of rat skin. *Endocrinology,* **93**, 311–15
27. Brincat, M., Versi, E., Moniz, C. F., Magos, A., de Trafford, J. and Studd, J. W. W. (1987). Skin collagen in postmenopausal women receiving different regimens of estrogen therapy. *Obstet. Gynecol.,* **70**, 123–7
28. Grosman, N. (1973). Study on the hyaluronic acid-protein complex, the molecular size of hyaluronic acid and the exchangeability of chloride in skin of mice and after oestrogen treatment. *Acta Pharmacol. Toxicol.,* **33**, 201–8
29. Grosman, N., Hvidberg, E. and Schou, J. (1971). The effect of oestrogenic treatment on the acid mucopolysaccharide pattern in skin of mice. *Acta Pharmacol. Toxicol.,* **30**, 458–64
30. Ho, K. K. Y. and Weissberger, A. J. (1992). Impact of short-term estrogen administration on growth hormone secretion and action: distinct route-dependent effects on connective and bone tissue metabolism. *J. Bone Mineral Res.,* **7**, 821–7
31. Rechler, M. W., Nissley, S. P., Podskalny, J. M., Moses, A. C. and Fryklund, L. (1977). Identification of a receptor for somatomedin-like polypeptides in human fibroblasts. *J. Clin. Endocrinol. Metab.,* **44**, 820–31
32. Cook, J. J., Haynes, K. M. and Werther, G. A. (1988). Mitogenic effects of growth hormone in cultured human fibroblasts. *J. Clin. Invest.,* **81**, 206–12
33. Clemmons, D. R. (1984). Multiple hormones stimulate the production of somatomedin by cultured human fibroblasts. *J. Clin. Endocrinol. Metab.,* **58**, 850–5
34. Weissberger, A. J., Ho, K. K. Y. and Lazarus, L. (1991). Contrasting effects of oral and transdermal routes of estrogen replacement therapy on 24-hour growth hormone (GH) secretion, insulin-like growth factor I, and GH-binding protein in postmenopausal women. *J. Clin. Endocrinol. Metab.,* **72**, 374–81
35. Marcus, R., Butterfield, G., Holloway, L., Gilliland, L., Baylink, D. J., Hintz, R. L. and Sherman, B. M. (1990). Effects of short term administration of recombinant human growth hormone to elderly people. *J. Clin. Endocrinol. Metab.,* **70**, 519–27
36. Ho, K. Y., Evans, W. S., Blizzard, R. M., Veldhuis, J. D., Merriam, G. R., Samojlik,

E., Furlanetto, R., Rogol, A. D., Kaiser, D. L. and Thorner, M. O. (1987). Effect of sex and age on the 24-hour profile of growth hormone secretion in man: importance of endogenous estradiol concentrations. *J. Clin. Endocrinol. Metab.,* **64**, 51–8

37. Fröhlander, N. and von Schoultz, B. (1988). Growth hormone and somatomedin C during postmenopausal replacement therapy with oestrogen alone and in combination with an antioestrogen. *Maturitas,* **9**, 297–302

38. Jorgensen, P. H., Andreassen, T. T. and Jorgensen, K. D. (1989). Growth hormone influences collagen deposition and mechanical strength of intact rat skin. *Acta Endocrinol.,* **120**, 767–72

41

The importance of extragenital symptoms in the menopause

M. Metka

A closer examination of a questionnaire recording climacteric symptoms (Figure 1), which is used in the out-patient department for climacteric disorders and prophylaxis of osteoporosis at the first department of gynecology and obstetrics, University of Vienna, reveals that about 95% of the effects of sexual hormones are extragenital, which means that the term 'sexual' in connection with sex hormones limits concepts of the function of these hormones. The technical term 'extragenital target organs' was chosen by us, since in the past 5 years the variety of target organs has become clear, and an increasing discussion of this problem is now taking place. The most important task is to carry out the necessary objective pathophysiological and epidemiological reappraisal of 'target organs', which up to now seemed to be practically of no importance. The great variety of the symptoms of the climacteric syndrome, and the numerous somatic effects of long-term estrogen deficiency, require a definition of sexual steroids going far beyond the term 'sexual'.

The term 'extragenital target organs' can be very helpful. For many of the concerned women, as well as for many colleagues, the effect of sexual hormones is understood too much in the sense of just sexual and genital. In a general review of problems in connection with the menopause at the World Congress of Osteoporosis in Hong Kong, a well-known expert mentioned, as well as postmenopausal osteoporosis and the possible athero-protective effect of estrogens, only vasomotor disorders, atrophic vaginitis and incontinence. To study the climacteric syndrome and postmenopausal estrogen deficiency symptoms, any examination has to

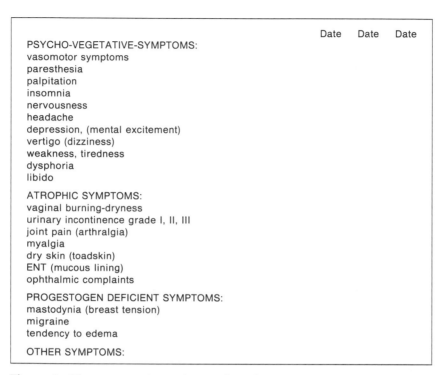

Figure 1 Menopause rating scale questionnaire

regard the patient as an entity. Many colleagues and concerned women reduce the problems of the menopause to vasomotor disorders, atrophic changes of the vagina and the vaginal tract, and to possible metabolic influences on the bone metabolism. This opinion is still widely held, but as far as we are concerned it is far too limited and has to be overcome. The variety of symptoms and the numerous consequences of long-term estrogen deficiency have to be demonstrated clearly. If we, the physicians, are aware of the variety of symptoms, we can give specific information and can use a broad spectrum of treatments.

An appropriate questionnaire (Figure 1), which offers for both the physician and the concerned woman a sufficient basis, is very well suited for this purpose. Generally, if less common climacteric symptoms appear alone or not in connection with the commonly acknowledged symptoms, these problems are passed onto another specialist. Palpitations, which often occur in connection with the changed hormonal environment in

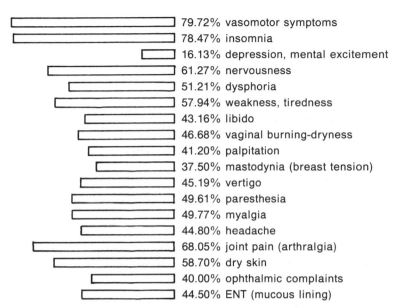

79.72% vasomotor symptoms
78.47% insomnia
16.13% depression, mental excitement
61.27% nervousness
51.21% dysphoria
57.94% weakness, tiredness
43.16% libido
46.68% vaginal burning-dryness
41.20% palpitation
37.50% mastodynia (breast tension)
45.19% vertigo
49.61% paresthesia
49.77% myalgia
44.80% headache
68.05% joint pain (arthralgia)
58.70% dry skin
40.00% ophthalmic complaints
44.50% ENT (mucous lining)

Figure 2 Statistical analysis of climacteric symptoms

the menopause, are often investigated and treated at length by internists. 'Arthropathia climacterica' is often at first treated orthopedically and only later with the appropriate substitution therapy with sex hormones.

A statistical analysis of patients attending our out-patient department for climacteric disorders shows that less well known symptoms are quite frequent (Figure 2). For instance, 40% of women report palpitations at the beginning of the menopause. In 15% of these women, palpitations were the only climacteric symptom; most of these women had already undergone prolonged differential diagnostic investigations, often including hospitalizations with numerous electrocardiograms and exercise electro-cardiograms. Palpitations are a symptom which has been neglected in connection with the climacteric syndrome. Much more intense etiological and epidemiological work is still to be done.

It is not only important for physicians to know about the extragenital symptoms and about the variety of symptoms, but it is our task and especially the task of colleagues in outstanding positions, to provide adequate information for the population about the variety of symptoms that can arise in the course of the endocrine changes during the menopause. The reasons for the consultations in 1986 – when our out-patient department was opened and when we had just started the information campaign – were vasomotor disturbances in 80% of patients, although a great variety of symptoms could be elicited by questioning. Seven years later the picture has changed completely. The concerned population is well informed and some women come to the out-patient department just for ocular complaints, which started with the menopause. This change in the reason for consultation shows that informing the population was of great importance, and that it had consequences. While for instance in 1986 no woman came to our out-patient department for 'prophylactic consultation', now 25% of the women come for this reason. These are women who have no climacteric symptoms and often still have a normal menstrual cycle.

A very important fact in connection with the problems of the extragenital target organs is that knowledge of these correlations is extremely helpful for compliance. Only if the patient is shown all her disturbances and if an adequate amelioration of all these disturbances is achieved with an eventual hormone substitution, will the woman be willing to start or continue with substitution therapy. There is a difference in whether a substitution just relieves menopausal flush or whether several different symptoms are targeted.

The influence of sexual hormones on the connective tissue is of great importance, since most of the extragenital symptoms and effects of hormone substitution can be explained by a positive effect of the hormones on the connective tissue – either in the joint capsule, in the intervertebral disc, in the musculoskeletal system as a whole, in the skin or in the eye.

The eye is also an extragenital target organ of the sexual hormones. Until 2 or 3 years ago there was no literature about this problem. By asking well directed questions we found that this symptom appears quite often.

The problem of arthropathia climacterica seems to be of great importance. In the last 20 years our way of looking at the musculoskeletal system and the fixing system of the connective tissue of the bones seems to have been too narrow regarding the influence of the sex hormones – concentrating only on the bone and especially on bone density. Obviously a very important reason for this is the ease with which bone density can be measured. In fact, the bones have kept together and moved and the joints should be studied in the same way. Some early studies show clearly that this system has a dependence on sexual hormones. Our medical forefathers knew very well that this problem has to be seen as an entity, and in 1938 they spoke not about osteoporosis, but about 'osteoarthrosis' in connection with postmenopausal estrogen deficiency.

Another important subject area is that of the skin: one of the reasons that the skin is of importance is that the positive reaction of this organ to a hormone substitution therapy can raise compliance considerably. A correctly applied systemic and/or local estrogen substitution can be the most effective cosmetic at the beginning of the menopause, and this often enables us to improve compliance for the prophylactic possibilities regarding the bones and circulation system.

For about 2 years our team in Vienna has emphasized the necessity of individual diagnosis, therapy and prophylaxis of the problem of ovarian insufficiency developing either postmenopausally, or for other reasons. If the problems are examined differentially and are individualized it must be a matter of concern for the physicians to check particularly the extragenital organs.

Section 8

Sex steroids and breast cancer

42

The importance of HRT for breast cancer: an introduction

I. Persson

This symposium, entitled 'the importance of HRT for breast cancer', is one of several sessions during this congress that deal with the issue of breast cancer and hormone replacement therapy. The topics of hormonal regulation of the normal breast and trends in breast cancer incidence and mortality have been explored in special interest group sessions that gave the opportunity for in-depth discussions on research issues. The controversies in our understanding of hormonal actions on the growth control of the normal breast are highlighted and debated among discussants in a special session.

The issue of HRT and its possible effect on breast cancer risk is important for many reasons. For example, the notion that HRT may alter the risk of breast cancer has, in the experience of many clinical doctors, a substantial impact. On the one hand, doctors may be concerned about prescribing HRT because of possible serious side-effects, such as breast cancer. Women who are in need of treatment, either because of symptoms or for preventive purposes, might themselves be unwilling to start or to continue HRT for the same reason.

It is likely that, as a consequence, HRT is also avoided by women who clearly have an indication for treatment and who would benefit by an improved quality of life. The counselling of patients on the treatment of climacteric symptoms is complex. One of the reasons for this is that our present knowledge on the relationships between HRT and breast cancer is incomplete, and data are, to say the least, controversial.

The purpose of this symposium is to discuss some of the more pertinent issues with regard to breast cancer, both in research and clinical settings. Important issues to discuss are:

(1) Is there a relationship between breast cancer risk and endogenous estrogens and progesterone? What can we learn from the various risk factors for breast cancer?

(2) Does HRT affect the occurrence of breast cancer? Are compounds, dose, duration and timing of exposure important in determining the risk? Does exposure to HRT interact with other factors in the patient or other exposures?

(3) What is the prognosis of HRT-related breast cancers? Are clinical properties of the tumors different? Is the mortality from breast cancer in HRT-exposed women different from that in women without exposure?

(4) How do the breast cancer and other risk effects balance against benefits associated with HRT? What is the expected overall impact on morbidity and mortality and life expectancy?

(5) How is the breast best monitored for safety during HRT? Can patients with breast cancer be treated with HRT?

43

Hormonal replacement therapy and incidence of breast cancer

M. Ewertz

INTRODUCTION

Breast cancer is the most frequent malignant disease among women in western parts of the world and incidence has been increasing worldwide[1]. Between 1981 and 1986 the cumulative incidence rate in those aged 0–75 years ranged from 5.5 to 7.3% in the Nordic countries, indicating that one in 14–20 Nordic women will develop breast cancer before the age of 75 years[2].

Use of hormonal replacement therapy (HRT) to relieve menopausal symptoms became widespread in the 1960s, and the uptake has varied between countries. In the United States, a survey showed that 32% of women aged 50–65 years currently use HRT[3]. In Northern Europe, ever-use of HRT seems to vary between 9 and 32% for women with a natural menopause, and between 30 and 55% for hysterectomized women[4,5].

It is evident that even a weak causal link between a disease as frequent as breast cancer and an exposure as common as HRT would have great public health impact. It is therefore important to examine the association between HRT and breast cancer risk.

EVER-USE

Since 1975, many studies have examined the relationship between HRT and breast cancer risk, but the results have not been consistent. Over the past 5 years, four meta-analyses have tried to reconcile the evidence[6–9].

Two[6,7] detected no increase in risk associated with ever-use of HRT, while the others[8,9] found small increases (6–11%) in breast cancer risk. However, the meta-analyses revealed significant heterogeneity between studies, leaving doubt as to whether it is wise to pool the results.

The heterogeneity between studies may relate to differences in meno-pause (status, type), which affects not only breast cancer risk but also the probability of exposure to HRT. Higher risks have been reported in studies including premenopausal women[7] and among women with a natural menopause[8]. Since bilateral oophorectomy reduces breast cancer risk, it might be expected that HRT would obliterate this protective effect. This was not reflected in ever-use[8].

Ever-use of HRT has also been examined in subgroups of women already at high risk, e.g. those with a positive family history, benign breast disease, or obesity, but no consistent pattern has emerged. The lack of consistency may be due to small numbers of HRT users within subgroups[10].

DURATION

Many studies have evaluated the trend in breast cancer risk with HRT use for 1–12 years, but evidence on more long-term use is limited[9,10]. As is the case for ever-use, results on risk with increasing duration of HRT are heterogeneous. Two meta-analyses[7,8] suggested some increase in risk with increasing duration of use, but others failed to confirm this[6,9]. It should be noted, however, that studies from Denmark and Sweden showed strong and consistent trends of increasing breast cancer risk with increasing duration of HRT[5,11].

Despite apparent inconsistencies, there seems to be a general consensus that HRT use for < 5 years does not increase the risk of breast cancer. Focusing on population-based case–control studies with a sufficient number of long-term HRT users, it may also be concluded that HRT use for ⩾ 10 years may be associated with a 30–80% increased risk[10].

TIMING OF USE

Assessment of the role of latency, i.e. time since first HRT use, is difficult, because the effect is strongly correlated with duration of use[5,11]. The majority of studies have found no association with latency[8,10].

Current use of HRT has been associated with an increased breast cancer risk in some studies, for instance in the Nurses' Health Study[12], where current users had a 33% increased risk (significant) compared with non-users. One meta-analysis[8] also reported increased risks associated with current use. The risk decreased with increasing time since last use (recency), but trends were not significant. Other studies have found no relation between recency and breast cancer risk[10].

DOSAGE AND TYPE OF HORMONES

Available evidence on dosage and type of hormones reflects the varying prescription practice between countries. In the United States, conjugated estrogens are most widely used[10], while usage of estradiol is more common in Europe and more often in combination with progestins[5,11].

Evidence on dosage is limited to conjugated estrogens. No consistent trends of increasing risk with increasing dosage have been observed[9,10].

Swedish data[11] suggest an increased risk associated with use of estradiol, but no increase in risk for other estrogens, mainly estriol. Other studies have included too few users of these compounds for a meaningful evaluation.

Three studies have shown increased risks associated with the combined use of estrogen and progestins, the relative risks being 1.36 for ever-use[5], 1.54 for current use[12], and 4.4 for $\geq$ 6 years of use[11]. A decreased risk has also been reported[13], but the methodology of this study may be questioned. Combined therapy with estrogen and androgens more than doubled the risk of breast cancer in two studies[5,12], while no increase in risk was detected in two others[14,15].

There is not sufficient evidence to evaluate the role of treatment with progestins alone without concomitant use of estrogens[5,12].

DISCUSSION

Although results from ample experimental, epidemiological and clinical studies indicate that estrogens play a fundamental role in the etiology of breast cancer, the literature has in general failed to provide clear and consistent evidence of a causal association between HRT and breast cancer. This may not be surprising, however, considering the methodological difficulties involved.

Many studies have included too few women to ensure a sufficient statistical power. If results of small as well as large studies were in the same direction, this problem should be overcome by meta-analyses. However, the meta-analyses revealed significant heterogeneity between studies, indicating that the observed inconsistencies were due to factors other than lack of statistical power. Such factors may relate to study design (cohort vs. case–control), length of follow-up in cohort studies, choice of controls in case–control studies (hospital vs. population) or inappropriate control for confounding factors, most notably menopause variables (status, type, age), and influence of bias (selection, surveillance, recall). Variation in these factors may have introduced sufficient 'noise' to obscure the detection of a fairly weak risk factor.

Methodological discrepancies are of minor concern regarding ever-usage of HRT, because this variable is artificial anyway – women use hormones for months or years. Therefore, duration of use is crucial in establishing a dose (duration)–response relationship.

Three reasonably well conducted studies (one cohort[11] and two case–control[5,14]) found consistent and significant trends of increasing breast cancer risk with increasing duration of HRT. However, a recent report from the Nurses' Health Study[12] failed to confirm a similar trend. Other important issues, such as type of hormone and dosage, have been addressed in few studies with a limited number of exposed women.

Thus, despite the large number of studies conducted, we still need to know more about the details of HRT in relation to breast cancer risk. It is important that future studies include a number of HRT users sufficiently large to ensure a reasonable statistical power of detecting relative risks in the order of 1.5–2.0. They should also concentrate on a proper assessment of HRT use, specifically start and end of treatment periods, type of hormone and dosage used. Furthermore, the information on HRT use should be validated, preferably from sources independent of the assessment method.

CONCLUSION

Available evidence suggests that use of HRT for < 5 years is not associated with an increased risk of breast cancer. Use for ≥ 10 years may be associated with a 30–80% increase in risk. Addition of progestins to estrogen treatment does not seem to lower breast cancer risk; on the contrary, it may increase the risk even more than therapy with estrogens alone. Some studies also suggest that therapy combining estrogens with androgens may be associated with particularly high risks of breast cancer.

REFERENCES

1. Miller, A. B. and Bulbrooke, R. D. (1986). UICC Multidisciplinary project on breast cancer: the epidemiology, aetiology and prevention of breast cancer. *Int. J. Cancer,* **37**, 173–7
2. Tulinius, H., Storm, H. H., Pukkala, E., Andersen, A. and Ericsson, J. (1992).

Cancer in the Nordic Countries, 1981–1986. *Acta Pathologica Microbiologica et Immunologia Scandinavica,* **100**, Suppl. 31

3. Harris, R. B., Laws, A., Reddy, V., King, A. and Haskell, W. L. (1990). Are women using postmenopausal estrogens? A community survey. *Am. J. Public Health,* **80**, 1266–8

4. Barlow, D. H., Grosset, K. A., Hart, H. and Hart, D. M. (1989). A study of the experience of Glasgow women in the climacteric ages. *Br. J. Obstet. Gynaecol.,* **96**, 1192–7

5. Ewertz, M. (1988). Influence of non-contraceptive exogenous and endogenous sex hormones on breast cancer risk in Denmark. *Int. J. Cancer,* **42**, 832–8

6. Armstrong, B. K. (1988). Oestrogen therapy after the menopause – boon or bane? *Med. J. Aust.,* **148**, 213–14

7. Steinberg, K. K., Thacker, S. B., Smith, J., Stroup, D. F., Zack, M. M., Flanders, W. D. and Berkelman, R. L. (1991). A meta-analysis of the effect of estrogen replacement therapy on the risk of breast cancer. *J. Am. Med. Assoc.,* **265**, 1985–90

8. Sillero-Arenas, M., Delgado Rodriguez, M., Rodrigues-Canteras, R., Bueno-Cavanillas, A. and Galvez-Vargas, R. (1992). Menopausal hormone replacement therapy and breast cancer: a meta-analysis. *Obstet. Gynecol.,* **79**, 286–94

9. Dupont, W. D. and Page, D. L. (1992). An overview of the effect of oestrogen replacement therapy on breast cancer risk. In Mann, R. D. (ed.) *Hormone Replacement Therapy and Breast Cancer Risk,* pp. 79–92. (Carnforth: Parthenon)

10. Brinton, L. A. and Schairer, C. (1993). Estrogen replacement therapy and breast cancer risk. *Epidemiol. Rev.,* in press

11. Bergkvist, L., Adami, H.-O., Persson, I., Hoover, R. and Schairer, C. (1989). The risk of breast cancer after estrogen and estrogen–progestin replacement. *N. Engl. J. Med.,* **321**, 293–7

12. Colditz, G. A., Stampfer, M. J., Willett, W. C., Hunter, D. J., Manson, J. E., Hennekens, C. H., Rosner, B. A. and Speizer, F. E. (1992). Type of postmenopausal hormone use and risk of breast cancer: 12-year follow-up from the Nurses' Health Study. *Cancer Causes Control,* **3**, 433–9

13. Gambrel, R. D., Maier, R. C. and Sanders, B. I. (1983). Decreased incidence of breast cancer in postmenopausal estrogen–progesterone users. *Obstet. Gynecol.,* **62**, 435–43

14. Brinton, L. A., Hoover, R. and Fraumeni, J. F., Jr. (1986). Menopausal oestrogens and breast cancer risk: an expanded study. *Br. J. Cancer,* **54**, 825–32

15. La Vecchia, C., DeCarli, A., Parazzine, F., Gentile, A., Liberati, C. and Francheschi, S. (1986). Non-contraceptive oestrogens and the risk of breast cancer in women. *Int. J. Cancer,* **38**, 853–8

44

Hormonal risk factors for breast cancer

B. S. Hulka

The female breast is subject to a lifetime of hormonal controls, whose impact is evident at the time of menarche and during the menstrual cycle, pregnancy and lactation. After the menopause, breast tissue becomes quiescent when circulating sex steroid hormone levels drop to low (estrogen) or unmeasurable levels (progesterone).

Epidemiologists have studied and recorded multiple risk factors for breast cancer, some of which are a reflection of hormonally mediated events. Evidence for the beneficial effect of surgical oophorectomy on risk of breast cancer was evident as early as 1956[1]. The earlier during reproductive life that oophorectomy is performed, the greater the benefit. This benefit is ascribed to the removal of the primary source of estrogen and progesterone production and reduction in life-time number of menstrual cycles[2-4].

Early menarche and late menopause have a modest impact on increasing breast cancer risk. Furthermore, it appears that the earlier the age of menarche, the earlier the onset of regular menstrual cycles[4,5]. The latter are generally accepted as indicators of normal ovarian function with respect to estrogen/progesterone production and cycling. Late menopause, variously defined as after age 50 or 52, has not been well characterized with respect to estrogen and progesterone production. Menstrual cycles are known to vary in length for some months or years prior to actual cessation of menses, and the duration of this variability is greater for women with late compared to early menopause[6].

Late age at first pregnancy and nulliparity both increase breast cancer risk. Risk decreases modestly with increasing number of pregnancies. Following a first birth, there is a short-term increase in the risk of breast

Table 1 Hormonally-related epidemiologic risk factors for breast cancer

Factor	Risk group		Relative risk[a]	Reference
	Low	High		
Gender	male	female	150	10
Oophorectomy	age < 35	no	2.5	11
Age at menarche	≥ 14	≤ 11	1.5	12
Age at first birth	< 20	≥ 30	1.9	13
Parity	≥ 5	nulliparity	1.4	12
Age at natural menopause	< 45	≥ 55	2.0	11
Obesity[b], postmenopausal	< 22.9	> 30.7	1.6	12
Oral contraceptive use	never	ever	1.0	15
	never	≥ 4 years use before first pregnancy	1.7	
Hormone replacement use	never	current	1.4	14
	never	15 + years	1.3	16

[a]Low risk group is the reference.
[b]Body mass index (kg/m^2)

cancer followed by a long-term reduction in risk relative to that of nulliparous women[7].

The biological explanations for these epidemiologic observations are several. With the onset of puberty and sex steroid hormone production, ductal epithelia in the breast proliferates; mitotic activity is prominent. An early pregnancy is not only associated with extensive proliferation of ductal, lobular and alveolar tissue, under the stimulus of high levels of estrogen and progesterone, but it also results in stem cell differentiation in the terminal ducts and lobules[8]. The reduction of omnipotent stem cells to more differentiated forms is thought to leave the breast permanently less susceptible to genotoxic insults. Subsequent pregnancies enhance this effect, but to a lesser extent than the first early pregnancy.

Obesity increases the risk of breast cancer in postmenopausal women. This effect is thought to be mediated by increased estrogenic stimulation of the breast. Androstenedione, derived from the adrenal gland, is the major endogenous source of estrogenic compounds in postmenopausal women, and adipose cells are a major site of aromatization of androstene-dione to estrone (the predominant postmenopausal estrogen). Serum levels of estrone are higher in postmenopausal obese women than thin women[9]. These hormonally related risk factors and the magnitude of the increased breast cancer risks are shown in Table 1[10–16].

Pike postulates that the epidemiologic risk factors are mediated through estrogenic and progestational effects on mitotic rates in the terminal ducts of the breast[17]. These rates are increased by estrogen in the follicular phase of the menstrual cycle and further enhanced by the addition of progesterone in the luteal phase. Hormonally-dependent mitotic rates could account for the decreased breast cancer risk after early surgical oophorectomy, early natural menopause and late menarche, since these events result in a decreased lifetime exposure to ovarian steroids. Obesity in postmenopausal women, resulting in increased extraglandular estrogen production, could increase breast-cell mitotic rate in the normally quiescent breast.

The effect of early age at first birth may be better explained by the hypothesis of Russo[8]. A combination of increased mitotic activity and stem cell differentiation during pregnancy results in a permanent decrease in the number of stem cells susceptible to genotoxic events and mitoses. Pregnancy, with resulting mammary gland development and differentiation, must occur early in reproductive life to minimize carcinogenic insults to undifferentiated terminal ducts. Thus, according to this theory, young age at first birth would reduce breast cancer risk[18].

These observations on indicators of endogenous hormonal events have led to intensive study of sources of exogenous hormones and their effect on breast cancer risk. Oral contraceptives during the reproductive years and hormone replacement therapy (HRT) in the peri- and postmenopausal years are the major sources. Numerous studies of each exposure have been conducted, but evaluating their results is complicated by the secular changes in hormonal composition, changing patterns with respect to duration of use and age at first use, and the secular changes in demographic characteristics of users. Hormonal use during both the reproductive and early postmenopausal years is extremely common. Estimates of ever-use of oral contraceptives vary by age group of respondent, but by age 40, 80% of American women have used oral contraceptives[19]. Patterns of HRT use vary by geographic region of the country, age and social class[20]. In 1985, use prevalence in the western United States was reported at 43% for women age 50–59 years, but only 15% for women on the east coast[21]. These figures are continually changing, in relation to media coverage of the health impact of hormones, physician recommendations, and women's perceptions of risks and benefits.

Studies of breast cancer risk are subject to methodologic problems such as non-comparability of groups using or not using the hormonal preparations, a particular problem with HRT. Users tend to be better educated, higher social class, thinner and generally healthier than non-

411

users[20]. The selection factors for use of oral contraceptives are different in that it is the never-users who differ with respect to health and personal characteristics relative to the majority population of users, making it difficult to define an appropriate reference population. Numerous reviews and meta-analyses exist on both topics[15,16,22,23] and still the summary risk estimates and conclusions are inconsistent as to whether or not oral contraceptives and HRT increase risk of breast cancer. Where positive associations appear, it is usually for subgroups of the study population and/or for specific use characteristics of the hormones.

The oral contraceptive literature focuses on several issues. A primary concern is that women who start oral contraceptive use at an early age (as teenagers, and/or before a first full-term pregnancy) may be at increased risk of developing early onset (before age 45) breast cancer. Since age-specific breast cancer rates are low for women aged < 45 years, an increased risk of 1.5 or 2-fold results in a small absolute number of hormone-induced breast cancers. More critical is what happens to this cohort of women as they move into older age groups, where the age-specific breast cancer rates are much higher. The CASH data show that women aged 45–54 years may actually experience a lower than expected number of breast cancers[24]. If this observation proves to be true, one might interpret the early increase in risk as a promotional effect of oral contraceptives on existing breast cancer, such that occult cancer becomes clinically manifest at an earlier age than it otherwise would. Oral contraceptives became available to American women in the early 1960s, and it is only now, some 30 years later, that the effects of these formulations in older women can be identified. This is an important rationale for the newly initiated National Institute for Child Health and Human Development (NICHD) study of breast cancer and oral contraceptives.

Table 2[24–37] summarizes some of the recent studies of breast cancer in young women, highlighting oral contraceptive use before a first full-term pregnancy. Where elevations in the risk estimates appear, they are mostly ≤ 2-fold, with variable dose–response relationships. The elevations are more evident in the studies where the age at diagnosis is < 45 years. In general, results have varied, some studies suggesting an increased risk with oral contraceptive use before first full-term pregnancy, others suggesting that the risk relates to long-term use at an early age[31,35,38] and still others finding total duration of use important[33]. Since this paper emphasizes hormonal relationships to breast cancer, studies evaluating use before first full-term pregnancy are shown.

As with oral contraceptives, numerous epidemiologic studies of HRT and breast cancer risk have been published over the past 20 years. Many

Table 2 Breast cancer risk estimates for oral contraceptive use before first full-term pregnancy

Study location	Reference	Age at diagnosis	Years of use	Relative risk[a]	95% confidence interval
USA	25	< 45	> 1–4	1.1	0.9–1.5
			> 4	1.2	0.9–1.6
Norway/Sweden	26	< 45	≥ 3	1.2	0.8–1.7
			4–7	1.0	0.6–1.7
			≥ 8	2.0	1.8–4.2
Northeastern USA	27	< 45	3–4	0.8	0.4–1.6
			5–6	1.5	0.6–4.0
			≥ 7	1.4	0.6–3.2
UK	28	< 45	1–4	2.0	1.0–3.8
			≥ 4	2.6	1.3–5.4
Seattle, WA	29	< 43	1–3	0.8	0.3–2.0
			≥ 4	1.3	0.3–4.6
Northern Italy	30	< 45	< 2	1.4	—
			≥ 2	1.2	—
Sweden	31	< 46	< 4	1.8	1.0–3.2
			4–7	2.1	1.1–3.8
			≥ 8	2.0	0.8–4.7
USA[b,c]	32	< 65	1–2	1.1	0.8–1.6
			≥ 3	0.8	0.4–1.7
UK[c]	33	< 36	1–4	1.0	
			> 4–8	1.5	
			> 8	1.4	
UK[b]	34	< 55	1–4	1.7	0.4–6.3
			≥ 4	1.2	0. 3–4.9
Global	35	< 62	< 2	0.8	0.6–1.1
			≥ 2	1.2	0.8–2.0
New Zealand	36	< 55	< 2	0.8	0.6–1.1
			2–5	0.7	0.5–1.0
			> 5	0.6	0.4–1.0
Long Island, NY	37	< 50	1–4	1.7	0.9–3.1
			> 4	2.1	0.8–5.3
USA	24	< 35	2–3	1.7	0.9–3.2
			4–5	1.5	0.7–3.2
			> 5	1.3	0.5–3.1

[a]Never use is the reference category; [b]Cohort studies; [c]Parous women. Malone, K.E. (1991). *Oral contraceptives and Breast Cancer*, Appendix A, pp. 75–101. (Washington, DC: National Academy Press)

of these are of high quality, exhibiting appropriate design and analytic strategies, and including large numbers of study subjects. Study findings, however, are not fully consistent; some show an increased breast cancer risk after long-term estrogen use, a few show increased risk with current or recent use and others show no association. When comparing results from the United States with European studies, higher risks appear in the latter, suggesting heterogeneity across geographic areas[14,39–50]. This could be a function of both the particular hormones used and the characteristics of women receiving them. In America, at least 70% of the estrogen product used is Premarin, composed of estrone sulfate and a mixture of other estrogens found in mare's urine (the source of Premarin)[51]. In Europe, estradiol and synthetic estrogens are more commonly used. Progestins and androgens have also been more frequently used in Europe. In America, progestin, mostly Provera, has been commonly used in addition to estrogen for little more than a decade. Studies currently in progress in America will evaluate the combined effect of estrogen plus progestins on the postmenopausal breast.

Another trans-Atlantic difference is the indication for HRT. In America, it is frequently prescribed for the prevention of osteoporosis and cardiovascular disease; essentially all postmenopausal women are candidates for its use. In Europe, at least until recently, hormones were more likely to be prescribed for indications associated with the perimenopausal period. Differences in the particular hormones used and the indications for prescribing them may have affected study results.

However one views the epidemiologic studies of HRT, it is evident that the risks incurred are modest: risk estimates of 1.3- to 2.0-fold, depending on duration and timing of use prior to diagnosis, chronological age and menopausal status of the user. Although most of the increased risk has been attributed to long-term use, the Nurses Health Study reports an adverse effect with current use of estrogen replacement therapy (ERT), an effect which increases with increasing age of the user[18]. Several American and European studies show an interaction between age at menopause and hormone use[42,47,49,52]. Hormone users with a late natural menopause exhibit an increased breast cancer risk. Recent studies also show an interaction between alcohol consumption and estrogen use; the increased breast cancer risk from ERT is predominantly among those who consume alcoholic beverages[16,18]. In all these associations, the high risk subgroups exhibit relative risk estimates of $\leqslant 2$.

Hormonal carcinogenesis is most certainly relevant to breast cancer etiology, and the epidemiologic risk factors commonly employed as proxy indicators for hormonal events are useful. However, the hormonal phenomena which these indicators represent should be clarified and more direct biological measurements applied. Furthermore, the ability to utilize epidemiologic risk factors in relation to molecular alterations representing disease susceptibility or pathogenesis can provide expanded opportunities for epidemiologic research. Although risk factors may exhibit secular variability in the magnitude of their effects on breast cancer risk, reproductive risk factors (hormonal surrogates) have persisted in their importance. Despite the obvious relevance of hormonal carcinogenesis to risk of breast cancer, a hormonal solution to breast cancer etiology has not emerged after many years of inquiry. Alternative and complimentary risk factors for breast cancer must also be sought.

REFERENCES

1. Lilienfeld, A. M. (1956). The relationship of cancer of the female breast to artificial menopause and marital status. *Cancer, 9*, 927–34
2. Kelsey, J. L. and Gammon, M. D. (1991). The epidemiology of breast cancer. *CA-A Cancer J. Clin., 41*, 146–65
3. Irwin, K. L., Lee, N. C., Peterson, H. B., Rubin, G. L., Wingo, P. A., Mandel, M. G. and The Cancer and Steroid Hormone Study Group (1988). Hysterectomy, tubal sterilization, and the risk of breast cancer. *Am. J. Epidemiol., 127*, 1192–201
4. Henderson, B. E., Ross, R. K., Judd, H. L., Krallo, M. D. and Pike, M. C. (1985). Do regular ovulatory cycles increase breast cancer risk? *Cancer, 56*, 1206–8
5. Apter, D. and Vihko, R. (1983). Early menarche, a risk factor for breast cancer, indicates early onset of ovulatory cycles. *J. Clin. Endocrinol. Metab., 57*, 82–6
6. Wallace, R. B., Sherman, B. M., Bean, J. A., Leeper, J. P. and Treolar, A. E. (1978). Menstrual cycle patterns and breast cancer risk factors. *Cancer Res., 38*, 4021–4
7. Kampert, J. B., Whittemore, A. S. and Paffenbarger, R. S. Jr. (1988). Combined effect of childbearing, menstrual events, and body size on age-specific breast cancer risk. *Am. J. Epidemiol., 128*, 962–79
8. Russo, J., Tay, L. K. and Russo, I. H. (1982). Differentiation of the mammary gland and susceptibility to carcinogenesis. *Breast Cancer Res. Treat., 2*, 5–73
9. Cauley, J. A., Gutal, J. P., Kuller, L. H., LeDonne, D. and Powell, J. G. (1989). The epidemiology of serum sex hormones in postmenopausal women. *Am. J. Epidemiol., 129*, 1120–31
10. Boring, C. C., Squires, T. S. and Tong, T. (1993). Cancer Statistics, 1993. *CA-A Cancer J. Clin., 43*, 7–26
11. Trichopoulos, D., MacMahon, B. and Cole, P. (1972). Menopause and breast cancer risk. *J. Natl. Cancer Inst., 48*, 605–13
12. Gapstur, S. M., Potter, J. M., Sellers, T. A. and Folsom, A. R. (1992). Increased risk of breast cancer with alcohol consumption in postmenopausal women. *Am. J. Epidemiol., 136*, 1221–31
13. White, E. (1987). Projected changes in breast cancer incidence due to the trend toward delayed childbearing. *Am. J. Publ. Health, 77*, 495–7
14. Colditz, G. A., Stampfer, M. J., Willett, W. C., Hennekens, C. H., Rosner, B. and

Speizer, F. E. (1990). Prospective study of estrogen replacement therapy and risk of breast cancer in postmenopausal women. *J. Am. Med. Assoc.*, **264**, 2648–53

15. Romieu, I., Berlin, J. A. and Colditz, G. (1990). Oral contraceptives and breast cancer. *Cancer,* **66**, 2253–63

16. Steinberg, K. K., Thacker, S. B., Smith, S. J., Stroup, D. F., Zack, M. M., Flanders, W. D. and Berkelman, R. L. (1991). A meta-analysis of the effect of estrogen replacement therapy on the risk of breast cancer. *J. Am. Med. Assoc.*, **265**, 1985–90

17. Pike, M. C., Bernstein, L. and Spicer, D. V. (1993). Exogenous hormones in breast cancer risk. In Niederhuber, J. E. (ed.) *Current Therapy in Oncology,* pp. 292–303. (St Louis, MO: Decker)

18. Russo, I. H., Calaf, G. and Russo, J. (1991). Hormones and proliferative activity in breast tissue. In Stoll, B. A. (ed.) *Approaches to Breast Cancer Development,* pp. 35–52. (The Netherlands: Kluwer Academic Publishers)

19. Committee on the Relationship between Oral Contraceptives and Breast Cancer, Institute of Medicine, Division of Health Promotion and Disease Prevention (1991). *Oral Contraceptives and Breast Cancer.* (Washington, DC: National Academy Press)

20. Matthews, K. A., Bromberger, J. and Egeland, G. (1989). Behavioral antecedents and consequences of the menopause. In Korenman, S. G. (ed.) *The Menopause: Biological and Clinical Consequences of Ovarian Failure: Evolution and Management,* pp. 1–10. (Nada, California, USA: Serono Symposia)

21. Hemminki, E., Kennedy, D. L., Baum, C. and McKinlay, S. M. (1988). Prescribing of noncontraceptive estrogens and progestins in the United States, 1974–1986. *Am. J. Publ. Health,* **78**, 1479–81

22. Sillero-Arenas, M., Delgado Rodriguez, M., Ridigues-Canteras, R., Bueno-Cavanillas, A. and Galvez-Vargas, R. (1992). Menopausal hormone replacement therapy and breast cancer: a meta-analysis. *Obstet. Gynecol.,* **79**, 286–94

23. Dupont, W. D. and Page, D. L. (1991). Menopausal estrogen replacement therapy and breast cancer. *Arch. Intern. Med.,* **151**, 67–71

24. Wingo, P. A., Lee, N. C., Ory, H. W., Beral, V., Peterson, H. B. and Rhodes, P. (1991). Age-specific differences in the relationship between oral contraceptive use and breast cancer. *Obstet. Gynecol.,* **78**, 161–70

25. Stadel, B. V., Rubin, G. L., Webster, L. A., Schlesselman, J. J. and Wingo, P. A. (1985). Oral contraceptives and breast cancer in young women. *Lancet, 2,* 970–3

26. Meirik, O., Lund, E., Adami, H. O., Bergstrom, R., Christofferson, T. and Bergsjo, P. (1986). Oral contraceptive use and breast cancer in young women. A joint national case–control study in Sweden and Norway. *Lancet, 2,* 650–4

27. Miller, D. R., Rosenberg, L., Kaufmann, D. W., Schottenfeld, D., Stolley, P. D. and Shapiro, S. (1986). Breast cancer risk in relation to early oral contraceptive use. *Obstet. Gynecol.,* **68**, 863–8

28. McPherson, K., Vessey, M. P., Neil, A., Doll, R., Jones, L. and Roberts, M. (1987). Early oral contraceptive use and breast cancer: results of another case–control study. *Br. J. Cancer,* **56**, 653–60

29. Jick, S. S., Walker, A. M., Stergachis, A. and Jick, H. (1989). Oral contraceptives and breast cancer. *Br. J. Cancer,* **59**, 618–21

30. LaVecchia, C., Parazzini, F., Negri, E., Boyle, P., Gentile, A., DeCarli, A. and

Franceschi, S. (1989). Breast cancer and combined oral contraceptives: an Italian case–control study. *Eur. J. Cancer Clin. Oncol.,* **25**, 1613–8

31. Olsson, H., Moller, T. R. and Ranstam, J. (1989). Early oral contraceptive use and breast cancer among premenopausal women: final report from a study in southern Sweden. *J. Natl. Cancer Inst.,* **81**, 1000–4

32. Romieu, I., Willett, W. C., Colditz, G. A., Stamfer, M. J., Rosner, B., Hennekens, C. H. and Speizer, F. E. (1989). Prospective study of oral contraceptive use and risk of breast cancer in women. *J. Natl. Cancer Inst.,* **81**, 1313–21

33. UK National Case–Control Study Group (1989). Oral contraceptive use and breast cancer risk in young women. *Lancet,* **8645**, 973–82

34. Vessey, M. P., McPherson, K., Villard-Mackintosh, L. and Yeates, D. (1989). Oral contraceptives and breast cancer: latest findings in a large cohort study. *Br. J. Cancer,* **59**, 613–17

35. WHO Collaborative Study of Neoplasia and Steroid Contraceptives (1990). Breast cancer and combined oral contraceptives: results from a multinational study. *Br. J. Cancer,* **61**, 110–19

36. Paul, C., Skegg, D. C. G. and Spears, G. F. S. (1990). Oral contraceptives and risk of breast cancer. *Int. J. Cancer,* **46**, 366–73

37. Weinstein, A. L., Mahoney, M. C., Nasca, P. C., Leske, M. C. and Varma, A. O. (1991). Breast cancer risk and oral contraceptive use: results from a large case–control study. *Epidemiology,* **2**, 353–8

38. Pike, M. C., Henderson, B. E., Krailo, M., Duke, A. and Roy, S. (1983). Breast cancer in young women and use of oral contraceptives: possible modifying effect of formulation and age of use. *Lancet,* **2**, 926–30

39. Brinton, L. A., Hoover, A. R. and Fraumeni, J. F. (1986). Menopausal oestrogens and breast cancer risk: an expanded case–control study. *Br. J. Cancer,* **54**, 825–32

40. McDonald, J. A., Weiss, N. S., Daling, J. R., Francis, A. M. and Polissar, L. (1986). Menopausal estrogen use and the risk of breast cancer. *Br. Cancer Res. Treatment,* **7**, 193–9

41. Wingo, P. A., Layde, P. M., Lee, N. C., Rubin, G. and Ory, H. W. (1987). The risk of breast cancer in postmenopausal women who have used estrogen replacement therapy. *J. Am. Med. Assoc.,* **257**, 209–15

42. Mills, P. K., Beeson, W. L., Phillips, R. L. and Fraser, G. E. (1989). Prospective study of exogenous hormone use and breast cancer in Seventh-Day Adventists. *Cancer,* **64**, 591–7

43. Kaufman, D. W., Palmer, J. R., de Mouzon, J., Rosenberg, L., Stolley, P. D., Warshauer, M. E., Zauber, A. G. and Shapiro, S. (1991). Estrogen replacement therapy and the risk of breast cancer: results from the Case–Control Surveillance Study. *Am. J. Epidemiol.,* **134**, 1375–85

44. Palmer, J. R., Rosenberg, J., Clarke, E. A., Miller, D. R. and Shapiro, S. (1991). Breast cancer risk after estrogen replacement therapy: results from the Toronto Breast Cancer Study. *Am. J. Epidemiol.,* **134**, 1386–95

45. Harris, R. E., Namboodiri, K. K. and Wynder, E. L. (1992). Breast cancer risk: effects of estrogen replacement therapy and body mass. *J. Natl. Cancer Inst.,* **84**, 1575–82

46. Hulka, B. S. (1990). Hormone-replacement therapy and the risk of breast cancer. *CA-A Cancer J. Clin.,* **40**, 289–96

47. LaVecchia, C., DeCarli, A., Parazzini, F., Gentile, A., Liberati, C. and Franceschi,

S. (1986). Non-contraceptive oestrogens and the risk of breast cancer in women. *Int. J. Cancer,* **38**, 853–8

48. Hunt, K., Vessey, M., McPherson, K. and Coleman, M. (1987). Long-term surveillance of mortality and cancer incidence in women receiving hormone replacement therapy. *Br. J. Obstet. Gynaecol.,* **94**, 620–35

49. Ewertz, M. (1988). Influence of non-contraceptive exogenous and endogenous sex hormones on breast cancer risk in Denmark. *Int. J. Cancer,* **42**, 832–8

50. Bergkvist, L., Adami, H.-O., Persson, I., Hoover, R. and Schairer, C. (1989). The risk of breast cancer after estrogen and estrogen-progestin replacement. *New Engl. J. Med.,* **321**, 293–7

51. Piper, J. M. and Kennedy, D. L. (1987). Oral contraceptives in the United States: Trends in content and potency. *Int. J. Epidemiol.,* **16**, 215–21

52. Hulka, B. S. and Schildkraut, J. M. (1992). North Carolina studies of oestrogens, oestrogen receptors and breast cancer. In Mann, R. D. (ed.) *Hormone Replacement Therapy and Breast Cancer Risk*, pp. 155–72. (Carnforth: Parthenon)

45

Antiestrogen action of progestogens on human breast cells

F. Kuttenn, C. Malet, E. Leygue, A. Gompel, R. Gol, N. Baudot,
C. Louis-Sylvestre, L. Soquet and P. Mauvais-Jarvis

INTRODUCTION

Many controversial studies have been published on the increased risk of breast cancer with the pill or with estrogen replacement therapy for menopause. It is unanimously accepted that estradiol stimulates breast cell multiplication; it can therefore increase the risk of errors arising at the time of cell replication and act as a 'promoter' of carcinogenesis. The role of progesterone is more disputed. Data obtained in experimental animals, and in *in vitro* and *in vivo* studies of breast cell growth and differentiation, and epidemiological data on hormonal risk factors in breast cancer, have caused most authors to conclude that progesterone slows down estradiol-induced cell multiplication and to stimulate functional maturation of cells.

However, the publication of discrepant results has thrown the medical community into confusion. It is therefore essential to gather as much information as possible on the hormone dependence of breast tissue and on the interactions of estrogens and progestogens. The stakes are high, since the conclusions have relevance for the estrogen/progestogen balance in contraceptive pills, the choices of treatment of menopause, and strategies for preventing breast cancer.

What is the role of estradiol and its interaction with progesterone, as deduced from physiological and experimental data on animals, *in vitro* and *in vivo* studies on human breast tissue and epidemiological studies of breast cancer?

EXPERIMENTAL STUDIES IN ANIMALS

Numerous animal experiments have clearly demonstrated the mitogenic effect of estradiol on the mammary gland[1-5]. Eisen[5] showed that administration of high doses of estrogen to mice successively leads to proliferation of the tubular system after 26 days, with dilatation of ducts, formation of cysts and fibrosis. After longer periods of estrogen administration, malignant tumors develop, in all stages from benign to malignant. Progesterone inhibits the development of these estradiol-induced tumors.

Many studies of mammary carcinogenesis in animals have used physical carcinogens (such as irradiation) or chemical carcinogens (dimethylbenz-anthracene or *N*-nitrosomethylurea known to raise the incidence of mutations in the Ha-*ras*-I oncogene) which have a role as initiators of carcinogenesis. Administration of estradiol to animals exposed to carcinogens increases the number, size and aggressiveness of the induced tumors, and shortens the time before tumor appearance. Estradiol has a role as a promoter of carcinogenesis. In contrast, pretreatment with progesterone prevents or decreases these effects of estradiol[6-9].

INTERACTION BETWEEN ESTRADIOL AND PROGESTERONE IN HUMAN BREAST TISSUE. PHYSIOLOGICAL AND EXPERIMENTAL DATA

The pubertal period

During the pubertal period, development of the breast tissue is estradiol-dependent: estradiol is secreted alone for several years. After the beginning of the ovulatory cycles, the breast is subjected to the alternate secretion of estradiol and progesterone.

During the menstrual cycle

In breast biopsies obtained at various times in the menstrual cycle, Vogel and colleagues[10] observed a proliferative aspect and numerous mitoses of the duct epithelium during the follicular phase; this aspect is similar to that observed in estrogen-treated animals[1]. During the luteal phase, there were very few mitoses; a secretory aspect was observed similar to that described after progestogen treatment of estradiol-pretreated animals[2,3].

Not only the epithelial cells are regulated by sex steroids. Under the influence of estrogen, the mesenchymatous component of the gland is transformed into intralobular connective tissue. The estrogens stimulate the production of an edematous substance, rich in mucopolysaccharides, which precedes hyalinization[11] and has an important role in the genesis of breast fibrocystic disease. Progesterone counteracts this effect of estrogen on the mesenchyma[12].

In breast cancer cell lines

Most studies of the hormone dependence of the human breast have been performed using cancer cell lines. Vignon and colleagues[13] and Horwitz and co-workers[14] have shown that the progestin R5020 clearly inhibits the growth of T47D cells.

In a recent paper, Musgrove and colleagues[15] showed that the progestin medroxyprogesterone acetate (MPA) slows the growth of breast cancer cell lines positive for estrogen and progesterone receptors. However, MPA has a biphasic effect: it causes a transient acceleration on cell cycles that have already started; it then blocks cells in the G_0/G_1 phase and prevents them from entering further cycles.

In normal breast cells

The stimulatory effects of estradiol and the inhibitory effects of progesterone on mitosis in human breast tissue have been demonstrated by the incorporation of [³H]thymidine in explants from normal or adenomatous breast tissue, maintained in culture from 2–8 days[16].

Longman and Buehring[17] showed that progesterone or progestins, when added alone, did not stimulate cell growth in explants of normal mammary tissue. When added to ethinylestradiol, which has the greatest stimulatory effect, progestins slow down cell growth.

It is interesting to note that the inhibitory effect of progestins is less marked in cancer cells than in normal cells. Cancer cells may escape from normal regulatory cell mechanisms and no longer respond to hormone action.

In our laboratory, we routinely obtain cultures of normal human breast cells established from samples obtained during reductive mammoplasty. In these cultures, it is possible to conduct separate studies of epithelial cells and fibroblasts[18]. We have focused on the interactions of estradiol and progestogens, especially on the epithelial cells. Ultrastructural characteristics of normal human breast epithelial (HBE) cells were examined by both scanning (SEM) and transmission (TEM) electron microscopy[19]. Under SEM, the cells exhibit a homogeneous pattern: they are large, polygonal and flattened. Microvilli are short and rare. Following estradiol treatment, the cells appear young and show extensive protrusions, with numerous bunches and blebs. Microvilli increase markedly in number and density, indicating intense replicative activity. However, the addition of the progestin promegestone (R5020) causes the cells to appear flattened without blebs; they are similar to control cells, with sparse microvilli. Parallel transmission electron microscopy reveals extensive Golgi apparatus and secretory activity under R5020 treatment.

Growth of these normal epithelial cells in culture was evaluated using daily cell counting and DNA assay. Growth was stimulated by estradiol in a dose-dependent manner and inhibited by the progestin R5020, also in a dose-dependent manner (Figures 1 and 2)[20-22]. Progesterone itself inhibits cell growth. [³H]thymidine incorporation after 4 days of treatment (i.e. during the exponential phase of cell growth) was higher following estradiol treatment than in control cells. Incorporation decreased when either progesterone or R5020 was added to estradiol, in a dose-dependent manner (Figure 3).

Interesting and comparable results on the interaction and effects of estradiol and progesterone on breast cell multiplication have recently been obtained *in vivo*[23]. A total of 32 patients was treated with either estradiol, progesterone or a placebo, applied locally to the breast during the follicular phase prior to surgery for benign breast diseases. The number of mitoses in the epithelial cells of the normal part of the breast was counted. After estradiol administration, both estradiol concentration in breast tissue and the number of mitoses were high. After progesterone administration, progesterone concentration in breast tissue was high, but the number of mitoses was low. These results support the conclusion that progesterone has an antimitotic effect.

Mechanisms of estradiol and progesterone antagonism in normal human breast cells

Two mechanisms underlying the progesterone regulation of estradiol action – also observed on breast fibroadenomas and cancer – have been characterized in normal human breast cells:

(1) Progesterone stimulates the enzyme 17β-dehydrogenase (E2DH) which converts estradiol, the active estrogen into estrone, its less active metabolite[18,20]; and

(2) Progesterone decreases the estradiol receptor (ER) content[24].

We had first studied these mechanisms in breast fibroadenomas, which are considered to be a good model since they offer a rich epithelial cell

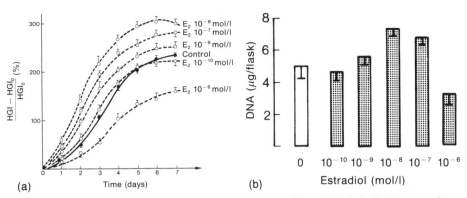

Figure 1 (a) Stimulatory dose-dependent effect of estradiol (E$_2$) on the growth of normal human breast epithelial cells in secondary culture. The study of cell growth was based on daily cell counting and determination of a histometric growth index (HGI). The results are expressed as percentage increase in HGI compared to the value on day 0 (HGI$_0$). (b) DNA values on day 7 (mean of triplicate flasks; bars, SD) (Reproduced from reference 22, with permission)

concentration, that still closely resembles normal tissue[25,26]. We then demonstrated that these mechanisms also operate in human breast cells in culture.

E2DH activity

This was measured as the production of estrone by cells incubated with [^{3}H]estradiol. E2DH activity was high and stimulated by progestins in epithelial cells, but low and not stimulated by progesterone in fibroblasts[18]. Consequently, E2DH was proposed as a marker of epithelial cells, of progesterone dependency and also of progesterone receptor (PR) operativity[20,27]. It therefore seemed interesting to compare the action of progestin on E2DH activity and on the DNA content of HBE cells. Progestin treatment lowered DNA content and stimulated E2DH activity in these cells. It thus slows down cell multiplication while favoring cell differentiation[20].

Steroid receptors

These are difficult to study in cultured normal breast cells due to their lower levels compared with cancer cells. Large numbers of cells are therefore required when using the classical biochemical methods for receptor assay. However, immunocytochemical studies using monoclonal

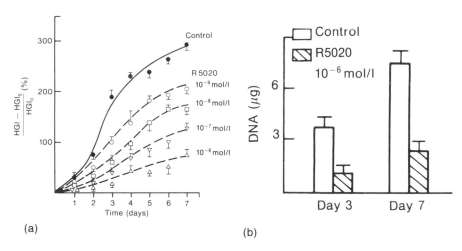

(a)   (b)

Figure 2 (a) Inhibitory effect of the progestin promegestone (R5020) on the growth of normal HBE cells in culture. The study of cell growth was based on daily cell counting and determination of a histometric growth index (HGI). The results are expressed as percentage HGI compared to the value on day 0 (HGI_0). (b) DNA values on day 3 and 7 in control cell cultures (no hormone addition) and cells cultured in the presence of R5020 (10^{-6} mol/l) (mean $\pm$ SD of determinations in triplicate flasks). (Reproduced from reference 20, with permission)

antibodies have enabled the characterization of ER and PR in these cells[24]. Immunostaining specific for ER has been observed in epithelial cells: it is nuclear, and varies from cell to cell in positivity and intensity. Moreover, it is enhanced in estradiol-treated cells and decreases after addition of the progestin R5020. PR was also detected with antibodies provided by Greene[24]. It is also hormone-modulated, increased by estradiol exposure and decreased by R5020.

In normal breast epithelial cells, therefore, estradiol stimulates both its own receptor and the progesterone receptor, whereas the progestin R5020 lowers the number of both ER and PR (Table 1). ER and PR are also present in fibroblasts, but at a lower level than in epithelial cells, and they are only weakly hormone-dependent, if at all[24].

C-myc *proto-oncogene expression HBE cells*

In breast cancer cell lines, the stimulatory effect of estradiol on cell growth can partly operate through the stimulation of proto-oncogene expression[28,29] and growth factor production.

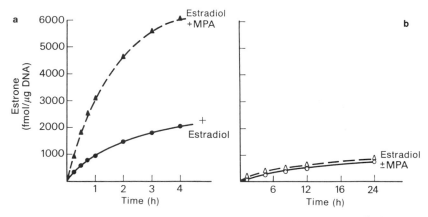

Figure 3 Time course of estrone formation after incubation with [^{3}H]estradiol (incubation medium 5 ml, final concentration = 2 nmol/l) in (a) normal human breast epithelial cells or (b) fibroblasts cultured in the presence of either estradiol (10^{-8} mol/l) alone (no difference from control), or estradiol + medroxyprogesterone acetate (MPA) (10^{-8} mol/l). (Reproduced from reference 18, with permission)

Table 1 Variations of estrogen receptor immunostaining in human breast epithelial cells cultured for 8 days in the absence of steroids (control) or in the presence of estradiol (10^{-8} mol/l), or estradiol (10^{-8} mol/l) + R5020 (10^{-7} mol/l) or R5020 (10^{-7} mol/l) alone. Reproduced from reference 24, with permission

Estrogen receptor immunostaining (% of stained cells)	Positive (%)	Negative (%)	Intensity of staining
Control	55	45	+ +
Estradiol	73	27	+ + +
Estradiol + R5020	44	56	+ +
R5020	35	65	+

The proto-oncogene c-*myc* is involved in the stimulation of cell replication and can itself be stimulated by numerous mitogens, including estradiol. Estradiol stimulation of c-*myc* was demonstrated in human breast cancer cell lines[28,29] and also in non-cancerous estradiol-dependent target tissues (uterus, chick oviduct)[30,31]. In contrast, progestins[32] and triphenylethylenic antiestrogens[29] inhibit c-*myc* expression.

We are investigating whether the foregoing mechanisms operate in normal breast cells. We have immunocytochemically demonstrated the presence of the c-*myc* protein[33]. The expression of this protein is exclusively nuclear, heterogeneous, and the intensity of staining varies from cell to cell. In addition, c-*myc* expression is hormone-modulated: the number of positive cells and intensity of staining increase following estradiol treatment and decrease after the addition of R5020 to estradiol.

Preliminary results from Northern blot studies confirm the interaction of estradiol with c-*myc* expression: early stimulation of mRNA occurred 30 min after estradiol treatment followed by later stimulation after 2 h. Interactions of progestins and c-*myc* are now being investigated.

HORMONAL RISK FACTORS FOR BREAST CANCER

As well as genetic susceptible factors in breast cancer, hormonal factors are most frequently mentioned, especially the effects of progesterone deficiency with unopposed estrogen administration. Considering these hormonal risk factors[34-38], nulliparity and late first pregnancy may be related to hypofertility and ovulatory disorders, early menarche and late menopause are responsible for prolonged anovulatory periods at each end of the reproductive life; periods when estradiol but no progesterone is secreted, and irregular menstrual cycles, as well as benign breast disease, are the consequences of ovulatory disorders with progesterone deficiency.

Interaction of estradiol and progesterone has also been observed in models of breast carcinogenesis in humans. The women of Hiroshima and Nagasaki who survived the 1945 atomic bomb[39] constitute a model for the study of cooperation between an initiator of carcinogenesis (irradiation) and a promoter (estradiol). Analysing the incidence of breast cancer among irradiated women by age at the time of the explosion, the risk was increased four or five times in women 11–14 years old at the time of irradiation, and doubled in women who were aged 15–19. The risk does not seem to be increased in women who were > 19 years old at the time of irradiation[39]. A similar observation was made among adolescent girls who were subjected to repeated radiological examination as part of antituberculosis treatment[40]. Breast cells therefore seem to be most susceptible to radiation-induced mutations in those young women who were irradiated during the para- or immediate post-pubertal period. This period is characterized by relative hyperestrogenism, anovulatory cycles, no progesterone secretion, and the greatest breast sensitivity to estradiol, consequently inducing rapid proliferation and development.

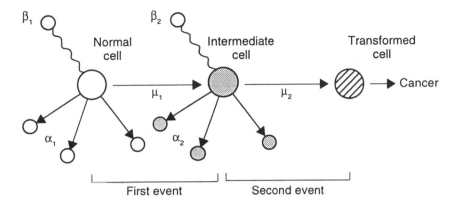

Figure 4 Scheme for two-step carcinogenesis according to Moolgavkar. (Reproduced from reference 41, with permission)

ROLE OF ESTRADIOL AND PROGESTINS IN THE TWO-STEP SCHEME FOR CARCINOGENESIS ACCORDING TO MOOLGAVKAR[41]

Considering the effects of estradiol and progestins on cell growth and differentiation, we can try to understand how they are involved in the process of carcinogenesis.

Moolgavkar has proposed a two-step scheme for carcinogenesis (Figure 4)[41]. This proposes that a normal cell has two possibilities: it either divides into new cells ($\alpha 1$) or it matures, differentiates ($\beta 1$ cell) and finally dies. However, if the normal cell is subjected to an initiator of carcinogenesis, it can evolve ($\mu 1$) into an intermediate (precancerous) cell. Intermediate cells can also either divide ($\alpha 2$) or differentiate ($\beta 2$) and die. But, if a second process of initiation intervenes ($\mu 2$), the cell definitely evolves into a cancer cell.

Cell division is a vulnerable phase for the cells with risks of errors of replication, oncogene activation, or exogenous carcinogen intervention. By stimulating cell multiplication, estrogens increase the risk of error at the time of replication. In this way, they can act as promoters of carcinogenesis. By orienting cells toward maturation, progesterone and progestins exclude them from the pool of vulnerable dividing cells and could be protective. Any situation characterized by an imbalance of endogenous or exogenous progesterone and estradiol with an unopposed estrogen effect should be avoided or corrected.

MIGHT PROGESTERONE BE A CARCINOGENIC FACTOR?

Progesterone itself and progestins have been presented as possible factors of carcinogenesis in a small number of controversial articles[42-44].

Ferguson and Anderson[42] claimed to have observed the greatest number of mitoses in the epithelial cells of normal breast tissue on days 24–25 of the cycle. They concluded that progesterone could have a mitogenic effect. However, their tissue samples came from women who had undergone surgery for benign breast diseases; these patients often suffer from anovulation or dysovulation. The occurrence of ovulation and the existence of a luteal phase were not confirmed by basal body temperature or by plasma progesterone assay. Although biopsies were carried out in the second part of the cycle, therefore, there was no guarantee of a luteal phase. It also seems that the mitotic index had been calculated by adding mitosis and apoptosis (i.e. dead cells).

In a further study of patients taking oral contraceptives, Anderson and co-workers[45] observed a correlation between the number of mitoses in breast tissue and the estrogen potency of the contraceptive (low, medium or high), but no correlation with the progestogen content of pills. They observed only a noticeable number of mitoses with progestogen micropills. However, in these contraceptives the progestogen dose is very low, and is frequently associated with endogenous hyperestrogenism.

Potten and colleagues[46] observed the highest rate of mitoses on day 21 of the cycle, which is too early in the luteal phase to be attributed to the cumulative effect of secreted progesterone. This high rate of mitoses could possibly reflect the cumulative effect of estradiol since the beginning of the cycle.

In an article published in 1983, Pike[43] suggested that oral contraceptives containing the highest doses of progestogen increased the risk of breast cancer. However, the Swyer test used to evaluate the progestogen potency of these pills has been criticized as non-specific. In particular, the pills that he claimed to contain the highest progestogen content were, in fact, the highest in estrogen.

The most recent and controversial article is by Bergkvist and co-workers[44], who evaluated breast cancer risk in postmenopausal women receiving estrogen replacement therapy. Whereas the global risk was 1.1, they found a relative risk of 4.4 when a progestogen was combined with estrogen in the treatment. However, this evaluation was based on only ten patients. The authors themselves declared that these results were not statistically significant and could be due to chance. The lay press echoed Bergkvist's findings but missed the last point, while his article was criticized in scientific journals. A detailed epidemiological review examining the questionable relationship between progestin exposure in contraceptive and hormone replacement therapies and breast cancer risk failed to find evidence of an association between progestins and breast cancer[47,48].

It is therefore essential to keep in mind the numerous experiments and data on the role of progesterone in controlling the action of estradiol:

(1) Extensive experimental studies on animals have demonstrated a proliferative effect of estradiol on breast tissue, whereas progesterone inhibits estradiol-induced proliferation and induces differentiation;

(2) Numerous studies have confirmed the respective effects of estradiol and progesterone on human breast tissue in cell cultures, explants and biopsies obtained at various times of the menstrual cycle or during estradiol or progesterone treatment;

(3) Clinical and epidemiological observations suggest that the hormonal profile in progesterone insufficiency and unopposed estrogenism seems to favor benign breast disease in the short term and increases the risk of breast cancer in the long term[34–37,49–52]; and

(4) There is an unequivocal beneficial effect of progestins in benign breast disease[53].

All of these data contradict the hypothesis of a carcinogenic effect of progesterone on breast tissue.

CONCLUSION

Normal human breast epithelial cells, which remain hormone-dependent in culture, constitute a useful tool for investigating the hormone-dependence of the normal human mammary gland. In this culture system, estradiol stimulates and progestins inhibit cell growth. In addition, progestins favor cell differentiation.

From these observations, as well as from the data obtained by many other authors, it appears that by stimulating cell proliferation, estradiol can act as a promoter of carcinogenesis. Any condition characterized by estrogen–progesterone imbalance with an unopposed estrogen effect should therefore be avoided or corrected. This should be taken into account in spontaneous anovulatory or dysovulatory menstrual cycles (puberty, perimenopause, hyperprolactinemia, polycystic ovaries, weight changes, stress: i.e., the 'estrogen-windows' of Korenman), the treatment of benign breast diseases and strategies for the prevention of breast cancer, and therapeutic choices for contraception and the menopause.

ACKNOWLEDGEMENTS

This work was supported by grants from Inserm, ARC, le Conseil Scientifique de la Faculté Necker.

REFERENCES

1. Bassler, R. (1970). Morphology of hormone induced structural changes in the female breast. *Curr. Top.,* **53**, 1–89
2. Benson, G. K., Cowie, A. T., Cox, C. P. and Goldzveig, S. A. (1957). Effects of oestrone and progesterone on mammary development in the guinea-pig. *J. Endocrinol.,* **15**, 126–44
3. Benson, G. K., Cowie, A. T., Cox, C. P., Folley, S. J. and Hosking, S. D. (1965). Relative efficiency of hoexestrol and progesterone as oily solution and a crystalline suspension in inducing mammary growth and lactation in early and late ovariectomized goats. *J. Endocrinol.,* **31**, 157–64
4. Lyons, W. R. and McGinty, D. R. (1941). Effects of estrone and progesterone on male rabbit mammary glands. I. Varying doses of progesterone. *Proc. Soc. Exp. Biol. Med.,* **48**, 83–9
5. Eisen, M. J. (1942). The occurrence of benign and malignant mammary lesions in rats treated with crystalline estrogen. *Cancer Res.,* **2**, 632–44
6. Segaloff, A. (1973). Inhibition by progesterone of radiation–estrogen-induced mammary cancer in the rat. *Cancer Res.,* **33**, 1136–8
7. Inoh, A., Kamiya, K., Fujii, Y. and Yokoro, K. (1985). Protective effect of progesterone and tamoxifen in estrogen-induced mammary carcinogenesis in ovariectomized w/Fu rats. *Jpn. J. Cancer Res. (Gann),* **76**, 699–704
8. Gottardis, M., Erturk, E. and Rose, D. P. (1985). Effects of progesterone administration on N-nitrosomethylurea-induced rat mammary carcinogenesis. *Eur. J. Clin. Oncol.,* **19**, 1479–84
9. Grubbs, C. J., Farnell, D. R., Hill, D. L. and McDonough, K. C. (1985). Chemo-prevention of N-nitro-N-methylurea-induced mammary cancers by pretreat-ment with 17β-estradiol and progesterone. *J. Natl. Cancer Inst.,* **74**, 927–30
10. Vogel, P. M., Georgiade, N. G., Setter, B. F., Vogel, S. and McCarty, K. (1981). The correlation of histologic changes in the human breast with the menstrual cycle. *Am. J. Pathol.,* **104**, 23–34
11. Ozello, L. and Speer, F. D. (1958). The mucopolysaccharides in the normal and diseased breast. Their distribution and significance. *Am. J. Pathol.,* **34**, 993–1009
12. Asboe-Hansen, G. (1958). Hormonal effects on connective tissue. *Physiol. Rev.,* **38**, 446–62
13. Vignon, D., Bardon, S., Chalbos, D. and Rochefort, H. (1983). Antiestrogenic effect of R5020, a synthetic progestin in human breast cancer cells in culture. *J. Clin. Endocrinol. Metab.,* **56**, 1124–30
14. Horwitz, K. B. and Freibenberg, G. R. (1985). Growth inhibition and increase

of insulin receptors in antiestrogen-resistant T47D$_{co}$ human breast cancer cells by progestins – implications for endocrine therapies. *Cancer Res., 45,* 167–73

15. Musgrove, E. A., Lee, C. S. L. and Sutherland, R. L. (1991). Progestins both stimulate and inhibit breast cancer cell cycle progression while increasing expression of transforming growth factor α1, epidermal growth factor receptor, c-*fos* and c-*myc* genes. *Mol. Cell. Biol., 11,* 5032–43

16. Welsch, C. W., McManus, M. J., Haviland, Th. J., Dombroske, S. E., Swim, E. L., Sharpe, S. and Conley, E. (1983). Hormone regulation of DNA synthesis of normal and hyperplastic human breast tissues *in vitro* and *in vivo.* In: Angeli, A. (ed.) *Endocrinology of Cystic Breast Diseases,* pp. 47–58. (New York: Raven Press)

17. Longman, S. M. and Buehring, G. C. (1987). Oral contraceptives and breast cancer. *In vitro* effect of contraceptive steroids on human mammary cell growth. *Cancer, 59,* 281–7

18. Prudhomme, J. F., Malet, C., Gompel, A., Lalardrie, J. P., Ochoa, C., Boué, A., Mauvais-Jarvis, P. and Kuttenn, F. (1984). 17β-Hydroxysteroid dehydrogenase activity in human breast epithelial cell and fibroblast cultures. *Endocrinology, 114,* 1483–9

19. Gompel, A., Chomette, G., Malet, C., Spritzer, P., Pavy, B., Kuttenn, F. and Mauvais-Jarvis, P. (1985). Estradiol-progestin interaction in normal human breast cells in culture. Ultrastructural studies. *Breast Disease, 1,* 149–56

20. Gompel, A., Malet, C., Spritzer, P., Lalardrie, J. P., Kuttenn, F. and Mauvais-Jarvis, P. (1986). Progestin effect on cell proliferation and 17β-hydroxysteroid dehydrogenase activity in normal human breast cells in culture. *J. Clin. Endocrinol. Metab., 63,* 1174–80

21. Mauvais-Jarvis, P., Kuttenn, F. and Gompel, A. (1986). Estradiol–progesterone interaction in normal and pathological breast cells. *Ann. N.Y. Acad. Sci., 464,* 152–67

22. Malet, C., Gompel, A., Spritzer, P., Bricout, N., Kuttenn, F. and Mauvais-Jarvis, P. (1988). Tamoxifen and hydroxytamoxifen isomers *versus* estradiol effects on normal human breast cells in culture. *Cancer Res., 48,* 7193–9

23. Barrat, J., de Lignières, B., Marpeau, L., Larue, L., Fournier, S., Nahoul, K., Linares, G., Giorgi, H. and Contesso, G. (1990). Effet *in vivo* de l'administration locale de progestérone sur l'activité mitotique des galactophores humains. *J. Gynecol. Obstet. Biol. Reprod., 19,* 269–74

24. Malet, C., Gompel, A., Yaneva, H., Cren, H., Fidji, N., Mowszowicz, I., Kuttenn, F. and Mauvais-Jarvis, P. (1991). Estradiol and progesterone receptors in cultured normal human breast epithelial cells and fibroblasts – immunocytochemical studies. *J. Clin. Endocrinol. Metab., 73,* 8–17

25. Kuttenn, F., Fournier, S., Durand, J. C. and Mauvais-Jarvis, P. (1981). Estradiol and progesterone receptors in human breast fibroadenomas. *J. Clin. Endocrinol. Metab., 52,* 1225–9

26. Fournier, S., Kuttenn, F., De Cicco, N., Baudot, N., Malet, C. and Mauvais-Jarvis, P. (1982). Estradiol 17β-hydroxysteroid dehydrogenase activity in human breast fibroadenomas. *J. Clin. Endocrinol. Metab., 55,* 428–33

27. Fournier, S., Brihmat, F., Durand, J. C., Sterkers, N., Martin, P. M., Kuttenn, F. and Mauvais-Jarvis, P. (1985). Estradiol 17β-hydroxysteroid dehydrogenase, a marker of breast cancer hormone dependency. *Cancer Res., 45,* 2895–9

28. Dubik, D. and Shiu, R. P. C. (1988). Transcriptional regulation of c-*myc* oncogene expression by estrogen in hormone responsive human breast cancer cells. *J. Biol. Chem.*, **253**, 12705–8
29. Santos, G. F., Scott, G. K., Lee, W. M. F., Liu, E. and Benz, C. (1988). Estrogen-induced post-transcriptional modulation of c-*myc* protooncogene expression in human breast cancer cells. *J. Biol. Chem.*, **263**, 9565–8
30. Murphy, L. J., Murphy, L. C. and Friesen, H. G. (1987). Estrogen induction of N-*myc* and c-*myc* protooncogene expression in rat uterus. *Endocrinology*, **120**, 1882–8
31. Weisz, A. and Bresciani, F. (1988). Estrogen induces expression of c-*fos* and c-*myc* protooncogenes in rat uterus. *Mol. Endocrinol.*, **2**, 816–24
32. Fink, K. L., Wieben, E. D., Woloschak, G. E. and Spelberg, T. C. (1988). Rapid regulation of c-*myc* protooncogene expression by progesterone in the avian oviduct. *Proc. Natl. Acad. Sci. USA*, **85**, 1796–800
33. Leygue, E., Louis-Sylvestre, C., Gol, R., Malet, C., Baudot, N., Cumins, C., Mowszowicz, I., Kuttenn, F. and Mauvais-Jarvis, P. (1993). Estrogen regulation of c-*myc* in normal human breast epithelial (HBE) cells in culture. Presented at *75th Annual Meeting American Endocrinology Society*, Las Vegas, June, Abstr. 1914
34. MacMahon, B., Cole P. and Brown, J. (1973). Etiology of human breast cancer: a review. *J. Natl. Cancer Inst.*, **50**, 21–42
35. Cowan, L. D., Gordis, L., Tonascia, J. A. and Jones, G. S. (1981). Breast cancer incidence in women with a history of progesterone deficiency. *Am. J. Epidemiol.*, **114**, 209–17
36. Korenman, S. G. (1980). The endocrinology of breast cancer. *Cancer*, **46**, 874–8
37. Sherman, B. M. and Korenman, S. G. (1974). Inadequate corpus luteum function: a pathophysiological interpretation of human breast cancer epidemiology. *Cancer*, **33**, 1306–12
38. Dupont, W. D. and Page, D. L. (1985). Risk factors for breast cancer in women with proliferative breast disease. *N. Engl. J. Med.*, **312**, 146–51
39. Tokunaga, M., Norman, J. E. and Agano, M. (1979). Malignant breast tumours among atomic bomb survivors Hiroshima and Nagasaki 1959–1974. *J. Natl. Cancer Inst.*, **62**, 1347–52
40. Miller, A. B., Home, G. R., Sherman, G. J., Lindsay, J. P., Yaffé, M. J., Dinner, P. J., Risch, H. A. and Preston, D. L. (1989). Mortality from breast cancer after irradiations during fluoroscopic examination in patients being treated for tuberculosis. *N. Engl. J. Med.*, **321**, 1285–9
41. Moolgavkar, S. H., Day, N. E. and Stevens, R. C. (1980). Two-stage model for carcinogenesis: epidemiology of breast cancer in females. *J. Natl. Cancer Inst.*, **65**, 559–69
42. Ferguson, D. J. P. and Anderson, T. J. (1981). Morphological evaluation of cell turnover in relation to the menstrual cycle in the resting human breast. *Br. J. Cancer*, **44**, 177–81
43. Pike, M., Henderson, B. and Krailo, M. (1983). Breast cancer in young women and use of oral contraceptives: possible modifying effect of formulation and age at use. *Lancet*, **2**, 926–30
44. Bergkvist, L., Adami, M., Persson, I., Hoover, R. and Schairer, C. (1989). The risk of breast cancer after estrogen and estrogen–progestin replacement.

N. Engl. J. Med., **321**, 293–7
45. Anderson, T. J., Battersby, S., King, R. J. B., McPherson, K. and Going, J. J. (1989). Oral contraceptive use influences resting breast proliferation. *Hum. Pathol.,* **20**, 1139–44
46. Potten, C. S., Watson, R. J., Willimas, G. T., Tickle, S., Roberts, S. A., Harris, M. and Howell, A. (1988). The effect of age and menstrual cycle upon proliferative activity on the normal human breast. *Br. J. Cancer,* **258**, 163–70
47. Staffa, J. A., Newschaffer, C. J., Jones, J. K. and Miller, V. (1992). Progestins and breast cancer: an epidemiologic review. *Fertil. Steril.,* **57**, 473–91
48. Clarke, C. L. and Sutherland, R. L. (1993). Progestin regulation of cellular proliferation: update 1993. *Endocrine Rev.,* **1**, 132–5
49. Mauvais-Jarvis, P., Sitruk-Ware, R., Kuttenn, F. and Sterkers, N. (1979). Luteal phase insufficiency: a common pathophysiological factor in development of benign and malignant breast diseases. In Bulbrook, R. D. and Taylor, D. J. (eds.) *Commentaries on Research in Breast Disease,* pp. 25–29. (New York: Alan R. Liss Inc.)
50. Vorherr, H. (1986). Fibrocystic breast disease: pathophysiology, pathomorphology, clinical picture and management. *Am. J. Obstet. Gynecol.,* **154**, 161–79
51. Sitruk-Ware, R., Thalabard, J. C., Benotmane, A. and Mauvais-Jarvis, P. (1989). Risk factors for breast fibroadenoma in young women. *Contraception,* **40**, 251–68
52. Plu-Bureau, G., Thalabard, J. C., Sitruk-Ware, R., Asselain, B. and Mauvais-Jarvis, P. (1992). Cyclical mastalgia as a marker of breast cancer susceptibility: results of a case–control study among French women. *Br. J. Cancer,* **65**, 945–9
53. Mauvais-Jarvis, P. and Kuttenn, F. (1993). Benign breast disease. In Bardin, C. W.(ed.) *Current Therapy in Endocrinology and Metabolism,* Vth edn. (Philadelphia: B.C. Decker Inc.), in press

46

Trends in breast cancer incidence and mortality by country, age, cohort and period: hypotheses on risk determinants

M. Ewertz

INTRODUCTION

In most developed countries, the incidence of female breast cancer has been increasing over the past 30 years, while mortality rates have remained more or less stable (Figure 1).

The Special Interest Group session focused in particular on two issues:

(1) Is the increase in breast cancer incidence a true increase, i.e. a result of an increasing prevalence of etiological factors, or due to an increasing diagnostic effort?

(2) The differing trends between incidence and mortality reflect an improved survival. Can this be attributed to an earlier diagnosis and/or to improvements in treatment of breast cancer?

Seven speakers were invited to address the above issues and to take part in the following discussion.

PRESENTATIONS

Trends in breast cancer incidence and mortality in the United States were presented by Professor Hulka (University of North Carolina, USA). She emphasized the role of screening in explaining the increase in breast

Number per 100,000 woman–years

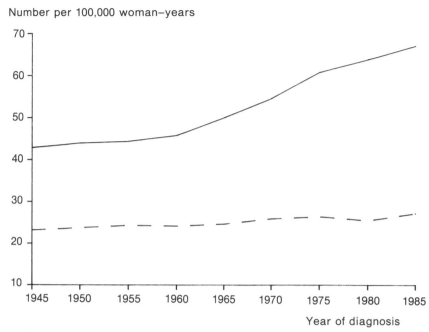

Figure 1 Age-standardized (world population) incidence (——) and mortality (------) of breast cancer in Denmark, 1943–89

cancer incidence. Data from the surveillance, epidemiology, and end results (SEER) registries, representing a 10% sample of the American population, showed that the increase in incidence was confined to *in situ* cancers, small tumors (up to 3 cm), and those with local spread. There was no increase in incidence of tumors > 3 cm or those with distant metastases.

Professor Mack (University of Southern California, USA) pointed out that in the USA increases in breast cancer incidence can be caused by presidential wives having breast cancer. Incidence and mortality rates from Los Angeles County were presented by race, year, and age at diagnosis. While the incidence increased in all but premenopausal latino women, mortality rates were stable or decreasing for white and latino women, but increasing among black women. It was suggested that the timeliness of treatment in black women lags behind that in white women.

Professor Tulinius showed trends in breast cancer incidence and mortality in Iceland. While mortality rates have been stable, pronounced increases in incidence have been observed. The overall 22% increase per decade comprised an increase for premenopausal women amounting to 11% per decade, and for postmenopausal 25% per decade.

Professor Hakulinen presented data from the Finnish Cancer Registry, pointing out that any cancer with an increasing incidence and improving survival, illustrated by colon cancer, would show similar trends in incidence and mortality to those seen for breast cancer. He elaborated on discrepancies between predicted and observed trends in breast cancer incidence, finding that the observed increase exceeded that predicted only in the age group 50–59 years.

Professor Lund (Norway) showed that the increase in breast cancer incidence has slowed down for young women, and that most of the increase in incidence observed in Norway could be ascribed to earlier diagnosis. He gave compelling evidence of the protective effect of parity on breast cancer risk.

Trends in breast cancer incidence and mortality in Sweden were presented by Professor Persson, who pointed out the strong cohort effect in incidence. An examination of average increase by age and year of diagnosis did not support that the use of oral contraceptives may influence breast cancer incidence. Mortality rates showed little change with time.

Finally, Dr Glud presented data from an ecological study performed in Denmark, addressing the role of prevalence of risk factors in relation to breast cancer incidence. Early fertility, average age at menarche, and use of exogenous hormones did not explain the increase in incidence. However, changes in dietary habits, evaluated by energy percentages of carbohydrate and fat and alcohol consumption, correlated well with the period-specific shift.

DISCUSSION

One of the key issues in the explanation of the increase in breast cancer incidence is the effect of early diagnosis. There was a consensus among the invited speakers that early diagnosis, through an increased awareness of breast cancer among women and doctors, an increased diagnostic effort in patients with breast lumps, particularly elderly women, and the implementation of mammography screening programs in more recent years, may have contributed substantially to the increase observed.

However, the strong cohort effect observed for breast cancer incidence in most countries also indicates a 'true' increase, caused by an increasing prevalence of breast cancer risk factors. Studies using population-based estimates of prevalence of such factors over time in relation to incidence have provided ambiguous results. Some have provided evidence in support, while others have failed to find an association between changes in breast cancer incidence and changes in hormonal factors, such as childbearing, age at menarche, and use of exogenous hormones. This contrasts with results obtained from studies based on individuals, where strong associations have been found between breast cancer risk, parity and age at first childbirth. It was mentioned in the discussion that the protective effect of childbirths may not be life-long, but may wear off with time. The data presented did not suggest that the use of oral contraceptives or exogenous hormones in general may have substantial influence on breast cancer risk, though minor effects cannot be ruled out entirely.

With respect to the influence of diet on breast cancer risk, the interpretation of ecological studies was cautioned, since such studies do not prove causality. Many cohort studies have failed to confirm any effect of fat intake on breast cancer risk. It is hoped that the Women's Health Initiative, a large intervention study to be conducted in the United States, will shed further light on this issue. In the discussion, it was also mentioned that we may have been looking at the wrong exposure window; diet during adolescence may be more important in relation to breast cancer risk than adult diet.

The question of the role of breast feeding on breast cancer risk was raised from the audience. The protective effect of breast feeding reported in studies predating the 1970s can be ascribed to lack of control for the effect of parity. Some later studies have found a protective effect of long-term breast feeding independent of parity, but this has not been confirmed by others. Thus, this issue still needs clarification.

The improved survival of patients with breast cancer was not discussed at great length, but the general opinion was that it was in accordance with more tumors being diagnosed at an earlier stage. Aspects of breast cancer treatment were not discussed.

CONCLUSION

A substantial part of the increase in breast cancer incidence can be explained by an increasing diagnostic effort over time, leading to more cancers being diagnosed at an early stage. This has also led to an improvement in survival of breast cancer patients over time. The strong cohort effect in breast cancer incidence suggests that part of the increase may be due to an increasing prevalence of breast cancer risk factors, although good quality data are lacking to support this.

47

Compliance with hormone replacement therapy: where we stand today

L. E. Nachtigall

To achieve optimal therapy with any drug regimen, both the physician and the patient must accept the therapy. Estrogen therapy requires acceptance not only by the patients and physicians, but, in addition, by the media, family, and friends. Hormone therapy has caught the attention of the media recently, and media reports constitute a large part of women's education about hormone therapy. A woman approaches estrogen therapy with this background, her inherent ability to comply, her expectations for help, her symptoms, and her level of formal education. The physician brings his or her education, factual information, and experience with hormone replacement. In addition, the physician must ensure that each patient receives an accurate risk–benefit analysis which should help the patient separate true complications from nuisance side-effects.

Several studies have shown particularly poor compliance with hormone replacement therapy (HRT)[1,2]. In the field study done by McKinlay[1], in some populations, compliance with HRT was among the worst ever reported. Of 2500 women of diverse backgrounds, aged 45–55 years, 70% had HRT prescribed at one time or another. However, 30% of these women never even obtained the treatment. In addition, 10% of those who did obtain the prescribed treatment reported only taking the medication sporadically. In Ravnikar's study, the overall rate of compliance in 600 patients was only 30%[2]. Because this appeared to be a low level of compliance, we were interested in assessing compliance in the Department of Obstetrics and Gynecology at New York University Medical Center, where we believed that an effort had been made to inform

Table 1 Reasons for discontinuation of treatment within 1 year among 220 menopausal out-patients receiving any type of hormone replacement therapy

Reason	No. of patients
Withdrawal bleeding	3
Irregular bleeding	5
Breast tenderness	3
Edema/fluid retention	2
Nausea	1
Headache	1
Total	15

patients thoroughly about hormone therapy, and where the doctors did not prescribe hormone therapy unless they were convinced of its benefits to the patient. We evaluated 220 middle-class women who were private patients, all of whom had received a prescription for hormone replacement therapy (any combination of estrogen and progestogen). The patients were 43–62 years old and each was menopausal, confirmed by an elevated follicle stimulating hormone level. At their 1-year visit, they were questioned about compliance in taking the medication. Only 7% had discontinued the therapy. Over half of those who discontinued it did so because of bleeding episodes and the remainder because of other side-effects[3] (Table 1).

We also re-evaluated compliance among women participating in a multivariate study on the efficacy and safety of transdermal estradiol prior to its FDA approval in the United States. Diaries had been kept both by the women and by the investigators and were available for analysis. This group included 1330 women (ages 46–58 years) from eight centers, all of whom received prescriptions for hormone replacement therapy in the form of transdermal estradiol and various progestogens. Only 5% discontinued therapy, most because of bleeding episodes (Table 2).

When looking at both these studies, it becomes readily apparent that, first, bleeding was the major reason for discontinuing estrogen therapy, and, second, if patients understand the benefits and are prepared for the side-effects of HRT before receiving a prescription, they are much more likely to obtain that prescription and take the medication correctly.

The benefits include relief of vasomotor instability, prevention of vaginal atrophy[4], and prevention of osteoporosis[5]. The risk factors for osteoporosis can be reviewed with the patient, to assess whether she is in a high-risk group. Bone mass measurements[6], if indicated, can provide a visual aid concerning her status. The role of estrogen replacement in the prevention

Table 2 Reasons for discontinuation of treatment within 1 year among 1330 menopausal out-patients receiving transdermal estradiol hormone replacement therapy

Reason	*No. of patients*
Withdrawal bleeding	23
Irregular bleeding	14
Breast tenderness	8
Edema/fluid retention	8
Nausea	1
Headache	1
Skin irritation from patch	12
Total	67

Table 3 Nuisance side-effects from hormone replacement therapy

Breakthrough bleeding	Headaches
Breast tenderness	Edema
Vaginal irritation	Menses
Local skin irritation (patch)	Nausea

of heart disease has not been established, but it is worthwhile mentioning studies that have shown beneficial effects of estrogen on lipid metabolism[7] and reduction in cardiovascular mortality.

Nuisance side-effects must be differentiated from complications: it is typically the nuisance side-effects, particularly bleeding, that cause patients to discontinue treatment (Table 3). The idea that every woman with postmenopausal bleeding has cancer unless proven otherwise, has to be changed with the advent of wider use of HRT. Estrogen replacement, unopposed by progesterone, clearly led to an eight-fold increase in adenocarcinoma of the endometrium[8]. This knowledge frightens the patient into discontinuing her medication, and frightens the doctor into performing too many biopsies. Subsequent studies have shown that the addition of a progestin for at least 6 days inhibits estrogen-induced endometrial DNA synthesis[9], reducing the endometrial cancer incidence to near zero and the endometrial hyperplasia incidence to 0.5%. A proportion of women taking progesterone for < 12 days will still have a proliferative endometrium on biopsy, particularly those women who bleed before the tenth day of progesterone administration[10]. However, since no hyperplasia has been found in biopsies from such patients, it seems that the antiestrogenic (antimitotic) effect of the progestin can exist without

Table 4 Ways to enhance patient compliance

Educate patients	Stress ease of taking medication
clear discussion	Use appropriate measures to reduce
booklets	nuisance factors
books	Know when to biopsy
indicate need for surveillance even	Demonstrate results/benefits
after hormone therapy	cholesterol level
give printed prescriptions and	vaginal examination
handouts	bone density

morphologic transformation of the endometrium to a full secretory phase. It is clear that we can completely remove the complication of endometrial cancer from HRT with adequate cyclic (10–14 days) administration of progestins. These will lead to a cyclic, planned menstrual bleed in 80% of women. When these women bleed according to plan very regularly there is no need to biopsy, and if there is no patient objection to the return of menses, the schedule is acceptable. For women who object not only to irregular bleeding, but to any bleeding at all, an attempt to oppose endometrial growth without a withdrawal response has led to the use of continuous combined HRT. A variety of regimens have been used, all of which include daily estrogen plus daily progestin. Although there is a high incidence of irregular bleeding during the first 3–4 months following initiation of continuum combined therapy, after 4 months the incidence drops to <25%.

Progestin therapy may cause headaches, abdominal bloating, edema, or breast tenderness. These symptoms can almost always be controlled with a change in the type, dose, or duration of the progestin. If all else fails, the patient may have to be treated with unopposed estrogens, with careful monitoring of the endometrium[11].

The doctor's role must be not only to help the individual patient decide whether the benefits of HRT outweigh the risks, but to enhance patient compliance (Table 4).

REFERENCES

1. McKinlay, S. (1986). *Massachusetts Woman's Health Survey.* Cambridge Research Center Report. (Boston)
2. Ravnikar, V. A. (1987). Compliance with hormone therapy. *Am. J. Obstet. Gynecol.,* **156**, 1332–4
3. Nachtigall, L. E. (1990). Enhancing patient compliance with hormone replacement therapy at menopause. *Obstet. Gynecol.,* **75**, 775–805
4. Nachtigall, L. E. and Utian, W. H. (1987). Comparative efficacy and tolerability

of transdermal estradiol and conjugated estrogens. In Lauritzen, S. (ed.) *Transdermal Estrogen Substitution.* (Lewiston, NY: Hans Huber)

5. Lindsay, R., Hart, D. M., Aitken, J. M., MacDonald, E. B., Anderson, J. B. and Clarke, A. C. (1976). Long-term prevention of postmenopausal osteoporosis by oestrogen: evidence for an increased bone mass after delayed onset of oestrogen treatment. *Lancet,* **1**, 1038–41

6. Slemenda, C. W., Hui, S. L., Longcope, C., Wellman, H. and Johnston, C. C. Jr. (1990). Predictors of bone mass in perimenopausal women: a prospective study of clinical data using photon absorptiometry. *Ann. Intern. Med.,* **112**, 96–101

7. Notelovitz, M., Gudat, J., Ware, M. D. and Dougherty, M. C. (1983). Lipids and lipoproteins in women after oophorectomy and the response to oestrogen therapy. *Br. J. Obstet. Gynaecol.,* **90**, 171–7

8. Weiss, N. S., Szekely, D. R., English, D. R. and Schweid, A. I. (1979). Endometrial cancer in relation to patterns of menopausal estrogen use. *J. Am. Med. Assoc.,* **242**, 261–4

9. Whitehead, M. I., Hillard, T. C. and Crook, D. (1990). The role and use of progestogens. *Obstet. Gynecol.,* **75**, 59–76S

10. Whitehead, M. I. and Fraser, D. (1989). The effects of estrogens and progestogens on the endometrium: modern approach to treatment. *Obstet. Gynecol. Clin. North Am.,* **14**, 299–317

11. Goldstein, S. R., Nachtigall, M. J., Snyder, J. R. and Nachtigall, L. E. (1990). Endometrial assessment by vaginal ultrasonography before endometrial sampling in patients with post menopausal bleeding. *Am. J. Obstet. Gynecol.,* **163**, 119–23

Section 9

Clinical aspects on hormone replacement therapy

48

Menopausal experience of users of hormone replacement therapy

*K. A. Matthews, L. H. Kuller, R. R. Wing, E. N. Meilahn and
J. T. Bromberger*

It is well documented that postmenopausal women who use hormone replacement therapy (HRT) are protected from coronary heart disease and osteoporosis[1,2]. It is also the case that, relative to non-users, users of HRT have more favorable cardiovascular risk factor profiles, including lipid, fibrinogen, fasting insulin and fasting glucose levels[3]. These observations are based on cohort studies of women, not on randomized clinical trials, and usually do not take into account or adjust for characteristics prior to the use of HRT. It is therefore important to examine the extent to which users of HRT differ from non-users prior to the use of hormones or prior to the menopause. This paper describes the initial biological and psychological characteristics of women who subsequently became HRT users in the peri- and postmenopausal period, and their subsequent menopausal experience in light of their initial characteristics.

The paper is based on data from the Healthy Women Study, a study of the biological and psychological changes in women as they experience the menopausal transition[4]. In 1983–84, 541 participants were recruited who at study entry had menstruated within the previous 3 months, were 42 to 50 years old, were not taking any regular medications that would interfere with tracking of biological risk factors (e.g. antihypertensive medications, insulin, HRT), had diastolic blood pressure < 100 mmHg, and had a driver's license. The last requirement was due to the fact that women were recruited from a list of women in Allegheny County who had driver's licenses. Participants were better educated than eligible non-participants; 60% of the eligible women agreed to participate.

At study entry, women underwent an extensive clinical evaluation, including measures of family history of disease, obstetric and gynecological history, blood pressure, lipids and lipoproteins, insulin, fasting glucose tolerance, height, weight, health behaviors, and psychological traits and stress. When women ceased menstruation for 12 months *or* ceased menstruation and used HRT in combination for 12 months, they were re-evaluated in a protocol almost identical to that above. At the same time, an age-matched premenopausal woman was re-evaluated. All women were evaluated after 3 years of study participation. Thereafter, women were evaluated in the clinic at years 1, 2, 5, and 8 after the cessation of menses.

CHARACTERISTICS AT STUDY ENTRY OF HRT USERS

Among the 353 women who had ceased cycling for at least 12 months, 184 had used HRT at some time. Most were using combination preparations. Comparisons of the characteristics of ever users and never users were made by χ^2 or *t*-test; a significance level of $p < 0.05$ is reported herein. Ever users and never users of HRT were of similar age and marital status at study entry. However, never users of HRT were less educated than ever users, with 37% vs. 21%, respectively, having a high school degree or less. The two groups had similar levels of low density lipoprotein (LDL-C) cholesterol and triglycerides. However, ever users of HRT had higher levels of high density lipoprotein (HDL) total and HDL-2, and lower levels of apolipoprotein B, compared to never users, indicative of a more favorable lipid profile prior to the use of HRT. Other biological characteristics at study entry also distinguished ever users of HRT: they had lower systolic and diastolic blood pressure levels and weighed less than had never users. Ever users of HRT also reported being more physically active in their leisure time and consuming more alcohol than did never users. Taken together, the results show that ever users of HRT were healthier prior to the use of HRT, suggesting that cohort studies might be over-estimating the beneficial effects of HRT.

Comparison of the psychological characteristics of ever and never users of HRT provides clues as to why women might have used HRT. Ever users had higher scores at study entry on measures of Type A (being aggressive and competitive) and private self-consciousness (being aware of private feelings and symptoms, being reflective) than did never users. Ever users were not more depressed or distressed at study entry than never users. Perhaps ever users were more likely to seek treatment for menopausal symptoms and for prevention of chronic diseases known to afflict elderly women because of their high educational attainment, their assertiveness, and their heightened awareness of feelings and symptoms.

CHANGES IN CHARACTERISTICS OF HRT USERS DURING THE MENOPAUSE

Because HRT users are healthier at the outset of the menopausal transition, they may not have the same menopausal experience as non-users. To address this possibility, changes in biological and psychological characteristics from study entry to follow-up approximately 3 years later, adjusted for level at study entry, were compared among women who became postmenopausal and did not use HRT, women who became postmenopausal and did use HRT, and age-matched premenopausal women[5]. The groups had a similar experience, with the exception of lipid levels. The groups had similar changes in weight, blood pressure, physical activity, and alcohol intake over the follow-up period[6]. Postmenopausal women who did not use HRT had twice the increase in LDL-C over time than did age-matched premenopausal women; women on HRT showed increases comparable to those of premenopausal women. Postmenopausal women who did not use HRT showed a significant decline in HDL-C, not experienced by either HRT users or premenopausal women. HRT users showed substantial increases in triglycerides, probably due to increased production of large triglyceride-rich very-low-density lipoproteins (VLDL) by the liver[7]. Further follow-up of more menopausal women has shown that the decline in HDL-C with the menopausal transition is not reliable. Menopause, in the absence of HRT use, does lead to a significant decline in HDL-2 levels, however. Taken together, our results show that the favorable effect of HRT on biological characteristics and health behaviors is restricted to levels of lipid and lipoproteins.

With regard to psychological characteristics, HRT did not lead to a more favorable psychological experience overall. Users did not differ from other postmenopausal women in reports of depressive symptoms or total menopausal symptoms experienced in the last 2 weeks; postmenopausal women not on HRT reported fewer stress symptoms (adjusted for initial symptom level) than did HRT users or premenopausal controls[8]. In fact, it appears that a subset of hormone users were vulnerable to depressive symptoms during the menopausal transition. These women were characterized at study entry as having low self-esteem and holding their anger in, and, if they experienced an important stressful event, being low in masculine traits. These findings may explain why many women still believe that the menopausal transition is a very difficult one: a subset of women with specific traits prior to the menopause and who use HRT have depressive symptoms (not clinical depression) during the menopausal period.

Given the high number of women taking HRT currently, and the current recommendations to use HRT to prevent coronary disease and osteoporosis, it will be important to evaluate the psychological effects of HRT, in light of women's pre-existing psychological traits.

SUMMARY

In our cohort study of middle-aged women, hormone users have a very different menopausal experience than non-users. Prior to the menopause, they are healthier, better educated, and more aggressive as well as self-reflective. They experience less adverse lipid changes due to the menopause, although they do experience elevated triglyceride levels. However, they do not benefit psychologically from using HRT and a subset of women who use HRT may be susceptible to increased depressive symptoms. Studies such as the Women's Health Initiative – a randomized clinical trial of HRT and a low fat diet – will permit evaluation of the overall benefits and risks of use of HRT in the general population of postmenopausal women.

ACKNOWLEDGEMENTS

This research was supported by grant HL28266 awarded by the National Institutes of Health to the first and second authors.

REFERENCES

1. Stampfer, M. J. and Colditz, G. A. (1991). Estrogen replacement therapy and coronary heart disease: a quantitative assessment of the epidemiologic evidence. *Prev. Med.*, **20**, 47–63
2. Cummings, S. R. (1990). Epidemiology of osteoporosis in women. In Korenman, S. G. (ed.) *The Menopause*, pp. 59–66. (Norwell, MA: Serono Symposia)
3. Nabulsi, A. A., Folsom, A. R., White, A., Patsch, W., Heiss, G., Wu, K. K. and Szklo, M. for the Atherosclerosis Risk in Communities Study Investigators (1993). Association of hormone-replacement therapy with various cardiovascular risk factors in postmenopausal women. *N. Engl. J. Med.*, **328**, 1069–75
4. Matthews, K. A., Kelsey, S. F., Meilahn, E. N., Kuller, L. H. and Wing, R. R. (1989). Educational attainment and behavioral and biologic risk factors for coronary heart disease in middle-aged women. *Am. J. Epidemiol.*, **129**, 1132–44
5. Matthews, K. A., Meilahn, E., Kuller, L. H., Kelsey, S. F., Caggiula, A. W. and Wing,

R. R. (1989). Menopause and coronary heart disease risk factors. *N. Engl. J. Med.,* **321**, 641–6

6. Wing, R. R., Matthews, K. A., Kuller, L. H., Meilahn, E. N. and Plantiga, P. L. (1991). Weight gain at the time of the menopause. *Arch. Intern. Med.,* **151**, 97–102

7. Walsh, B. W., Schiff, I., Rosner, B., Greenberg, L., Ravnikar, V. and Sacks, F. M. (1991). Effects of postmenopausal estrogen replacement on the concentrations and metabolism of plasma lipoproteins. *N. Engl. J. Med.,* **325**, 1195–204

8. Matthews, K. A., Wing, R. R., Kuller, L. H., Meilahn, E. N., Kelsey, S. F., Costello, E. J. and Caggiula, A. W. (1990). Influences of natural menopause on psychological characteristics and symptoms of middle-aged healthy women. *J. Cons. Clin. Psychol.,* **58**, 345–51

49

Continuous combined HRT: a possible way to avoid uterine bleeding?

L.-Å. Mattsson

Evidence regarding the positive effects of hormone replacement therapy (HRT) is accumulating. The benefits of HRT for the treatment of genital atrophy and for the prevention of osteoporosis in postmenopausal women are well established[1,2]. In addition, a number of reports have documented beneficial effects on the cardiovascular system in women taking estrogens in the climacteric period[3,4]. Combinations of estrogens and progestogens have been advocated to protect the endometrium from hyperplasia and possible malignancies. Conventionally, progestogens are added to the estrogen treatment either sequentially or cyclically for at least 10 days each treatment month. However, such combinations lead to withdrawal bleeding in almost 90% of treated women.

Many women receiving HRT are distressed by uterine bleeding: this may be one of the reasons why few women start therapy and a large number discontinue prematurely[5,6]. Evidence suggests that only 30% of patients are compliant with therapy. This is a problem, especially when long-term treatment is needed for the prevention of bone loss and coronary heart disease (CHD). A treatment period of at least 5–10 years is desirable, but until now only a minority of women have continued HRT for such a long period. Long-term treatment with estrogens and progestogens given on a continuous basis may increase compliance: a number of investigators have found that these preparations are fairly well accepted by postmenopausal women[7–9].

TREATMENT REGIMENS AND ROUTES OF ADMINISTRATION

When continuous combined HRT was introduced, more than 10 years ago, the main objective was to reduce bleeding disturbances and therefore increase compliance. Progestogens given cyclically may induce premenstrual-like symptoms: reduced daily dose of progestogens in continuous combined therapy can avoid such side-effects in most women.

During the last decade a number of different estrogens and progestogens in different doses have been tested, aiming to find the ideal combination (Table 1). The main objective of treatment should be amenorrhea with a minimum of subjective and metabolic side-effects. In spite of various dose combinations of estrogens and progestogens in the formulations tested, most investigators have reported a gradual reduction in bleeding disturbances during treatment. However, it should be noted that bleeding episodes have not been defined consistently in various trials[10].

Most investigators have used oral administration for continuous combined therapy, although a few pilot studies have been conducted using transdermal application of both estrogens and progestogens. Due to the limited number of patients only preliminary conclusions can be drawn, but this route of administration may be an option for the future[11-13]. In one study the progestogen component was administered via the uterine cavity[14]. The authors reported beneficial effects in perimenopausal women when estradiol valerate 2 mg/day was given orally in combination with an intrauterine device (IUD) releasing levonorgestrel at a dose of 20 μg/24 h. This combination was compared to orally administered estradiol valerate 2 mg in 3-week periods in combination with 250 μg of levonorgestrel during the last 10 days. In the IUD group 15 of 18 women became amenorrheic after 12 months of treatment while all women in the group given cyclical treatment orally had regular withdrawal bleedings. No endometrial proliferation could be detected in any of the women after 12 months.

Obviously, many treatment alternatives can be used as continuous combined therapy. However, the impact on variables such as bleeding patterns, bone and lipid metabolism has to be considered. The effects on these variables are important factors when deciding which preparations are to be recommended for women on long-term therapy.

BLEEDING PATTERNS AND HISTOPATHOLOGY

A number of studies of different continuous combined HRT formulations have been undertaken in attempts to reduce the stimulation of the

Table 1 Studies of continuous combined hormone replacement therapy with a duration of $\geqslant$ 12 months

| Reference | Estrogen | Progestogen | | Duration (months) | n | Bleeding (%) | | Dropouts (% of recruited) |
		Type	Dose (mg)			3–4 months	12 months	
7	E_2-17β + E_3	NETA	0.5–2.0	6–52	265	18	4	30
8	E_2-17β + E_3	NETA	1.0	12	28	54	31	11
16	CEE	NETA	0.35–2.1	6–29	95	33–58	5	35
9	E_2-17β	NETA	1.0	12	15	47	14	7
			0.5	12	15	73	9	33
18	CEE	MPA	2.5	12	46	57	18	38
		MPA	5	12	46			15
24	E_2-17β	P	200–300	12	11	40	0	9
22	E_2-17β	NETA	1.0	60	18	25 (6 months)	0	25
14	E_2V	LNG	0.02	12	18	56	17	0
12	CEE	NETA	0.7	18	46	45	25	62
		MPA	5	18	28	45	38	

E_2-17β, estradiol; E_3, estriol; CEE, conjugated equine estrogens; E_2V, estradiol valerate; NETA, norethisterone acetate; MPA, medroxyprogesterone acetate; P, micronized progesterone; LNG, levonorgestrel

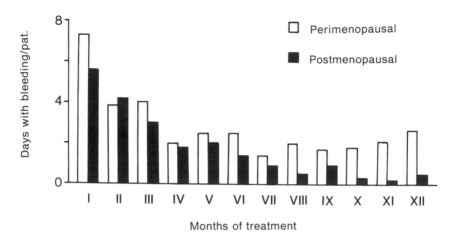

Figure 1 Comparison of the number of days with bleeding per patient in perimenopausal (□) and postmenopausal (■) women during 1 year of continuous combined estrogen/progestogen treatment

endometrium and to minimize bleeding disturbances. In our first study, 26 peri- and postmenopausal women were followed for 1 year[8]. All were given one tablet daily containing 2 mg 17β-estradiol, 1 mg estriol and 1 mg norethisterone acetate. The number of bleedings recorded was higher in perimenopausal than in postmenopausal women (Figure 1). Most of the postmenopausal women experienced no bleeding at all, except for spotting at the beginning of the treatment period. Endometrial samples were found to be atrophic even in women with bleeding, and vaginal bleeding was felt to be an unreliable indicator of endometrial histopathology. Lipoprotein metabolism during treatment was also evaluated in these women[15]. Low density lipoprotein (LDL) decreased both at 3 and 12 months of therapy, concomitant with a decrease in high density lipoprotein (HDL) cholesterol at the same intervals. However, no change in the ratio of HDL/LDL was detected during treatment compared to the baseline values.

In a study by Magos and associates[16] 95 postmenopausal women were treated with a continuous combined regimen consisting of conjugated estrogens (0.625–1.25 mg daily) and norethisterone (0.35–2.1 mg daily) and monitored for up to 2.5 years. The main objective in this study was to induce amenorrhea: in some women doses of progestogens were increased during the course of treatment to obtain amenorrhea in all patients. After 1 year of therapy about 5% of patients still in the study experienced bleeding episodes. The authors reported a drop-out rate of about 35%, mostly because of bleeding disturbances. After 6 months of continuous combined therapy endometrial biopsy specimens showed an atrophic endometrium in more than 50% of the patients. No abnormal histology was noted in this study after 18 months of treatment. Patients given the higher dose of estrogen experienced a higher frequency of bleeding disturbances and the authors recommended that patients should start on a lower dose of estrogen for better control of bleeding, especially during the first treatment period.

In a second study from our group the main objective was to determine whether the dose and the type of the progestogen given had any clinical and metabolic impact[9]. Sixty postmenopausal women, mean age 55.4 years, were randomly allocated to one of four treatment groups: a continuous estrogen/progestogen regimen consisting of 2 mg 17β-estradiol daily in combination with either norethisterone acetate 1 mg and 0.5 mg or megestrol acetate 5 mg or 2.5 mg. Irregular uterine bleeding was almost entirely confined to the early phase of the study and was substantially less with the formulation containing 1 mg norethisterone acetate compared to the other treatment groups during the first 4 months. After the initial treatment phase the clinical efficacy was the same irrespective of the type and the dose of progestogen administered. The proportion of women with amenorrhea was higher in the group of patients receiving 1 mg norethisterone acetate and we stated that it might be an advantage to administer a relatively high dose of progestogen at the beginning of treatment to minimize bleeding disturbances. Many women may otherwise discontinue therapy during this period. The ratio of estrogen and progestogen given obviously influences bleeding patterns at least during the first 3–4 months of therapy (Figure 2). Significant reductions of LDL cholesterol and HDL cholesterol levels were found but no differences could be demonstrated between the groups during treatment as assessed by analysis of variance[17].

Weinstein and colleagues conducted a trial in which 92 women were given 0.625 mg of conjugated equine estrogens with either 2.5 or 5 mg of medroxyprogesterone acetate taken continuously for 1 year[18]. In this study a decrease in vaginal bleeding was demonstrated after 13 weeks and a further decrease after 26 weeks of therapy. About 9% of the women discontinued therapy because of bleeding disturbances. A favorable lipoprotein profile was also found during treatment. The authors suggested that treatment should start with 2.5 mg of medroxyprogesterone acetate and 0.625 mg conjugated equine estrogens, the progestogen being increased to 5 mg if heavy or persistent uterine bleeding occurred.

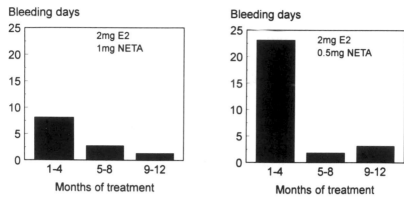

Figure 2 The mean number of days with bleeding during three 4-month periods, in women treated with two different types of orally administered continuous combined hormone replacement therapy. E2 = estradiol; NETA = norethisterone acetate. The figure illustrates the importance of an appropriate ratio between the estrogen and progestogen component to obtain bleeding control in the beginning of the treatment

In an 18-month study, Hillard and co-workers followed 79 postmeno-pausal women switched over from sequential estrogen–progestogen treatment to continuous combined estrogen–progestogen therapy[19]. The latter treatment comprised conjugated equine estrogens 0.625 mg daily with either norethisterone acetate 0.35 mg twice daily or medroxyproge-sterone acetate 2.5 mg twice daily. Only 38% of the patients completed the study, which is a very high drop-out rate. The main reason for discontinuing therapy was chronic irregular bleeding. Persistent amenor-rhea was achieved by only approximately one-third of the patients who started continuous combined estrogen–progestogen therapy. However, it is not known how many of the patients would have become amenorrheic if they had remained in the study for the whole treatment period. The authors conclude that women with persistent early bleeding on continuous combined therapy should be changed to a sequential treatment and that regular endometrial sampling is advised.

CONTINUOUS COMBINED HRT – RECOMMENDATIONS

Irrespective of the type of continuous combined HRT used, some of the recommendations below may be useful for the physician.

Careful patient selection

In a number of studies, the number of bleedings recorded during therapy has been lower in postmenopausal than in perimenopausal women. In a study by Sporrong and co-workers, it was found that women who had been postmenopausal for > 5 years before starting therapy had fewer bleeding episodes compared to other postmenopausal women[20]. Accordingly, women best suited for this type of therapy are those who are at least 2 years postmenopausal.

Information and motivation

All patients should be informed about the possibility of irregular bleeding during the first 3–4 months of treatment. Most bleeding episodes will be spotting, but these can be annoying to some women, who have to be informed that amenorrhea will probably occur if they continue therapy. The physician should encourage and motivate the patient to continue therapy despite irregular bleeding during the initial period. Most investigators have reported that the majority of patients become amenorrheic after 6 months. A number of studies have also shown that the continuation rate is very much dependent on the frequency of bleeding disturbances at the beginning of treatment[9,18].

Atrophic endometrium

It seems to be important for the endometrium to be atrophic before the start of the treatment. Some studies in which women have changed from sequential therapy directly to continuous combined therapy have found a high percentage of withdrawals[16,19]. Accordingly, a treatment-free period may be recommended before continuous combined therapy is initiated. Another possibility may be to give progestogens for 10–14 days to induce withdrawal bleeding and to achieve a thin endometrium before the continuous combined HRT is started.

Estrogen–progestogen ratio

It is important to emphasize the relevance of the ratio between the estrogen and the progestogen component in the formulation prescribed. This ratio is of special importance at the beginning of the treatment to obtain an acceptable bleeding pattern. Unpublished data by Dr Stadberg in our group showed that about 80% of women given 1 mg estradiol along with 0.5 mg norethisterone acetate were amenorrheic after 2 months of treatment. A relatively low dose of estrogen or a high dose of progestogen during the initial period may avoid unnecessary bleeding disturbances. Doses of estrogens and progestogens may need to be changed during the course of therapy to suit the needs of each individual.

Endometrial surveillance

Although most investigators have found the endometrium to be atrophic during continuous combined therapy at least one study has reported malignancies during such therapy[21]. It is therefore important to realize that bleeding disturbances occurring $\geqslant 6$ months after initiation of therapy should be dealt with according to conventional clinical practice. The endometrium should be examined either by endometrial biopsy or by vaginal ultrasonography. If sonography is used as a screening method an endometrial biopsy should be performed if the endometrial thickness exceeds 4 mm. It may also be prudent to perform an endometrial examination before therapy, at least in women at high risk for endometrial malignancies.

CONCLUSIONS

To prevent bone loss and coronary atherosclerosis HRT should be taken by postmenopausal women for at least 5–10 years. Most elderly women dislike uterine bleeding. In a number of studies[7–9,14,18,20,22–24] continuous combined HRT has induced amenorrhea and been well accepted by many women. Provided that certain guidelines are followed by the physician prescribing estrogens and progestogens on a continuous basis, this type of therapy can be advocated for postmenopausal women and will probably increase compliance, which is mandatory if the long-term beneficial effects of HRT are to be achieved.

REFERENCES

1. Mattsson, L.-Å., Cullberg, G., Eriksson, O. and Knutsson, F. (1989). Vaginal administration of low-dose oestradiol – effects on the endometrium and vaginal cytology. *Maturitas,* **11**, 217–22
2. Lindsay, R., Hart, D. M. and Clarc, D. N. (1984). The minimum effective dose of estrogen for prevention of postmenopausal bone loss. *Obstet. Gynecol.,* **63**, 759–63

3. Barrett-Connor, E. and Bush, T. L. (1991). Estrogen and coronary heart disease in women. *J. Am. Med. Assoc.*, **265**, 1861–7
4. Stampfer, M. D., Colditz, G. A. and Willett, W. C. (1991). Postmenopausal estrogen therapy and cardiovascular disease. Ten year follow-up from the nurses health study. *N. Engl. J. Med.*, **325**, 756–62
5. Hahn, R. G. (1989). Compliance considerations with estrogen replacement: withdrawal bleeding and other factors. *Am. J. Obstet. Gynecol.*, **161**, 1854–8
6. Ryan, P. J., Harrison, R., Blake, G. M. and Fogelman, I. (1992). Compliance with hormone replacement therapy (HRT) after screening for postmenopausal osteoporosis. *Br. J. Obstet. Gynecol.*, **99**, 325–8
7. Staland, B. (1982). Continuous treatment with a combination of estrogen and gestagen – a way of avoiding endometrial stimulation. *Acta Obstet. Gynecol. Scand.*, **130** (Suppl.), 29–35
8. Mattsson, L.-Å., Cullberg, G. and Samsioe, G. (1982). Evaluation of continuous combined oestrogen/progestogen regimen for climacteric complaints. *Maturitas*, **4**, 95–102
9. Sporrong, T., Hellgren, M., Samsioe, G. and Mattson, L.-Å. (1988). Comparison of four continuously administered progestogen plus oestradiol combinations for climacteric complaints. *Br. J. Obstet. Gynecol.*, **95**, 1042–8
10. Whitehead, M. I., Hillard, T. C. and Crook, D. (1990). The role and use of progestogens. *Obstet. Gynecol.*, **75**, 59–76S
11. Uvebrant, M., Mattsson, L. Å. and Sandin, K. (1990). Continuous transdermal administration of combined oestrogen/progestogen for climacteric symptoms. *Sixth International Congress on the Menopause*, Bangkok. Abstract No. 247
12. Hillard, T., Ellerington, M., Witcroft, S., Godfree, V., Pryse-Davies, J. and Whitehead, M. (1990). Effect of low-dose transdermal continuous combined oestrogen and progestogen on breast tenderness, vaginal bleeding and endometrial stimulation. An ideal treatment for the 'older woman'? *Sixth International Congress on the Menopause*, Bangkok. Abstract No. 87
13. Keller, P. J., Hotz, E. and Imthurn, B. (1992). A transdermal regimen for continuous combined hormone replacement therapy in the menopause. *Maturitas*, **15**, 195–8
14. Andersson, K., Mattsson, L.-Å., Rybo, G. and Stadberg, E. (1992). Intrauterine release of levonorgestrel – a new way of adding progestogen in hormone replacement therapy. *Obstet. Gynecol.*, **79**, 963–7
15. Mattsson, L.-Å., Cullberg, G. and Samsioe, G. (1984). A continuous estrogen–progestogen regimen for climacteric complaints: effects on lipid and lipoprotein metabolism. *Acta Obstet. Gynecol. Scand.*, **63**, 673–7
16. Magos, A. L., Brincat, M., Studd, J. W. W., Wardle, P., Schesinger, P. and O'Dowd, T. (1985). Amenorrhea and endometrial atrophy with continuous oral estrogen and progestogen therapy in postmenopausal women. *Obstet. Gynecol.*, **65**, 496
17. Sporrong, T., Hellgren, M., Samsioe, G. and Mattsson, L.-Å. (1989). Metabolic effects of continuous estradiol–progestin therapy in postmenopausal women. *Obstet. Gynecol.*, **73**, 754
18. Weinstein, L., Bewtra, C. and Gallagher, J. (1990). Evaluation of a continuous combined low-dose regimen of oestrogen–progestin for treatment of the menopausal patient. *Am. J. Obstet. Gynecol.*, **156**, 1534–9
19. Hillard, T. C., Siddle, N. C., Whitehead, M. I., Fraser, D. I. and Pryse-Davies,

J. (1992). Continuous combined conjugated equine estrogen–progestogen therapy: effects of medroxyprogesterone acetate and norethindrone acetate on bleeding patterns and endometrial histological diagnosis. *Am. J. Obstet. Gynecol.*, **167**, 1–7

20. Sporrong, T., Samsioe, G., Larsen, S. and Mattsson, L.-Å. (1989). A novel statistical approach to analysis of bleeding patterns during continuous hormone replacement therapy. *Maturitas*, **11**, 209–15

21. Leather, A. T., Savvas, M. and Studd, J. W. W. (1991). Endometrial histology and bleeding patterns after 8 years of continuous combined estrogen and progestogen therapy in postmenopausal women. *Obstet. Gynecol.*, **78**, 1008

22. Christiansen, C. and Riis, B. J. (1990). Five years with continuous combined oestrogen/progestogen therapy. Effects on calcium metabolism, lipoproteins and bleeding pattern. *Br. J. Obstet. Gynecol.*, **97**, 1087–92

23. Bewtra, C., Kable, W. T. and Gallagher, J. C. (1988). Endometrial histology and bleeding patterns in menopausal women treated with estrogen and continuous or cyclic progestin. *J. Reprod. Med.*, **33**, 205

24. Hargrove, J., Maxon, W., Wentz, A. and Burnett, L. (1989). Menopausal hormone replacement therapy with continuous daily oral micronized estradiol and progesterone. *Obstet. Gynecol.*, **73**, 606–12

50

Long-cyclic hormonal cycle therapy in postmenopausal women

A. David, B. Czernobilsky and L. Weisglass

INTRODUCTION

Cyclic withdrawal bleeding is often induced by postmenopausal sequential hormonal therapy as a result of the addition of a progestogen for 10–13 days to the estrogens to prevent endometrial hyperplasia. Such bleeding is considered a nuisance by more than 57% of the postmenopausal population[1,2].

The response of the postmenopausal intrauterine endometrium to the cyclic sequential regimen displays the same characteristic morphologic changes observed in the premenopausal endometrium exposed to endogenous cyclic steroids. The sole difference is the timetable, which is stretched. Under the former there is a long gap between stimulation and the proliferative response, which may be due to the presence of various degrees of fibrosis at the basal endometrium or the amount of stroma surrounding scarce epithelial glands. Following this luteal phase secretory pattern, withdrawal bleeding occurs in 80–90% of patients.

We expected that the most attractive aspect of the more recent combined continuous hormonal regimen would be the absence of withdrawal bleeding. However, this was misleading[3-7]. The unpredictable, irregular breakthrough bleeding associated with the latter was even more distressing to our patients[8], especially to orthodox Jewish women who are restricted socially and sexually when bleeding. It was also unfortunate that patients suffered these effects at the beginning of their 'journey' with these treatments, impairing their compliance despite our many

463

Table 1 Bleeding patterns during continuous combined hormonal regimens: 17β-estradiol (2 mg) + norethisterone acetate (1 mg/tablet/day) or conjugated estrogens (0.625 mg/tablet) + medroxyprogesterone acetate (2.5 or 5 mg/tablet)

Months	Patients with bleeding (%) (n = 50)	Duration of bleeding		Recurrent episodes (days/month)
		< 4 months	> 4 months	
1	96			
2	96	31	17	
3	90			
4	34			
5	24			
6	22.6			
7*	40.6			1–6
8*	34.6			1–11
9*	34.6			1–6
10	16			
11†	26.6			3–8
12†	10.6ᵃ			

*Bleeding recurrences in those patients who bled for <4 months
†Bleeding recurrences in those patients who bled for >4 months.
Amount of bleeding varied from spotting to 6–8 pads/day
ᵃOne patient bled all year; also includes those who bled for >4 months

explanations and promises of a better future.

According to our studies (Table 1), the incidence of irregular bleeding episodes decreased from 96% of patients in the 1st month of treatment to 34% in the 4th month, and to 22.6% in the 6th month. Bleeding recurrences were considered significant, particularly their duration.

In 1984 we began a pilot study with unopposed estrogen. The aim of the study was to determine the time of onset of cystic glandular hyperplasia and to determine at what stage progestogen should be added so as to eliminate undesired endometrium.

MATERIAL AND METHODS

The pilot study consisted of 50 postmenopausal patients. After informed consent was obtained, all patients underwent hysteroscopy followed by endometrial biopsy. Biopsy was initially performed with the Novak curette; when this proved to be rather painful, vision-guided biopsy was performed with flexible forceps. Patients then began the hormonal regimen, receiving three cycles of unopposed 17β-estradiol (2 mg/tablet/day) for 21 consecutive days followed by one medication-free week. Hysteroscopy and biopsy were repeated after each cycle. A fourth cycle of 17β-estradiol for 11 days was followed by the progestogen norethisterone acetate (1 mg/tablet/ day for 10 days) in addition to the 17β-estradiol. Endometrial biopsy was performed 1 day after the end of this sequential cycle, and hysteroscopy was performed at the end of the withdrawal bleeding which usually followed this fourth cycle. On the whole, each patient underwent four series of the four-cycle treatment described, giving a total of 16 cycles.

From 1986 to 1992, as part of a national program for prevention of osteoporosis and cardiovascular accidents, 1350 patients followed this regimen. Of these, 528 agreed to be examined twice yearly using hysteroscopy supplemented by endometrial biopsy. The rest of the patients enrolled were interviewed for any side-effects and compliance.

RESULTS

Before treatment, hysteroscopy showed the uterine cavity to have smooth, pale, clear walls and no mucosa. At biopsy 52.1% of the patients showed no tissue or unidentified tissue with strips of surface epithelium and mucus; 43.5% had an atrophic endometrium, with thin, low, cuboidal epithelium and a few scattered, very narrow, glands (Table 2). After the first unopposed treatment cycle, typical proliferative endometrium was found in only 15.2–21.7% of cases, increasing only after the second and third cycle of treatment (Table 2). Hysteroscopy showed the slow progress of proliferation, which began in all patients with tiny bud formation in the cornua surrounding the tubes ostia, sometimes bilaterally but usually unilaterally (see Figure 1). The proliferation first covered the fundus, then spread to the lateral walls and ended at the anterior and posterior walls.

Cystic glandular hyperplasia changes appeared only after the third cycle as a new formation. In contrast to the uniform proliferation, hyperplasia bursts occurred as irregular patches in unpredictable sites, all over the walls and fundus of the uterine cavity. Diffuse hyperplasia was noted in 2.1–8.7% of patients, and focal hyperplasia in 4.3–13% (Table 2).

The hyperplasia was asymptomatic. No atypical hyperplasia was seen in any patient after the unopposed cycles and during the entire 16 months of the four series of cycles. The same results were encountered in the 528 patients followed for 6 years.

After the fourth sequential combined treatment, the endometrium was shed completely in a secretory phase. Complete sloughing of the mucosa was observed at the end of this withdrawal bleeding, by hysteroscopy (Table 2).

Of the 1350 patients, 135 (10%) discontinued the treatment: 2.5% for

Table 2 Results of the endometrial biopsies, before treatment and after the first, second and third cycles of unopposed 17β-estradiol 2 mg/day for 21 days. After the fourth cycle consisting of 17β-estradiol 2 mg/day for 11 days followed by a 10-day combination of 17β-estradiol (2 mg) and 1 mg norethisterone acetate (1 mg/tablet) secretory glands are seen and no hyperplasia. Numbers in parentheses are percentages

	Atrophic endometrium	'No' curettings	Proliferative endometrium	Normal secretory endothelium	Cystic glandular hyperplasia	
					Diffuse	Focal
Before HRT						
	20 (43.5)	24 (52.1)	2 (4.3)	0	0	0
After 1st treatment cycle[a]						
I	35 (76.1)	4 (8.7)	7 (15.2)	0	0	0
II	32 (69.6)	5 (10.9)	9 (19.6)	0	0	0
III	33 (71.7)	6 (13.0)	7 (15.2)	0	0	0
IV	31 (67.3)	5 (10.9)	10 (21.7)			
After 2nd treatment cycle[a]						
I	6 (13.0)	2 (4.3)	38 (82.6)	0	0	0
II	5 (10.8)	1 (2.17)	40 (86.9)	0	0	0
III	6 (13.0)	1 (2.17)	39 (84.8)	0	0	0
IV	8 (17.3)	1 (2.17)	37 (80.4)	0	0	0
After 3rd treatment cycle[a]						
I	2 (4.3)	0	37 (80.4)	0	3 (6.5)	4 (8.7)
II	1 (2.1)	1 (2.1)	36 (78.2)	0	2 (4.3)	6 (13.0)
III	2 (4.3)	0	38 (82.6)	0	1 (2.1)	5 (10.8)
IV	3 (6.5)	0	37 (80.4)	0	4 (8.7)	2 (4.3)
After 4th treatment cycle[a]						
I	2 (4.3)	8 (17.4)	2 (4.3)	34 (73.9)	0	0
II	0	8 (17.4)	1 (2.1)	37 (80.4)	0	0
III	2 (4.3)	6 (13.0)	1 (2.1)	37 (80.4)	0	0
IV	1 (2.1)	7 (15.2)	2 (4.3)	36 (78.2)	0	0

[a]I–IV, number of treatments (each treatment covers four cycles)

no particular reason or after being discouraged by friends; 1% because of recurrent symptomatic complaints during the rest periods; 0.5% because of breast tension, increased body weight and nervousness; and 1.5% because of cancerophobia or other side-effects (itching, recurrent moniliasis, hypermucorrhea and erythema nodosum). Bleeding episodes were reported in 0.33%. Among the 528 closely followed patients, 4.5% bled: breakthrough bleeding in 0.7% and withdrawal bleeding in 3.8%, after the 21 days of unopposed estradiol.

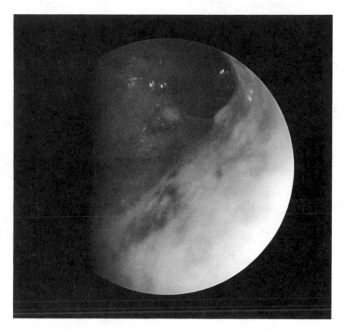

Figure 1 Hysteroscopic panoramic view of the uterine cavity after a 1-month unopposed cycle treatment. Note two tiny endometrial buds – proliferative state – next to the right tubal ostium

DISCUSSION

When estrogens such as 17β-estradiol (2 mg/tablet/day) or conjugated estrogens (0.625 mg/tablet/day) are given in combination with either 1 mg norethisterone acetate or 2.5 or 5 mg medroxyprogesterone acetate continuously, the action of estrogen on the endometrium is counteracted by the progestogens. This process was found to be unsynchronous, with an imbalance between the glandular epithelium and the stroma. This resulted in atrophy at only one site with vascular fragmentation and hemorrhage in the adjacent stroma with pseudodecidualization, while secretory epithelial glands were not seen (Figure 2).

Hysteroscopy displayed in the same cavities low endometrium and small endometrial elevations. Guided biopsies of these irregularities showed prominent vessels, with blood leakage and interstitial hemorrhage. In the same area of endometrium we found complete disorder with cystic hyperplastic glands, proliferative and atrophic glands, mingled together (Figure 3). It is this lack of synchronization between epithelium and

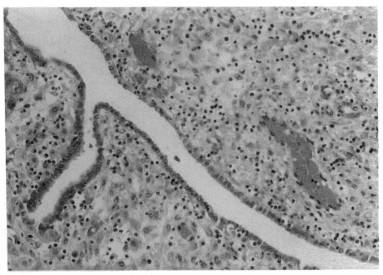

Figure 2 Endometrium after 3 months of a continuous combined hormonal regimen. The stroma is in a pseudodecidual state, presence of blood in the vessels and atrophic epithelial glands (hematoxylin–eosin × 128)

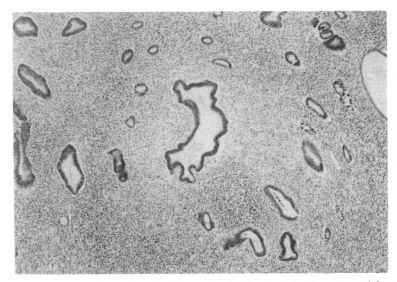

Figure 3 Endometrium showing hyperplastic gland with adjacent proliferative and atrophic glands (hematoxylin–eosin × 50)

stroma that apparently triggers the irregular bleeding of the continuous combined regimens.

After a 4-month 'insult' to these endometria, the gap between the estrogenic and progestogenic effects narrows, and the endometrial system becomes more stabilized, displaying atrophic changes. However, as indicated by the not uncommon episodes of recurrent bleeding, the mechanism is unpredictable, with wide interpatient variations in endometrial response.

The long-cyclic hormonal cycle regimen eliminates these irregular bleedings and is able to minimize withdrawal bleedings to three periods per year, following the fourth sequential combination of estrogen and progestogen.

From the results presented here, 63 days – or 77 days, if the 7-day rest periods are taken into account – are needed for unopposed 17β-estradiol to promote hyperplastic endometrial growth in 2.1–13% of patients, most of it in a focal distribution. These rates were within the range expected in this postmenopausal age group (mean age 55.3 years) without any hormonal treatment. Moreover, after the first 49–56 days (including rest periods), only endometrial proliferation was found. The addition of 1 mg/day of norethisterone acetate for 10 days is needed only after the 3rd month of unopposed estrogens, resulting in a regular withdrawal bleeding in 80.4% of the patients. This long-cyclic hormonal cycle regimen can be restarted from zero with the same endometrial results.

The compliance in the entire group of 1350 patients was excellent, 90% after 6 years of treatment. The reduced number of withdrawal bleedings per year and the almost complete abolition of irregular bleeding were the main contributors to the high compliance.

CONCLUSION

Based on the results of hysteroscopy and endometrial biopsy of the uterine cavity, postmenopausal women may be safely given unopposed 17β-estradiol for three consecutive cycles. Following three cycles, the development of cystic hyperplasia is possible; administration of a fourth cycle of sequential–combined estrogen-progestogen is therefore required. This therapeutic strategy leads to a well-shed uterine cavity, is well accepted by postmenopausal women and should be considered as part of national programs for prevention of osteoporosis and cardiovascular accidents.

REFERENCES

1. David, A., Reif, A. and Weisglass, L. (1987). Cyclic and combined hormonal treatment regimen in postmenopausal women: hysteroscopic findings. In Fiorretti, P., Flamigni, C., Jasoni, V. M. and Melis, G. B. (eds). *Postmenopausal Hormonal Therapy: Benefits and Risks*, pp. 77–81. (New York: Raven Press)
2. Hemminki, E., Brambilla, D. J., MacKinlay, S. M. and Posner, J. C. (1991). Use of estrogens among middle-aged Massachussets women. *Drug Intelligence and Clinical Pharmacy*, **25**, 418–23
3. Staland, B. (1981). Continuous treatment with natural estrogens and progestogens. A method to avoid endometrial stimulation. *Maturitas*, **3**, 145–56
4. Mattson, L.-A., Cullberg, G. and Samsioe, G. (1982). Evaluation of a continuous estrogen–progestogen regimen for climacteric complaints. *Maturitas*, **4**, 95–102
5. Sporrong, G. T., Samsioe, G., Larsen, S. and Mattson, L.-A. (1989). A novel statistical approach to analysis of bleeding patterns during continuous hormone replacement therapy. *Maturitas*, **11**, 209–15
6. Christiansen, C. and Riis, B. J. (1990). Five years with continuous combined estrogen/progestogen therapy. Effects on calcium metabolism, lipoproteins and bleeding pattern. *Br. J. Obstet. Gynecol.*, **97**, 1087–92
7. Weinstein, L., Bewtra, C. and Gallagher, J. C. (1990). Evaluation of a continuous combined low dose regimen of estrogen progestin for treatment of the menopausal patient. *Am. J. Obstet. Gynecol.*, **162**, 1534–42
8. David, A., Tajchner, G. and Czernobilsky, B. (1993). Comparison of two estrogen–progestogen continuous combined regimens for treatment of the menopausal patient. *Maturitas*, in press

51

Hormonal therapy and menstrual bleeding

J. Sciarra and L. Nachtigall

Since menstrual bleeding often accompanies hormone replacement therapy, this symposium was directed at a discussion of the mechanisms of menstrual bleeding, compliance with hormone replacement therapy, and various solutions to monitor and to manage patients with bleeding problems.

The program participants arrived at the following conclusions:

(1) In patients on hormone replacement therapy, compliance is enhanced by explanations of the reasons for therapy and by decreasing nuisance factors, such as spotting, breast tenderness, and fluid retention.

(2) Because of the fact that mechanisms of bleeding in the pre- and the perimenopausal period are not clearly understood, there needs to be a concerted effort to understand the mechanisms whereby exogenous steroids regulate and maintain the endometrial vasculature.

(3) Cyclic treatment may be a solution to overcome irregular bleeding. Compliance of women is related to many factors, but the patient–doctor relationship is the most important factor in the patient continuing on therapy.

(4) Continued combined hormone replacement therapy will probably increase compliance in postmenopausal women, provided careful information is given to them about bleeding disturbances, and what kind of bleeding they can anticipate at the beginning of the treatment program.

(5) Endometrial assessment using transvaginal ultrasound is now a possibility. Ultrasound is a non-invasive procedure that can exclude significant pathology in about 50% of women with bleeding abnormalities, and should be considered as part of the examination of peri- and postmenopausal women.

52

Hormone replacement therapy in a risk–benefit perspective

E. Daly, M. P. Vessey, D. Barlow, A. Gray, K. McPherson and M. Roche

INTRODUCTION

The use of hormone replacement therapy (HRT) by postmenopausal women has been recommended for many years for the relief of menopausal symptoms and the prevention of osteoporosis. More recently, there has been good evidence that HRT has a role in the prevention of coronary heart disease and, less convincingly, in the prevention of stroke. Weighing against these benefits is the possibility that the long-term use of HRT may increase the risk of developing breast cancer. There is evidence that for non-hysterectomized users the increased risk of endometrial cancer associated with estrogen therapy can be eliminated by the use of a progestogen for ⩾ 10 days of each cycle[1]. However, since it appears that estrogen exerts its cardioprotective effect partially through a lipid-mediated mechanism, it has been postulated that the concurrent use of progestogen will attenuate or reverse this effect[2]. No evidence exists to support this hypothesis; indeed, the recently published results of one follow-up study show similar cerebrovascular disease profiles in users of unopposed estrogen and combined therapy users[3]. Until more conclusive evidence becomes available, it is recommended that the lowest possible dose of progestogen which provides endometrial protection be used[4]. In addition, newer less androgenic progestogens, which do not appear to reverse the beneficial effects of estrogen on serum lipid profiles, have been developed for use in combined preparations in an attempt to overcome this potential problem[5].

Several recent publications have reviewed the published literature on the benefits and risks of long-term HRT[6-12] but up-to-date cost-effectiveness studies on this topic are scarce[13-16]. Weinstein and Schiff concluded that, overall, estrogen–progestogen therapy appeared to be cost-effective relative to estrogen only therapy, except in women who considered the adverse effects of continued menstruation to offset the relief of menopausal symptoms[13]. However, this study included no assumptions about the effect of HRT on cerebrovascular disease. As a consequence of the lack of published data on many aspects of HRT use, especially the long-term effects of combined therapy, it has been necessary to make assumptions about treatment effects. Such assumptions are derived from a review of the epidemiological literature and represent the authors' best estimates. We have taken a cautious view which may please neither the optimists nor the pessimists. Sensitivity analyses have been performed to evaluate the impact of each assumption on the final results, although not all are presented here due to limitations of space.

METHODS

Structure of the model

A cost-effectiveness framework in the form of a computer model was established to study the impact of long-term HRT use in hypothetical cohorts compared with untreated control groups. Cost-effectiveness was defined as the ratio of the net increase in health care costs to the net effectiveness in terms of increased life expectancy and quality of life[17].

Two main treatment strategies were considered throughout the analysis:

(1) Treating hysterectomized women with estrogen only therapy (ORT); and

(2) Treating non-hysterectomized women with combined estrogen and progestogen replacement therapy (CRT).

In our standard analysis women received treatment for 10 years starting at age 50, and full compliance was assumed. Treatment and control groups were taken to be identical with respect to uterine status. Current users were assumed to see their GP on two extra occasions each year for monitoring.

Four consequences of treatment were considered:

(1) Mortality induced or prevented by HRT;

(2) Morbidity induced or prevented by HRT;

(3) Changes in quality of life following relief of menopausal symptoms; and

(4) Health care costs associated with treatment.

Age-specific mortality and morbidity rates (in 5-year age bands) for each disease end-point were used to calculate the expected numbers of deaths and hospital admissions occurring each year from age 50 until the end of follow-up. For the hypothetical treatment cohorts, mortality and morbidity rates were modified by applying appropriate relative risk estimates. Age-specific hospital admission costs for each disease of interest were applied to the annual difference in admissions between the treated and untreated groups. Annual costs and savings thus calculated were appropriately discounted (6% per annum). Summing the annual cost/cost saving for each disease of interest over the total period of follow-up yields a total cost/cost saving associated with admissions induced/prevented among the treatment group. Costs to the NHS of providing health care during the extended lifetime of women on HRT were estimated using age-specific annual health care costs per capita. Combining the above costs and savings with drug and monitoring costs enabled a treatment cost per user to be calculated. To examine the effect of treatment on mortality, the number of life years gained (LYG) was calculated by summing the differences between the number of survivors in the comparison cohort and the treatment cohort at the end of each year. The cost per life year gained is given by dividing the discounted treatment cost per user by the discounted LYG per user.

Health effects

Disease endpoints considered in this analysis included (ICD9 3 digit codes in brackets):

(1) Endometrial cancer (179,182);

(2) Breast cancer (174);

(3) Fractured neck of femur (820, 821);

(4) Fractured wrist (814);

(5) Fractured vertebra (805);

(6) Ischemic heart disease (410–414); and

(7) Cerebrovascular disease (430–438).

In addition, the impact of treatment on a woman's risk of undergoing a hysterectomy (OPCS operation codes 690–694 or 696) or dilatation and curettage (D & C) (OPCS codes 703, 704) was considered. Mortality and morbidity rates for all other causes were assumed to be identical in the treatment and control groups.

Data sources

For the untreated control group, current population mortality and morbidity rates for the UK were assumed to apply – this seems a reasonable assumption, given the very low levels of long-term HRT use in this country[18,19]. Mortality rates used were taken from national mortality figures for 1990[20]. Since national statistics are thought to underestimate the true mortality (and morbidity) associated with fractured neck of femur, we used an overall case-fatality rate of 25% applied to incidence rates for this condition.

For most of the diseases of interest, hospital admission rates, taken from the most recent Hospital Inpatient Enquiry (HIPE)[21], were regarded as a good proxy for morbidity. However, for the three types of fracture considered, different sources of data were used. Incidence rates published by Boyce and Vessey[22] were used as a measure of hip fracture morbidity, although average length of hospital stay data from HIPE were used in our costing calculations for this disease. Fractured wrist incidence rates were taken from a community survey by Donaldson and co-workers[23]. Since hospital admission data are unhelpful in estimating morbidity associated with vertebral fractures, incidence rates were derived from the results of a survey by Melton and colleagues[24].

Assumptions about disease risk

A review of the epidemiological literature enabled best estimates to be made of the changes in disease risk following the use of ORT and CRT. Our standard assumptions about disease risk following 10 years' treatment are summarized below. Lack of space prevents the inclusion of the literature review which led to the derivation of these figures (Oxford HRT Study Group, report to the UK Department of Health, 1992, unpublished).

Endometrial cancer

It was assumed that CRT users are at no increased risk of developing endometrial cancer.

Breast cancer

It is assumed that 5 years' use of either ORT or CRT is not associated with any increased risk of breast cancer. Risk is assumed to increase by 30% following 10 years' use (of either ORT or CRT) and 50% following 15 years' use, the risk remaining elevated after discontinuation of treatment for a period equal to the period of treatment.

Osteoporotic fractures of the hip, wrist and vertebrae

We assumed a 20% reduction in fracture risk during the first 5 years' use of ORT or CRT, followed by a 60% reduction where treatment is continued. After discontinuation of treatment, this reduction in risk was assumed to persist for a period equal to the period of treatment.

Ischemic heart disease

We assumed ischemic heart disease risk to decrease by 25% following 5 years' use of ORT and by 50% following 10 years' use, with risk remaining reduced after discontinuation of treatment for a period equal to the period of treatment. For CRT, we assumed a halving of the cardioprotective effect.

Cerebrovascular disease

We assumed a 25% reduction in the risk of stroke following the use of ORT and a 12.5% reduction following the use of CRT. These assumptions are less well founded than those for ischemic heart disease; however, sensitivity analyses have been performed using a range of risk assumptions.

Hysterectomy and dilatation and curettage

Since any unexpected bleeding in a woman on HRT (ORT or CRT) is likely to be thoroughly investigated, there are grounds for supposing increased gynecological intervention rates among women undergoing treatment. We assumed a 25% increase in the risk of undergoing a hysterectomy or D & C among women receiving CRT. The effect is assumed to last only during the period of treatment.

Health care costs

In the health sector, the cost-effectiveness of a particular intervention can be defined as the ratio of the net change in costs to the net change in health outcomes.

The health care costs resulting from therapy can be broken down into the following components:

(1) Expected lifetime cost of therapy, including monitoring and maintenance costs;

(2) Expected costs of treating side-effects;

(3) Expected savings in costs from reduced morbidity; and

(4) Expected costs of treating patients during any increased life expectancy.

Expected lifetime costs of therapy

The main component of the expected lifetime costs of therapy is the annual retail cost of providing HRT drug preparations to women in the treated cohort, and the annual cost of routine GP consultations associated with therapy. These annual costs were calculated over the full period of treatment, discounted to present values. Direct costs to the NHS accounted for in this analysis included (i) an annual cost of £24 per woman treated with ORT (Premarin 0.625 mg)[25] and £53 per woman treated with CRT (Prempak-C 0.625 mg), and (ii) the cost of two extra GP consultations per year of use. We estimated that at 1992/93 prices the cost of an average GP consultation was £22.63 (£9.10 excluding any drugs prescribed). An average cost per out-patient attendance in acute non-teaching hospitals of £42.75 was used[26].

Expected costs of treating side-effects and expected cost savings from reduced morbidity

Indirect costs to the NHS incurred or averted as a result of treatment include the costs of treating side-effects and cost savings from reduced morbidity. In estimating these costs and savings the four main areas of health service activity in which significant costs arise must be considered.

These include primary care consultations; medicines dispensed by general practitioners; hospital in-patient care; and hospital out-patient care.

Wrist fractures and vertebral fractures Savings from wrist fractures prevented were estimated based on the assumption that management of such a fracture would include, on average, three out-patient attendances and two GP consultations (based on calculated ratio of GP consultation rate[27] for wrist fracture, to wrist fracture incidence rate), yielding a cost per wrist fracture case of £170 (1992/93 prices). Savings associated with a reduction in the incidence of vertebral fractures were based on recently published evidence from a study of the incidence of clinically diagnosed vertebral fractures. This population-based study estimated that one-third of all vertebral fractures come to medical attention and that as many as 8% require admission to hospital[28]. In our costings it was assumed that each case coming to medical attention resulted in two GP visits and two out-patient visits. Hospital admission costs were calculated based on age-specific in-patient lengths of stay for vertebral fracture (ICD9 code 805) derived from data published in the Hospital In patient Enquiry (HIPE)[21]. Age-specific costs averaged over both symptomatic and asymptomatic cases thus calculated ranged from £170 to £420.

Hysterectomy and dilatation & curettage Data from the UK Department of Health[29] gave an average cost per in-patient day for acute non-teaching hospitals in England in 1986/87 of £102. Using the health-specific inflation index this becomes £157 at 1992/93 prices. In estimating hospital admission costs for hysterectomy and D & C, we assumed that age-specific in-patient lengths of stay[21] multiplied by the average cost per in-patient day of £157 would be sufficiently accurate. This yields average costs per admission for hysterectomy ranging from £1610 (age 50–54) to £3810 (age 85–89). Estimated admission costs for D & C range from £350 to £1300.

Breast cancer, heart disease, stroke and hip fracture For the other four diseases of interest information on routine treatment procedures was obtained from interviews with clinicians working in non-teaching hospitals. This involved obtaining data on the estimated average frequency of out-patient attendances per case (both before admission and following discharge), average length of stay, readmission rates, radiotherapy treatment, physiotherapy, drug therapy, and frequency of GP consultation.

Table 1   Range of health service costs* (£, 1992/93) per hospital admission (per case for fractures)

Breast cancer	1 950–6 910
Ischemic heart disease	1 540–4 750
Cerebrovascular disease	4 000–12 010
Hysterectomy	1 610–3 810
Dilatation and curettage	350–1 300
Hip fracture	2 230–6 210
Vertebral fracture	170–420
Wrist fracture	170

*Includes in-patient costs, out-patient costs, radiotherapy, physiotherapy, GP consultations, and drug cost

This enabled us to construct typical treatment paths for each of the four diseases, and from this a cost per case was calculated.

To price the in-patient component of the total cost, we used data on average age-specific length of stay[21] multiplied by an average cost per in-patient day of £157. The cost per radiotherapy fraction of £32 estimated by Goddard and Hutton[30] was updated to £45 (1992/93 prices) and used in our costings for breast cancer. In calculating the cost per hip fracture case, a physiotherapy session was costed as an outpatient visit at £43. Table 1 details the range of health service costs per in-patient admission for the main diseases of interest (except for fractures for which an average cost per case is shown).

Expected costs of treating patients during their increased life expectancy

If the net consequence of a health care intervention such as HRT is to extend a person's life expectancy, it is desirable in a cost-effectiveness study to take account of the cost of treating that person during their extra lifetime. One way of approaching this is to calculate the average annual age-specific per capita health care expenditure. Age-specific costs per capita for all Hospital and Community Health and Family Health Service Authority services were estimated to range from £361 (age 45–64) to £2363 (age ⩾85) in 1992/93 terms (Oxford HRT Study Group, report to the UK Department of Health, 1992, unpublished).

Using the QALY in cost-effectiveness studies

Life years gained is not an adequate measure of outcome if a health care program makes an important impact on morbidity, or extends life expectancy at less than full health. The quality-adusted life year (QALY) is an attempt to address this problem. This approach involves attaching utilities or weights (between zero and one) to years of life in different health states. If a treatment delays death by 6 months but leaves the patient in pain or bedridden then that 0.5 of an additional life year is weighted, so that in units of QALYs it becomes <6 months. Similarly, if a treatment improves physical status or reduces the duration of pain or disability, the change in weights will result in an increased number of QALYs.

The case for and against the use of QALYs in the allocation of resources has been hotly debated[31–35]. There is some concern about the increasing use of league tables to compare costs per QALY for various health care interventions derived from different sources. Those concerned argue that since different sets of valuations for health states have been used in their calculation, these costs per QALY are not comparable[36]. The conclusion of those appreciating both the advantages and shortcomings of the QALY system is that it can only serve as an aid to, and not a replacement for, responsible discussion about the most efficient use of scarce resources.

Quality adjustments for menopausal symptom relief

Since many women on HRT achieve relief from distressing menopausal symptoms, accounting for this improvement in quality of life is important in an assessment of the benefits and risks of treatment. In order to assess the impact of menopausal symptoms on women's overall quality of life, some fieldwork was undertaken which involved administering a questionnaire to a sample of 63 women, aged between 45 and 60 years, attending a specialist menopause clinic and two general practices in Oxford (Oxford HRT Study Group, in preparation). Eligible women who agreed to participate were given a short non-technical description of mild and severe menopausal symptoms. They were then asked to indicate their quantitative judgement of the effect these symptoms would have on their overall quality of life. This enabled the calculation of utility values for health states with mild and severe menopausal symptoms. As a measure of the benefit obtained from treatment in relation to relief of symptoms we calculated average quality of life (QoL) gains per HRT user. In the main analysis, QoL gains were added to the life years gained (LYG)

Table 2 Deaths and hospital admissions (to age 69 years) per 1000 women treated for 10 years with estrogen only (ORT) or estrogen plus progestogen (CRT) replacement therapy

	Control (no uterus)	ORT cohort	Control (with uterus)	CRT cohort
Deaths	171	−11 (6%)*	176	−5 (3%)
Admissions	1 908	−22 (1%)	2 080	+22 (1%)

*% change in parentheses

component (i.e. actual increase in life expectancy) in order to calculate the cost/QALY associated with treating women with menopausal symptoms.

We assumed that 90% of users experience relief from symptoms[37], 5% experience side-effects, and the other 5% experience no change in overall quality of life. We assumed that the 5% who experience side-effects remain on treatment for 6 months. With regard to duration of symptoms, it has been reported that 56% of women experience acute menopausal symptoms for between 1 and 5 years, and that 26% of women have symptoms for >5 years[38]. For the purpose of this analysis, we assumed that on average, women experience symptoms for 5 years, and that HRT users who obtain relief do so for the same period.

RESULTS

Standard assumptions about disease risk

Table 2 summarizes the estimated numbers of deaths induced or prevented (to age 69) per 1000 women treated for 10 years. Since with our standard assumptions, all relative risks of disease return to 1 at the age of 70, the difference in the number of deaths in the two groups (treated and untreated) peaks at age 69. Both treatment strategies show an overall decrease in deaths, with a reduction of 6% among hysterectomized women and 3% among women receiving CRT. Similarly, in terms of life years gained, greatest benefit is seen in the hysterectomized cohort treated with ORT, with an average of 0.23 life years (3 months) gained per woman. The corresponding figure for non-hysterectomized women treated with CRT is 0.10 years (1 month).

Figure 1 shows that the greatest impact on mortality is seen in relation to a reduction in the risk of ischemic heart disease (IHD), with 11 deaths prevented (to age 69) per 1000 women treated for 10 years with ORT, and six deaths prevented per 1000 women treated for 10 years with CRT.

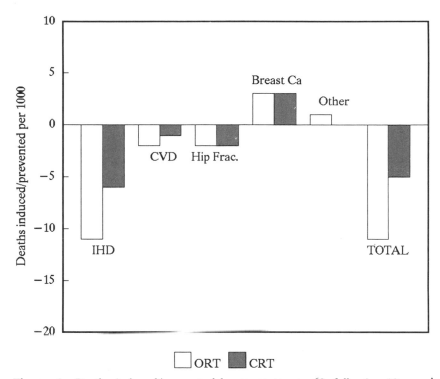

Figure 1 Deaths induced/prevented by cause to age 69, following 10 years' treatment with estrogen only (ORT) or estrogen plus progestogen (CRT) replacement therapy. IHD, ischemic heart disease; CVD, cerebrovascular disease; breast Ca, breast cancer; hip frac., hip fracture

The excess number of 'other' deaths among women treated for 10 years with ORT is a cohort effect and reflects the higher number of survivors in the treatment group compared with the control group.

Figure 2 shows expected life years gained (LYG) for different treatment periods. In general, we have assumed that following cessation of therapy, effects persist for a period equal to the period of treatment. Based on these assumptions, an average increase of about 1 year would be expected per hysterectomized woman treated for 20 years with unopposed therapy, while 5 years' treatment has relatively little impact on mortality in either of the treatment groups.

Hospital admissions (to age 69) induced or prevented per 1000 women treated for 10 years are shown in Figure 3. An overall reduction of 22 admissions is seen per 1000 hysterectomized women treated with ORT, with most of the benefit resulting from the cardioprotective effect of

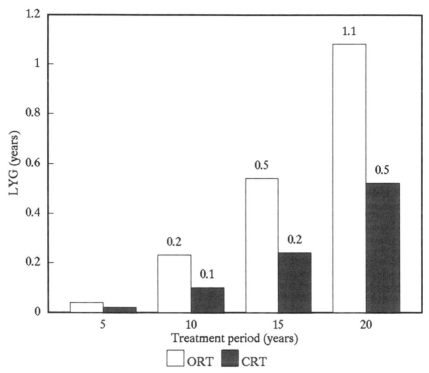

Figure 2 Average life years gained (LYG) per woman for different periods of treatment with estrogen only (ORT) or estrogen and progestogen (CRT) replacement therapy

treatment, representing a reduction of about 1% on the baseline number of admissions. Excess admissions for other causes among this group underline the fact that even a small net increase in life expectancy (3 months) poses an increased burden for the NHS in terms of both workload and cost. For the non-hysterectomized treatment group an overall increase in admissions is seen, mainly accounted for by hysterectomy and D & C.

In both groups, a total of 103 hip, wrist and vertebral fractures are preventable per 1000 women (to age 69), representing an overall reduction of 40% on the baseline figure of 260. Vertebral fractures account for two-thirds of all fractures prevented, while hip fractures account for only 7%, reflecting the relative unimportance of hip fracture as a cause of morbidity among women below the age of 70.

In Table 3 average discounted treatment costs per woman are shown for each treatment strategy. The main bulk of the average treatment cost

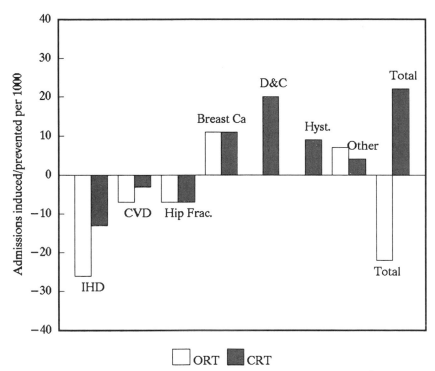

Figure 3 Hospital admissions induced/prevented by cause to age 69 following 10 years' treatment with estrogen only (ORT) or estrogen plus progestogen (CRT) replacement therapy. IHD, ischemic heart disease; CVD, cerebrovascular disease; hip frac, hip fracture; breast Ca, breast cancer; hyst., hysterectomy

per woman is accounted for by the direct costs of drugs and monitoring. For hysterectomized women another important cost component is that of providing health care during the period of added life expectancy.

Figure 4 shows cost per discounted life year gained (DLYG) for different treatment periods. For both treatment strategies, cost per DLYG decreases as the treatment period increases, reflecting our assumptions about the duration of health effects after treatment is discontinued. A reduction of approximately 30% is seen in the cost per LYG when the period of treatment is increased from 10 to 15 years, and likewise from 15 to 20 years, suggesting that it is more cost-effective to treat asymptomatic women for longer periods of time.

Table 3 Average cost/saving to the health service per woman treated for 10 years (followed up until death) (£)

	Estrogen only treatment	Estrogen plus progestogen treatment
Direct costs		
drug	184	407
monitoring	140	140
Indirect costs		
hospital admissions and associated costs (net)	(41)	(6)
vertebral fractures	(11)	(12)
wrist fractures	(3)	(3)
cost of providing health care to survivors	46	21
Total cost	316	547

Figures in parentheses are savings; all costs/savings are discounted at 6% per annum

Effect of different assumptions about disease risk

Breast cancer

The effect of varying assumptions about breast cancer risk following treatment is shown in Figure 5. We performed a large number of sensitivity analyses, varying both the magnitude of increased risk and the duration of effect, but have shown only a selection of results here. A two-fold increase in breast cancer risk prevailing for 10 years would substantially reduce the net life years gained per user, and for the CRT cohort, the excess mortality from breast cancer would swamp all benefits in relation to cardiovascular disease and hip fracture mortality. If this relative risk is assumed to last indefinitely, then for both treatment strategies, a net loss of life of between 6 and 12 weeks (undiscounted) per woman treated is predicted. Similarly, other assumptions compare the effects of a 30% increase in breast cancer risk prevailing for a period of 10 years or indefinitely. With a permanently elevated relative risk of 1.3, the balance is tipped on the benefit side, with a net increase in life expectancy per woman of between 3 and 9 weeks. Assuming no elevated risk of breast cancer following 10 years' treatment, overall LYG figures are predicted at 8 weeks for the non-hysterectomized cohort and 15 weeks for the hysterectomized cohort.

Ischemic heart disease and stroke

Figure 6 shows the effect of varying assumptions about ischemic heart

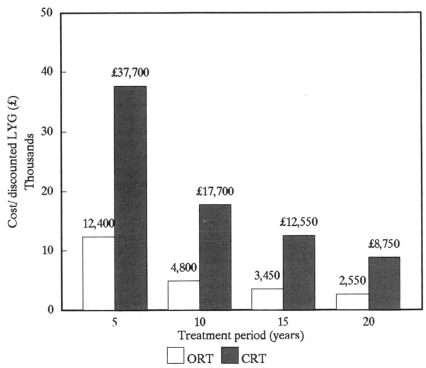

Figure 4 Cost per discounted life year gained (LYG) for different periods of treatment with estrogen only (ORT) or estrogen plus progestogen (CRT) replacement therapy

disease risk. It appears that altering assumptions about the duration of effect has a marked impact on LYG for both treatment groups. Varying assumptions about IHD risk leads to LYG figures ranging from 1 week (no reduction in IHD risk) to 1.16 years (permanent 50% reduction in risk) per hysterectomized ORT user. Note that using the same assumption about risk for both treatment cohorts gives comparable overall LYG figures, the difference being entirely due to the standard assumptions used about cerebrovascular disease risk in the two groups (since all other disease risk assumptions are the same).

Figure 7 demonstrates the effects of varying assumptions about the risk of stroke following 10 years' treatment. Altering assumptions about the duration and magnitude of effect has less impact on LYG figures than that seen when IHD risk is varied, although this reflects the narrower range of relative risk assumptions tested. For a particular stroke risk assumption, any difference between LYG figures for the hysterectomized and non-

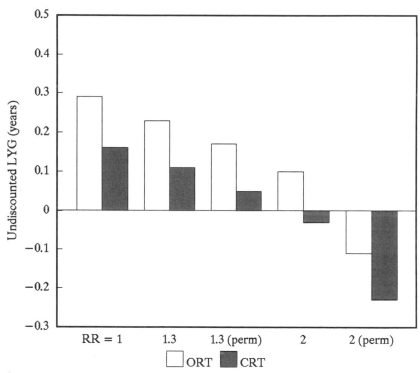

Figure 5 Life years gained (LYG) per woman treated for 10 years with estrogen only (ORT) or estrogen plus progestogen (CRT) using different assumptions about breast cancer risk. RR, relative risk; perm, permanent

hysterectomized cohorts reflects our standard assumptions about IHD risk. Assuming a lasting beneficial effect on stroke risk (relative risk = 0.75) leads to overall gains of about 5–6 months per user.

Treating symptomatic women

Figure 8 shows cost per QALY figures for mildly symptomatic women treated for different periods of time with ORT or CRT. It is assumed that symptomatic women on treatment obtain, on average, 5 years of symptom relief. Costs per QALY range from £310 for hysterectomized (symptomatic) women treated with ORT for 5 years to £1250 for symptomatic CRT users treated for 20 years. What is clearly apparent is the dramatic reduction in cost per life year gained when adjustments are made for symptom relief. For combined therapy users (10 years' treatment) the

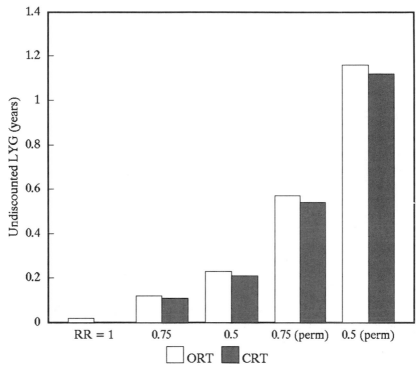

Figure 6 Life years gained (LYG) per woman treated for 10 years with estrogen only (ORT) or estrogen plus progestogen (CRT) using different assumptions about ischemic heart disease risk. RR, relative risk; perm, permanent

cost falls from £17 700 for an unquality-adjusted life year (Figure 4), to less than £1000 when adjustments are made for quality of life improvements. While long-term treatment of asymptomatic women appears to be more cost-effective than short-term treatment (Figure 4), the cost-effectiveness of treating symptomatic women appears to decrease with increasing treatment period. This is due to the LYG figures being swamped by the QoL gains resulting from menopausal symptom relief.

DISCUSSION

The results of our analysis consistently underline the potential benefits of long-term estrogen therapy for hysterectomized women, particularly in relation to a reduction in cardiovascular disease. Our model predicts an increase in life expectancy of about 1.5 years when a lasting 50%

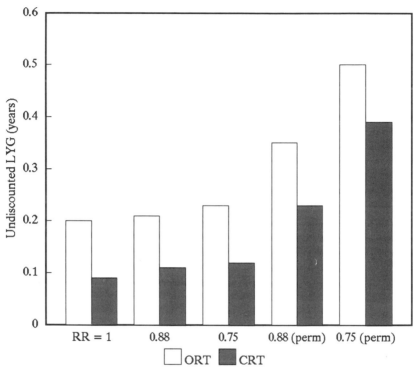

Figure 7 Life years gained (LYG) per woman treated for 10 years with estrogen only (ORT) or estrogen plus progestogen (CRT) using different assumptions about cerebrovascular disease risk. RR, relative risk; perm, permanent

reduction in IHD risk and a lasting 25% reduction in CVD risk is assumed. Assuming, in addition, permanent benefit with respect to fracture risk, gives a figure of 1.7 years, while a lasting 30% increase in breast cancer risk decreases this figure marginally to 1.6 years. Several reviews have also suggested that a halving of cardiovascular mortality following estrogen use would overshadow all other treatment effects[39–42].

Given that by the age of 50, up to 18% of the female population of England will have had a hysterectomy[43], a strategy aimed at this group alone would have major public health implications. Offering treatment to this group of women and to those with menopausal symptoms would be an effective way of targeting a substantial proportion of the perimenopausal population. When more conclusive evidence of the benefits of treatment in relation to cardiovascular disease becomes available, a recommendation for the treatment of women at high risk of coronary heart disease might also be appropriate. Whether less cardioprotection will be seen with

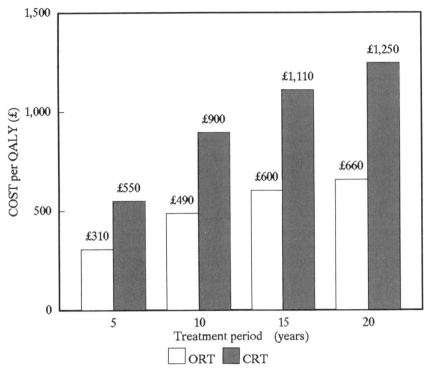

Figure 8 Cost per quality-adjusted life year (QALY) for different periods of treatment with estrogen only (ORT) or estrogen plus progestogen (CRT), assuming 5 years of relief from mild symptoms

combined therapy than with unopposed estrogen remains the most important unanswered question. If progestogens do reduce the cardioprotective effect of estrogen, this raises the issue of whether women with intact uteri might be given unopposed estrogen[44], since the data suggest that this would prevent a much greater volume of cardiovascular morbidity and mortality than the endometrial morbidity it would cause[15].

It has been argued that only randomized controlled trials will provide conclusive evidence of the cardioprotective effect of estrogen and the effect of adding a progestogen[8,44–46]. The observational studies from which the majority of evidence on the long-term effects of treatment has been obtained, have been criticized for their inability to ensure comparability between users and non-users[47], and for the possibility that selection bias is operating. It has been suggested that part of the beneficial effect on total mortality observed in long-term HRT users may be associated with their higher income, higher social class, and more intensive use of medical services[48,49]. The argument for a true protective effect is supported by evidence that cardiovascular disease risk is elevated in women with a premature menopause and that this is reduced by estrogen treatment[50,51]. In addition, ORT has been shown to reduce mortality in women with proven coronary artery disease[52].

An important question concerns the optimum length of treatment. Treating women with menopausal symptoms appears to be very cost-effective regardless of the treatment period, but our results suggest that it is more cost-effective to treat asymptomatic women for extended periods of time. This is because the benefits derived in terms of life years gained and averted costs are not so great for the shorter treatment periods; however, this is dependent on the assumptions we have used about disease risk. A reduction of approximately 30% is seen in the cost per discounted LYG when the period of treatment is increased from 10 to 15 years. The argument for long-term therapy of up to 20 years has already been made for those women in whom treatment is clearly beneficial and devoid of side-effects[53,54]. The treatment period currently recommended in this country is 5–6 years, as this is thought to be the minimum period for achieving bone protection[55]. However, results reported elsewhere[15] suggest that a reduction in fracture risk following long-term HRT, even if permanent, would not have a substantial impact on mortality.

If long-term therapy is required to reap the full benefits of HRT, compliance becomes an important issue. While many women will take short-term HRT to relieve menopausal symptoms, compliance with long-term therapy has been shown to be poor. Studies have found that among combined therapy users, problems associated with the progestogen element of treatment are most often given as reasons for abandoning treatment[56], while other contributing factors include reluctance to continue with long-term therapy in the absence of specific conditions, confusion about the long-term benefits and risks, and the fear of breast cancer. Although the small increase in breast cancer risk which may be associated with long-term use is unlikely to overwhelm the benefits of treatment, this potential side-effect of treatment may heavily influence the overall balance of benefits and risks as perceived by women. Wilkes and Meade found during recruitment to a pilot trial which was undertaken to compare HRT use with no treatment, that for some women, any risk of breast cancer is too great for them to consider HRT, particularly if they do not have any symptoms[45].

Notwithstanding, there appears to be growing interest in taking HRT among menopausal women in the UK. Whereas only 1–3% of

Table 4 Cost per quality-adjusted life year (QALY) for different health interventions (£, 1992/93)

10 years' estrogen replacement therapy (severe menopausal symptoms)	200
Advice by GP to stop smoking[60]	300
10 years' estrogen replacement therapy (mild menopausal symptoms)	500
10 years' estrogen plus progestogen replacement therapy (mild menopausal symptoms)	900
Coronary artery bypass grafting for severe angina (left main disease)[61]	1750
Action by GPs to control hypertension	2850
15 years' estrogen replacement therapy (no menopausal symptoms)	3450
Breast cancer screening program[62]	5550
Heart transplantation[61]	8350

postmenopausal British women were using HRT 10 or 15 years ago[57,58], a recent survey estimated that about 8–9% of women aged 40–64 were receiving HRT[59]. The financial implications for both general practice and the NHS in meeting this growing demand may be considerable. Comparing our results with costs per QALY for other health care interventions (see Table 4) suggests that the cost-effectiveness of treating women with menopausal symptoms is comparable to that of a GP giving advice to stop smoking, and offers very good value for money. Long-term prophylactic treatment of hysterectomized women, on the basis of our assumptions, also compares favorably with currently accepted health interventions, including screening for breast cancer. However, it is acknowledged that while comparison of cost per QALY results within a particular study gives some indication of the relative cost-effectiveness of the different treatment strategies considered, comparison of cost per QALY figures obtained from different studies may not always be valid given that different methods may have been used to measure quality of life.

In summary, it appears that HRT may have an important role to play in preventing premature mortality and reducing morbidity in selected groups of women. Our results suggest that long-term prophylactic treatment of hysterectomized women is relatively cost-effective, while treatment of symptomatic women for any period of time offers very good value for money. However, these results are dependent on the assumptions used, must not be viewed in isolation, and should be seen as decision-aiding information rather than decision-taking yardsticks. Until better data become available, decisions about treatment must be taken at the level of the individual patient.

ACKNOWLEDGEMENTS

The authors gratefully acknowledge the financial support of the Department of Health. Thanks must also be extended to those at the Anderson Clinic in the John Radcliffe Maternity Hospital, and to those at the Jericho Health Centre and Beaumont Street general practices. We are also grateful to those consultants who kindly supplied information on treatment procedures.

REFERENCES

1. Persson, I., Adami, H.-O., Bergkvist, L., Lindgren, A., Pettersson, B., Hoover, R. and Schairer, C. (1989). Risk of endometrial cancer after treatment with oestrogens alone or in conjunction with progestogens: results of a prospective study. *Br. Med. J.,* **298**, 147–51
2. Ross, R. K., Pike, M. C., Henderson, B. E., Mack, T. M. and Lobo, R. A. (1989). Stroke prevention and oestrogen replacement therapy. *Lancet,* **1**, 505
3. Falkeborn, M., Persson, I., Adami, H.-O., Bergstrom, R., Eaker, E., Lithell, H., Mohsen, R. and Naessen, T. (1992). The risk of acute myocardial infarction after oestrogen and oestrogen–progestogen replacement. *Br. J. Obstet. Gynaecol.,* **99**, 821–8
4. Jensen, J. and Christiansen, C. (1987). Dose–response effects on serum lipids and lipoproteins following combined oestrogen–progestogen therapy in post-menopausal women. *Maturitas,* **9**, 259–66
5. Siddle, N. C., Jesinger, D. K., Whitehead, M. I., Turner, P., Lewis, B. and Prescott, P. (1990). Effect on plasma lipids and lipoproteins of postmenopausal oestrogen therapy with added dydrogesterone. *Br. J. Obstet. Gynaecol.,* **97**, 1093–100
6. Hunt, K. and Vessey, M. (1991). The risks and benefits of hormone replacement therapy: an updated review. *Curr. Obstet. Gynaecol.,* **1**, 21–7
7. Hillard, T. C., Whitcroft, S., Ellerington, M. C. and Whitehead, M. I. (1991). The long-term risks and benefits of hormone replacement therapy. *J. Clin. Pharm. Ther.,* **16**, 231–45
8. Adami, H.-O. (1992). Long-term consequences of estrogen and estrogen–progestin replacement. *Cancer Causes Control,* **3**, 83–90
9. Jacobs, H. S. and Loeffler, F. E. (1991). Postmenopausal hormone replacement therapy. *Br. Med. J.,* **305**, 1403–8
10. Barrett-Connor, E. (1992). Risks and benefits of replacement estrogen. *Annu. Rev. Med.,* **43**, 239–51
11. Grady, D., Rubin, S. M., Petitti, D. B., Fox, C. S., Black, D., Ettinger, B., Ernster, V. L. and Cummings, S. R. (1992). Hormone therapy to prevent disease and prolong life in postmenopausal women. *Ann. Intern. Med.,* **117**, 1016–37
12. Session, D. R., Kelly, A. C. and Jewelewicz, R. (1993). Current concepts in estrogen replacement therapy in the menopause. *Fertil. Steril.,* **59**, 277–84
13. Weinstein, M. C. and Schiff, I. (1983). Cost-effectiveness of hormone replacement therapy in the menopause. *Obstet. Gynecol. Survey,* **38**, 445–55
14. Roche, M. and Vessey, M. P. (1990). Hormone replacement in the community:

risks, benefits and costs. In Drife, J. O. and Studd, J. W. W. (eds.) *HRT and Osteoporosis*, pp. 363–72. (London: Springer-Verlag)

15. Daly, E., Roche, M., Barlow, D., Gray, A., McPherson, K. and Vessey, M. (1992). Hormone replacement therapy: an analysis of benefits, risks and costs. *Br. Med. Bull.*, **48**, 368–400

16. Cheung, A. P. and Wren, B. G. (1992). A cost-effectiveness analysis of hormone replacement therapy in the menopause. *Med. J. Aust.*, **156**, 312–16

17. Weinstein, M. C. and Stason, W. B. (1977). Foundations of cost-effectiveness analysis for health and medical practices. *N. Engl. J. Med.*, **296**, 716–21

18. Spector, T. D. (1989). Use of oestrogen replacement therapy in high risk groups in the United Kingdom. *Br. Med. J.*, **299**, 1434–5

19. Barlow, D. H., Brockie, J. A. and Rees, C. M. P. (1991). Study of general practice consultations and menopausal problems. *Br. Med. J.*, **302**, 274–6

20. Office of Population Censuses and Surveys. (1992). *Mortality Statistics: Cause 1990*. (London: HMSO)

21. Department of Health and Social Security and Office of Population Censuses and Surveys. (1987). *Hospital Inpatient Enquiry 1985*. (London: HMSO)

22. Boyce, W. J. and Vessey, M. P. (1985). Rising incidence of fracture of the proximal femur. *Lancet*, **1**, 150–1

23. Donaldson, L. J., Cook, A. and Thomson, R. G. (1990). Incidence of fractures in a geographically defined population. *J. Epidemiol. Comm. Health*, **44**, 241–5

24. Melton, L. J., Kan, S. H., Frye, M. A., Wahner, H. W., O'Fallon, W. M. and Riggs, B. L. (1989). Epidemiology of vertebral fractures in women. *Am. J. Epidemiol.*, **129**, 1000–11

25. British National Formulary Number 25 (March 1993). (London: British Medical Association and the Royal Pharmaceutical Society of Great Britain)

26. Social Services Select Committee (1989). 8th report (London: HMSO)

27. Department of Health and Social Security and Office of Population Censuses and Surveys. (1986). *Morbidity Statistics from General Practice, Third National Study 1981–1982*. (London: HMSO)

28. Cooper, C. and Melton, L. J. (1992). Vertebral fractures: how large is the silent epidemic? *Br. Med. J.*, **304**, 793–4

29. Health and Personal Social Services Statistics (1989). (London: HMSO)

30. Goddard, M. and Hutton, J. (1988). *The Costs of Radiotherapy in Cancer Treatment*. Discussion Paper No. 48. (University of York: Centre for Health Economics)

31. Cubbon, J. (1991). The principle of QALY maximisation as the basis for allocating health care resources. *J. Med. Ethics*, **17**, 181–4

32. Harris, J. (1991). Unprincipled QALYs: a response to Cubbon. *J. Med. Ethics*, **17**, 185–8

33. Wade, D. T. (1991). The 'Q' in QALYs. *Br. Med. J.*, **303**, 1136–7

34. Editorial (1991). Quality of life. *Lancet*, **338**, 350–1

35. Smith, A. (1987). Qualms about QALYs. *Lancet*, **1**, 1134–6

36. McTurk, L. (1991). A methodological quibble about QALYs. *Br. Med. J.*, **302**, 1601

37. Hunt, K. (1988). Perceived value of treatment among a group of long-term users of hormone replacement therapy. *J. Roy. Coll. Gen. Pract.*, **38**, 398–401

38. McKinlay, S. M. and Jefferys, M. (1974). The menopausal syndrome. *Br. J. Prev. Soc. Med.*, **28**, 108–15
39. Hillner, B. E., Hollenberg, J. P. and Pauker, S. G. (1986). Postmenopausal estrogens in prevention of osteoporosis. Benefit virtually without risk if cardiovascular effects are considered. *Am. J. Med.*, **80**, 1115–27
40. Ross, R. K., Paganini-Hill, A., Mack, T. M. and Henderson, B. E. (1987). Estrogen use and cardiovascular disease. In Mishell, D. R., Jr. (ed.) *Menopause: Physiology and Pharmacology*, pp. 209–23. (Chicago: Year Book Medical Publishers)
41. Sitruk-Ware, R. and de Palacios, P. I. (1989). Oestrogen replacement therapy and cardiovascular disease in post-menopausal women. A review. *Maturitas*, **11**, 259–74
42. Miller, A. B. (1991). Risk/benefit considerations of antiestrogen/estrogen therapy in healthy postmenopausal women. *Prev. Med.*, **20**, 79–85
43. Coulter, A., McPherson, K. and Vessey, M. P. (1988). Do British women undergo too many or too few hysterectomies? *Soc. Sci. Med.*, **27**, 987–94
44. Meade, T. W. and Berra, A. (1992). Hormone replacement therapy and cardiovascular disease. *Br. Med. Bull.*, **48**, 276–308
45. Wilkes, H. and Meade, T. W. (1991). Hormone replacement therapy in general practice. *Br. Med. J.*, **303**, 416–17
46. Goldman, L. and Tosteson, A. N. A. (1991). Uncertainty about postmenopausal estrogen: time for action, not debate. *N. Engl. J. Med.*, **325**, 800–2
47. Vandenbrouke, J. P. (1991). Postmenopausal oestrogen and cardioprotection. *Lancet*, **337**, 833–4
48. Coope, J. (1991). Postmenopausal oestrogen and cardioprotection. *Lancet*, **337**, 1162
49. Coope, J. and Roberts, D. (1990). A clinic for the prevention of osteoporosis in general practice. *Br. J. Gen. Pract.*, **40**, 295–9
50. Rosenberg, L., Hennekens, C. H., Rosner, B., Belanger, C., Rothman, K. J. and Speizer, F. E. (1981). Early menopause and the risk of myocardial infarction. *Am. J. Obstet. Gynecol.*, **139**, 47–51
51. Colditz, G. A., Willett, W. C., Stampfer, M. J., Rosner, B., Speizer, F. E. and Hennekens, C. H. (1987). Menopause and the risk of coronary disease in women. *N. Engl. J. Med.*, **316**, 1105–10
52. Sullivan, J. M., Vander Zwaag, R., Hughes, J. P., Maddock, V., Kroetz, F. W., Ramanathan, K. B. and Mirvis, D. M. (1990). Estrogen replacement and coronary artery disease. Effect on survival in postmenopausal women. *Arch. Intern. Med.*, **150**, 2557–62
53. Whitehead, M. and Studd, J. (1988). Selection of patients for treatment: which therapy and for how long? In Studd, J. W. W. and Whitehead, M. I. (eds.) *The Menopause*, pp. 116–29. (Oxford: Blackwell Scientific Publications)
54. Hammond, C. B. (1989). Estrogen replacement therapy: what the future holds. *Am. J. Obstet. Gynecol.*, **161**, 1864–8
55. Coope, J. (1991). Management of the menopause in the community. *Br. J. Fam. Planning*, **16** (Suppl.), 42–5
56. Randall, S. (1990). Problems encountered by long-term hormone replacement therapy users. *Br. J. Fam. Planning*, **16**, 101–5
57. Thompson, S. G., Meade, T. W. and Greenberg, G. (1989). The use of hormonal replacement therapy and the risk of stroke and myocardial infarction in

women. *J. Epidemiol. Comm. Health,* **43**, 173–8

58. Adam, S., Williams, V. and Vessey, M. P. (1981). Cardiovascular disease and hormone replacement treatment: a pilot case–control study. *Br. Med. J.,* **282**, 1277–8

59. Wilkes, H. C. and Meade, T. W. (1991). Hormone replacement therapy in general practice: a survey of doctors in the MRC's general practice research framework. *Br. Med. J.,* **302**, 1317–20

60. Williams, A. (1987). Screening for risk of CHD: is it a wise use of resources? In Oliver, M., Ashley-Miller, M. and Wood, D. (eds.) *Screening for Risk of Coronary Heart Disease,* pp. 97–105. (Chichester: Wiley)

61. Williams, A. (1985). Economics of cornary artery bypass grafting. *Br. Med. J.,* **291**, 326–9

62. Department of Health and Social Security (1986). *Breast Cancer Screening.* A report to the health ministers of England, Wales, Scotland and Northern Ireland by a working group chaired by Sir Patrick Forrest. (London: HMSO)

53

Helping women decide about hormone replacement therapy: approaches to counselling and medical practices

L. Sarrel and P. M. Sarrel

We have come to appreciate the tremendous intellectual and emotional energy many women put into the question of hormone replacement therapy (HRT) – whether to start and, if they do start, whether or not to continue. There is a lot of ambivalence, confusion and angst about this treatment among women over 40 or 45 years of age.

Menopause healthcare could and should be more responsive to women's struggles over the HRT decision. The ultimate goal is to enable women to decide about their own menopause healthcare, based on the best available information from a number of sources, with as little confusion and anxiety as possible, and with full consideration of their personal values and feelings.

With these goals in mind, we want to focus on four areas:

(1) The role of one-to-one or group counselling, utilizing psychotherapeutic strategies;

(2) The need to shift away from the word 'compliance' and its pejorative implications;

(3) Use of the Health Belief Model; and

(4) Structuring medical care delivery to provide crucial follow-up individualization of care and ongoing opportunities to discuss healthcare decisions.

ONE-TO-ONE COUNSELLING, USING PSYCHOTHERAPEUTIC STRATEGIES

How can one-to-one interviews or group discussions help a woman trying to decide about HRT? They can serve some of the same functions as good psychotherapy – helping a woman to understand herself better; making clear what was fuzzy; perhaps making conscious what was pre-conscious. Sometimes a woman recognizes that her reasoning has been skewed by psychological defense mechanisms, denial of her personal vulnerability to aging, illness, and death being most common.

Psychotherapists employ many different 'tools', some of which can be adapted to HRT counselling either by specialized counsellors or by doctors who have the time and the inclination to do this. What is the difference between a typical medical approach and a psychotherapeutic one? At the risk of being simplistic, a psychotherapeutic process focuses less on the external and the observable and more on the internal and the subjective. It strives to elicit a woman's feeling and to understand the meanings that she gives to her feelings and to the events in her life, including her symptoms.

The following are two brief examples of a dialog between a woman and a healthcare provider in which psychotherapeutic strategies were used.

Rita G. is a 55-year-old woman whose last period was at age 53 and who has been agonizing over the question of HRT for 2 years. A male doctor friend of hers, who she respects very much, said 'You're making a *big* mistake by not taking hormones'. In the interview, she asked, 'Why do I feel so strongly that I shouldn't take it? In a way, my head says yes but my heart says no. My body seems to be doing OK on its own. I have some symptoms – like not much sex drive and some hot flashes – but I can live with those. Can't I just trust my own body?'

She was asked a favorite psychotherapy question – 'Does this remind you of anything you've been through before?' A pause, 'Yes – come to think of it, I can see the scene; I'm 22, pregnant (married to my first husband) and my gynecologist is coming towards me with this syringe, telling me that, since I'm spotting, this will help me hold onto the pregnancy. I said 'What's in that?' He said, 'DES (diethylstilbestrol), a natural female hormone.' I had an immediate gut reaction. 'No', I said, 'I don't want it. Let's just see what my body does on its own'. At the end of the interview she spontaneously commented that it was very helpful to remember that earlier story about DES. She was at least clearer about why she had such mistrustful feelings about taking hormones.

Jane M. is a nurse whose last period was 1 year ago. When I asked her whether she had considered HRT, she said, 'Oh, I'm feeling OK. I don't want HRT because of the breast cancer risk.' Another classic psychotherapy tool is repeating or paraphrasing the person's statement as a question.

Interviewer: 'So, you're most afraid of breast cancer?'

Jane: 'Well, I know there's some concern about osteoporosis if I don't take HRT and no one in my family has had breast cancer. To tell you the truth, I think what I'm really afraid of is more my own feelings. I'd probably get so stressed just *thinking* about breast cancer that I'd get, well, maybe a little crazy. And I can't go crazy. I have to function'. Jane explained that she had a lot of personal responsibilities just now. She was planning a large wedding for her daughter; her husband had severe asthma with some incapacitating attacks; her mother, who lived nearby, had severe diabetes. Jane added, 'Come to think of it – I feel I can't even take the time to think it all out and decide what to do; maybe after my daughter's wedding'.

If this sounds depressingly familiar it may be because it is a common female pattern. Sociologists tell us that there is a tendency for women to value service to and for others, particularly their family, above their own needs. Jane was encouraged to make her own health a high priority, for herself and for her family!

It has been observed that some women need to take HRT for a few months simply to make them feel well enough to think clearly about the question of HRT. Sometimes counselling alone can help to relieve stress and anxiety sufficiently for clear thinking. Educators and psychologists know that learning can be blocked by anxiety. Some anxiety is needed for motivation, but too much can lead to mental paralysis, to an inability to think clearly or to act.

Part of using psychotherapeutic strategies successfully includes paying attention to oneself in one's professional role. Healthcare practitioners sometimes bring beliefs, their own ways of thinking and speaking to or about patients, which actually discourage the sense of trust and openness which is so important to good medical care and to good psychotherapy.

In the HRT literature, at conferences and symposia, one hears words which are not at all facilitative. Women's symptoms of weight gain, irregular bleeding, even headache may be called 'nuisance symptoms'. To women experiencing them, these symptoms may be very serious. Similarly, women's feelings about menopause or HRT are often called 'irrational' in a dismissive way. Psychotherapists believe that no feelings are 'wrong' or 'bad' or irrelevant. A feeling is a fact about the person who feels it; it is as important and worthy of interest as more objective facts such as signs and symptoms.

WORDS THAT SHOULD NOT BE USED, FOR EXAMPLE 'COMPLIANCE'

By the mid-1980s, health psychologists were noting a shift away from the term compliance, which connotes patient obedience, to the term adherence, which suggests a more voluntary effort by the individual[1].

The *Random House Unabridged Dictionary* defines compliance as: 1. the act of conforming, acquiescing or yielding; 2. a tendency to yield readily to others, especially, in a weak or subservient way; 3. conformity; accordance; 4. cooperation or obedience, e.g., 'The compliance of all French citizens'. The word compliance is demeaning and, some might argue, sexist when applied to HRT. It is interesting to note that the *Index Medicus* does not use the term; the reader is referred to 'cooperative behavior'. In much recent literature the word adherence has replaced compliance. Adherence is defined by the dictionary as fidelity or steady attachment. It seems to imply more choice and mutuality in the planning and implementing of healthcare. We believe that, when referring to HRT, the most neutral word would be 'continuance'. Continuance is a simple descriptor of behavior, unencumbered by implications.

THE HEALTH BELIEF MODEL AS IT MIGHT APPLY TO DECISIONS ABOUT HRT

Writings on 'compliance' with HRT tend to reflect the clinical experience of the individual practitioner. Bibliographies show familiarity with previous literature about 'compliance' with HRT, but not with the extensive literature from the fields of public health, health education or health psychology which could inform and advance attitudes regarding how people think and act and make choices about their own health.

Since the development of the Health Belief Model by social psychologists in the early 1950s, it has been used extensively to study both preventive health behaviors and sick-role behaviors, both prospectively and retrospectively. There is substantial empirical support for the Health Belief Model, which is a conceptual model, using information about individuals to understand, identify, and predict their potential for changing health-related behaviors. It can determine the likelihood of action or the possibility of behavior change by an individual confronted with a health issue (Figure 1)[2].

Reviews of the literature on the Health Belief Model have found three of its variables to be particularly useful as predictors of behavior. The first of these is 'perceived susceptibility', which is of most use in predicting preventive health behavior. A person's perceived susceptibility is understood by determining the extent to which they believe that they are at risk for a particular condition. The following case illustrates a common misunderstanding about risk which can lead to muddled decision-making about HRT.

A very intelligent and educated 58-year-old woman who had decided not to take HRT told us, 'I don't need it for my health because my mother is 78 and straight and tall, so I don't worry about osteoporosis'. This woman believed that the absence of one important risk factor meant that she is risk-free. Health professionals need to be very clear about what 'risk factor' actually means: it is all too easy to misuse this concept in the service of wishful thinking about one's perceived susceptibility to a disease.

The second variable in the Health Belief Model which has been found to be strongly predictive is 'perceived seriousness'. If a woman is considering HRT to prevent osteoporosis, does she know what this condition can mean? Does she know that it can seriously affect both the quality and length of her life? Does she know, for example, that in the USA last year as many women died of the complications of hip fracture as died of breast cancer?

Of all the factors in the Health Belief Model, 'perceived barriers' has been shown repeatedly to exert the most powerful influence on health behavior. Societal and institutional barriers to the use of HRT include the cost of seeing the doctor, the cost of the medication, and the doctor's negative belief about HRT. A study performed in England in 1990[3] found some surprising perceived barriers. Some women sought no medical attention for menopause because they thought that the doctor was too busy, they did not want to worry the doctor. Some perceived barriers relate to the nature of the treatment. Women may not start HRT because they are hesitant to embark on a very lengthy, possibly life-long, regimen, or they may see possible side-effects as a barrier.

We believe that understanding the Health Belief Model would help doctors and others who counsel women about HRT. It would be interesting to design a study to determine whether or not this is so.

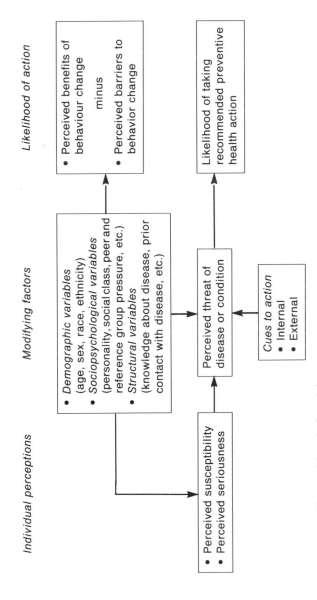

Figure 1 The Health Belief Model

A STRUCTURED APPROACH TO MENOPAUSE HEALTHCARE BASED ON AN UNDERSTANDING OF THE BIOLOGICAL AND PSYCHOLOGICAL ISSUES INVOLVED

A structured approach to menopause healthcare has been developed in the Department of Obstetrics and Gynecology at Yale University School of Medicine during the past decade. An initial series of visits aims to develop an understanding of the patient, evaluating her medically and psychologically, and implementing hormone replacement therapy when indicated. Continuing visits are subsequently timed and structured to support the initial healthcare program.

The initial phase of the program is usually made up of four visits over 12 weeks. The first visit lasts 1 h, the next three visits last for 30 min each. Each visit has specific goals determined to constitute a rational sequence. The over-riding objective of these visits is to establish a working relationship between a woman and her healthcare providers, in which there is mutual respect and trust.

The goals of the first visit are to determine the meanings and significance in the woman's life of the biological changes of the menopause, to be sensitive and responsive to the questions a woman asks, to perform a physical examination and obtain specimens for laboratory studies, and to help a woman start the process of self-awareness and thoughtful decision-making.

At the start of the first visit, each woman completes a self-administered questionnaire, the Menopause Symptom Index (MENSI) (Figure 2). Symptoms are clustered with reference to the different body systems (vascular, nervous, genitourinary) which can be affected by altered hormone production at menopause. The frequency of each symptom during the past month and whether or not it represents a problem to the woman is elicited. The MENSI serves to introduce the patient to the variety of issues that the program is designed to address, and to help her start to think more definitely about her personal experiences of the menopause.

Interaction with the program nurse or physician usually begins with a review of the problem symptoms identified by the woman. In reviewing symptoms with our patients we ask for a fuller description of the personal meaning of that symptom for the woman. For example, sleep disturbance may be having a major effect on the quality of her life. Women who have not had a good night's sleep for months, or even years, describe their problems of chronic fatigue, irritability and anger. Change in memory can be terrifying, triggering fears of major brain disturbance. Chest pressure and pain frequently lead to multiple physician visits, with many evaluative

Clinical MENSI – initial/return visit questionnaire

The questions should be asked, 'In the last month did you experience...?'
Indicate by circling the numbered response for the first part of each question.
Code for the Questions: 0 = No, 1 = Occasionally, 2 = Yes, on a regular basis.
The reply to the second part of the question, 'Is it a real problem for you?' should be indicated by circling Y
for Yes or N for No.

SAMPLE QUESTION:
'In the last month did you experience hot or warm flushes?'   0   1   2
'Was it a real problem for you?'   Y   N

0 = No   1 = Occasionally   2 = Yes, regularly

1. Hot or warm flushes? 0 1 2	11. Anxiety? 0 1 2
Anxiety? Y N	Problem? Y N
2. Palpitations? 0 1 2	12. Depressions? 0 1 2
Problem? Y N	Problem? Y N
3. Headaches? 0 1 2	13. Fear of being alone in public? 0 1 2
Problem? Y N	Problem? Y N
4. Sleep disturbance? 0 1 2	14. Loss of urinary control? 0 1 2
Problem? Y N	Problem? Y N
5. Chest pressure or pain? 0 1 2	15. Vaginal dryness? 0 1 2
Problem? Y N	Problem? Y N
6. Shortness of breath? 0 1 2	16. Loss of sex desire? 0 1 2
Problem? Y N	Problem? Y N
7. Numbness 0 1 2	17. Pain w/intercourse? 0 1 2
Problem? Y N	Problem? Y N
8. Weakness or fatigue? 0 1 2	18. Disrupted function: Home? 0 1 2
Problem? Y N	Problem? Y N
9. Pain in bone joints? 0 1 2	19. Disrupted function: Work? 0 1 2
Problem? Y N	Problem? Y N
10. Memory loss? 0 1 2	20. Other symptoms:
Problem? Y N	

MENSI SCORE (0–38)
NUMBER OF 'YES' ANSWERS

Figure 2   The Menopause Symptom Index (MENSI)

procedures showing no evidence of disease. The fear of having a heart attack remains and the failure of doctors to provide an explanation leads to even deeper anxiety, frustration and anger. Vaginal dryness, dyspareunia and loss of libido can lead to a sense of loss of femininity, marital discord or depression. At the initial visit we feel it appropriate to elicit these feelings and start to indicate their possible connection with hormone deficiency.

As in other counselling, the airing of feelings with an understanding listener is almost always helpful and almost never hurtful. Our patients are asked about the questions that worry them. Most common are questions concerning the risk of taking hormones. We try our best to provide up-to-date information about breast and endometrial cancer. At the same time, we also start to provide an understanding of how hormones work and of the potential benefits which balance potential risks. The medical evaluation includes a complete physical examination and indicated laboratory studies.

In the last part of the first visit we create a diary based on the symptoms the woman has described as most troublesome. The women are asked to evaluate their symptoms on a 0–4 scale each day (from 'none' to 'severe'). Such daily diary entries help to motivate a woman to become self-aware, so that she will subsequently be better able to judge whether taking hormones is truly helpful to her well-being. No medication is prescribed at the first visit.

The second visit begins with the diary review. It is rare for a woman not to return for the follow-up visits and it is unusual for her to fail to maintain the daily diary, which is a measure of motivation. Failure to keep the diary signals the need for a discussion of what has been happening in the woman's life since her last visit, and how she is feeling about her menopause symptoms and the initiation of hormone treatment. When ambivalence about starting hormone treatment is expressed, the discussion focuses on the issues involved.

For about one in five women it is decided at the second visit that hormone treatment is not indicated. Laboratory studies may show adequate estrogen levels and measures of estrogenicity. When that is the case we usually suggest waiting to see whether the situation changes, and recommend a second evaluation in 6–9 months.

If a decision is made to start hormone replacement therapy we prescribe estrogen alone during the first cycle. This allows the woman to adjust to the estrogen. It is important to assess its effects before starting progestin. We inform the woman of side-effects that may occur in the first cycle; an increase in vasomotor symptoms is not unusual, nor is breast tenderness.

We try to reassure her that these effects will be transitory and that her symptoms will probably be markedly reduced by the next visit.

At visit three, 4 weeks later, our goal is to determine the effectiveness of treatment, to assess side-effects, and to evaluate continuing motivation. The diary is reviewed. We wish to be sure that symptoms are being reduced: if this is not the case, consideration is given to increasing the estrogen dose. If the woman feels her needs are being met, and if she has a uterus, we then describe the need for progestin to prevent endometrial hyperplasia and carcinoma. Our routine is to prescribe estrogen to be taken every day with the progestin to be taken in the evening on days 1–12 of each calendar month. Menstruation is to be expected at some time between days 11 and 17, and is regarded as a sign of adequacy of hormone replacement.

At the last visit of the initial phase we want to know about the effects of taking the progestin. Did menstruation occur when expected? Were there any side-effects? Our main concerns are if chest pain or headache was induced by the progestin or if the addition of the hormone caused any psychological reactions such as depression. If there were no or minimal side-effects we then recommend visits every 6 months. Most women voluntarily maintain their diaries. They have learned to recognize signals of when the hormones are working and when they are not, and have established a pattern of administration and body response which they understand and appreciate. It is not surprising that continuance rates for more than 5 years are >80%.

This article has covered an apparent diversity of subjects. The common thread is our desire to stress an approach to menopause care which focuses on helping women to participate actively in their own healthcare, using concepts borrowed from psychotherapy and health psychology as well as a thoughtfully designed structured series of clinical visits. The specific use of the MENSI incorporates a number of these strategies.

Optimal menopause care requires time, sensitivity to women's needs, an absence of patriarchal attitudes or chauvinism, and a willingness to view healthcare decision-making as an ongoing dialogue between a woman and her healthcare provider. The provider should strive to fulfill this requirement.

REFERENCES

1. Rodin, J. and Salovey, P. (1989). Health psychology. *Annu. Rev. Psychol.*, **40**, 533–79
2. Becker, M. H. (ed.) (1974). *The Health Belief Model and Personal Health Behavior*. (Thorofare, NJ: Charles B. Stack)

3. Draper, J. and Roland, M. (1990). Premenopausal women's views on taking hormone replacement therapy to prevent osteoporosis. *Br. Med. J.,* **300**, 786–8

Section 10

Non-hormonal management of the
menopause

54

Non-hormonal management of the menopause

M. Notelovitz

WHY WOMEN CHOOSE NOT TO TAKE HORMONAL THERAPY

The session on the non-hormonal management of the menopause was introduced by Janine O'Leary Cobb who discussed why women choose not to take hormone therapy.

A large proportion of women do not take hormones. Estimates of the incidence of hormone therapy in geographical regions of Italy, France, Germany, Denmark, South Australia, the UK and the USA range from 3% (Italy) to 32% (California). Substantial numbers of women also start hormone therapy and stop within a few months: according to one resource, the average duration of such therapy is only 9 months. In short, the majority of peri- and postmenopausal women do not seek or accept hormone therapy and, of those who do start treatment, up to two-thirds will abandon it within 1 year.

Some women who elect not to take hormonal therapy are less likely to view menopause as a medical condition, or even as an event of importance, although the intensity of symptoms may over-ride this attitude for some women. In one on-going study (personal communication: O'Leary Lobb) of 344 middle class, mostly White women between the age of 35 and 65 (mean age 47) only 17% are current users of hormones. Of those choosing not to take hormones, 85% say they 'don't need to'; 28% 'don't like the idea'; and 6% cited contraindications.

The data relating to the attitude of women are influenced by the source of information. For example, some reasons cited by women who subscribe to a lay journal, *A Friend Indeed*, who elect not to take hormones include: menopause is a natural transition to non-reproductive status; osteoporosis is not a serious threat; unwillingness or inability to tolerate side-effects; hormone supplementation is regarded neither as 'preventive' or as 'safe'; many are frightened of breast cancer; given a choice some women prefer to die of heart disease; prolongation of life is not a high priority; and because experience has taught that strong drugs should be treated with great caution.

Physicians are more likely to see, and to be asked to treat, women who undergo an induced menopause, who face an unexpected and very early menopause, or who have unusually severe vasomotor or psychological symptoms. These women constitute a minority in North American, and an even smaller minority in other societies. Ms. Cobb concluded that if physicians are to attract women to take hormone therapy, they need to understand and appreciate the reasoning of those women who have chosen not to take it.

BEHAVIORAL TREATMENT OF MENOPAUSAL HOT FLASHES

The behavioral treatment of menopausal hot flashes was discussed by Dr Freedman. He noted that menopausal hot flashes consist of substantial peripheral vasodilation and sweating, with reports of internal warmth. Hot flashes accompany the estrogen withdrawal of menopause, but their occurrence is not correlated with plasma or urinary estradiol levels. Further, although LH pulses occur with 70% of hot flashes, hot flashes can occur without LH pulses (isolated gonadotropin deficiency) and LH pulses can occur without hot flashes (hypothalamic amenorrhea).

Since clonidine, a centrally acting α_2-adrenergic agonist which lowers central sympathetic activation, has been shown to ameliorate hot flashes, he hypothesized that menopausal estrogen withdrawal sensitizes a central noradrenergic mechanism. Menopausal women with and without hot flashes were prescreened with ambulatory sternal skin conductance monitoring. Intravenous infusions of clonidine HCl and yohimbine HCl (an α_2-adrenergic antagonist) were given blind to both groups (yohimbine under basal conditions, while clonidine was given during peripheral heating). Yohimbine provoked hot flashes and clonidine ameliorated heat-induced hot flashes in symptomatic women, but there were no effects in asymptomatic women.

MHPG (3-methoxy-4-hydroxyphenylglycol) is the main metabolite of brain norepinephrine. Plasma MHPG levels in menopausal women with and without hot flashes were measured under basal conditions and during peripheral heating. Basal levels of MHPG were significantly higher in symptomatic than the asymptomatic women, and increased significantly further during hot flashes. This supports the hypothesis of elevated noradrenergic activation in women with menopausal hot flashes.

Based on the above work, Freedman hypothesized that reducing central nervous system activation with relaxation therapy would ameliorate hot flashes. A pilot study was performed on 14 women who received either muscle relaxation plus deep breathing or α-electroencephalographic (EEG) biofeedback (control group). Relaxation ameliorated heat-induced hot flashes in the laboratory ($p < 0.01$) and decreased the reported frequency of hot flashes by about 50% ($p < 0.01$). EEG biofeedback had no effect. The relaxation group also decreased their respiration rate during heat challenge ($p < 0.01$), whereas the biofeedback group did not. It was then hypothesized that slow, deep breathing was the active component of the behavioral treatment. Three groups were studied: a paced respiration (PR) group, a progressive muscle relaxation group (PMR) and an α-EEG biofeedback group (control). Hot flashes were objectively defined with ambulatory sternal skin conductance monitoring for 24 h before and after treatment. Respiration rate (RR) and tidal volume (TV) were measured before and after treatment with a Beckman metabolic cart. The PR group showed a significantly reduced hot flash frequency ($p < 0.02$), decreased RR ($p < 0.02$), and increased TV ($p < 0.03$) whereas the other two groups showed no significant effects. These results show that slow, deep breathing can be effective behavioral treatment for menopausal hot flashes.

MANAGEMENT OF MENOPAUSE WHEN ESTROGEN IS CONTRAINDICATED

Clinicians frequently need to treat menopausal women who are unable to take estrogen because of absolute or strong relative contraindications. Ronald Young noted that in the United States breast cancer alone excluded 10% of all women from taking estrogen. Because of this and other diseases, therapies are needed to help menopausal women. The following therapeutic modalities were suggested.

Vaginal dryness/dyspareunia

Polycarbophil is a relatively new moisturizing agent that has distinct advantages over the more traditionally used water-soluble jellies. A lowering of vaginal pH and improved blood flow is achieved with its use.

European data indicate that low doses of estradiol (10–25 μg) applied intravaginally achieve a positive local effect without any significant systemic uptake. Monitoring of serum levels of estradiol is advised.

Hot flashes and other vasomotor symptoms

Naproxen may produce a 50% reduction in hot flashes, but most clinicians conclude that it has little other than placebo effect. Clonidine is an α-adrenergic drug that works both centrally and peripherally. It is best suited to hypertensive patients, as normotensive women may develop severe orthostatic complaints as well as headaches, fatigue and nausea. The dose is 0.1 mg twice daily. Veralipride, a centrally acting antidopaminergic compound, eliminates symptoms in 60–80% of patients. Return of symptoms may occur after 6 months. Side-effects are predictable and include breast tenderness and galactorrhea. Metaclopramide and sulpiride are related compounds with similar effects. The dosage of veralipride is 100 mg/day. Progestational agents are effective in curtailing hot flashes. Physicians, however, face the dilemma of dealing with overlapping warnings and contraindications shared by these agents and estrogens. Medroxyprogesterone acetate (MPA) is the most commonly used progestin in the United States and is employed both orally and parenterally in standard doses. Beta blockers such as Sotalol are most effective in treating hot flashes, but are less effective for insomnia and anxiety. Although good control studies are still lacking, methyldopa (250–500 mg/day) is effective in many women. Naloxone is an opiate receptor agonist with mixed results in the treatment of hot flashes. The need for high doses and parenteral administration limits its practical use. OD 14 (Liviol) has mixed estrogenic, androgenic and progestational properties. It effectively reduces hot flashes while lowering luteinizing hormone and follicle stimulating hormone levels. The standard dose is 2.5 mg/day.

OSTEOPOROSIS

Various studies have indicated that sufficient calcium or calcium plus vitamin D intake may provide adequate protection; others maintain that the best a positive calcium balance can accomplish is to lower the daily requirements of estrogen. All of these measures appear to have their maximum impact if begun prior to the onset of the menopause. To these one must add avoidance of tobacco and alcohol, attention to dosages of prescription medications, particularly thyroid drugs, steroids and heparin, and measures to prevent fracture-causing trauma in the elderly. Progestins may actually promote new bone formation, perhaps through androgenic/ anabolic properties; there is also concern about potential untoward effects on lipids and lipoproteins. Doses include 5–20 mg of oral MPA daily and 100–200 mg of MPA every 2–3 months. Some investigators have suggested that sodium fluoride, while protecting against early fractures in trabecular bone, may be associated with later increases in cortical bone fracture. High doses in a micronized pill have been reported to be effective, but the initial success of this regimen could not be duplicated. Tamoxifen is widely used in breast cancer therapy; studies in both animals and human subjects have demonstrated its efficacy in the prevention of bone loss. Calcitonin is available as a subcutaneous injection and intranasally (in Europe). Initially it was thought that resistance to therapy developed after 1 year, but prolonged use is now common. Many reports have tested the efficacy of this agent. Side-effects include nausea, facial flushing, and anorexia. The standard dose is 20–100 IU subcutaneously three times weekly, or daily. Other drugs being evaluated include OD 14, androgens and ergocalciferol.

Originally, sodium etidronate was used in so-called coherence therapy regimens, but it is now employed as an episodic medication on its own. The recommended dose is 400 mg/day orally for 2 weeks followed by a 6-week pause. The regimen is repeated cyclically.

Lipids and lipoproteins

There is no real substitute for the reputed beneficial effects of estrogen replacement in reducing lipids. Dietary manipulation and cholesterol lowering drugs are alternatives.

Dr Young concluded by noting that, as an alternative to not prescribing estrogen therapy, the proscription against estrogen needs to be discussed with the patient. Most patients with a prior history of diabetes, hypertension, thromboembolic episodes, myocardial infarction, stroke, leiomyomata and endometriosis, among many other disorders, are no longer felt to be non-candidates for estrogen replacement. Former uterine cancer patients take estrogen and increasing numbers of breast cancer patients are now taking estrogens.

ROLE OF KAMPO (HERBAL) MEDICINE FOR THE MANAGEMENT OF POSTMENOPAUSAL WOMEN IN JAPAN

There is a great deal of interest in the use of traditional or home remedies, for the management of menopause-related problems. Takao Koyama

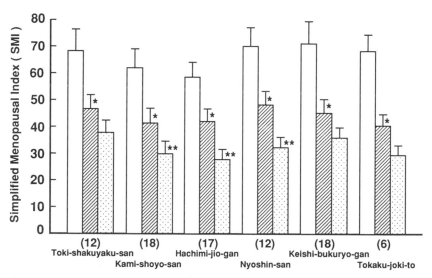

Figure 1 Symptoms during the climacteric period before (☐) and after 4 weeks (▨) and 8 weeks (⬚) of treatment with Kampo preparations. Numbers in parentheses are the number of patients. $^*p < 0.05$ (vs. before treatment); $^{**}p < 0.05$ (vs. at 4 weeks of treatment)

summarized his experience with Kampo (Chinese herbal) medicine amongst Japanese women. A simplified menopausal index was first developed as a guide for the use of Kampo medicine. Six varieties were prescribed on the basis of the simple menopause index questionnaire: Toki-shakuyaku-san, Kami-shoyo-san, Hachimi-jio-gan, Nyoshin-san, Keishi-bukuryo-gan and Tokaku-joki-to. Climacteric disorders improved significantly in all cases treated with these preparations (Figure 1). The various Kampo medicines can be selectively targeted according to the primary cluster of symptoms. For example, Toki-shakuyaku-san or Kami-shoyo-san was prescribed for paler, thin and feeble patients with 'negative signs', while Keishi-bukuryo-gan was used for rather healthy-looking, sturdy patients with 'positive signs'. Decreases in scores on the simple menopausal index correlated with a decrease in clinical complaints such as irritability, shoulder stiffness, hot flashes and insomnia. Kampo medicine is thought by the author to be suitable for the early treatment or prophylaxis of disorders associated with the menopause, and also for diseases of old age and senility. Further research is being undertaken.

EXERCISE AND HOT FLASHES

If impairment of central opioid activity is one factor in provoking hot flashes, mechanisms that increase central opioid activity might diminish the frequency of hot flashes. Regular physical activity is known to effect an increase in central opioid activity and might, according to Hammer and co-workers, decrease the incidence of hot flashes.

All women aged 52–54 years of age ($n = 1246$), living in the community of Linköping, were sent a questionnaire concerning items such as age at menopause, use of hormonal treatment and surgery. They were also asked to grade hot flashes subjectively from none to severe, according to the extent to which they influenced daily activities and sleep at night. The same questions were sent to 142 women between 50 and 58 years of age, who were registered as active members of a local gymnastic club. In addition, they were asked questions about how many hours per week they took part in physical exercise.

The relative number of women suffering from moderate or severe hot flashes was significantly lower amongst those postmenopausal women who were physically active compared to the non-selected group ($p < 0.01$) (Figure 2). When the women were divided into groups by years since menopause, the difference was still obvious amongst women 1 year after menopause ($p < 0.01$). Very few of the physically active women suffered from severe hot flashes; only one (6%) regarded her symptoms as severe. Among the unselected women, 25% regarded their symptoms as severe and 75% as moderate.

The number of hours per week exercised varied among the women in the gymnastic club between 1 and 10, with an average of 3/week. Those physically active women who did not experience any hot flashes spent slightly longer each week undergoing physical activity than did the women within the same group who suffered from moderate to severe hot flashes ($p < 0.05$).

The lower prevalence of hot flashes amongst physically active women may be due to selection of healthy, positive women with no somatic or psychosomatic problems. Since the fees for taking part in fitness class were very low, however, there was probably no socioeconomic bias between the selected and non-selected groups. One of the mechanisms that could be responsible for improvement could be increases in central opioid activity, which may thus approach the levels that exist before menopause or during estrogen replacement therapy. Physical exercise is also helpful for general well-being, reducing muscle tension, insomnia and anxiety.

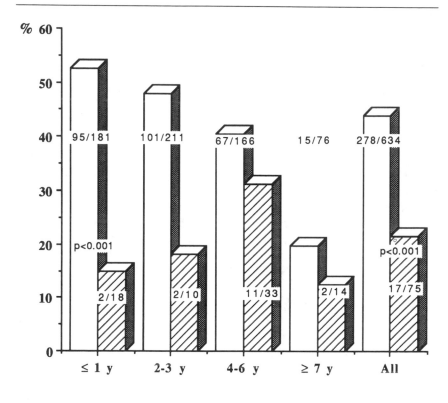

years after menopause

Figure 2 Moderate to severe vegetative symptoms among non-selected 52- and 54-year-old women (□) and physically active postmenopausal women (▨) in Linköping, Sweden

EXERCISE AND ITS EFFECT ON CARDIOVASCULAR HEALTH AND OSTEOPOROSIS

The issue of physical fitness and its role in the health of postmenopausal women was reviewed by Dr Notelovitz, drawing largely from the experience and research at the Center for Climacteric Studies (University of Florida) and more recently from the research division of the Women's Medical and Diagnostic Center in Gainesville, Florida.

Numerous studies have confirmed a progressive decline in the physical fitness in women (as measured by VO_{2max}) with time, a factor that has been attributed both to the natural process of age-related deterioration and a decrease in activity. This change is not related to the menopause *per se*. A comparison of age-matched women (46–55 years), some of whom were menstruating and remained menopausal, revealed no difference in the mean oxygen uptake studies – 27.4 ± 6.3 ml/kg/min vs. 26.3 ± 4.7 ml/kg/min, respectively.

Exercise stress testing is the only appropriate method of evaluating the physical fitness level of women. The method commonly used was originally designed for young men. Based on the evaluation of 163 healthy climacteric women, aged 35–75 years, a modified Balke method (using direct calorimetry) was developed that allowed appropriate physical fitness testing with a very low incidence of false positive electrocardiographic tracings. In order to make this method more practical for everyday clinical use, a subsequent study developed a predictive maximal oxygen uptake test, utilizing the same protocol but substituting the formula $10.4 + 1.29$(exercise time) for the direct measurement of oxygen uptake, thus removing the need for a metabolic cart. The test was validated both for untrained women and after 6 and 12 months of aerobic exercise training.

Recent studies have confirmed that as physical fitness of women improves, so the risk for all cause mortality, especially death from cardiovascular disease and cancer, decreases. The maintenance of compliance thus becomes a major issue. The preliminary results of a 2-year study comparing the physical fitness profile (VO_{2max} and total exercise time) in four groups of women (control; variable resistance muscle exercise; bicycle ergometer and treadmill walking) were presented. Significant improvement in physical fitness was achieved within 6 months in both aerobically trained groups, and maintained for the entire duration of the study. VO_{2max} was unaffected in the muscle strengthening group but the total exercise time did improve over time – not to the same extent as the aerobic exercises, however. Despite the improvement in VO_{2max}, there was no alteration in the lipid profile as measured by total plasma cholesterol, triglycerides, high density lipoprotein (HDL) cholesterol and low density lipoprotein (LDL) cholesterol. The values were no different at 2 years when compared with the baseline means.

Other studies have shown that intensity of aerobic exercise influences the HDL cholesterol level in women. The duration of exercise may also be important. Subsequent studies, with maintenance of the intensity of exercise (70–80% of maximum heart rate) but increase in the duration of exercise (from 20 to 30 min/session), resulted in measurable and significant decreases in total cholesterol and improvement in the HDL/LDL ratio. The changes observed were equivalent to those noted in a simultaneous studied group of women taking 0.625 mg of conjugated equine estrogens. The measured alteration in lipids is too small to account

55

Why women choose not to take hormone therapy

J. O'Leary Cobb

It has been recognized for some years that a large proportion of women in midlife choose not to take hormones. Estimates of use of hormone therapy in various geographical regions range from 3% (Italy) to 32% (California)[1-4], but the reasons for this variation are largely conjectural.

In addition, substantial numbers of women start on hormone therapy (HRT) and stop within a few months[5-7]. The medical director of Wyeth-Ayerst has admitted that the average duration of such therapy is 9 months[8]. The problem of compliance has received some consideration in the literature[9-14], giving us some idea about why women choose to discontinue HRT, but this falls short of dealing with women who refuse HRT at all. The majority of women currently in perimenopause and postmenopause therefore choose not to seek or to accept HRT. Of those who do start HRT, as many as two-thirds abandon it within a year.

There has been remarkably little interest in this phenomenon. There is some evidence that women who choose not to take hormone therapy are less likely to view menopause as a medical condition, or even as an event of importance[15-18], although the intensity of current symptoms may apparently occasionally over-ride this decision[19].

One or two studies, using small numbers of women, have looked at women's attitudes towards hormone therapy[20,21], and there may be more in progress, but the bulk of the information we have is anecdotal. I have some 7000 letters sent to my publication, *A Friend Indeed*, a newsletter for women in midlife or menopause, by women in Canada, the USA, and eight other countries. The letters are not, of course, representative of all

menopausal women. Not all women write letters. An estimated 10–15% of women have no problem with the menopause; for them, it is a non-event; another 5–10% have chosen hormone therapy and are happy with their choice. Nor do I hear from women who cannot afford HRT, even if it is prescribed. These women have been overlooked, and continue to be overlooked, by health care systems in many countries, including my own. I have no way of estimating their numbers.

The letters we have on file are from women who are thinking about asking for HRT, or who have been prescribed hormones, but who have reservations, usually to do with something they have read or heard about in the media. Reservations are less often due to side-effects that they themselves have experienced, or to tales told them by other women.

I would argue that the reluctance to use HRT is nearly always based on knowledge, not ignorance. It may be inadequate or accurate information, but it is rarely discussed with the physician, who has no time; and frankly, few physicians are receptive to their patients' opinions.

I have heard from a handful of women who refuse HRT simply because they do not want to put 'chemicals into their bodies', ignoring the fact that everything they ingest consists of chemicals. My experience is that this kind of irrational thinking is rare.

Why do so many women choose not to take hormones? When I was testifying in Washington 2 years ago, a gynecologist on the panel told the Congressional Subcommittee that non-compliance was to be expected because daily administration of any medication is difficult. I would submit that it is not that simple. Remember, these are the same women who took oral contraceptives for months, years, sometimes even decades. The taking of a daily pill is not the obstacle.

Based on my mail, I can outline nine reasons why women choose not to take hormones.

1. They view menopause as a natural transition, one that may impose temporary aggravations such as hot flushes or mood swings, but one which they are willing to tolerate. Many women go to a doctor simply for confirmation that menopause is the cause of their complaints; they want nothing more than reassurance.

2. Osteoporosis is not perceived as a personal threat. Ten years ago, very few women knew about the dangers of osteoporosis and even fewer recognized that estrogen halted loss of bone. Thanks to convincing campaigns mounted by drug companies and the dairy industry, most women are now aware of the relationships between calcium, estrogen and bone mass. Many women are familiar with their own risks of

osteoporosis either because of a family history or because of counseling received in conjunction with gynecological surgery. HRT certainly has a place for women at risk, but many women feel that estrogen therapy is being promoted like a vaccination. If they are not likely to be at risk, they are not interested. They know that the projections commonly used are based on an older generation whose habits of living may have been quite different[22]. They may also recognize that the estimated incidence of osteoporosis (which varies, according to the source, from 1 in 4 to 1 in 2) includes a range of effects, some serious, some less so, and that predictions about individual vulnerability are still remarkably unreliable. Many are also aware that newer medications, that actually build bone, are likely to be on the market within a decade or two.

3. Women who experience side-effects, or who see side-effects experienced by their friends, are less likely to persist with hormones. This would seem self-evident but there is a strong tendency to discount the intensity or importance of side-effects. I am not talking just about monthly bleeds, which are becoming more avoidable, or breast tenderness, or headaches, or weight gain. Side-effects also include subtle changes that are difficult for a woman to verbalize, that make her feel like a stranger to her own body. I get many letters about doctors who say, 'None of my other patients has ever complained of that' while the patient facing him is thinking, 'No, they just stop taking it and never come back'. Physicians who are unwilling to experiment with different products, dosages or regimens, who trivialize or dismiss complaints about side-effects, increase the number of women not taking HRT.

4. To convince women of the benefits of HRT, many physicians (taking their cue from pharmaceutical advertising) refer to it as 'preventive'. Many women have difficulty with this concept. Preventive strategies for general good health are a healthy diet, a modicum of personal hygiene and regular physical exercise. Prevention of osteoporosis means building healthy bone. Prevention of heart disease requires aerobic exercise, and a low-fat, high-fiber diet. Hormone supplementation is not viewed as preventive, it is viewed as treatment. This may seem to be merely semantics but it is responsible for a lot of passive resistance to hormone therapy.

5. Women often object to the insistence that estrogen is 'safe'. 'What you need,' says the doctor, 'is hormone therapy. I'll be glad to give you a

prescription. But first let's check your blood pressure, cholesterol and lipid levels, and then we'll do a quick review of your family and medical history. I'd like to know about any tendencies to blood clots, fibroids or gallstones. I'll order you a mammogram and, once that's over with, you've got your prescription'. If it's so safe, why this battery of tests?

6. Women are frightened of breast cancer and there is considerable evidence that estrogen therapy adds to existing risk[23]. This is particularly relevant as women age. Mammograms, while reassuring, merely reveal tumors that have already been in existence for some years. In the opinion of many women, mammograms and breast examinations cannot provide adequate safeguards against the increased risks which result from extended use of hormone therapy.

7. Breast cancer, women are told, is insignificant compared to the potential for postmenopausal heart disease[24]. What about the facts that (a) heart disease is on the decrease while breast cancer is on the rise, and (b) breast cancer strikes younger women than does heart disease? Will hormone therapy permit us to live long enough to develop breast cancer? This has happened to the mothers of a few of my subscribers. Based on the women that they know, and the pain they have witnessed, many women choose heart disease over breast cancer.

8. At the present time, estrogen therapy is being promoted as a way of prolonging life. This is disputed in a couple of recent meta-analyses, one of which tells us that the average woman of 50, with pre-existing heart disease, might extend her life an average of 11 months if she took estrogen therapy for 30 years[25]. The real point – and I cannot say this forcefully enough – is that most women do not consider the extension of life a priority. We all have to die sometime and perhaps 30–40% of death certificates indicate that some form of cardiovascular disease is responsible. But autopsy is not routine, and we cannot know how accurate each death certificate is. For many women, dying of heart disease is infinitely preferable to a car accident or to breast cancer. It is not the quantity of life that concerns them; it is the quality of life left to live.

9. Since 1945, we have witnessed the introduction of myriad 'miracle drugs' which have immediate and positive benefits, but which usually entail unexpected adverse effects, short- or longterm, including increasing tolerance or dependency. The very potency of estrogen suggests caution. We know, based on experience, that anything that can make a person feel so well so quickly must have a catch. We know

that menopausal complaints are not universal, that in many cultures menopause simply marks a quiet transition to non-reproductive status (as it does, indeed, for 10% of women in Western society).

Many women regard it as common sense to look first to gentler remedies – healthier foods, more exercise, perhaps herbal teas or vitamin and mineral supplements. This is not to say that herbs or vitamin supplements are innocuous, but they do offer the option of personally controlling the amounts used, of charting gradual improvements, and thus of managing one's own menopause. The side-effects of this kind of regimen are likely to be increased self-knowledge and increased self-confidence.

It is a woman's sense of loss of control that is often the most difficult aspect of menopause. If physicians would support and encourage the woman's efforts to deal with her own menopausal complaints, and be ready with an offer of hormones if all else fails, perhaps women would not be flocking in such numbers, behind their doctors' backs, to complementary health care providers[26].

Since I started *A Friend Indeed* in 1984, I have read and heard the laments of many British and European gynecologists about the low rates of hormone use in their own countries as compared to the United States. But North American women have at least twice and often three times the rate of hysterectomy, compared to Japan, the UK, Germany, Sweden and almost every other European country[27,28], despite equivalent rates of mortality and morbidity. Women who have undergone hysterectomy and/or oophorectomy are five times more likely to be prescribed estrogen therapy and twice as likely to continue taking it[7,29].

If doctors want to convince women about the benefits of estrogen therapy, all they have to do is increase the rate of unnecessary gynecological surgery. High rates of surgery ensure a continuing roster of candidates for HRT. I have yet to see this phenomenon on the agenda at meetings like this.

Women like me – health activists without medical training – are often considered to be irrationally 'anti-hormone'. I do not think this is fair. I receive many, many letters from women who have been hysterectomized, who are contending with unexpected and very early menopause, who seem to be at high risk for osteoporosis, or who are suffering intolerable hot flashes and night sweats. I answer every letter and I urge each of them to see a doctor and, with his or her counsel, to seriously consider taking hormones. For those with severe vasomotor or psychological symptoms, I suggest that HRT might put them back on their feet so that they can make rational choices to implement other health-giving activities.

Those experiencing menopause as a result of surgery or chemotherapy, those under 40, and those few in great distress constitute the women that doctors see most often. For these women, HRT may be truly a panacea. But these women are not all women.

The majority of women are able to tolerate the flashes (or flushes), the sleeplessness, the irritability. They don't have a family history of heart disease or osteoporosis. The jolt of menopause is a jolt of reality, motivating them to rethink what they want out of life and how they want to spend their old age. In choosing not to take HRT, many women are affirming their right to the full experience of menopause – the ups, the downs, and the self-knowledge that comes to be viewed as a blessing.

Is it possible that mother nature, in her wisdom, has allowed our estrogen levels to diminish so that we would be less vulnerable to the hyperplastic changes that multiply with age? I would like to think so.

REFERENCES

1. Harris, R. B., Laws, A., Reddy, V. M., King, A. and Haskell, W. D. (1990). Are women using postmenopausal estrogens? A community survey. *Am. J. Publ. Health,* **80**, 1266–8
2. MacLennan, A. H., MacLennan, A. and Wilson, D. (1993). The prevalence of oestrogen replacement therapy in South Australia. *Maturitas,* **16**, 175–83
3. Oddens, B. J., Boulet, M. J., Lehert, P. and Visser, A. P. (1992). Has the climacteric been medicalized? A study on the use of medication for climacteric complaints in four countries. *Maturitas,* **15**, 171–81
4. Køster, A. (1990). Hormone replacement therapy: use patterns in 51-year-old Danish women. *Maturitas,* **13**, 345–56
5. Kaufert, P. L. (1986). The menopausal transition: the use of estrogen. *Can. J. Publ. Health,* **77** (Suppl. 1), 86–91
6. McKinlay, J. B., McKinlay, S. M. and Brambilla, D. J. (1987). Health status and utilization behavior associated with menopause. *Am. J. Epidemiol.,* **125**, 110–21
7. Hemminki, E., Brambilla, D. J., McKinlay, S. M. and Posner, J. P. (1991). Use of estrogens among middle-aged Massachusetts women. *Drug Intelligence and Clinical Pharmacy,* **25**, 418–23
8. Sheehy, G. (1992). *The Silent Passage: Menopause,* p. 20. (New York: Random House)
9. Nachtigall, L. E. (1990). Enhancing patient compliance with hormone replacement therapy at menopause. *Obstet. Gynecol.,* **75**, 77S–80S
10. Ryan, P. J., Harrison, R., Blake, G. M. and Fogelman, I. (1991). Compliance with hormone replacement therapy (HRT) after screening for postmenopausal osteoporosis. *Br. J. Obstet.,* **99**, 325–8
11. Hahn, R. G. (1989). Compliance considerations with estrogen replacement: withdrawal bleeding and other factors. *Am. J. Obstet. Gynecol.,* **161**, 1854–8

12. Hahn, R. G., Nachtigall, R. D. and Davies, T. C. (1984). Compliance difficulties with progestin-supplemented estrogen replacement therapy. *J. Fam. Practice,* **18**, 411–14

13. Ravnikar, V. A. (1987). Compliance with hormone therapy. *Am. J. Obstet. Gynecol.,* **156**, 1332–4

14. Wulf, U. Promoting compliance with HRT: a roundtable discussion. *Menopause Management,* **11**, 10–13, **16**, 35–37

15. Cowan, G., Warren, L. and Young, J. (1985). Medical perceptions of menopausal symptoms. *Psychol. Women Q.,* **9**, 3–14

16. Delorey, C. (1989). Women at midlife: women's perceptions, physicians' perceptions. *J. Women Aging,* **1**, 57–69

17. Ferguson, K. J., Hoegh, C. and Johnson, S. (1989). Estrogen replacement therapy: a survey of women's knowledge and attitudes. *Arch. Intern. Med.,* **149**, 133–6

18. Leiblum, S. R. and Swartzman, L. C. (1986). Women's attitudes toward the menopause: an update. *Maturitas,* **8**, 47–56

19. Schmitt, N., Gogate, J., Rothert, M., Rovner, D., Holmes, M., Talarcyzk, G., Given, B. and Kroll, J. (1991). Capturing and clustering women's judgment policies: the case of hormonal therapy for menopause. *J. Gerontol.,* **46**, 92–101

20. Mansfield, P. K. and Voda, A. M. (1992). Factors influencing midlife women's decisions regarding hormone therapy. Poster presentation, *North American Menopause Society Meetings,* Cleveland, Ohio, September 1992

21. Mansfield, P. K., Voda, A. M. and Seery, B. (1993). To take or not to take: midlife women's decisions about HRT. Presented at the *Meeting of the Society for Menstrual Cycle Research,* Boston, June 11, 1993

22. Hanssen, M. A., Hassager, C., Jensen, S. B. and Christiansen, C. (1992). Is heritability a risk factor for postmenopausal osteoporosis? *J. Bone Min. Res.,* **7**, 1037–43

23. Steinberg, K. K., Thacker, S. B., Smith, S. J., Stroup, D. F., Zack, M. M., Flanders, W. D. and Berkelman, R. L. (1991). A meta-analysis of the effect of estrogen replacement therapy on the risk of breast cancer. *J. Am. Med. Assoc.,* **265**, 1985–90

24. Stampfer, M. J., Colditz, G. A., Willet, W. C., Mansan, J. E., Rosner, B., Speizer, F. E. and Hennekens, C. H. (1991). Postmenopausal estrogen therapy and cardiovascular disease. *N. Engl. J. Med.,* **325**, 756–62

25. Grady, D., Rubin, S. M., Petitti, D. B., Fox, C. S. and Black,D. (1992). Hormone therapy to prevent disease and prolong life in postmenopausal women. *Ann. Intern. Med.,* **117**, 1016–37

26. Eisenberg, D., Kessler, R. C., Foster, C., Norlock, F. E., Calkins, D. R. and Delbanco, T. L. (1993). Unconventional medicine in the United States: prevalence, costs and patterns of use. *N. Engl. J. Med.,* **328**, 246–52

27. McPherson, K., Strong, B., Epstein, A. and Jones, L. (1981). Regional variations in the use of common surgical procedures: within and between England and Wales, Canada and the U.S.A. *Soc. Sci. Med.,* **15A**, 273–8

28. Coulter, A., McPherson, K. and Vessey, M. (1988). Do British women undergo too many or too few hysterectomies? *Soc. Sci. Med.,* **27**, 987–94

29. Cauley, J. A., Cummings, S. R., Black, D. M., Mascioli, S. R. and Seeley, D. G.

(1990). Prevalence and determinants of estrogen replacement therapy in elderly women. *Am. J. Obstet. Gynecol.*, **165**, 1438–40

30. Hemminki, E., Brambilla, D. J., McKinlay, S. M. and Posner, J. G. (1991). Use of estrogens among middle-aged Massachusetts women. *DICP*, **25**, 18–23

56

Mechanisms and behavioral treatment of menopausal hot flushes

R. R. Freedman

ETIOLOGY OF MENOPAUSAL HOT FLUSHES

Menopausal hot flushes consist of substantial peripheral vasodilation and sweating, with reports of internal warmth[1]. Although hot flushes accompany the estrogen withdrawal of menopause, their occurrence is not correlated with plasma or urinary estradiol levels[2]. Luteinizing hormone (LH) pulses occur with 70% of hot flushes but hot flushes can occur without LH pulses (as in isolated gonadotropin deficiency) and LH pulses can occur without hot flushes (as in hypothalamic amenorrhea)[3].

Increased norepinephrine turnover in the hypothalamus is one mechanism thought to be responsible for the activation of central thermoregulatory mechanisms and may trigger the peripheral events of the hot flush that are characteristic of a heat dissipation response[4]. Clonidine, an α_2-adrenergic agonist, acts centrally to reduce norepinephrine turnover[5] and has been shown to ameliorate hot flushes in some clinical studies[6-8]. Conversely, yohimbine, an α_2-adrenergic antagonist which acts in the central nervous system to increase norepinephrine turnover, elevates central sympathetic activation[9]. We used clonidine and yohimbine as complementary pharmacologic probes to determine the involvement of a central α_2-adrenergic mechanism in the initiation of menopausal hot flushes[10].

α_2-Adrenergic mechanism in menopausal hot flushes

Hot flushes were objectively defined using skin conductance levels recorded from the sternum. A computer was programmed to detect any sternal skin conductance increase of at least 2μmho in 30 s. We had previously shown that the agreement between this criterion and patients' self-reports was 95% for spontaneous hot flushes recorded in the laboratory, 86% for those recorded during ambulatory monitoring, and 89% for those provoked by peripheral heating. Additionally, this response did not occur in premenopausal women recorded in the same conditions[11].

Nine postmenopausal women, aged 43–63 years, served as subjects. They were prescreened with ambulatory monitoring of sternal skin conductance levels (SCL) to have at least five hot flushes in a 24-h period. Six asymptomatic women, aged 46–61 years, served as a comparison group. They were prescreened by ambulatory monitoring to have no hot flushes in a 24-h period. All women were in good health and had been amenorrheic for $\geqslant 2$ years.

In two blind laboratory sessions, subjects received either intravenous clonidine HCl 1μg/kg or placebo followed by a 60-min waiting period and then by 45 min of peripheral heating. In two additional blind sessions, subjects received yohimbine HCl (0.032–0.128μg/kg intravenously) or placebo. Clonidine significantly ($p = 0.01$) increased the length of heating time needed to provoke a hot flush compared to placebo (40.6 ± 3.0 min vs. 33.6 ± 3.6) and reduced the number of hot flushes that did occur (2 vs. 8) (Figure 1). In the symptomatic women, six hot flushes occurred during the yohimbine sessions and none during the corresponding placebo sessions, a statistically significant difference ($p < 0.015$). No hot flushes occurred in the asymptomatic women during either session (Figure 2).

These data support the hypothesis that α_2-adrenergic receptors within the central noradrenergic system are involved in the initiation of hot flushes and suggest that brain norepinephrine may be elevated in this process. Animal studies have shown that yohimbine increases norepinephrine release by blocking inhibitory presynaptic α_2-adrenergic receptors[9,12]. These autoreceptors mediate the turnover of norepinephrine through a feedback mechanism, and a reduction in their number and/or sensitivity would result in increased norepinephrine release[12].

This mechanism is consistent with human studies showing that yohimbine elevates and clonidine reduces plasma levels of 3-methoxy,4-hydroxyphenylglycol (MHPG), the main metabolite of brain norepinephrine[13–15]. Therefore, the yohimbine provocation, and clonidine inhibition of hot flushes, in symptomatic women may reflect a deficit in inhibitory α_2-adrenergic receptors not seen in asymptomatic women.

Additionally, the injection of clonidine into the hypothalamus reduces body temperature and activates heat conservation mechanisms, effects that are blocked by yohimbine[16]. Thus, α_2-adrenoceptors in the hypothal-

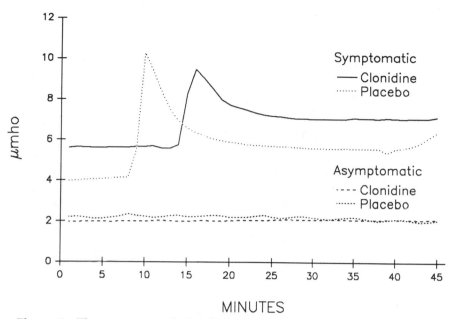

Figure 1 The occurrence of a hot flush during body heating was delayed after 1 μg/kg clonidine, compared with placebo. No hot flushes occurred in an asymptomatic woman. The heating pads were applied at time 0; clonidine or placebo was injected 60 min before this (1 μmho = 10^6 ohm)

amus may be responsible for the events of the hot flush that are characteristic of a heat dissipation response.

There is considerable evidence demonstrating that estrogens modulate adrenergic receptors in many tissues. It is possible, therefore, that hypothalamic α_2-adrenergic receptors are affected by the estrogen withdrawal associated with the menopause[17]. As noted above, a decline in inhibitory presynaptic α_2 receptors would lead to increased central norepinephrine levels and this is consistent with evidence from animal studies.

Central sympathetic activation in menopausal hot flushes

Previous studies have shown that plasma levels of MHPG, the major metabolite of brain norepinephrine[14], are reduced by clonidine and increased by yohimbine[13,15]. In the present study, we therefore measured plasma MHPG levels during spontaneous hot flushes and during those induced by peripheral heating.

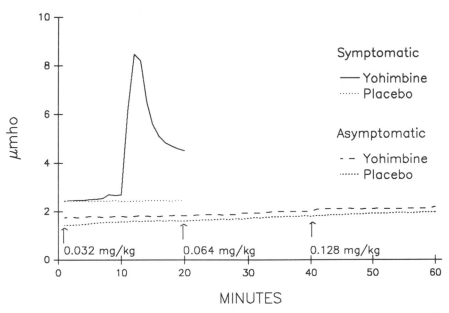

Figure 2 A hot flush, indicated by a sternal skin conductance response, occurred after intravenous infusion of 0.032 mg/kg yohimbine in a menopausal woman with hot flushes. No such responses occurred in the matched placebo session or in an asymptomatic woman given higher doses (1 μmho = 10^6 ohm)

Thirteen symptomatic and six asymptomatic postmenopausal women were prescreened with ambulatory sternal skin conductance monitoring using the methods described above. They were supine in a room at 23°C, and an intravenous line was placed to enable 10 ml blood samples to be drawn at the beginning and end of a 60-min period and at the point of any SCL-defined hot flush that occurred. Patients were then heated for 45 min, as in the prior study. Blood samples were again taken at the beginning and end of this period and during SCL-defined hot flushes. Blood samples were drawn from the asymptomatic women at time points comparable to those of the symptomatic women. Samples were centrifuged and stored at −70°C and MHPG levels were subsequently determined by gas chromatography/mass spectrometry.

In the symptomatic women, six hot flushes occurred in the resting period and seven during the heating period. No hot flushes occurred in the asymptomatic women during either period. MHPG levels were significantly higher in symptomatic than in asymptomatic women at all

Table 1 Plasma MHPG (ng/ml) during resting and heating periods in symptomatic and asymptomatic women

Symptomatic women		Asymptomatic women	
Resting		*Resting*	
Basal	3.5 ± 0.2	Basal	2.6 ± 0.1
Hot flush	4.3 ± 0.2	Hot flush	2.7 ± 0.2
Recovery	3.8 ± 0.2	Recovery	2.5 ± 0.2
Heating		*Heating*	
Basal	3.4 ± 0.2	Basal	2.3 ± 0.2
Hot flush	3.9 ± 0.3	Hot flush	2.1 ± 0.1
Recovery	3.4 ± 0.2	Recovery	2.2 ± 0.2

time points ($p < 0.0001$, Table 1). In the symptomatic women MHPG levels increased significantly ($p < 0.001$) during resting and heat-induced hot flushes. There were no significant MHPG changes in the asymptomatic women.

These data demonstrate that resting levels of plasma MHPG are significantly higher in symptomatic than in asymptomatic menopausal women, consistent with the hypothesis that basal levels of central sympathetic activation are higher in the former than in the latter group. These findings also show that MHPG levels increase significantly during spontaneous and heat-induced hot flushes. However, the temporal resolution of our experimental methods does not permit conclusions to be drawn regarding the causal relationship, if any, between MHPG levels and hot flushes. The data are consistent with the notion that α_2-adrenoceptor responsiveness is altered in women with menopausal hot flushes.

BEHAVIORAL TREATMENT OF MENOPAUSAL HOT FLUSHES

Although hormone replacement therapy is an effective treatment for hot flushes, it may be contraindicated for some women who have an increased risk of cancer. We have presented evidence that central sympathetic activation is increased in women with hot flushes. Behavioral relaxation methods have been shown to reduce sympathetic activity in normal subjects[18] and in some clinical populations[19].

In a pilot investigation we treated seven menopausal women with hot flushes using a combination of progressive muscle relaxation exercises and slow deep breathing[20]. Seven additional women were assigned to receive a control procedure, α_2-electroencephalographic biofeedback. The latter procedure was chosen because it elicits subjective reports of relaxation without its physiological effects[21]. Hot flushes were assessed by physiological responses to peripheral heating and by diaries. Subjects were randomly assigned to receive six, once-weekly 1-h sessions of training in either the experimental or the control procedure.

The latency to hot flush onset during peripheral heating was used as the objective physiologic outcome measure. Prior to treatment there was no significant difference between the two groups in their latency of hot flush onset during heating. Following treatment, the latency to hot flush onset was significantly prolonged in the experimental group ($p < 0.01$) but remained unchanged in the control group. Prior to treatment the reported daily hot flush frequency was not different in the experimental (6.6 ± 4.6 SD) and control (5.9 ± 2.7) groups. At the end of treatment, hot flush frequency was significantly ($p < 0.01$) reduced in the experimental subjects (3.0 ± 2.4), but not in the controls (7.0 ± 1.9). At 6-month follow-up, the improvement in reported daily symptom frequency was maintained in the experimental subjects, whereas the controls remained unchanged.

Physiological recordings of skin conductance level, heart rate, peripheral temperature and respiration rate were performed during the treatment sessions. Analyses of these data showed that respiration rate was significantly slowed in the experimental subjects, but not in the controls. There were no significant effects for any other physiological measure.

This investigation demonstrates that a combination of muscle relaxation exercises and slow deep breathing significantly reduced hot flush frequency in a small group of subjects. However, since two treatment procedures were combined, it was not possible to determine which component was responsible for the therapeutic effect. The physiological data showed that respiration rate was the only recorded variable which was significantly altered during training. Therefore, a second study was performed in which one group of subjects received slow deep breathing alone, another group received muscle relaxation exercises alone, and a third group received α-wave electroencephalographic biofeedback[22].

Thirty-three postmenopausal women were recruited from newspaper advertisements requesting women for participation in a research study of behavioral treatments for hot flushes. All women reported having at least five hot flushes per day and had been amenorrheic for at least 1 year. None had received estrogen during the year prior to study. The women were randomly assigned in equal numbers to receive one of the three behavioral treatment procedures. These were conducted during eight, 1-h biweekly treatment sessions.

Patients who received paced respiration training had abdominal and thoracic chest excursions recorded using strained gauges and a polygraph.

Table 2 Hot flush frequency during 24-h ambulatory monitoring (mean ± SD)

	Treatment group		
	Paced respiration	*Muscle relaxation*	*α-Wave feedback*
Pre-treatment	15.7 ± 8.1	14.2 ± 9.8	10.3 ± 7.3
Post-treatment	9.6 ± 6.2*	13.6 ± 10.6	12.0 ± 10.2

*$p < 0.02$, significantly different from pre-treatment value

A research assistant observed the polygraph tracings and instructed the patient to breath at 6–8 cycles/min and to increase the amplitude of the abdominal tracing. Patients learning muscle relaxation were trained according to the method of Bernstein and Borkovec[23]. Patients receiving α-electroencephalographic biofeedback received visual feedback for the production of 8–13 Hertz EEG activity, using previously published methods[20].

Before and after treatment, all women underwent 24-h ambulatory monitoring of sternal skin conductance level to detect hot flushes[11]. Before and after treatment, each patient also received a test of her ability to voluntarily relax. After a 10-min rest period, the patient was instructed to relax as deeply as possible for 5 min, followed by a second 10-min rest period. During the entire session, the patient's respiration rate and tidal volume were recorded.

Before treatment, there were no significant differences among the three groups in hot flush frequency (Table 2). Following treatment, the paced respiration group significantly reduced their hot flush frequency ($p < 0.02$) but the other two groups did not significantly change. There were no group differences in respiration rate or tidal volume during the pretreatment voluntary relaxation test. Following treatment, the paced respiration group significantly increased their tidal volume ($p < 0.05$) and reduced their respiration rate ($p < 0.015$), but the other two groups did not significantly change.

This study demonstrates that training in slow deep breathing alone will result in a significant reduction in the occurrence of menopausal hot flushes. This effect was documented by 24-h monitoring of an objective measure of hot flushes and, therefore, is not subject to the limitations of self-report data. Moreover, our recordings were performed over a 24-h period and, therefore, detected both sleeping and waking hot flushes. This technique may be useful for women with hot flushes who are unable to receive hormone replacement therapy.

CONCLUSION

Research in our laboratory has demonstrated that hot flushes can be objectively detected by laboratory and ambulatory monitoring of sternal skin conductance changes[11]. These changes bear a close correspondence with patient's self-reports of hot flushes, but do not occur in premenopausal women under comparable recording conditions. Using complementary pharmacologic probes, we then demonstrated that clonidine, a centrally acting α_2-agonist, ameliorated hot flushes and that yohimbine, an α_2-adrenergic antagonist, induced hot flushes[10]. These findings support the theory that a deficit in central, inhibitory α_2-adrenergic receptors is involved in the initiation of menopausal hot flushes. We then showed that plasma levels of MHPG, the main metabolite of brain norepinephrine, are elevated under basal conditions in women with hot flushes and further increase significantly during the hot flush itself[17]. These elevations do not occur in asymptomatic postmenopausal women.

Using these findings, we developed a behavioral relaxation method to treat symptomatic menopausal women who are unable to receive hormone replacement therapy. Eight 1-hour sessions of training in slow deep abdominal breathing significantly reduced hot flush frequency determined by objective methods, whereas plausible control procedures had no such effects. We hypothesized that the slow deep breathing exercises act in some way to modulate the increased central sympathetic activation and, thereby, reduce the frequency of hot flushes. Cross-sectional studies have demonstrated that slow deep breathers have high alveolar CO_2 levels and that fast shallow breathers have low CO_2 levels[24]. The former group had slower resting heart rates, reduced adrenal cortical activity, and decreased autonomic responses as compared with the latter group, although measures of central sympathetic activation were not obtained. Thus, it is possible that voluntary control of respiratory function reduces the elevated central arousal that initiates hot flushes.

In conclusion, we have presented evidence that menopausal hot flushes are triggered through elevated central sympathetic activation and can be ameliorated by a simple behavioral procedure. However, the mechanism(s) of action of the relaxation technique upon hot flushes remains to be determined through further research.

ACKNOWLEDGEMENT

Research conducted by the author was supported by Research Grant AG05233, National Institute on Aging.

REFERENCES

1. Sturdee, D. W., Wilson, K. A., Pipili, E. and Crocker, A. D. (1978). Physiological aspects of the menopausal hot flush. *Br. Med. J.,* **2**, 79–80
2. Casper, R. F. and Yen, S. S. C. (1985). Neuroendocrinology of menopausal flushes: an hypothesis of flush mechanism. *Clin. Endocrinol. (Oxf.)*, **22**, 293–312
3. Gambone, J., Meldrum, D. R., Laufer, L., Chang, R. J., Lu, J. K. H. and Judd, H. L. (1984). Further delineation of hypothalamic dysfunction responsible for menopausal hot flashes. *J. Clin. Endocrinol. Metab.,* **59**, 1097–102
4. Tataryn, I. V., Lomax, P., Bajorek, J. G., Chesarek, W., Meldrum, D. R. and Judd, H. L. (1980). Postmenopausal hot flushes: a disorder of thermoregulation. *Maturitas,* **2**, 101–7
5. Schmitt, H. (1977). The pharmacology of clonidine and related products. In Gross, E. (ed.) *Antihypertensive Agents*, pp. 299–396. (New York: Springer-Verlag)
6. Laufer, L. R., Erlik, Y., Meldrum, D. R. and Judd, H. L. (1982). Effect of clonidine on hot flushes in postmenopausal women. *Obstet. Gynecol.,* **60**, 583–9
7. Clayden, J. R., Bell, J. W. and Pollard, P. (1974). Menopausal flushing: double blind trial of a non-hormonal medication. *Br. Med. J.,* **1**, 409–12
8. Schindler, A. E., Muller, D., Keller, E., Goser, R. and Runkel, F. (1979). Studies with clonidine (Dixarit) in menopausal women. *Arch. Gynecol.,* **227**, 341–7
9. Goldberg, M. and Robertson, D. (1983). Yohimbine: a pharmacological probe for study of the α_2-adrenoceptor. *Pharmacol. Rev.,* **35**, 143–80
10. Freedman, R. R., Woodward, S. and Sabharwal, S. C. (1990). α_2-Adrenergic mechanism in menopausal hot flushes. *Obstet. Gynecol.,* **76**, 573–8
11. Freedman, R. R. (1989). Laboratory and ambulatory monitoring of menopausal hot flashes. *Psychophysiology,* **26**, 573–9
12. Starke, K., Gothert, M. and Kilbringer, H. (1989). Modulation of neuro-transmitter release by presynaptic autoreceptors. *Physiol. Rev.,* **69**, 864–989
13. Charney, D. S., Heninger, G. R. and Sternberg, D. E. (1982). Assessment of α_2 adrenergic autoreceptor function in humans. Effects of oral yohimbine. *Life Sci.,* **30**, 2033–41
14. Maas, J. W. (1983). *MHPG: Basic Mechanisms and Psychopathology.* (New York: Academic Press)
15. Leckman, J. F., Maas, J. W., Redmond, D. E. and Heninger, G. E. (1980). Effects of oral clonidine on plasma MHPG in man. *Life Sci.,* **26**, 2179–85
16. Zacny, E. (1982). The role of α_2-adrenoceptors in the hypothermic effect of clonidine in the rat. *J. Pharm. Pharmacol.,* **34**, 455–6
17. Insel, P. A. and Motulskey, H. J. (1987). Physiologic and pharmacologic regulation of adrenergic receptors. In Insel, P. A. (ed.) *Adrenergic Receptors in Man*, pp. 201–36. (New York: Marcel Dekker)
18. Hoffman, J. W., Benson, H., Arns, P. A., Stainbrook, G. L., Landsberg, G. L., Young, J. B. and Gill, A. (1981). Reduced sympathetic nervous system responsivity associated with the relaxation response. *Science,* **215**, 190–2
19. Benson, H. (1977). Systemic hypertension and the relaxation response. *N. Engl. J. Med.,* **296**, 1152–6
20. Germaine, L. M. and Freedman, R. R. (1984). Behavioral treatment of meno-

pausal hot flashes: evaluation of objective methods. *J. Consult. Clin. Psychol.*, **52**, 1072–9

21. Plotkin, W. B. and Rice, K. M. (1981). Biofeedback as placebo: anxiety reduction facilitated by training in either suppression or enhancement of alpha brainwaves. *J. Consult. Clin. Psychol.*, **49**, 590–6

22. Freedman, R. R. and Woodward, S. (1992). Behavioral treatment of menopausal hot flushes: evaluation by ambulatory monitoring. *Am. J. Obstet. Gynecol.*, **167**, 436–9

23. Bernstein, D. A. and Borkovec, T. D. (eds.) (1973). *Progressive Relaxation Training: A Manual for the Helping Professions.* (Champaign, Illinois: Research Press)

24. Schaefer, K. E. (1958). Respiratory pattern and respiratory response to CO_2. *J. Appl. Physiol.*, **13**, 1–14

Section 11

The aging male – is there an andropause?

57

The aging male

W.-B. Schill, F.-M. Köhn and G. Haidl

INTRODUCTION

Andrology, usually considered to be the care of men in their reproductive years who suffer from infertility, has so far neglected the aging male. This is due to the fact that men older than 50 are rarely seen because of impaired fertility, but more often consult a doctor for erectile dysfunction. Thus, in contrast to increasing knowledge about the menopause which terminates the reproductive period in women, knowledge about the aging male has been limited. From a clinical point of view, however, specific male problems that are associated with advancing age, leading to organic diseases such as benign prostatic hyperplasia (BPH) and prostatic carcinoma, are well covered by urology and other medical disciplines.

The demographic development in the industrialized countries means that more consideration will in future be given to the aging male. Germany may serve as an example of the 'aging' population resulting from increased expectation of life and falling birth rate. Of 38.8 million men living in Germany territory on December 31, 1991, 11.8 million were >50 years old, and 4.1 million were >65 years old[1]. On January 1, 1990, the European Community numbered 50.5 million men aged 20–39 years, 39.5 million aged 40–59, and 26.6 million men >60 years old[2]. Projections for the year 2000 suggest a slight decrease in the number of men aged 20–39 years to 49.4 million, an increase in those aged 40–59 years to 43.1 million, and an increase in those >60 years old to 30.6 million[2]. The proportion of men older than 60 in the year 2000 will be significantly higher than it is today.

Increasing expectations of life, involving claims for satisfactory living conditions even in old age, will stimulate the acquisition of knowledge, diagnosis and therapy of medical problems of the aging male. Results obtained in women cannot be transferred to men. In contrast to the relatively well-defined aging of the female gonads, the process of aging in the male is retarded and shows great interindividual variation. Nevertheless, old age is accompanied by clinical signs of reduced virility such as decreases in muscle mass and strength, in sexual hair growth and in libido, indicating diminished androgen levels.

An age-related decline in androgen secretion and plasma testosterone levels might suggest the possibility of androgen substitution. While medical geriatricians, internists, urologists, orthopedists and dermatologists are concerned with the aging male, this problem has not yet become a central point of interest to the andrologist in clinic and research.

The following review will focus on andrological aspects and related problems of the aging male; para-aging and well-known diseases that are not primarily within the field of andrology (e.g. treatment of fractures or diabetes mellitus in old age) are not covered.

Before the various aspects of the aging male are discussed, the theories of aging in man should be briefly recalled[3]:

(1) *Genetic program theory.* This concept is largely theoretical, and postulates that the process of aging is directed by a programmed sequence of genetically based signals.

(2) *Genetic mutation theory.* Accumulation of genetic damage during the process of aging results in disturbed cellular functions.

(3) *Waste product theory.* Waste products of cellular metabolism (e.g. lipofuscin in post-mitotic cells) that cannot be removed accumulate in cells and interfere with their normal function.

(4) *Cross-linking of macromolecules theory.* Complexes of small molecules within macromolecules such as nucleic acids or structural proteins (e.g. collagen) affect cellular function.

(5) Neuroendocrine theory. The basis of this concept is that neuroendocrine functioning with the hypothalamic–pituitary–peripheral endocrine system maintains the proper equilibrium of the organism. Changes in the function of the neuroendocrine system are thought to be responsible for the process of aging.

(6) *Free radical theory.* Nucleic acids and structural proteins are progressively affected by free radicals which interfere with normal cellular function and contribute to the process of aging.

(7) *Immune theory.* An impaired immune system with aging results in decreased host defense and autoimmunity.

(8) *Metabolic theory.* Studies demonstrating an inverse correlation between life span and metabolic rate gave rise to the theory that high metabolic activity with increasing age leads to disturbed cellular function.

FERTILITY STATUS AND TESTICULAR ALTERATIONS

There is growing interest in aging and its effect on the reproductive potential of men, since an increasing number of couples wish to have children in their late reproductive years, when the reproductive system is no longer operating optimally. Fertility in men usually persists well into old age, and a sudden fall in either Leydig cell or seminiferous tubular function does not occur. However, as is the case for other organs, there is considerable interindividual variation in age-dependent changes of the testes[4-6]. One-third of men over the age of 60 and 50% of those over 80 are completely infertile[7]. In principle, however, spermatogenesis may be retained well into senescence. Children have been fathered by men >90 years old[8].

In a study of 200 patients aged 65–93 years, Holstein[9] demonstrated intact spermatogenesis, including the development of mature spermatids, in 90% of testes. Comparing the daily sperm production of men aged 21–50 years with that of men aged 55–80 years, the younger group showed a 30% higher sperm production[10]. Single degenerative germ cells can be demonstrated in the testes of any adult fertile man. However, men >65 years old show additional kinetic disorders such as disturbed spermatogoniogenesis, disturbed meiosis or spermatid malformations[9], which parallel a highly significant decrease in daily sperm production. This indicates a gradual decline of fertility with increasing age, although alterations in sperm quality may be minimal. Most frequently, a decrease in motility and in the percentage of spermatozoa with normal morphology can be demonstrated[11,12].

Several studies have shown that a significant drop in fertility is only observed in couples where the female partner is >39 years old; the age of the male partner does not appear to play a significant role in infertility.

With advancing age, the seminiferous tubules gradually become atrophic as a result of decreasing germinal epithelium. These changes do not affect the entire testes in like manner, but may initially occur focally. There is a conspicuous increased desquamation of partly immature germ cells into the lumen of the seminiferous tubules. The basal layers of the germinal epithelium are also disorganized. Pale type spermatogonia leave the basal region, forming stratified layers. Dark type spermatogonia are sometimes completely missing. There is no further differentiation of spermatocytes or spermatids. Spermatogenesis is disturbed with regard to both kinetics and quality. Spermatogonia show morphological changes, including occurrence of electron-dense particles in the cytoplasm or cytoplasmic inclusions in the nuclear membrane. After the leptotene stage of meiosis, spermatocytes do not develop further, but form so-called megalospermatocytes, which form groups and later disintegrate[9]. In men >65 years old, the majority of spermatids show morphological changes, with no typical pattern. So-called giant spermatids may be present. Sertoli cells are also affected, with an increased lipid content as they incorporate increasing numbers of degenerated germ cells. Altered Sertoli cell function leads to increased secretion of follicle stimulating hormone. Serum inhibin levels in elderly men are also lower than those in young people[13], supporting the decline in Sertoli cell function with aging. Further age-dependent alterations affect the tunica propria, which may show fibrosis (tubular sclerosis) and, finally, tubular hyalinization. Other typical age-dependent defects of the seminiferous tubular structures include diverticula with evagination of the germinal tissue into the interstitium. The structure is filled with type I spermatocytes and Sertoli cells, but no lumen is present. The lamina propria shows only one layer of myofibroblasts. Diverticula can be observed in up to 80% of testicular biopsies in old men[9].

Apart from the age-dependent alterations of spermatogoniogenesis, disturbed meiosis and spermatid malformations, macrophages are frequently seen in the tubuli seminiferi or in the epididymis. These are large cells which have incorporated numerous spermatozoa. They are also called spermatophages and are found in increasing numbers in the testes of old men[9].

To compensate for the reduced synthetic activity of the Leydig cells, gonadotropin releasing hormone (GnRH) and luteinizing hormone (LH) are increasingly released via the negative feed-back mechanism of the pituitary–gonadal axis, finally resulting in an increase in size (hyperplasia) of the Leydig cells. The number of Leydig cells declines with advancing age: about 700 million Leydig cells are present in a 20-year-old man, decreasing by 6–7 million/year during the further process of aging[14].

In old age, lymphocytic and plasmacytic infiltrates are observed in the peritubular tissue. This may be due to immunological processes resulting from degenerated germinal epithelium. The rete testis is often dilated.

GENETIC RISKS IN CHILDREN OF OLD FATHERS

Controversy exists regarding the relationship between increased paternal age and the incidence of chromosome anomalies. The American Association of Tissue Banks has established an upper age limit of 40 years for semen donors; the limit set by the American Fertility Society is 50 years[15]. However, the results of earlier studies demonstrating an increased occurrence of trisomy 21 (Down syndrome) in children of fathers >55 years old could not be confirmed by later investigations. Structural chromosome anomalies do, however, seem to be more frequent in spermatozoa of older men. Martin and co-workers[16] observed the highest incidence of structural chromosome anomalies in men >44 years old, with approximately 13% of spermatozoa showing chromosomal damage. So far, however, there is no evidence from studies of live newborns or prenatally diagnosed fetuses that older fathers have an increased frequency of offspring with *de novo* (non-inherited) structural chromosomal anomalies[15].

Genetic mutations result from errors in DNA replication and can be passed to the next generation as a single gene defect. Therefore, the effect of advanced paternal age has been extensively studied in association with new cases of single gene defects. It was suspected that increased paternal age can lead to autosomal dominant mutations. This theory is now widely accepted, and increased paternal age has been associated with a variety of autosomal dominant diseases, including achondroplasia, aniridia, hemophilia A, Lesch-Nyhan syndrome, Marfan syndrome, neurofibromatosis, polycystic kidney disease, poliposis coli and progeria. In addition, a paternal age effect, acting at the level of the maternal grandfather, has been suggested for X-linked recessive disorders[15].

The risk of a man >40 years fathering a child with an autosomal dominant mutation is comparable with the risk of trisomy 21 in a child whose mother is aged 35–40 years. Friedman[17] has established risk estimates for increased paternal age and its contributions to new autosomal dominant mutations. His estimates are 0.2/1000 at a paternal age of <29; 1.1/1000 at paternal ages 30–34; 1.3/1000 at paternal ages 35–39; 4.5/1000 at paternal ages 40–44; and 3.7/1000 at paternal ages >45 years. Friedman suggests that approximately one-third of children with autosomal dominant mutations were fathered by men over the age of 40. Lian[18] found that paternal age > 40 years was related to a 20% increased occurrence of birth defects.

In summary, based on the available data, men >45 years must be viewed cautiously with regard to potential genetic risks. It is recommended that fathers should have their children before this age. There is only one argument in favor of advanced paternal age: the literature and studies of high school boys have indicated that descendants of older fathers, and particularly of paternal grandfathers, have a higher intelligence[19].

ENDOCRINOLOGICAL ALTERATIONS

Changing sex hormone concentrations in aging men are due to functional disturbances of the Leydig cells, the feedback mechanism of the pituitary–gonadal axis and the bioavailability of hormones. Decreases in sex hormone concentrations become manifest as early as the fifth to sixth decade of life. However, due to great interindividual variability, testosterone levels in older men may well be within the normal range for younger men. An age-associated decrease of testosterone becomes statistically relevant only after the seventh decade of life[20]. With advancing age there is a progressive decline in the synthesis of testosterone by Leydig cells, accompanied by an increase in LH levels. Several investigators have clearly demonstrated that the decrease in testosterone is of primarily testicular origin. Leydig cells seem to be less responsive to stimulation by LH[21]; this is apparently not due to a reduction in LH receptors on Leydig cells. Decreased responsiveness to LH is probably caused by a diminished reserve of testosterone in the Leydig cells, which is parallel to a significant decrease of the total steroid content in the testes of elderly men. A shift in testicular androgen biosynthesis has also been reported, favoring synthesis and secretion of Δ4-steroids over Δ5-steroids in old age, Δ5-steroids being the precursors of testosterone in the biosynthetic chain[20]. The primarily testicular origin of decreased androgen secretion in senescence is further supported by the reduction of Leydig cells in elderly men. There have also been reports of diminished testicular perfusion in aging testes, with a decrease in the number of capillaries pointing to a reduced oxygen supply in testicular tissue of old men[20].

Apart from the primarily testicular origin of decreased plasma androgen levels, additional alterations occur at the hypothalamo–pituitary level. Despite elevated LH plasma concentrations, which partly compensate for the reduced synthetic activity of the Leydig cells, the frequency of high amplitude LH pulses from the pituitary gland is significantly decreased, whereas the amplitude of LH pulses remains unchanged[22]. In addition, although GnRH stimulation reveals a large secretory reserve capacity of the gonadotrophs, LH levels do not increase enough to produce normal free testosterone levels[23]. While the pituitary content of FSH in older men remains constant, pituitary LH content is reduced.

Bremner and co-workers[24], as well as Deslypere and Vermeulen[25], observed disappearance of the circadian testosterone rhythm in elderly men, while serum androgen levels in young men demonstrated nyctohemeral variations with high testosterone concentrations in the early morning. This is probably the consequence of a decreased LH rhythm, suggesting an alteration at the hypothalamo–pituitary level.

In other studies, Vermeulen[20] investigated the sensitivity of gonadotrophs, particularly LH, to the feedback effect of plasma sex hormone levels. Transdermal application of dihydrotestosterone (DHT) gel produced similar levels of DHT in young and elderly men; however, the decrease in LH levels was significantly greater in the elderly men than in the young adults. As a consequence, the decrease in serum testosterone levels was also more pronounced in the elderly, indicating a greater sensitivity of the gonadotrophs to the androgen feedback.

Similar findings were observed when estrogen-containing gels were applied transdermally. GnRH tests during the period of pharmacologically increased sex hormone levels suggested that DHT would act at the hypothalamic level, whereas estrogens would mainly act at the pituitary level, blocking LH release. It is suggested that the changes in the hypothalamo–pituitary function in elderly men may be secondary to changes in neurotransmitter or neuromodulator systems such as hypothalamic dopamine, noradrenaline or opioid concentrations[26,27].

At the testicular level, a decline in intratesticular testosterone concentrations cannot be avoided, despite increased serum LH levels. Reduced intratubular testosterone concentrations, however, may affect spermatogenesis, which, together with the effects of age on the germ cells, results in elevated serum FSH levels. Furthermore, there is evidence that LH and FSH molecules undergo age-related changes, resulting in reduced bioactivity.

Stress may also play a role in age-associated changes in plasma testosterone levels. As far as testicular function is concerned, elderly men are less sensitive to stress than are young adults. Vermeulen and co-workers showed that hypoglycemia induces a significant decline in testosterone levels in young but not in elderly men. Interestingly, other environmental factors such as diet, moderate physical activity or life style had no effect on plasma testosterone levels[20].

Because of their hydrophobic nature, steroid hormones such as testosterone are bound to plasma proteins, including albumin and sex hormone binding globulin (SHBG). Only 2% of testosterone is unbound and thus biologically active. Above the age of 70 serum SHBG levels are increased[28], resulting in decreased concentrations of free testosterone. Thus, in addition to decreased synthesis of testosterone, increased binding capacity of the testosterone binding globulin determines the availability of biologically active free testosterone molecules.

Elevated SHBG concentrations are due to an increase in free estradiol. Serum estrogen levels in elderly men are higher as a result of increased aromatization of androgens, especially in the peripheral fatty tissue which is increased during aging. Declining free testosterone levels in plasma are accompanied by a decrease in tissue testosterone and/or its active metabolite, DHT. Deslypere and Vermeulen[29,30] demonstrated a highly significant decline in both testosterone and DHT concentrations in different tissues with age. In elderly men, Vermeulen[31] also observed altered testosterone metabolism, characterized by a decreased ratio of 5α to 5β metabolites, in parallel with a decline of 5α-reductase activity with increasing age. Despite diminishing serum testosterone levels, testosterone levels in the accessory glands such as the prostate remain constant because of α-reductase activity[29].

The aforementioned data are supported by epidemiologic studies during the past few years which have focused on plasma hormone changes in the aging male[32].

IS THERE A MALE CLIMACTERIC?

The term 'climacterium virile' was created in 1939 by Wermer[33], who described men at or beyond the fifth decade of life who suffered from vegetative complaints and a number of symptoms such as impaired memory, lack of concentration, tiredness, nervousness, and lowered resistance to stress. In analogy to the female climacteric, a sudden reduction in plasma testosterone levels and rapid senile involution of the testes were initially thought to be responsible. Later studies, however, showed that hormonal changes and morphological processes of aging in the male gonads were significantly different from those in aging women. The decline in testosterone levels observed in old age is gradual, and although the germinal epithelium shows age-related changes, there is great interindividual variability: functioning germ cells are found even in men over 80 years. The existence of a male climacteric is therefore questionable, and the existence of a relationship between climacterium virile and changes in the plasma testosterone levels is doubtful. Improvement of subjective symptoms by administration of androgen derivatives is not contradictory to this, but may reflect the psychotropic effects of androgens[34]. None of the symptoms attributed to the male climacteric has been demonstrated to be of statistically significant prevalence in men at the fifth or sixth decade of life. Only three constellations of two symptoms have occurred more frequently than by chance in men of this age group:

(1) Loss of potency, hyperhidrosis;

(2) Impaired potency and increased nervousness; and

(3) Obstipation and impaired memory[35].

In summary, while there is evidence of 'climacteric complaints' in the male, these do not occur as frequently and inevitably as in women and are rather of psychosociological origin[36,37]. The frequently used synonym 'midlife crisis' appears to be more appropriate than 'male climacteric'.

SEXUALITY, LIBIDO, IMPOTENTIA COEUNDI

Sexual activity involving intercourse diminishes, especially between the ages of 50 and 70 years[38]. High sexual activity in young years is usually maintained up to the age of 65[39]. A similar correlation has been observed with regard to masturbation and erotic stimulation. Tenderness (not involving sexual intercourse) is preferred by most people beyond the age of 65, while coitus is paramount in the sexual desire of those aged 45–65 years. In a small number of cases, sexual activity increases with advancing age[40]. Likewise, elderly people are often receptible to sexual practices previously not experienced. However, in pertinent studies it must be considered that sexual activity in a relationship depends on the wants and needs of two individuals. Sexual desire in aging men is different from that in aging women. While 15% of men over 59 years deny having sexual interest, the corresponding rate in women is 57%[41]. In this connection it must also be recognized that for significantly more men than women satisfactory sex life is determined by intercourse[42].

In various investigations, 80–90% of men >60 years and 60–70% of women over 60 continue sexual activity[43,44]. Apart from sex, other sociologic and medical factors are responsible for these differences in sexual behavior[40]. Sexual intercourse is performed most frequently by married people and least frequently by single persons. This is explained by the so-called 'disuse theory' assuming that sexual activity in old age is achieved the better the more frequently it is performed. Other factors influencing sexuality are the general state of health and hormonal factors.

Results of studies on the correlation between serum testosterone levels and sexual activity in elderly men have been controversial[31]. Cardiovascular or metabolic diseases, commonly noted during advancing age, can directly or indirectly affect sexual potency. Erectile problems are reported by 30–60% of younger men with diabetes mellitus[45] and by 95% of diabetic men older than 75 years[46]. In these cases, erectile failure can be attributed to the diabetic neuropathy. Erectile disturbances occur in up to 90% of those with renal insufficiency[47].

Smokers and patients with impaired fat metabolism suffer more frequently from impotence than do healthy men of the same age. Apart from quantitative alterations in the sexual behavior of aged people there are also qualitative changes. Erection and ejaculation are delayed or weakened, while postcoital detumescence occurs more rapidly[38] and the refractory period is elongated[48]. The incidence of erectile impotency is reported to be 2% in men below the age of 40 and 19% in those aged 50–60 years[49]. Impaired arterial circulation plays the most important role in erectile dysfunction, with a prevalence of 50%[46]. Drugs account for approximately 25% of erectile impotency; antihypertensive agents such as β-blockers, guanethidine, hydralazine, prazosin, reserpine, methyldopa and angiotensin-converting enzyme inhibitors most frequently cause erectile problems, particularly in the elderly. Conversely, sequelae of hypertonia, e.g. obstructive vascular diseases, may also cause erectile disturbances. Other drugs that may adversely affect potency include psychopharmacological agents, antiandrogens, antihistamines, diuretics, lipid-lowering agents, anti-inflammatory agents and cytostatics.

Apart from a careful medical history, the investigation of impotence should include blood count, creatinine, liver-specific enzymes, bilirubin, glucose, thyroid hormones, testosterone, free testosterone, sex hormone binding globulin, prolactin, estradiol, FSH and LH. After physical examination, pharmacological tests with intracavernosal injection of vasoactive drugs and detection of the arterial pulses by ultrasound Doppler sonography can be performed. Neurologic examinations, including determination of the bulbocavernous reflex time, may provide additional information. Nocturnal penile tumescence can be monitored by special devices; this allows distinction between organic and psychogenic causes of erectile dysfunction. A psychologic examination should be offered if necessary.

THERAPY OF ERECTILE DYSFUNCTION

In general, internal diseases such as hypertension, diabetes mellitus, hyperproteinemia and thyroid dysfunction should be adequately treated by drugs or diet. It should be noted that drugs in themselves may contribute to erectile dysfunction. For therapy of hypertension associated with erectile problems, the calcium antagonist nitrendipine is an encouraging agent which has shown positive effects in preliminary clinical studies[50]. Impotence in association with hyperprolactinemia can be treated causally with bromocriptine. In elderly patients showing premature involution of cerebral structures and evidence of Leydig cell insufficiency (testicular size, testosterone), combined treatment with an androgen (e.g. mesterolone) and pirazetam, a non-steroidal compound, is recommended. However, the importance of evaluating the prostate prior to androgen therapy in this age group is emphasized. Positive effects of the α-blocking agent yohimbine, especially in patients with psychogenic impotence, have been reported[51]. Men with vascular or neurogenic impotence who cannot undergo surgery or in whom surgery has been unsuccessful may respond to corpus cavernosum injection: up to two injections of prostaglandin E_1 per week are made by the patient himself. This requires high compliance, because the man commits himself to recording and regular controls. The latter also serves for the detection of cavernosal fibrosis.

Impaired arterial circulation can be treated by various surgical procedures; success rates as high as 80% have been reported[52]. In approximately 55% of cases, venous cavernosal insufficiency can be corrected by resection of the deep dorsal vein[53].

Penile prostheses are implanted when erectile failure cannot be treated by causal therapy or corpus cavernosum injections. Semirigid and hydraulic prostheses are available[54]; the latter function by means of shifting fluid from a reservoir. The adverse effects of the semirigid devices are mechanical complications and non-physiological conditions caused by the persistent erection. Alternative devices for achievement of penile erection are manual vacuum pumps which create negative pressure and induce tumescence, which is maintained by placing a constricting band at the base of the penis. Such devices may be recommended to patients who refuse prostheses. A problem that may occur is local ischemia of the skin resulting from improper use of the constricting band.

Psychotherapy continues to play an important role, although psychogenic factors of erectile failure have been diagnosed less frequently during the past few years.

CHANGES IN MUSCLES AND BONES

Aging of muscles and bones, manifest as loss of function and substance, begins at the age of approximately 30 years[55]. Factors contributing to these changes are genetic disposition, endocrinological factors, nutritional changes, and immobilization. Age-related involution of muscles and bones may be asymptomatic or may lead to subjective complaints. Senile muscular wasting becomes manifest as a reduction in the amount of muscles and diminished physical strength. In addition to decreased absorption of potassium, inadequate exercise, neuronal degeneration and a reduced amount of protein result in senile muscular disorders. With advancing age, changes are also observed in the skeleton. Starting at the age of 30, there is a continuous reduction in the amount of bone[55], approximately 30% of the original bulk being lost during the following 40 years. Compared to the aging process in women, loss of bone in men is less dramatic. The occurrence of osteoporosis is probably dependent on the original bulk of bone during the third decade of life. The risk of osteoporotic fracture is significantly lower in men than in women[56]. Even though osteoporosis is less common in men than in women, one in every six men will have suffered a fractured hip by the age of 90, an event associated with mortality and serious morbidity rates of 15% and 50%, respectively[57].

Hypogonadism is a major risk factor for osteoporosis not only in women, but also in men. As early as in 1948, Albright and Reifenstein[58] reported that eunuchs developed osteoporosis. However, the effects of androgen on bone metabolism are still poorly understood. In adults, bone density at a given age is determined by the peak bone mass achieved at sexual maturity and the subsequent amount of bone loss. Androgens affect both of these processes and they are a major determinant of bone mass in men. Several studies have demonstrated the important effect of pubertal increase in androgens on bone mass. The pubertal rise in testosterone secretion is followed closely by an increase in alkaline phosphatase activity and subsequently of cortical bone density. Peak cortical and trabecular bone mass is reached in men during their mid-twenties. Thereafter, bone density declines linearly with age, trabecular bone being lost more rapidly than cortical bone. It is suggested that a decline of gonadal function in the aging male may be responsible for bone loss; however, further prospective studies are needed to determine whether the modest testosterone decrease that occurs during aging is a significant factor in age-associated bone loss.

In young men after castration, progressive bone loss is observed with increasing years after orchidectomy. It is possible that gonadal steroids directly act on osteoblasts to stimulate bone formation, since androgen and estrogen receptors have been recently demonstrated in osteoblasts. Androgens may also affect bone metabolism by interaction with calcium regulatory hormones such as calcitonin. In addition, testosterone can be converted to dihydrotestosterone in human bone cultures, indicating the possibility that DHT is the active androgen in bone. However, the effect of androgens on osteoblasts may require its aromatization into estrogens.

Finally, there seems to be evidence that locally active cytokines, including prostaglandins, transforming growth factor-β and the local production of insulin-like growth factor-I (IGF-I), which stimulates collagen production by osteoblasts, also play an important role in bone metabolism.

BENIGN PROSTATIC HYPERPLASIA

BPH is a common and typical finding in elderly men, with an incidence of 70% in men aged 60–70 years, 80% in those aged 70–80 years, and 90% in those >80 years[59]. The prostate weighs 18–20 g at the age of 20, and progressively grows, reaching 50–60 g at the eighth decade of life[60]. Contrary to adenoma, BPH represents not only an increase in glandular tissue, but hyperplasia of the glandular and connective tissue of the periurethral glands (so-called inner glands).

Clinically, BPH is characterized by functional disturbances of micturition[59]. Initially, the patient merely notices decreased force of the urinary stream and frequent voiding. The second stage is characterized by urine retention, which is followed by the state of decompensation and incontinence with overflow. Urine is discharged involuntarily, but may also be retained in the upper urinary tract, resulting in urinary tract infections or renal insufficiency. Usually, the patient requires much effort for the first morning micturition, because the prostate is additionally enlarged due to increased engorgement with blood occurring at night[60]. This condition is called prostatic congestion. Complete obstruction of the bladder outlet and overstraining of the muscles resulting from urinary retention leads to acute anuria with an urgent desire to urinate.

Another complication of BPH is hematuria as a result of bleeding from prostatic varices. Progressive vesicular obstruction causes muscular hypertrophy with the formation of trabeculae. When disturbed passage cannot be compensated by increased muscular action, pseudodiverticula occur at the wall of the bladder[60]. BPH is thought to be related to alterations in the internal hormonal environment[59]. The growth of the prostate is influenced by androgens; progressively declining plasma testosterone levels in elderly men cannot therefore be responsible for BPH. However, hormone concentrations in the prostatic tissue itself are characterized by an increased level of 5-α-DHT[61] and elevated 5-α-reductase activity[62] in the hyperplastic stroma. Methodological errors have caused some authors to doubt the increased levels of 5-α-DHT[63]. Apart from androgens, estrogens and estrogen receptors also seem to be involved in BPH[60]. Estrogen concentrations in the prostate are higher than those in the plasma[64]. However, whether estrogen levels in benign prostatic hyperplasia are different from those in normal prostatic glands, where estrogens originate from, and the influence they might have on benign prostatic hyperplasia have not been determined. Animal studies have shown that combined administration of 17β-estradiol and DHT can induce prostatic hyperplasia.

For elderly men suspected of having BPH, the first diagnostic step is rectal examination. However, palpation does not allow definite statements about prostatic size and parts that are rectally not evaluable. Quantifiable methods of examination include uroflowmetry, sonographic determination of postvoid residual urine, ultrasound scanning of the upper urinary tract, urethrocystoscopy, tonometry of bladder and urethra, urethrocystography, micturition urethrocystography, and laboratory findings of urinary retention and serum electrolytes. Therapeutic measures differentiate between conventional and surgical procedures[60]. While enlargement of the prostate cannot be treated therapeutically, congestion and subjective complaints may be influenced at early stages. Recommended are general measures such as a diet for regulation of the bowels, avoidance of hard alcoholic drinks and hot spices. Drugs of herbal origin are used primarily, e.g. serenoa (sabal fruit), hypoxis rooperi, willow-herb, pumpkin seed, nettle, and pollen extracts. In patients with recurrent urinary retention, major postvoid residuum, macrohematuria or severe subjective complaints, surgical treatment is indicated.

While as many as 80–90% of patients with prostatic hyperplasia were treated by suprapubic, transvesical surgical procedures 20 years ago, today's therapy of choice is transurethral resection of the prostate. The mortality rate is less than 1%[65]. Potency is retained in >95%, urinary continence in 99%[65]. If surgery is contraindicated in patients with severe urinary retention, an indwelling catheter can be used.

Recent approaches to therapy, which are still experimental, include GnRH analogs, 5-α-reductase inhibitors, and aromatase inhibitors[66].

CHRONIC PROSTATITIS

Chronic prostatitis is more common before the age of 50 years[65], while older men are primarily affected by urinary tract infections caused by obstruction due to BPH. Clinically, the following entities are differentiated: acute bacterial prostatitis, chronic bacterial prostatitis, non-bacterial prostatitis, and prostadodynia (vegetative urogenital syndrome). Patients with chronic prostatitis usually complain about pain in the genital or perineal area, and may experience painful ejaculation or hematospermia (particularly when prostatitis is associated with vesiculitis). The most commonly involved organisms are *Escherichia coli, Klebsiella, Proteus* and *Pseudomonas*[65].

While chronic prostatitis is not primarily a problem of the aging man, differential diagnosis is required because of the non-specific symptoms, particularly with regard to psychosomatic complaints (masked depression).

PROSTATIC CARCINOMA

Prostatic carcinoma is the most common cancer in men today. In American males, it accounted for 21% of non-skin cancer diagnoses in 1989 and is more frequent than lung cancer[67]. Its incidence is 30 000/100 000 population >50 years, although only 23/100 000 die each year[67]. The initial stages of prostatic carcinoma are usually asymptomatic. Later, urinary obstruction, pain due to metastases, enlargement of lymph nodes and functional disturbances of the affected organs can be observed. Rectal examination usually reveals an irregular surface and indurated areas of the prostate. Definite diagnosis requires transrectal sonography and sonographically controlled puncture followed by histologic examination. The accuracy of these measures is approximately 85–90%[65].

Radical prostatectomy can be performed by the perineal or retropubic approach. The mortality rate is 0–2%[67]. Moderate incontinence occurs in 0–4%[67]; impotence, however, is observed in up to 60% of patients[65]. Hormonal therapy of prostatic cancer includes castration and administration of antiandrogens. According to recent studies, GnRH analogs (antagonists) also appear suitable for treatment of androgen-related diseases in the aging man[68].

POSSIBLE HORMONAL SUPPLEMENTATION IN OLD AGE

Initial attempts to treat age-related disturbances endocrinologically were reported by Brown-Sequard[69] who described his self-experiments to the Societé de Biologie in Paris. After injection of canine testicular suspension he observed increased libido and potency, later demonstrated to be a placebo effect[68].

As discussed above, total testosterone concentrations are lowered in men >60 years old, without, however, falling below the average values observed in healthy adult men. Therefore, testosterone supplementation is considered a useful therapy for aging men. However, there is scant information about whether androgen supplementation in older men might be beneficial, in terms of improving bone density or muscle mass and strength, or whether potential benefits might be outweighed by negative effects on lipid profiles, hematological parameters, or the prostate. In a double blind, placebo-controlled cross-over study, Tenover[70] recently investigated the effect of testosterone enanthate (100 mg/week) in 13 healthy men aged 57–76 years. Body weight, body fat, biochemical parameters of bone metabolism, hematological parameters, blood fats, prostate markers and hormone levels were determined before therapy and after the end of the 3-month study. Injection of testosterone enanthate resulted in elevated concentrations of both total testosterone and free testosterone in all men, the levels ranging within median normal limits. Prior to therapy, total testosterone levels had been within normal levels, and those of free testosterone below normal. Testosterone treatment increased libido or aggressiveness in business transactions in some men. In others, a general increase in sense of well-being was reported. All men showed an increase in weight, but not in body fat. Urinary excretion of hydroxyproline decreased, indicating delayed bone absorption. Positive effects of testosterone enanthate were also observed in the hematological parameters. Hematocrit, hemoglobin and red blood cell count increased, while total cholesterol and low density lipoprotein (LDP) were reduced during therapy with testosterone enanthate. In addition, there were no significant changes in prostate size and residual urine; however, a significant increase in prostate specific antigen was observed, 30% of the men showing elevated levels even at 3 months after cessation of therapy. Changes in liver function, skin, testicular size and hair pattern were not observed. In summary, short-term therapy with physiological levels of testosterone enanthate had positive effects on both fat and bone metabolism and on hematopoiesis in all men. However, no definite statement can be made about potential adverse effects on the prostate during long-term therapy.

In principle, testosterone supplementation in old patients may produce the following side-effects:

(1) Changes in fat metabolism (possible changes of LDL/HDL ratio = cardiovascular risk?);

(2) Stimulation of erythropoiesis with a risk of polycythemia;

(3) More rapid development of benign prostatic hyperplasia; and

(4) Stimulation of subclinical prostatic carcinoma.

In any case, when testosterone supplementation is considered in old age, these men should be carefully screened and monitored periodically to avoid any risk of a more rapid development or exacerbation of pre-existing BPH or prostatic cancer. Androgen therapy in aging men is still controversial, and large prospective studies on the beneficial and undesired effects of testosterone administration aimed at life quality are urgently needed. So far, androgen therapy in aging men can only be recommended for the substitution of manifest testosterone deficiency[71].

Another therapeutic attempt, which is still experimental, is the administration of growth hormone (GH). Total GH secretion, GH secretory pulses and growth hormone releasing hormone-induced GH secretion decline with advancing age, resulting in lower serum IGF-I levels[72]. Reduced GH secretion is thought to be related to senile osteoporosis, muscular atrophy and sleep disturbances. Initial placebo-controlled studies in small patient groups, including old men and those deficient in IGF-I, showed that IGF-I levels, bone density and body weight increased during therapy, while body fat was reduced[73]. At present, however, it is too early to draw any conclusions as to whether this treatment will significantly contribute to physical and psychological improvement of processes that are involved in senescence.

From the presented data and the review of the literature it is evident that many questions about physiology and pathophysiology of the aging male are still open. However, increased research in this field will be mandatory in the near future to meet the requirements of the aging population.

REFERENCES

1. Bevölkerungsstatistik (1991). Tab B15. Statistisches Bundesamt, Wiesbaden
2. Bevölkerungsstatistik (1992). Statistisches Bundesamt, Berlin
3. Murray, S. S. (1992). Theories of biological aging. In Morley, J. E. and Konenman, S. G. (eds.) *Endocrinology and Metabolism in the Elderly*, pp. 3–22. (Cambridge: Blackwell)
4. Greeve, J. and Bichler, J. (1987). *Sexualhormone und Altern.* (Eppelheim: VOD)
5. Holstein, A. F. and Hubmann, R. (1981). Spermatogonia in old age. *Fortschr. Androl.,* **8**, 108–17
6. Holstein, A. F. (1983). Zur Spermatogenese im Senium. *Verh. Anat. Ges.,* **77**, 379–80
7. Harman, S. M. (1978). Clinical aspects of aging of the male reproductive system. In Schneider, E. L. (ed.) *The Aging Reproductive System*, pp. 29–58. (New York: Raven)

8. Silber, S. J. (1991). Effects of age on male fertility. *Semin. Reprod. Endocrinol.,* **9**, 241–8

9. Holstein, A. F. (1986). Spermatogenese im Alter – ein Grenzgebiet zwischen normaler und pathologischer Anatomie. *Urologe (A),* **25**, 130–7

10. Johnson, L., Petty, C. S. and Neaves, W. B. (1984). Influence of age on sperm production and testicular weights in men. *J. Reprod. Fertil.,* **70**, 211–18

11. Nieschlag, E., Lammers, U., Freischem, C. W., Langer, K. and Wickings, E. J. (1982). Reproductive functions in young fathers and grandfathers. *J. Clin. Endocrinol. Metab.,* **55**, 676–81

12. Schwartz, D., Mayaux, M. J., Spira, A., Moscato, M. L., Jouannet, P., Czyglik, F. and David, G. (1983). Semen characteristics as a function of age in 833 fertile men. *Fertil. Steril.,* **39**, 530–5

13. Tenover, J. S., McLachlan, R. I., Dahl, K. D., Burger, H. C., de Kretser, D. M. and Bremner, W. J. (1988). Decreased serum inhibin levels in normal elderly men: evidence for a decline in Sertoli cell function with aging. *J. Clin. Endocrinol. Metab.,* **67**, 455–9

14. Neaves, W. B., Johnson, L., Porter, J. C., Parker, C. R. and Petty, C. S. (1984). Leydig cell numbers, daily sperm production and serum gonadotropin levels in aging men. *J. Clin. Endocrinol.,* **59**, 756–63

15. Bordson, B. L. and Leonardo, Y. S. (1991). The appropriate upper age limit for semen donors: a review of the genetic effects of paternal age. *Fertil. Steril.,* **56**, 397–401

16. Martin, R. H. and Rademaker, A. W. (1987). The effect of age on the frequency of sperm chromosomal abnormalities in normal men. *Am. J. Hum. Genet.,* **41**, 484–92

17. Friedman, J. M. (1981). Genetic disease in the offspring of older fathers. *Obstet. Gynecol.,* **57**, 745–9

18. Lian, Z.-H., Zack, M. M. and Erickson, J. D. (1986). Paternal age and the occurrence of birth defects. *Am. J. Hum. Genet.,* **39**, 648–60

19. Dietz-Helmers, A. (1974). On correlation between the generation age of fathers and grandfathers and the intelligence of the descendants. *Experientia,* **30**, 567–9

20. Vermeulen, A. (1988). Alteration of Leydig cell function and its mechanism in the aging male. In Holstein, A. F., Leidenberger, F., Hölzer, K. H. and Bettendorf, G. (eds.) *Carl Schirren Symposium: Advances in Andrology,* pp. 82–5. (Berlin: Diesbach)

21. Hartmann, S. H. and Talbart, G. B. (1985). Reproductive aging. In Finch, C. E. and Hanflicks, L. (eds.) *Handbook of the Biology of Aging,* 2nd edn., pp. 457–510. (New York: van Nostrand Reinhold)

22. Winters, S. J. and Troen, P. (1982). Episodic luteinizing hormone (LH) secretion and the response of LH and follicle-stimulating hormone to LH-releasing hormone in aged men: evidence for coexistent primary testicular insufficiency and an impairment in gonadotropin secretion. *J. Clin. Endocrinol. Metab.,* **55**, 560–5

23. Wide, L. (1985). Median charge and charge heterogeneity of human pituitary FSH, LH and TSH: II. Relationship to sex and age. *Acta Endocrinol.,* **109**, 190–7

24. Bremner, W. J., Vitiello, M. V. and Prinz, P. N. (1983). Loss of circadian

rhythmicity in blood testosterone levels with aging in normal men. *J. Clin. Endocrinol. Metab.*, **56**, 1278–81

25. Deslypere, J. P. and Vermeulen, A. (1984). Leydig cell function in normal men: effect of age, life style, residence, diet and activity. *J. Clin. Endocrinol. Metab.*, **59**, 955–61

26. Simpkins, J. W. (1983). Changes in hypothalamic hypophysiotropic hormones and neurotransmitters during aging. In Meites, J. (ed.) *Neuroendocrinology of Aging*, pp. 41–61. (New York: Plenum Press)

27. Peng, M. T. (1983). Changes in hormone uptake and receptors in the hypothalamus during aging. In Meites, J. (ed.) *Neuroendocrinology of Aging*, pp. 61–71. (New York: Plenum Press)

28. Baker, H. W. G. and Hudson, B. (1983). Changes in the pituitary–testicular axis with age. In de Kretser, B. M., Burger, H. G. and Hudson, B. (eds.) *The Pituitary and Testis. Clinical and Experimental Studies. Monographs on Endocrinology 25*, pp. 71–82. (Berlin, Hamburg, New York: Springer)

29. Deslypere, J. P. and Vermeulen, A. (1981). Aging and tissue androgens. *J. Clin. Endocrinol. Metab.*, **53**, 430–4

30. Deslypere, J. P. and Vermeulen, A. (1985). Influence of age on steroid concentration in skin and striated muscle in women and in cardiac muscle and lung tissue in men. *J. Clin. Endocrinol. Metab.*, **60**, 648–53

31. Vermeulen, A. (1990). Androgens and male senescence. In Nieschlag, E. and Behre, H. M. (eds.) *Testosterone*, pp. 261–76. (Berlin, Heidelberg: Springer)

32. Simon, D., Preziosi, P., Barrett-Connor, E., Roger, M., Saint-Paul, M., Khalil, N. and Papoz, L. (1992). The influence of aging on plasma sex hormones in men: The Telecom study. *Am. J. Epidemiol.*, **135**, 783–91

33. Wermer, A. A. (1939). The male climacteric. *J. Am. Med. Assoc.*, **119**, 1441–3

34. Kaiser, E., Kies, N., Maas, G., Schmid, H., Beach, R. C., Bormacher, K., Horrmann, W. M. and Richle, E. (1978). The measurement of the psychotropic effects of an androgen in the aging male with psychovegetative symptomatology: a controlled double blind study mesterolone versus placebo. *Prog. Neurol. Psychopharmacol.*, **2**, 505–15

35. Nieschlag, E., Benkert, C., Comhaire, F., Doerr, P., Schmidt, H. and Serio, M. (1978). The male climacteric. Workshop report. In van Keep, P. A., Serr, D. M. and Greenblatt, R. B. (eds.) *Female and Male Climacteric. Current Opinion*, pp. 133–39. (Lancaster: MTP Press)

36. Greeve, J. (1987). Das sogenannte Klimakterium virile. In Greeve, J. and Bichler, J. (eds.) *Sexualhormone und Altern*, pp. 91–3. (Eppelheim: VOD)

37. Featherstone, M. and Hepworth, M. (1985). The male menopause: lifestyle and sexuality. *Maturitas*, **7**, 235–46

38. Schneider, H. D. (1991). Sexualität. In Oswald, W. D., Herrmann, W. M., Kanowski, S., Lehr, U. M. and Thomae, H. (eds.) *Gerontologie*. (Stuttgart, Berlin, Köln: Kohlhammer)

39. Gaunitz, F. (1987). Altern und Sexualität. In Greeve, J. and Bichler, J. (eds.) *Sexualhormone und Altern*, pp. 101–5. (Eppelheim: VOD)

40. Schneider, H. D. (1989). Sexualität im Alter. In Platt, D. (ed.) *Handbuch der Gerontologie, Bd. 5: Neurologie, Psychiatrie*, pp. 445–52. (Stuttgart, New York: Gustav Fischer Verlag)

41. Verwoerdt, A., Pfeiffer, E. and Wang, H. S. (1969). Sexual behavior in senescence. *Geriatrics*, **24**, 137–54

42. Trummers, H. (1976). *Sozialpsychologische Aspekte der Sexualität im Alter.* (Köln: Böhlau)

43. Starr, B. D. and Weiner, M. B. (1982). *Liebe und Sexualität in reiferen Jahren.* (Bern: Scherz)

44. Brecher, E. M. (1984). *Love, Sex and Aging.* (Boston: Little, Brown & Co.)

45. Finkle, A. L. (1983). Sexual function during advancing age. In Platt, D. (ed.) *Geriatrics 2*, pp. 189–99. (Berlin, Heidelberg, New York: Springer)

46. Kaiser, F. E. (1992). Impotence in the elderly. In Morley, J. E. and Konenman, S. G. (eds.) *Endocrinology and Metabolism in the Elderly*, pp. 262–71. (Cambridge: Blackwell)

47. Graf, H. and Ludvik, G. (1989). Niereninsuffizienz und Sexualstörungen. *Sexualmedizin, 18*, 160–6

48. Krause, W. (1990). Hormonelle Altersveränderungen aus der Sicht des Andrologen. *Fortschr. Med., 108*, 371/31–374/34

49. Porst, H. (1987). *Erektile Impotenz.* (Stuttgart: Ferdinand Enke Verlag)

50. Haidl, G. (1989). Effekt von Nitrendipin auf die vaskulär bedingte erektile Dysfunktion. *Med. Welt, 40*, 1258–9

51. Reid, K., Morales, A., Harris, C., Surridge, D. H. C., Condra, M., Owen, J. and Fenemore, J. (1987). Double-blind trial of yohimbine in treatment of psychogenic impotence. *Lancet, 1*, 421–3

52. Hauri, D. (1989). Operative Möglichkeiten in der Therapie der vaskulär bedingten erektilen Impotenz. *Urologe (A), 28*, 260–5

53. Weidner, W., Weiske, W. H. and Rudnick, J. (1989). 'Leakage'-Korrektur durch Resektion der Vena dorsalis penis profunda. *Urologe (A), 28*, 217–22

54. Greim, K., Noll, F. and Schreiter, F. (1989). Die Behandlung der erektilen Dysfunktion mit Penisprothesen. *Urologe (A), 28*, 266–70

55. Perschel, W. T. (1987). Altersbedingte Veränderungen der Muskulatur und der Knochen. In Greeve, J. and Bichler, J. (eds.) *Sexualhormone und Altern,* pp. 94–100. (Eppelheim: VOD)

56. Nordin, B. E. C. and Need, A. G. (1990). Prediction and prevention of osteoporosis. In Bergener, M., Ermini, M. and Stähelin, H. B. (eds.) *Challenges in Aging,* pp. 249–65. (London: Academic Press)

57. Finkelstein, J. S. and Klibanski, A. (1990). Effects of androgens on bone metabolism. In Nieschlag, E. and Behre, H. M. (eds.) *Testosterone*, pp. 204–18. (Berlin, Heidelberg: Springer)

58. Albright, F. and Reifenstein, E. C. (1948). Metabolic bone disease: osteoporosis. In Albright, F. and Reifenstein, E. C. (eds.) *The Parathyroid Glands and Metabolic Bone Disease*, pp. 145–204. (Baltimore: Williams and Wilkins)

59. Greeve, J. (1987). Die benigne Prostatahyperplasie – eine altersbedingte Endokrinopathie? In Greeve, J. and Bichler, J. (eds.) *Sexualhormone und Altern,* pp. 106–11. (Eppelheim: VOD)

60. May, P. (1992). Die Prostatahyperplasia. In Platt, D. (ed.) *Handbuch der Gerontologie, Bd. 4/2 Urologie, Orthopädie*, pp. 3–16. (Stuttgart, Jena, New York: Gustav Fischer Verlag)

61. Siiteri, P. K. and Wilson, J. D. (1970). The formation and content of dihydrotestosterone in the hypertrophic prostate of man. *J. Clin. Invest., 49*, 1737–45

62. Krieg, M., Bartsch, W., Thomsen, M. and Voigt, K. D. (1983). Androgens and

estrogens: their interaction with stroma and epithelium of human benign hyperplasia and normal prostate. *J. Steroid Biochem.*, **19**, 155–61

63. Walsh, P. C. (1984). Human benign prostatic hyperplasia: etiological consideration. In Kimball, F. A., Buhl, A. E. and Carter, D. B. (eds.) *New Approaches to the Study of Benign Prostate Hyperplasia.* (New York: Alan R. Liss Inc.)

64. Kozak, J., Bartsch, W., Krieg, M. and Voigt, K. D. (1982). Nuclei of stroma: site of highest estrogen concentration in human benign prostatic hyperplasia. *Prostate,* **3**, 433–8

65. Basso, A. (1984). The prostate in the elderly. In Platt, D. (ed.) *Geriatrics 3*, pp. 193–212. (Berlin, Heidelberg, New York, Tokyo: Springer)

66. Krieg, M. and Tunn, S. (1990). Androgens and human benign prostatic hyperplasia (BPH). In Nieschlag, E. and Behre, H. M. (eds.) *Testosterone*, pp. 219–44. (Berlin, Heidelberg: Springer)

67. Moon, T. D. (1992). The aging prostate: prostate cancer. In Morley, J. E. and Konenman, S. G. (eds.) *Endocrinology and Metabolism in the Elderly*, pp. 272–92. (Cambridge: Blackwell)

68. Tenover, J. S., Dahl, K. D., Vale, W. W., Rivier, J. E. and Bremner, W. J. (1990). Hormonal responses to a potent gonadotropin hormone-releasing hormone antagonist in normal elderly men. *J. Clin. Endocrinol. Metab.*, **71**, 881–8

69. Brown-Séquard, C. E. (1989). Expérience démonstrant la puissance dynamogénique chez l'homme d'un liquide extrait de testicules d'animaux. *Arch. Physiol. Norm. Pathol.*, **5**, 651–8

70. Tenover, J. S. (1992). Effects of testosterone supplementation in the aging male. *J. Clin. Endocrinol. Metab.*, **75**, 1092–8

71. Jackson, J. A., Waxman, J. and Spiekerman, M. (1989). Prostatic complications of testosterone replacement therapy. *Arch. Intern. Med.*, **149**, 2365–6

72. Hoffmann, A. R., Liebermann, J. A. and Ceda, G. P. (1992). Growth hormone therapy in the elderly: implications for the aging brain. *Psychoneuroendocrinology,* **17**, 327–33

73. Rudman, D., Feller, A. G., Nagraj, H. S., Gergans, G. A., Lalitha, P. Y., Goldberg, A. F., Schlenker, R. A., Cohn, L., Rudman, I. W. and Mattson, D. E. (1990). Effects of human growth hormone in men over 60 years old. *N. Engl. J. Med.*, **323**, 1–6

58

Andropause, fact or fiction?

A. Vermeulen

Although the life expectancy of a human male is about 8 years less than that of a woman, male aging, and more specifically aging of the male reproductive system, has attracted much less interest than aging in women. The concept of a male equivalent to the menopause, the andropause, is still the subject of debate. The special interest group session 'Andropause, fact or fiction?' was therefore most welcome.

The first paper in this session was given by Dr J. B. McKinlay of the New England Research Institute in Massachusetts and was entitled *Medical and psychological correlates of the erectile dysfunction (impotence) in normal aging men*. He reported results from the Massachusetts Male Aging Study, a large epidemiologic survey of 1700 men, aged 40–70 years, randomly sampled from the community. Potency was determined from subjects' responses to a self-administered questionnaire, the statistical validity of this approach having been established by cross-validation with data from over 300 patients attending a Urology Clinic. Some degree of impotence, varying from minimal to complete was found in 51% of the sample. The prevalence of complete impotence tripled between the ages of 40 and 70, from 5 to 15%. Among the important determinants of this impotence were diabetes and heart disease (Figures 1, 2); cigarette smoking exacerbated the risk of impotence associated with diabetes, heart disease and hypertension (Figure 3).

As expected, depression was strongly associated with impotence; the same applies to other psychological factors such as low level of dominance and anger, whether expressed outward or directed inward. Surprisingly, however, of the 17 different hormones measured, including testosterone, only dehydroepiandrosterone sulfate level significantly predicted impo-

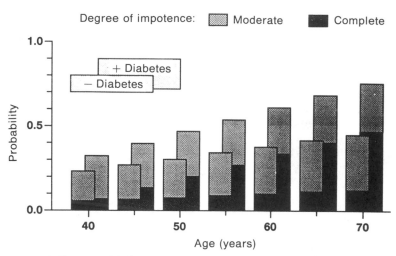

Figure 1 Influence of diabetes on impotence. Source: Massachusetts Male Aging Study, New England Research Institute (NERI), Watertown, MA. Age-controlled effect of diabetes statistically significant ($p < 0.0001$)

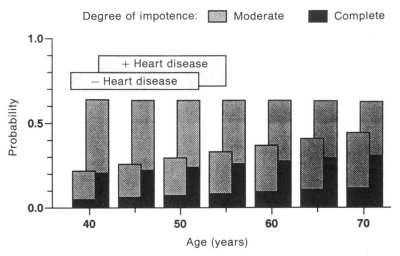

Figure 2 Association of heart disease with impotence. Source: Massachusetts Male Aging Study, New England Research Institute (NERI), Watertown, MA. Age-controlled effect of heart disease statistically significant ($p < 0.0001$)

tence. Neither obesity nor moderate alcohol consumption showed any significant correlation with impotence.

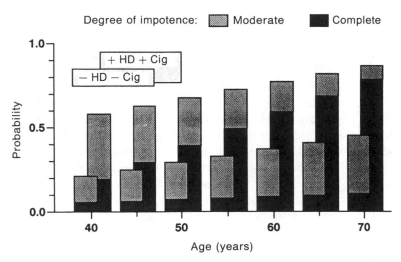

Figure 3 Combined influence of heart disease and cigarette smoking on impotence. Source: Massachusetts Male Aging Study, New England Research Institute, Watertown, MA. Age-controlled interaction of heart disease with cigarette smoking statistically significant ($p < 0.0005$)

Another rather unexpected finding was that aging men did not evidence increased sexual dissatisfaction as a result of decreasing erectile function. It appears from this study that the sexual expectations of men decline with age and their level of sexual satisfaction may reflect the normative expectations held by specific age groups. It should be recalled that this study did not involve a group of self-selected subjects, but a random sample from the community.

The author concluded that the multiplicity of potential determinants suggests that impotence is not only associated with age but that modifiable para-aging phenomena play an important role. This finding should have important implications for the clinical management of and public health policies toward factors associated with impotence.

The next lecture, given by Professor K. Carlstrom, from Huddinge University Hospital, Sweden, dealt with the topic of the Adrenopause.

It is not generally realized that steroid secretion by the adrenal gland is greatly influenced by age. The adrenal cortex secretes three types of steroids: mineralocorticoids (e.g. aldosterone) by the zona glomerulosa, glucocorticoids (e.g. hydrocortisone) by the zona fasciculata and androgens (e.g. dehydroepiandrosterone and its sulfate) by the zona reticularis and fasciculata. The secretion of androgens and hydrocortisone are both regulated by adrenocorticotropin (ACTH), which is secreted by the pituitary.

The adrenal cortex secretes weak androgens, the Δ4 steroid, androstene-dione, and the 3β-hydroxy-5-ene steroids, dehydroepiandrosterone, its metabolite 5-androstene 3β,17βdiol and dehydroepiandrosterone sulfate (DHEAS). The latter three steroids may be considered as 'primitive' steroids, very close to the parent product of all steroid hormones, cholesterol. Androstenedione is the major precursor of estrogens formed in peripheral tissues. Androst-5ene3β,17βdiol is estrogenic by itself and binds to the estrogen receptor, whereas dehydroepiandrosterone and its sulfate may be estrogenic, through their conversion to androst-5ene-3β,17βdiol; however, they are also androgenic as they may be transformed into testosterone in peripheral tissues.

It should be recalled that the adrenal androgens contribute 50% of total estrogenic activity in men and 95% of estrogenic activity in postmeno-pausal women. They are also responsible for > 50% of androgenic activity in women, their contribution to androgenic activity in men being negligible.

DHEAS circulates in plasma at a concentration which is about ten times that of cortisol: its circulating level is by far the highest of all steroids, and its blood production rate is also the highest of all steroid hormones. It is surprising, therefore, that this steroid does not appear to have a well defined function and patients without adrenal androgen secretion, such as those with Addison's disease, when adequately substituted with cortisol, show no sign of hormone deficiency. Although DHEAS has been connected with immune processes, has been considered to be an anti-obesity hormone, and to have anti-atherogenic activities, its exact role remains enigmatic.

Cortisol production, expressed per m^2 body surface, and plasma levels remain constant during life, but DHEAS levels show important variations with age (Figure 4). Levels are extremely low during the first years of life, increasing almost exponentially in the prepubertal years, to reach their highest concentration around the age of 20–30. They then decrease almost linearly with age to levels which are only about 20% of the highest levels. Levels of dehydroepiandrosterone show similar variations, whereas variations in androstenedione levels are much less pronounced, showing a decrease around age 50 and varying very little thereafter (Figure 5).

Similarly, whereas the response to ACTH stimulation does not vary with age for cortisol and increases for 17-hydroxyprogesterone, the response of dehydroepiandrosterone to ACTH is significantly lower in elderly persons than in young subjects. Professor Carlstrom suggests the ratio of

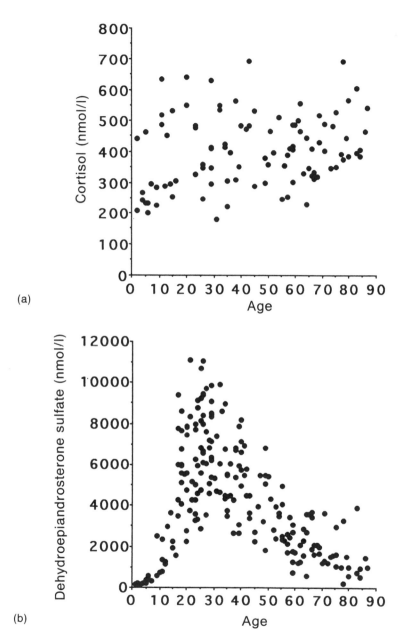

Figure 4 Changes in basal levels of (a) cortisol and (b) dehydroepiandrosterone sulfate with age

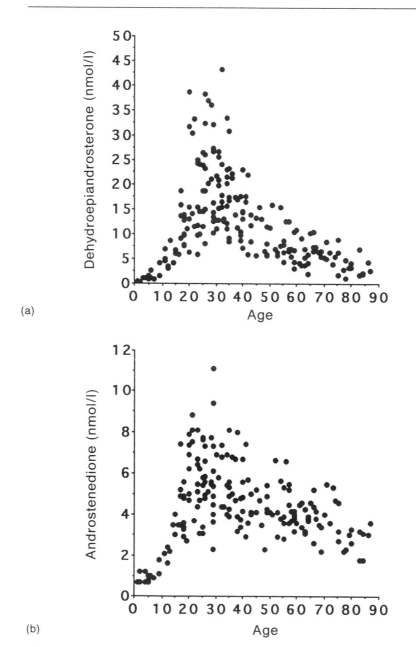

Figure 5 Changes in basal levels of (a) dehydroepiandrosterone and (b) androstenedione with age

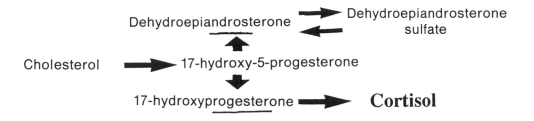

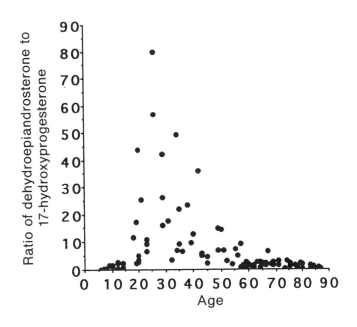

Figure 6 The adrenocortical 'senility index'

the increase in DHEA to the increase in 17-hydroxyprogesterone upon ACTH stimulation may be a 'senility' index (Figure 6).

The mechanisms by which these age-dependent variations in dehydro-epiandrosterone secretion are brought about are not completely understood. The age-dependent decrease in the rate of metabolic clearance of cortisol which results, via a feedback mechanism, in reduced ACTH secretion, may explain a 25% decrease in dehydroepiandrosterone levels, but it cannot account for the much greater decrease observed. Modulation by gonadal hormones can be excluded, but the existence of a specific pituitary peptide which stimulates androgen secretion is questionable. The possibility of modulation of androgen secretion by growth factors remains a possibility.

Professor Carlstrom suggests that the primitive and harmless 3β-hydroxysteroids may be the adrenal safety valve: a reduced supply of 17-hydroxypregn-5-enolone, the common substrate to both the cortisol and the androgen pathway, would result in shunting of biosynthesis towards cortisol production. Finally, Professor Carlstrom provided some data on androgen levels in patients with benign prostatic hyperplasia (BPH) or prostatic carcinoma. In both conditions total plasma testosterone and non-specifically bound testosterone levels are increased compared to age-matched normal controls. In BPH patients, dehydroepiandrosterone levels and their response to ACTH are also higher than in controls. He concludes that patients with prostatic disease are endocrinologically younger than age-matched controls.

The last speaker in this session was Professor Vermeulen, from Ghent, Belgium, who discussed Leydig cell function in elderly men and its clinical implications. In middle-aged men, in distinction to middle-aged women, reproductive capacity does not come to an abrupt end, fertility persisting until a very old age. Although elderly men do not experience a sudden decrease in sex hormone secretion, in distinction to menopausal women, there is, nevertheless, an age-dependent decrease in Leydig cell secretion, causing a progressive decline in plasma and tissue levels of testosterone. This decrease is more pronounced for bioavailable testosterone, as indicated by the greater decrease in free testosterone than total testosterone levels, a consequence of an age-associated increase in sex hormone binding globulin.

Whereas all 'normal' postmenopausal women have very low plasma estrogen levels, compared to those during reproductive life, (free) testosterone levels in elderly men show important interindividual variations: some men in their eighties have levels considered normal in young men. Some authors have even questioned whether the lower testosterone levels observed in elderly men are a consequence of the aging process *per se*, or are rather the sequelae of prior illnesses. Although the latter certainly accelerate and accentuate the decrease in testosterone levels in elderly men, it is nevertheless now generally accepted that perfectly healthy elderly men have lower free testosterone levels than young men.

This decrease appears to have largely a primary testicular origin, as evidenced by the decreased number of Leydig cells, the decreased response to human chorionic gonadotropin alterations in the biosynthesis of androgens, increased luteinizing hormone levels as measured both by immuno- or bioassay and the normal response of gonadotrophs to a pharmacological dose of gonadotropin releasing hormone (GnRH). Nevertheless, there is also evidence for alterations at the hypothalamo–pituitary pole of the gonadal axis, as shown by the absence of normalization of the (free) testosterone levels despite an adequate secretory reserve capacity of both gonadotrophs and Leydig cells, the disappearance of circadian variations in plasma testosterone levels in elderly men, the decrease in amplitude of luteinizing hormone pulses in elderly men, and the absence of any increase in either amplitude or frequency of the pulses in response to anti-opioids. As the response of the gonadotrophs to minimal, physiological doses of GnRH appears to be preserved, the data suggest a decrease in the mass of GnRH secreted at each pulse, possibly the consequence of a decrease of the cellular mass of the pulse generator.

DO THE DECREASED ANDROGEN LEVELS IN ELDERLY MEN HAVE ANY CLINICAL SIGNIFICANCE?

Aging in men is, without doubt, accompanied by clinical signs of decreased virility, such as decreased sexual body hair and growth rate, requiring less frequent shaving, decreased muscle mass and strength, decreased bone mass, decreased vigor, and decreased libido and sexual activity, which, together with signs of neurovegetative dystonia, nervousness and insomnia suggest the existence of a male equivalent to the endocrine menopausal syndrome. Not all these signs and symptoms, however, are only the consequence of decreased androgen levels. It is evident, for example, that many factors play a role in the age-associated decrease in sexual activity: fear of failure, prolonged unavailability of sexual partners and long periods of forced abstinence, boredom with the same sexual partner, impaired perfusion of the corpora cavernosa secondary to atherosclerosis, and senile polyneuritis resulting in decreased tactile sensitivity of the penis, may all play a role. Nevertheless, androgens do play a role in the age-associated decrease in sexual activity and several authors found a weak but significant correlation between plasma testosterone levels and frequency of sexual activity. It seems, however, that above a certain threshold value, testosterone levels no longer affect sexual activity.

Of primary importance to the clinician is the problem of whether the age-associated decrease of androgen levels warrants any androgen substitution in (some of) these elderly men. In other words, can androgen substitution reverse the symptoms of decreased virility without risk of severe side-effects. Androgen substitution obviously is not required in elderly men with normal androgen levels, whatever their complaints may be. In hypogonadal males, androgen substitution rapidly reverses the signs and symptoms of androgen deficiency.

Androgen substitution in elderly males has been the subject of few controlled studies. It is common experience that, in elderly men with low androgen levels, androgen substitution improves physical and mental well-being, together with a modest, but significant increase in hematocrit, red cell mass and hemoglobin. Androgens also increase lean body and muscle mass, although the decrease in elderly men may be related more to the lack of physical activity than to androgen deficiency. Finally, androgens seem to stimulate osteoblastic activity, as shown by a decrease in hydroxyproline excretion and an increase in alkaline phosphatase and osteocalcin levels. The effects of androgens on impotence are disappointing; however, this is not surprising as androgen deficiency is seldom the major cause of impotence.

With respect to the side-effects of androgen therapy, the major risk concerns the activation of subclinical prostatic carcinoma, which is found in about 50% of males over 70 years old. The overwhelming majority of these carcinomas do not manifest clinically during the lifetime of the subject, but, as the majority of these are androgen dependent, it is reasonable to believe that androgen substitution might accelerate their growth. Androgen substitution in elderly males should therefore only be performed under strictly controlled conditions, after exclusion of all detectable carcinomas.

Other side-effects, such as unfavorable effects on lipid levels, are of less concern, particularly since the effects of substitutive doses of natural androgens on the plasma profile are controversial: several studies have reported favorable effects.

In conclusion, the answer to the question 'Andropause, fact or fiction?', is a matter of semantics. Strictly speaking, the male equivalent of the menopause, with its sudden definitive end of reproductive capacities and a sudden decrease in sex hormone levels, does not occur in males. However, in the great majority, if not all, elderly men there is clearcut evidence for an age-associated, progressive decline both in fertility and in plasma androgen levels, responsible for the clinical signs of decreased virility. Many of these signs and symptoms of androgen deficiency regress upon androgen substitution, but, in view of the risk of severe side-effects and the lack of well controlled clinical studies concerning the balance between the risks and benefits, generalized use of androgen substitution has to await the results of such studies and therefore cannot be recommended at the moment.

Section 12

Sexuality around menopause

59

Survey research on the menopause and women's sexuality

N. L. McCoy

A considerable number of studies have surveyed women around the time of the menopause, but only a few have investigated the relationship of menopause to sexuality. Early surveys of sexual behavior discounted or ignored the menopause.

Kinsey and his colleagues[1] found that 48% of 127 menopausal women felt that menopause had resulted in a decrease in their sexual response and that 53% believed that it had resulted in a decreased frequency of sexual activity. Their data showed a steady decrease in median frequency of total outlet to orgasm associated with time in years from menopause. Nevertheless, they did not believe that these declines were a consequence of menopause. Because the median frequency of total sexual outlet to orgasm among active married and single women stayed 'more or less on a level until 55 or 60 years of age', they concluded that the decline was due to aging processes in the male. If, however, one examines their data for percentage of single women who were active at each 5-year age period, an entirely different picture emerges. Between the ages of 26 and 45, the percentage of single women who were active during each 5-year period was >65%; at 46–50, this figure changes to 61%, at 51–55, 52%, and at 56–60, only 44% of single women were active, revealing a clear decrease in sexual activity commencing in the late 40s.

In another project examining aging and sexuality, Pfeiffer and colleagues[2] studied 261 white men and 241 white women ranging in age from 46 to 71 and found large sex differences from the age of 46. The percentages of those indicating 'no interest in sex' at 46–50 were 0% of men and 7% of women, increasing to 11% of men and 51% of women at 61–65. Similar figures for 'no sexual intercourse' at 46–50 were 0% of men and 14% of women, increasing to 20% of men and 61% of women at 61–65. These authors made no mention of menopause or of the possibility that menopause might have played a role in these differences.

A key study in this area is that of Hallstrom[3], who first proved that it was menopause and not simply aging that was associated with a decline in women's sexuality. He studied a random sample of 800 women selected from the Census Register in Goteborg, Sweden, and invited them to undergo a comprehensive health examination. Data were obtained in a 1–2 h semi-structured interview which was part of the examination. Women were intact, not taking hormones, either married or living with a man, and either 38, 46, 50 or 54 years old. The women were divided into four groups on the basis of climacteric phase: premenopausal, perimenopausal, early postmenopausal and late postmenopausal. The sexual variables of sexual interest, change in sexual interest, change in capacity for orgasm, coital frequency and change in coital frequency were all significantly related to age, but when climacteric phase was held constant, all relationship to age disappeared; sexual interest and coital frequency significantly decreased across climacteric phase and changes in sexual interest, coital frequency and capacity for orgasm were also significantly related to climacteric phase.

An Italian study by Bottiglioni and Aloysio[4] with similar findings included 756 women volunteers between the ages of 40 and 65 who were interviewed at a menopause clinic. Women were considered to be premenopausal if they were between 40 and 45 and had not cycled for 6 months, or were between 46 and 50 and had irregular cycling, or were ⩾ 50 and still cycling. Early postmenopausal women were within 5 years and late postmenopausal women were more than 5 years from the last cycle. For women aged 50–65, the authors determined change in sexual variables by comparing each woman's report of her current sexual status with that of the previous decade. Although no statistical evaluation was carried out, the percentage of women with a negative change in sexual satisfaction, sexual drive, and frequency of orgasmic response, markedly increased from pre- to early postmenopause. The percentage of women reporting a decreased frequency of sexual intercourse increased systematically across the three menopausal phases.

In another Swedish study, Hagstad[5] randomly selected a sample of 1746 women aged 37–66 from the Census Register in Goteborg, Sweden. Of the 1431 women who participated, 1188 were intact and not using hormones. Information was obtained from questionnaires. The only sexual variable was vaginal dryness which was significantly less common in both pre- compared with perimenopausal as well as in peri- compared with postmenopausal women.

In a British study, Hunter and co-workers[6] conducted a postal survey of women by recruiting through newspaper advertisements and a radio program. Of 1090 volunteers, 850 returned usable questionnaires. Of those, 682 respondents were intact and not using hormones and ranged in age from 45 to 65 (mean 52.3 years). Women were classified as premenopausal if they had cycled regularly, perimenopausal if they had cycled irregularly, and postmenopausal if they had not cycled during the past 12 months. Seventy percent of all women reported being sexually active. Sexual interest was significantly decreased in peri- and postmenopausal women, and vaginal dryness was significantly more common among postmenopausal women. While 45% of postmenopausal women reported vaginal dryness, only 26% of the other women did so. Roughly 84% of women indicated satisfaction with their sexual relationships. Sexual functioning factor scores, which consisted of responses to the 'sexual interest', 'vaginal dryness' and 'dissatisfaction with sexual partner' items, were also best predicted by menopausal status.

In a follow-up of the previous study, Hunter[7] contacted 56 premenopausal women from the first survey who had agreed to continue. Of the 47 women who responded, 36 had had a natural menopause and were not using hormones. Their mean age was 48.5 in the first survey and 51.4 in the second. Only 58% (21) of these women were sexually active and completed all three sexual items. For these women, there were essentially no changes from the first to the second survey in the percentage reporting loss of sexual interest, vaginal dryness, or dissatisfaction with sexual relationships. In a previous report of these data[8], the author concluded that there were too few complete responses to assess.

Holte and Mikkelsen[9,10] conducted a survey in which 2349 women, 45–55 years of age, were randomly selected from the population register of the municipality of Oslo. Of the 1886 women who completed the postal questionnaire, 1566 were intact and not using hormones and had a mean age of 50.7 years. Women who cycled regularly and within the last 2 months were classified as premenopausal, women who cycled irregularly or had cycled at least once in the last 6 months as perimenopausal, those not cycling for 6–12 months as early postmenopausal, and those not cycling for ≥ 1 year as late postmenopausal. Vaginal dryness was the only sexual variable, and was clearly related to menopausal development across the phases. The highest percentage of women reporting vaginal dryness were 3 years from their last cycle. It is interesting to note that Hagstad[5] also found a peak in reported vaginal discomfort at 3 years postmenopause.

In a follow-up study, Holte[11] randomly selected 200 premenopausal subjects from his original survey to participate in a 5-year longitudinal study. Every 12 months during the study, each subject completed a 3–4 h semi-structured interview, psychological testing, and a gynecological examination. All subjects were intact and not using hormones. Of 193 who agreed to participate, 177 completed all parts of the study. Of those, 118 did not meet criteria for inclusion in the final analyses, and the final sample consisted of 59 subjects. The mean age of the final sample at the beginning of the study was 51.1 years with a range of 47–56. As in the earlier study, the only sexual variable reported was vaginal dryness. Data revealed that vaginal dryness was significantly increased from pre- to postmenopause, as was vaginal dryness over the past 12 months. Increase in distress caused by vaginal dryness from pre- to postmenopause was only marginally significant ($p < 0.07$).

A longitudinal study of the menopause transition specifically addressing sexuality was conducted by McCoy and colleagues[12,13]. Of 155 initial volunteers recruited through TV, radio and newspapers, 43 perimenopausal subjects who were intact and not using hormones agreed to continue beyond the initial phase of the study. Women were considered perimenopausal if they had experienced sustained changes in cycle length and menstrual bleeding within the last year and had menstruated at least once during the last 12 months. For the first 6 months, each woman was seen at 3-month intervals and after that at 4-month intervals, during the first 5 days of her cycle if she was cycling. Each woman recorded menstrual and sexual activity daily on monthly calendars and completed a sexuality questionnaire and a modified Kupperman Test of Menopausal Distress[14] at each interview; 20 ml of blood was also drawn for assay. In an early report[12] from this study covering the first two interviews, subjects were called early perimenopausal if they were still cycling at least once within 30 days or late perimenopausal if they cycled less than that. The average age was 49.1 years (range 41–56). Analyses of calendar records of sexual intercourse revealed a significantly higher rate of sexual intercourse among the early compared with the late perimenopausal women. Early and late perimenopausal subjects were having intercourse an average of roughly twice a week and once a week, respectively.

A later report[13] from this study involved 16 intact women with sexual partners who were not using hormones and who had continued in the study for at least 1 year past their last cycle. The average age of menopause was 52 (range 47–56). Number of days with sexual intercourse from daily calendars declined significantly from pre- to postmenopause. Questionnaire data revealed that women showed a significant decrease in sexual interest as reflected in sexual thoughts and fantasies, an increase in the frequency of vaginal dryness, and decreased satisfaction with their partner as a lover from pre- to postmenopause. There were no significant differences in dyspareunia or reported frequency of orgasm. Testosterone was the hormone most consistently associated with coital frequency.

A series of studies by Bachmann and Leiblum and their colleagues[15-17] focused on sexuality and looked particularly at the relationship between sexual activity and vaginal atrophy. Subjects in all studies were at least 1 year postmenopausal, intact, and not using hormones, and were interviewed and underwent a gynecological examination. In the 1991 study[15], 59 women in their 60s (mean age 63.9) were recruited through a hospital-based gynecologic practice. Subjects' ratings of their premenopausal sexual desire were significantly higher than current sexual desire ratings; 56% reported diminished sexual interest. In the 1984 study[16], subjects were 69 women who ranged in age from 50 to 65 (mean 56.6) and were recruited from newspaper advertisements and community education lectures. Of these women, 51 who had partners reported a significant decline in coital frequency from pre- to postmenopause. A 1983 study[17] had a sample of 52 women who ranged in age from 50 to 65 (mean 56.8) and were recruited in the same way as the previous study. In all three of these studies[15-17], active women had significantly less vaginal atrophy than inactive women. While it is tempting to assume that sexual activity prevents vaginal atrophy, we really cannot do so on the basis of these data. In the 1984 study[16], active women had significantly higher levels of luteinizing hormone (LH) than inactive women and in the 1983 study[17], women with less vaginal atrophy had significantly higher mean levels of follicle stimulating hormone and LH as well as of androstenedione and testosterone. These androgens accounted for more variance than current frequency of intercourse. Whether the major causal variable in the relationship between hormones, sexual activity and vaginal atrophy is hormones or sexual activity or both is, as yet, an unanswered question.

In summary, the most studied sexual variables have been coital frequency, vaginal dryness and sexual interest. Of the six survey studies[1,3,4,12,13,16] that examined coital frequency in relationship to menopausal phase, all six found a decrease in relationship to increasing menopausal phase. The same is true for all five studies[5,6,9,10,13] examining vaginal lubrication, and all five studies[3,4,6,13,15] that investigated sexual interest. There is much less comparable knowledge on capacity for orgasm[3,4,13] or vaginal discomfort[5,13] but the trend is the same. Nevertheless, using these results and our current knowledge about hormones and

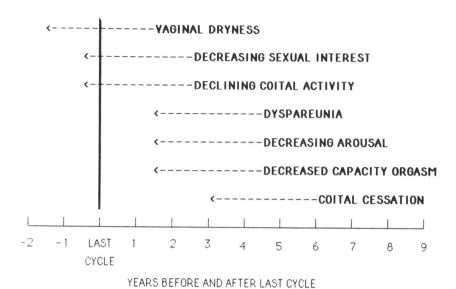

Figure 1 Sequential changes in women's sexuality arising from menopausal hormone levels

sexuality[18], I have constructed a schematic (Figure 1) representing the way in which low levels of androgens and estrogens associated with the menopause may affect sexuality over time. Our efforts in this area, thus far, have been focused on group averages; we know comparatively little about the considerable variations among women and their sources. Clearly, we are just beginning to find answers and can only hope that more studies of the menopausal transition will include sexual variables.

REFERENCES

1. Kinsey, A. C., Pomeroy, W. B., Martin, C. E. and Gebhard, P. H. (1953). *Sexual Behavior in the Human Female*. (Philadelphia: W. B. Saunders)
2. Pfeiffer, E., Verwoerdt, A. and Davis, G. C. (1972). Sexual behavior in middle life. *Am. J. Psychiatr,* **128**, 1262–7
3. Hallstrom, T. (1979). Sexuality of women in middle age: the Goteborg Study. *J. Biosoc. Sci.,* **6** (Suppl.), 165–75
4. Bottiglioni, F. and De Aloysio, D. (1982). Female sexual activity as a function of climacteric conditions and age. *Maturitas,* **4**, 27–32
5. Hagstad, A. (1988). Gynecology and sexuality in middle-aged women. *Women Health,* **13**, 57–80
6. Hunter, M., Battersby, R. and Whitehead, M. (1986). Relationships between

psychological symptoms, somatic complaints and menopausal status. *Maturitas,* 8, 217–28

7. Hunter, M. (1992). The South-East England longitudinal study of the climacteric and postmenopause. *Maturitas,* 14, 117–26

8. Hunter, M. S. (1990). Somatic experience of the menopause: a prospective study. *Psychosom. Med.,* 52, 357–67

9. Holte, A. and Mikkelsen, A. (1991). Psychosocial determinants of climacteric complaints. *Maturitas,* 13, 205–15

10. Holte, A. (1991). Prevalence of climacteric complaints in a representative sample of middle-aged women in Oslo, Norway. *J. Psychosom. Obstet. Gynaecol.,* 12, 303–15

11. Holte, A. (1992). Influences of natural menopause on health complaints: a prospective study of healthy Norwegian women. *Maturitas,* 14, 127–41

12. McCoy, N., Cutler, W. and Davidson, J. M. (1985). Relationships among sexual behavior, hot flashes, and hormone levels in perimenopausal women. *Arch. Sex. Behav.,* 14, 384–95

13. McCoy, N. L. and Davidson, J. M. (1985). A longitudinal study of the effecs of menopause on sexuality. *Maturitas,* 7, 203–10

14. Kupperman, H. S., Wetchler, B. B. and Blatt, M. H. G. (1959). Contemporary therapy of the menopausal syndrome. *J. Am. Med. Assoc.,* 171, 1627–37

15. Bachmann, G. A. and Leiblum, S. R. (1991). Sexuality in sexagenarian women. *Maturitas,* 13, 43–50

16. Bachmann, G. A., Leiblum, S. R., Kemmann, E., Colburn, D. W., Swartzman, L. and Shelden, R. (1984). Sexual expression and its determinants in the postmenopausal woman. *Maturitas,* 6, 19–29

17. Leiblum, S., Bachmann, G., Kemmann, E., Colburn, D. and Swartzman, L. (1983). Vaginal atrophy in the postmenopausal woman: the importance of sexual activity and hormones. *J. Am. Med. Assoc.,* 249, 2195–8

18. McCoy, N. L. (1992). Menopause and sexuality. In Sitruk-Ware, R. and Utian, W. (eds.) *The Menopause and Hormonal Replacement Therapy: Facts and Controversies* (Clinical Gynecology Series), pp. 73–100. (New York: Marcel Dekker)

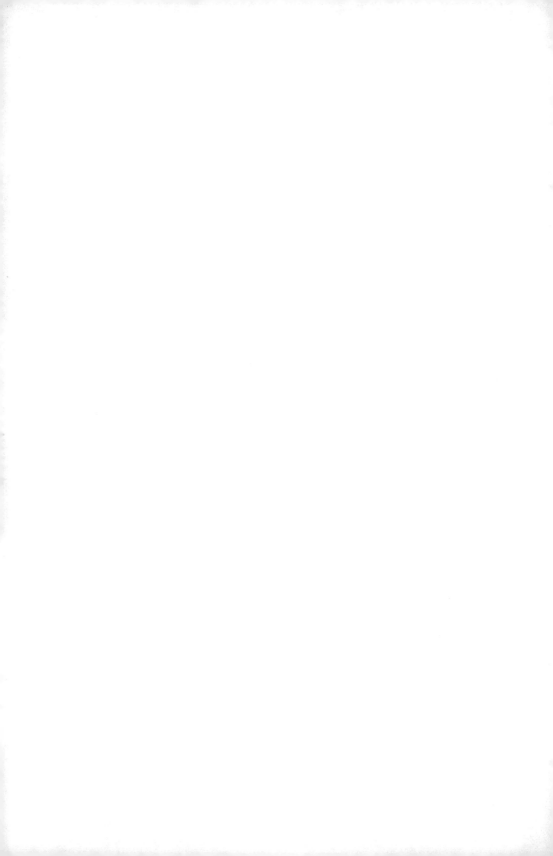

60

Hormonal influences on sexuality in the postmenopause

B. B. Sherwin

Still in 1993, a great deal of mythology concerning sexual functioning in postmenopausal women prevails. Although a myriad of factors combine to determine the quality of sexual life following the menopause, the role of hormonal alterations at this time have received relatively little attention. This chapter will focus on the hormonal determinants of aspects of sexual functioning in postmenopausal women in the attempt to elucidate the specificity of hormone–behavior relationships in aging women.

HORMONAL CHANGES AT MENOPAUSE

Before reviewing the relevant findings of clinical studies on hormones and female sexuality, it is useful to recall the changes in sex hormone production around the time of menopause. In premenopausal women, the ovary secretes 95% of the estradiol that enters the circulation[1]. After menopause, the ovary virtually stops producing estradiol and estrone, a much weaker estrogen, becomes the predominant estrogen that arises from peripheral conversion from androstenedione[2]. Although it used to be thought that the drastic decrease in ovarian estradiol secretion at the time of menopause was due solely to follicle depletion and ovarian senescence, it is now clear that age-related alterations in hypothalamic function also occur[3]. Thus, the transition to menopause is a multifactorial process involving both neural and ovarian factors.

In women, both the adrenal and the ovary contain the biosynthetic pathways necessary for androgen synthesis and secretion. The ovary produces approximately 25% of plasma testosterone, 60% of androstene-dione and 20% of dehydroepiandrosterone, whereas the adrenal produces 25% of circulating testosterone, 40% of androstenedione, 50% of dehydro-epiandrosterone and 90% of dehydroepiandrosterone sulfate (DHEAS). The remainder of circulating androgens in the female are thought to arise through peripheral conversion, which likely accounts for the production rate of 50% of testosterone and 25% of dehydroepiandrosterone[4]. Several investigators have reported that plasma testosterone levels are lower in naturally postmenopausal women compared to younger women whose blood was sampled during the follicular phase of the menstrual cycle[5,6]. Moreover, there is some evidence that the decrease in the ovarian production of testosterone occurs prior to the menopause and that values remain stable for some time thereafter. Roger and colleagues[7] reported that plasma testosterone levels were lower in menstruating women over 40 years of age compared to values in cycling women less than 40 years old, but that values in women over 40 did not differ from those of naturally postmenopausal women. Similarly, in a study of peri- and postmenopausal women, although plasma testosterone levels did not decline with increas-ing time since the last menstrual cycle, levels were significantly lower than in younger, normal women during the early follicular phase of the menstrual cycle[8].

In order to investigate residual ovarian production of steroids after the menopause, the concentration of hormones was measured in blood samples taken from the ovarian artery and the ovarian vein at the time of abdominal surgery. The presence of a concentration gradient across the ovary shows that the ovary is secreting steroids. Two such studies found that the ovary continues to secrete appreciable amounts of testosterone in about 50% of postmenopausal women[9,10]. In a third investigation, the ovarian vein values of testosterone were significantly lower in postmenopausal women than in a control group of young women during the periovulatory phase of the cycle[11]. However, caution should be exercised in interpreting the results of the cross-ovarian gradient studies since testosterone levels in the general circulation may have been inflated as a consequence of increased adrenal androgen output in response to the stress of surgery. Notwithstanding this caveat, the available evidence suggests that whereas the postmenopausal ovary continues to secrete testosterone in about 50% of women, the concentrations produced are significantly lower than those produced during the menstrual cycle in younger women. Moreover, in 50% of naturally postmenopausal women, no significant ovarian testosterone production is evident.

NEUROBIOLOGICAL EFFECTS OF ESTROGEN AND ANDROGEN

In order to account for an effect of a sex hormone on sexual behavior, one needs to assume that they are capable of exerting effects on the brain. Autoradiographic studies have established that specific receptors for estradiol are found in specific areas of the brain, predominantly in the pituitary, the hypothalamus, limbic forebrain and the cerebral cortex[12]. Testosterone receptors are concentrated in the preoptic area of the hypothalamus and also occur in smaller numbers in the limbic system and in the cerebral cortex[12]. Moreover, it has also been established that sex hormones may have two modes of action on brain function; they can alter the expression of genetic information by interacting with the genome[13] and/or they can change the permeability of cell membranes leading to direct effects on cellular function[14]. Thus, sex hormones exert both direct and indirect effects on neuronal activity in areas of the brain that subserve emotion and sexuality.

PERIPHERAL EFFECTS OF ESTROGEN

Because the integrity of the tissues of the female reproductive tract is dependent on estrogen, degenerative changes in these structures ensue when levels of estrogen decrease after the menopause. The vaginal epithelium of postmenopausal women who do not receive estrogen therapy becomes attenuated and appears pale due to a decrease in vascularity. Marked atrophic changes may result in atrophic vaginitis. In this condition, the vaginal epithelium is very thin and may become inflamed or even ulcerated[15]. These changes, in turn, may lead to a severe diminution in vaginal lubrication and/or dyspareunia.

There is some evidence that estrogen may also affect touch perception[16]. Furthermore, several lines of evidence indicate that estrogens exert direct physiologic effects on blood vessel walls, resulting in an increase in blood flow[17]. Therefore, the known effects of estrogen on peripheral tissues make it likely that the very low levels of circulating estrogen in untreated postmenopausal women may have a negative impact on sexual functioning. Specifically, there is a high probability that decreased vaginal lubrication, decreased genital vasocongestion and possible dyspareunia will occur in postmenopausal women with increasing time since the last menstrual cycle.

Various research methodologies have been used to investigate the concomitants and possible etiology of declining sexual function in peri-

and in postmenopausal women. Research findings from correlational and hormone replacement therapy studies have been particularly informative.

CORRELATIONAL STUDIES

Several investigators have tested the association between circulating levels of the sex steroids and aspects of sexual behavior in postmenopausal women. Bachman and co-workers[18] found that neither estradiol nor testosterone levels discriminated between sexually active and inactive untreated postmenopausal women but that sexually active women had less vaginal atrophy than the inactive women. In a longitudinal study, cycling perimenopausal women were followed for at least 1 year beyond the cessation of their menstrual cycles. Compared with their premeno-pause data, the women had fewer sexual thoughts or fantasies and experienced less vaginal lubrication during sex after menopause. While estradiol and testosterone levels both showed significant declines from pre- to postmenopause, testosterone showed the more consistent association with coital frequency[19]. Because 38% of subjects dropped out of the study before its completion, because they became highly symptomatic and needed to begin estrogen replacement therapy, it is likely that the decline in aspects of sexual functioning was underestimated in this biased sample.

Perimenopausal women with irregular menstrual cycles between the ages of 44 and 52 years failed to report significant deficits in sexual desire, response or satisfaction, although those whose estradiol levels were low did report a decrease in coital activity[20]. The relationships between testosterone levels and aspects of sexual behavior were not reported in that study.

HORMONE REPLACEMENT THERAPY STUDIES

The paradigm that is perhaps most powerful for the study of the specificity of the sex steroids on female sexuality involves administering hormone replacement therapy to women who have undergone total abdominal hysterectomy (TAH) and bilateral salpingo-oophorectomy (BSO). When both ovaries are removed from premenopausal women, circulating testosterone levels decrease significantly within the first 24–48 h postoperatively[4,6]. The fact that women are deprived of ovarian androgen production following this surgical procedure has provided a rationale for administering both estrogen and androgen as replacement therapy.

In Britain and Australia, subcutaneous implantation of pellets containing estradiol and testosterone has been used as a treatment for menopausal symptoms for several decades. This route of sex steroid administration results in a slow, constant release of the sex hormones over a period of at least 6 months. In a single-blind study, both surgically and naturally menopausal women who complained of loss of libido (undefined) despite therapy with conjugated equine estrogen were implanted subcutaneously with pellets containing estradiol 40 mg and testosterone 100 mg[21]. By the third month after implantation, patients reported a significant increase in libido, in enjoyment of sex as well as in the frequency of orgasm and of initiation of sexual activities. These changes occurred concurrent with a significant increase in plasma testosterone levels.

In another single-blind study, a group of premenopausal women (mean age 44.5 years) and a group of naturally and surgically menopausal women (mean age 53.3 years) were implanted with subcutaneous pellets containing estradiol 50 mg and testosterone 100 mg[22]. Loss of libido was a presenting symptom in over 80% of patients in both groups and hormone implant therapy reversed the symptom in two-thirds of the patients.

Twenty women who had experienced a severe loss of libido despite treatment with oral estrogens and progestins that adequately relieved other symptoms such as hot flashes and vaginal dryness randomly received subcutaneous implants of either estradiol 40 mg or of a combined pellet containing estradiol 40 mg and testosterone 50 mg[23]. Self ratings of various aspects of sexual functioning were carried out after implantation. After 6 weeks, the loss of libido in the single implant group remained whereas the combined group showed significant symptomatic relief. The mean peak testosterone concentrations after testosterone implantation slightly exceeded the upper limit of the normal female range.

Although these implant studies were single-blind, in two of them patients were preselected on the basis of loss of libido that had been unresponsive to estrogen alone[21,22] and the third study contained an estrogen alone control group as a basis for comparison. Even bearing in mind the methodologic flaws, results of these studies strongly suggest that testosterone and not estrogen is of primary importance for libido or sexual desire in women.

During the past decade, several prospective, controlled studies of general and sexual effects of combined estrogen–androgen parenteral preparations in surgically menopausal women were carried out. In all of them, premenopausal women who needed to undergo TAH and BSO for benign disease were randomly assigned to one of four treatment groups postoperatively. Those who received an estrogen–androgen (E–A) preparation or androgen alone (A) intramuscularly following surgery had a greater energy level and sense of well-being than those who received estrogen alone (E) or placebo (PL)[24]. Administration of the androgen-containing preparations (E–A and A) were also associated with lower somatic and pyschological symptom scores than E or PL[25]. Moreover, all women treated with hormones following surgery had more positive moods than those given PL[26].

Androgenic effects on sexual behavior were also investigated in these studies of women who had all been happily married for at least 5 years. It was also assured that they and their husbands were in good general health. The women monitored several aspects of their sexual behavior daily for a total of 8 months; 1 month preoperatively, and during two 3-month postoperative treatment phases that were separated by a placebo month. All drugs were given intramuscularly every 28 days. One dose of the E–A combined preparation we used contained testosterone enanthate 150 mg, estradiol dienanthate 7.5 mg and estradiol benzoate 1 mg. Women who received either of the androgen-containing drugs reported an enhancement of sexual desire and arousal, and an increase in the number of sexual fantasies compared with those treated with E or PL[27]. Ratings of women treated with androgen did not differ from those of a second control group comprised of women who had undergone TAH but whose ovaries had been retained (CON). This occurred even though patients in the CON group were an average of 10 years younger than the oophorectomized women. However, the frequencies of coitus or orgasm did not differ as a response to the various hormonal treatments. Sherwin and colleagues[28] subsequently confirmed these findings with E–A combination long-term, compared with a group that received long-term E alone and a third group that remained untreated following their TAH and BSO at least 2 years earlier.

Taken together, the findings from both studies using subcutaneous implant pellets and those using intramuscular hormonal preparations provide compelling evidence that the addition of testosterone to an estrogen replacement regimen is associated with an enhancement of sexual desire, interest, and enjoyment of sex in postmenopausal women. These findings also allow the conclusion that in women, as well as in men[29], testosterone has its major effect on the cognitive motivational, or libidinal aspects of sexual behavior such as desire and fantasies and not on physiological responses. Moreover, studies of non-human primates suggest that testosterone probably exerts this effect on sexual desire via mechanisms that impact directly on the brain rather than by any effect on peripheral tissues[30].

Of course it is also the case that following the menopause, progesterone, normally secreted by the developing corpus luteum, also falls to very low levels. The practice of administering synthetic progestins along with estrogen to postmenopausal women in order to protect against endometrial hyperplasia allowed for the investigation of possible progestational effects on female sexuality. In a retrospective study, Dennerstein and co-workers[31] reported a dampening effect of progestins on libido when compared to estrogen alone, although the effect was seen only in the monthly interview and not in the daily ratings data. In a recent prospective study of naturally menopausal women, Sherwin[32] monitored various aspects of sexual behavior by daily reports. No adverse effects on sexual desire were observed when a modest dose of a progestin was added to the oral sequential estrogen replacement regimen. Although progesterone decreases the amount of bioavailable androgen[33] and dampens sexual desire when administered in large doses to male sex offenders[34], the administration of small doses with estrogen to postmenopausal women does not seem to have a demonstrable effect on sexual desire. However, there is evidence to suggest that a higher progestin/estrogen ratio is more likely to dampen well-being[35] and mood[32] in postmenopausal women.

CONCLUSION

There is now considerable evidence to suggest that changes in the endocrine milieu that occur at the time of menopause are causally related to disturbances in one or more aspects of sexual functioning that are reported by approximately one-third to one-half of women at this time. Low levels of circulating estrogen result in atrophy of estrogen-dependent urogenital tissues, including the vaginal epithelium which, in turn, can cause dyspareunia. These estrogen-dependent symptoms are largely reversible with postmenopausal estrogen replacement therapy.

On the other hand, some women, particularly those who have undergone a surgical menopause, experience a decrease in sexual desire or libido that is not affected by the administration of estrogen alone. When the onset of this decrease in desire can be related in time to the peri- or postmenopausal period in a spontaneously menopausal woman or to the postoperative period in a surgically menopausal woman, the addition of testosterone to an estrogen replacement regimen is effective in restoring previous levels of sexual desire in most women.

ACKNOWLEDGEMENT

The preparation of this manuscript was supported by a grant (#MT-11623) from the Medical Research Council of Canada awarded to B. B. Sherwin.

REFERENCES

1. Lipsett, M. B. (1986). Steroid hormones. In Yen, S. S. C. and Jaffe, R. B. (eds.) *Reproductive Endocrinology, Physiology, Pathophysiology and Clinical Management*, pp. 140–53. (Philadelphia: W. B. Saunders)
2. Longcope, C. (1981). Metabolic clearance and blood production rates of estrogen in postmenopausal women. *Am. J. Obstet. Gynecol.*, 111, 779–85
3. Wise, P. M., Weiland, N. G., Scarborough, K., Sortino, M. A., Cohen, I. R. and Larson, G. H. (1989). Changing hypothalamopituitary function: its role in aging of the female reproductive system. *Horm. Res.*, 31, 39–44
4. Longcope, C. (1986). Adrenal and gonadal steroid secretion in normal females. *J. Clin. Endocrinol. Metab.*, 15, 213–28
5. Longcope, C. (1974). Steroid production in pre- and postmenopausal women. In Greenblatt, R., Mahesh, V. and Mcdonough, E. (eds.) *The Menopausal Syndrome*, pp. 6–11. (New York: Medcom Press)
6. Vermeulen, A. (1976). The hormonal activity of the postmenopausal ovary. *J. Clin. Endocrinol. Metab.*, 42, 247–53
7. Roger, M., Nahoul, K., Scholler, R. and Bagrel, D. (1980). Evolution with aging of four plasma androgens in postmenopausal women. *Maturitas*, 2, 171–7
8. Longcope, C., Franz, C., Morello, C., Baker, R. and Johnson, C. Jr. (1986). Steroid and gonadotropin levels in women during their peri-menopausal years. *Maturitas*, 8, 189–96
9. Longcope, C., Hunter, R. and Franz, C. (1980). Steroid secretion by the postmenopausal ovary. *Am. J. Obstet. Gynecol.*, 138, 564–70
10. Lucisano, A., Acampora, M. G., Russo, N., Maniccia, E., Montemurro, A. and Dell'Acqua, S. (1984). Ovarian and peripheral plasma levels of progestogens, androgens and oestrogens in post-menopausal women. *Maturitas*, 6, 45–53
11. Botella-Llusia, J., Oriol-Bosch, A. and Sanchez-Garrido, F. (1979). Testosterone and 17-β-oestradiol secretion of the human ovary. II. Normal postmenopausal women, postmenopausal women with endometrial hyperplasia and postmenopausal women with adenocarcinoma of the endometrium. *Maturitas*, 2, 7–12
12. McEwen, B. S., Davis, P., Parsons, B. and Pfaff, D. (1979). The brain as target for steroid hormone action. *Annu. Rev. Neurosci.*, 2, 65–74
13. Luine, V. N., Khylchevskaya, R. I. and McEwen, B. (1975). Effect of gonadal steroids on activities of monoamine oxidase and choline acetylase in rat brain. *Brain Res.*, 86, 293–306
14. Kelly, M. J., Moss, R. L., Dudley, C. A. and Fawcett, C. P. (1977). The specificity of the response of preoptic-septal area neurons to estrogen: 17β-estradiol vs 17α-estradiol and the response of extrahypothalamic neurons. *Exp. Brain Res.*, 30, 43–50
15. Bergman, A. and Brenner, P. F. (1987). Alterations in the urogenital system.

In Mishell, D. R. (ed.) *Menopause: Physiology and Pharmacology*, pp. 67–75. (Chicago: Year Book Medical Publishers Inc.)

16. Sarrel, P. (1990). Sexuality and menopause. *Obstet. Gynecol.*, **75**, 26–31

17. Semmens, J. P. and Wagner, G. (1982). Estrogen deprivation and vaginal function in postmenopausal women. *J. Am. Med. Assoc.*, **248**, 445–8

18. Bachman, G., Leiblum, S. R., Kemmann, E., Colburn, D. W., Swartzman, L. and Shelden, R. (1984). Sexual expression and its determinants in the post-menopausal women. *Maturitas*, **6**, 19–29

19. McCoy, N. L. and Davison, J. M. (1985). A longitudinal study of the effects of menopause on sexuality. *Maturitas*, **7**, 203–10

20. Cutler, W. B., Garcia, C. R. and McCoy, N. (1987). Perimenopausal sexuality. *Arch Sex. Behav.*, **16**, 225–34

21. Burger, H. G., Hailes, J., Menelaus, M., Nelson, J., Hudson, B. and Balazs, N. (1984). The management of persistent menopausal symptoms with oestradiol-testosterone implants: clinical, lipid and hormonal results. *Maturitas*, **6**, 351–8

22. Cardozo, L., Gibb, D. M. F., Tuck, S. M., Thom, M. H., Studd, J. W. W. and Cooper, D. J. (1984). The effects of subcutaneous hormone implants during the climacteric. *Maturitas*, **5**, 177–84

23. Burger, H., Hailes, J., Nelson, J. and Menslaus, M. (1987). Effect of combined implants of oestradiol and testosterone on libido in postmenopausal women. *Lancet*, **294**, 936–7

24. Sherwin, B. B. and Gelfand, M. M. (1984). Effects of parenteral administration of estrogen and androgen on plasma hormone levels and hot flushes in surgical menopause. *Am. J. Obstet. Gynecol.*, **148**, 552–7

25. Sherwin, B. B. and Gelfand, M. M. (1985). Differential symptom response to parenteral estrogen and/or androgen administration in the surgical meno-pause. *Am. J. Obstet. Gynecol.*, **151**, 153–60

26. Sherwin, B. B. and Gelfand, M. M. (1985). Sex steroids and affect in the surgical menopause: a double-blind cross over study. *Psychoneuroendocrinology*, **10**, 325–35

27. Sherwin, B. B., Gelfand, M. M. and Brender, W. (1985). Androgen enhances sexual motivation in females: a prospective cross-over study of sex steroid administration in the surgical menopause. *Psychosom. Med.*, **7**, 339–51

28. Sherwin, B. B. and Gelfand, M. M. (1987). The role of androgen in the maintenance of sexual functioning in oophorectomized women. *Psychosom. Med.*, **49**, 397–409

29. Bancroft, J. and Wu, F. C. W. (1983). Changes in erectile responsiveness during androgen replacement therapy. *Arch. Sex. Behav.*, **12**, 59–66

30. Everitt, B. J. and Herbert, J. (1975). The effects of implanting testosterone propionate in the central nervous system on the sexual behavior of female rhesus monkeys. *Brain Res.*, **86**, 109–20

31. Dennerstein, L., Burrows, G. D., Wood, C. and Hyman, G. (1980). Hormones and sexuality: effect of estrogen and progestogen. *Obstet. Gynecol.*, **56**, 316–22

32. Sherwin, B. B. (1991). The impact of differential doses of estrogen and progestin on mood and sexual behavior in postmenopausal women. *J. Clin. Endocrinol. Metab.*, **72**, 336–43

33. Baulieu, E. E. and Jung, I. (1970). A prostatic cytosol receptor. *Biochem. Biophys. Res.*, **38**, 599–606
34. Berlin, F. S. and Meinecke, C. F. (1981). Treatment of sex offenders with antiandrogenic medication. *Am. J. Psychiatry*, **138**, 601–7
35. Sherwin, B. B. and Gelfand, M. M. (1989). A prospective one-year study of estrogen and progestin in postmenopausal women: effects on clinical symptoms and lipoprotein lipids. *Obstet. Gynecol.*, **73**, 759–66

61

Being 50 in the 1990s: sexual life, everyday life

M. Lachowsky

Being 50 in the 1990s means having already used two-thirds of one's possible life span. It might also mean that one-third of the pages in one's ledger are still blank, waiting to be filled – and why not fulfilled. However, whichever way one looks at it, it means getting older, and that seems to have become increasingly difficult in our times. Troubled as they may be, with so many men and women dying young, killed through love or hate by their own fellowmen, one would like to imagine that staying on earth a little longer should be greeted as a feat and not as a defeat.

Young is beautiful, slim is beautiful. Maybe we lost or misplaced our sense of beauty somewhere along the line of scientific and medical progress. So let us turn to our sense of humor, and try to accept two other simple truths: first that menopause is another of life's poisoned gifts to womankind, but also a landmark man must do without, and second, that sexuality is one of the bridges between the two genders, one of life's gifts to man and woman alike, one of the ways to make use of all those differences and inequalities never to be erased, and as such worthy of our medical interest. Why is it never too easy to think or to talk of sexual life after a certain age, age which varies with the speaker's own age?

When, as children, we first hear about making love, usually from our schoolmates, we have trouble connecting our own parents to such strange situations. Then comes the time when, full of knowledge and certainties, we credit them with one intercourse per child. A little later, the discovery of our young body and of its possibilities is so passionately intriguing that it leaves no time for speculating over their patently old bodies. Finally, as we arrive at an adult parental stage, their sexuality is of no concern to us, except if, too present to be ignored, it disturbs or at least surprises us.

I do believe that our way of considering (or maybe of not considering) sexuality in the menopausal years proceeds from the same train of thought. Of course we are concerned by the subject of medical research, which is the main topic of our symposium: 'Does age with its hormonal changes affect sexuality and, if so, how can we amend and treat these disorders?' Underneath that very scientific question looms the human and sociological factor. The disturbing question every woman is bound to voice to her inner self someday is 'is it still possible to have a sexual life in the menopause?' This may vary, depending on her own status, age and anxiety, from 'can one have a sexual life when in menopause?' to 'how can one still have a sexual life when in menopause, and with whom?'.

Sexuality and the menopause are both individual, intimate affairs. Sexuality is not easily gauged and measured; no standard can be set either by biology or by statistics. Although both are part of human physiopathology, the media and fashion seem to be more concerned about it than doctors, especially in our times of crude technicality. Letters to the specialized editor demand solutions to difficulties with sex-life rather than love-life, giving fresh ideas to some readers and sad regrets to others.

In France, every year, more than 300 000 women 'enter' the menopause, under the eyes of older and younger women who have their own ideas and experiences of the menopause, their daughters and their mothers, the men who surround them in their professional as well as their private life, the medical world and the world of the press. Let us consider what happens to a woman at that special moment of her life. It is the end of menstruation, she will not 'see' anymore, as the current saying goes in French.

The blood from the 'inside' of woman impregnates all the mythologies, from the most ancient to the most recent, through all folk-lores. It makes her different, a rhythmical being. How then can she remain a woman without that rhythm and its ritual, without those periods which for months and years have regularly been proof that she was young and fertile, a full-blooded woman, with a body designed for giving love and giving life, a lover's and a mother's body. We all know that expressed in our medical words, all this is nothing but the result or the revelation of the exhaustion of the stock of ovocysts and of the great change in the hypothalamo–pituitary–ovarian system, both of which are responsible for the end of reproductive function. But for most women, and for their men, even if they did know it was on their program, menopause does not need so many learned words; it is simply a succession of 'nevermore' announcing the descent towards less and less beautiful years, towards winter.

Is there not a difference nowadays, in the era of women's liberation and contraceptive pills, when sexuality can be enjoyed without its ancestral reproductive aim, so much so that reproduction can do without sexuality? For many women, at least unconsciously, the end of their fertility is the death-toll of their femininity. They imagine that it leaves the same impression on men, which is often true. In the eyes of others, they see the alteration of their face, of their body, the claws of age. They feel hurt and shamed by their new image, and they discover the loss of their seductiveness in the eyes of men, who simply do not see them anymore.

All these losses, these depreciations, create another reality. Their sexuality has to adjust to their new bearings, as it adapted in their youth to those too small breasts or too heavy legs, to all those imperfections that never prevented women from having and giving pleasure, from loving and being loved. To feel worthy of another's love and desire, we need self-esteem, we must have made peace with the difference between our actual body and our imaginary one, between the image in the mirror and the one in our head. We all know how demanding that may be: how difficult it can be, and sometimes how disappointing, to recognize our image on a photograph, or our voice on a tape. This is made all the more uneasy by the cruel fact that menopause has the good taste – or perhaps the bad taste? – to happen around the middle of life, announcing a kind of second coming of age. This envelope in which woman had had so much trouble moulding herself at puberty had finally become quite hospitable, and suddenly, here come the treasons of menopause, more or less rapidly apparent, more or less bearable.

How indeed can today's woman cope with the weight of age when youth with its unwrinkled face and unsagging body has become the necessary passport to our world, the world of love and the world of money, with no time and no place for those who do not compare with the triumphant model? It is precisely on that social image, her external appearance, that the menopause is going to put its mark, the seal of the change of age. That turn of age, that returning age as we say in French 'le retour d'âge', has always cast a dim light on a woman's life, and especially on her sexual life. It is a turning point in a couple's life.

The man may play the leading part, but as often as not mothers and grandmothers have handed down their stories. 'My mother told me that after her menopause, IT never worked well again!' After that piece of

601

wisdom, do not imagine she will find much solace in our treatments, the dice are cast.

Of course, love and libido are a troublesome pair, and both are needed in a couple to keep the flame burning, even if it is no longer an Olympic flame. The man's role is capital: if he accepts his own aging image, if he can bear with his own losses, apparent or unapparent, he will read with equanimity the passing of time on his companion and thus tolerate it for both of them. If he recoils before the signs shown by the calendar and the mirror, if he attempts to deny them, the tell-tale signs on the woman will be too much for him. That perpetual reminder of additions turning into subtractions leaves them no choice: whether he goes or stays, he will throw back to his companion a dramatically devaluated image of herself, especially full of risks for her self-esteem and deprecating for her sex appeal.

Sexual disturbances in the menopause also arise from organic causes. We are all aware that hormonal replacement therapy is easier to administer than is psychological bolstering, but it is also quite true that some women blithely accept those difficulties to put an end to an already unsatisfying sex life. The menopause is then an excuse, revealing a discordant or at least indifferent state of affairs in the couple. However, sexuality cannot be reduced to a simple equation of hormonal balance. A desired and desiring woman may enjoy a gratifying love- and sex-life far into her menopausal years. Some arrangements are not to be neglected, as that charming old lady once told me with relish: 'You know, I did "cheat" on my husband when my menopause started. I used to pretend I was unavailable once a month as usual, I faked my periods and it was quite a feat as I had never been so sharp on the calendar! And how we enjoyed our encounters after those abstemious days! That is how I remained young in his eyes...longer than the fatal date.' For her, the idea of menopause was far worse than its concrete manifestations, the scarecrow being the word rather than the reality, which should not come as a surprise for us. Some words weigh more than others on the scales of life, as we gynecologists learn, even if we do not always find the light ones.

Not all women have, at that fragile moment in their life, a companion full of love and able to prove it! If no hormonopause officially exists for men, other pauses, other failures may happen. Some couples make do with them, warm tenderness and companionship often taking passion's place, all the more so when their common past is food for their present, and even for their future. One climbs upstairs less nimbly, one needs stronger glasses or newspapers are really badly printed nowadays, one makes love less frequently, one gets older, but together. For some others, the visible evidence of age is the worst of degradations and the husband of many years or the new companion will attempt to redeem his failing virility with much younger women, or by putting the blame on his mate, complaining of her loss of charm or her lack of libido. Women usually respond in one of two opposite modes: either they feel those appreciations or rather depreciations quite justified, caused by their 'turn of age'. 'I thought it was always the case, I expected it. Men keep their appetite much longer than we do...' said with resignation one of my patients. Or they may also discover a new life, sometimes with a much younger partner, and thoroughly enjoy such transgression as life's unexpected present. 'Now or never, or it will be too late' is not only a masculine credo!

The 'change of life', the menopause, is also a crisis, as even Hippocrates knew, fraught with dangers, bringing the risks of cancer and cardiovascular diseases nearer. The greater the longevity offered by medicine, the deeper the fear of illness, pain, solitude and death. Every woman needs to negotiate that turning point in her heart of hearts. Although her world is quite different from her grandmother's and even her mother's, she still recognizes herself in their tales, knowing full well the game is her own, and that no two people have the same cards in their hands. I wonder if medical people haven't somewhere appropriated this original and intimate event?

Family life is also generally changing at that period: both parents and children are getting older, both take their leave sometime, death taking the preceding generation and life the next one. But both may also make the house too full, leaving no privacy, causing quarrels and bickering. Nowadays women often suffer less from the 'empty nest syndrome' than from their children's love-making under her roof. Rivalry or renouncement, voyeurism or complicity, how can she find her place as a mother, as a woman?

Times of nevermore and of now or never, change and urgency, bends to negotiate, the menopause is essentially a narcissic wound. No woman stays unscathed but it will heal quite differently between one woman and another, depending also on her environment, be it personal, sentimental or socioprofessional. Well inserted in life, in her microcosm, our patient of about 50 will look 10 years younger, and her sexuality even less. Unemployed, abandoned and lonely, she will feel rejected and dejected, and she will forsake her sexuality along with her femininity rather than seeing it mocked or denied by others.

Where do gynecologists come in, what part have we to play in our patients' sex-lives? It is of common knowledge that we always talk sex and sexuality, whatever the given motive of consultation may seem. But sometimes we are less discrete, and may ask some of those questions women may have trouble voicing aloud. Let us try and help them to talk about 'that thing', 'cette chose-là' as Hélène Michel-Wolfromm used to name sexuality in her patients' words. Shame, fear of ridicule are still often part of the image of menopause, and as they prevent an honest answer they certainly modify the impressive statistics on sexuality in menopausal women. Our respect, our full attention is already therapeutic, showing them there is no age limit either for our interest or for love and sexuality, making their complaints as worthy of our medical attention as any other somatic problems. No age limit, but maybe some ways to give and find pleasure even with backaches or hip problems, with all parts of man's and woman's body.

Hormonal replacement treatment will be explained, the best strategy for that particular patient defined. We have all heard women refusing to be 'branded like cattle' by a patch, others feeling happy by not having to swallow a 'drug', and others again choosing the cream as a beneficial ointment to preserve their body. No need to stress here the important part that such therapy plays in vaginal dryness, which can hurt so much, on the lubrication which comes slower with age, and less abundantly. So why not insist on the need of time and gentleness for the preludes, why not take our time to tell those facts of life to the companion of our patient.

Why not prescribe the application of estrogens on the pubis, to slow the depilation which is so unpleasant for some of our patients? Hormonal therapies usually have a rapid effect on mood, on tiredness and listlessness, helping all appetites to revive. As always, however, let us be modest: it is the woman's idea of menopause, what she expected, what she heard from her mother and friends, from doctors and newspapers, and her own way of considering feminine destiny which will color her menopause. The men in her life have quite a responsibility too!

TO CONCLUDE

Local and general hormone replacement, psychological support, technical advice and family counselling: the approach of sexuality in the menopause requires all that and even more. So let us reassure our patients – and ourselves – by reminding them, with Pascal, that 'There is no age for love, love is always a rebirth,' and with Wladimir Yankelevitch that 'Sexuality is reading always anew a text already read, read for a thousand times'.

62

Some aspects of sexuality during the normal climacteric

A. Oldenhave

INTRODUCTION

In 1920, Helene Deutsch stated that women stopped being 'real women' after the menopause and should be considered as the 'third sex'[1]. Sexuality was considered suitable only for reproduction. Because of the sexual revolution and the women's movement, ideas about sexuality in middle-aged and older women changed radically. Instead of 'dying as a sexual being', it was stressed that mature women had in fact a great potential for enjoying sex. The climacteric was looked upon as a liberation for further sexual development, since fear of unwanted pregnancy and menstrual problems would no longer interfere with sexual enjoyment. Gloria Bachman, however, believes that these optimistic ideas have gone a little too far and that the ideal of the mature woman as a 'sexual lioness' may be just as much a burden for women as the 'asexual being' of the former days[2].

METHODS AND DEFINITIONS

All 10 598 women aged aged 39–60 residing in the municipality of Ede (The Netherlands) received a postal questionnaire in April 1987. The study was presented as a survey on 'Health and Well-being'. In the accompanying letter, sex, the climacteric and hysterectomy were not stressed as the main subjects of the study. Altogether, 7256 usable replies were received, representing a 71% response rate. The following women were excluded from the analysis: women without a steady partner, hysterectomized and/or oophorectomized women and users of oral contraceptives. A total of 4788 women was included. Almost all (96.2%) of the women with a partner were married, 1.7% were divorced, 0.5% were widowed and in 0.1% the civil status was unknown. Climacteric status was classified into 13 categories according to menstrual pattern characteristics and the number of months or years since the last menstrual bleeding before the questionnaire was completed. Women with a regular menstrual pattern in the year preceding the survey formed one group. Women with irregular menstrual cycles in the preceding year were categorized into four premenopausal groups according to the number of *months* since the last menstrual bleeding, i.e. less than or equal to 1 months, greater than 1 but less than or equal to 3 months, greater than 3 but less than or equal to 6 months, and greater than 6 but less than or equal to 12 months. Women whose last menstrual bleeding had occurred over 12 months previously were categorized into eight postmenopausal groups according to the number of *years* since the last menstrual bleeding, i.e. 1, 2, 3, 4, 5, 6–7, 8–9 and greater than or equal to 10 years. The size of the study population enabled the study of the effect of climacteric status in women in a limited age group (range 45–49 years). The results from women with a regular menstrual pattern were compared with those of women who had not menstruated for at least 6 months before the survey. *Within* this age range, the effect of climacteric status was adjusted for age.

The severity of vaginal dryness and pain during coitus, experienced in the month preceding the survey, was assessed on a four-point scale: absent, slight, moderate and severe. The question 'How much pleasure do you usually experience in sex?' could be answered with 'I don't engage in sex (anymore)', 'I mostly enjoy it', 'I sometimes enjoy it', 'Actually I don't really enjoy it' and 'no pleasure'.

RESULTS

Pleasure in sex

The majority of women engaged in sex, the proportion decreasing from 98% in regularly menstruating women to 84% of those whose last menstrual bleeding had occurred 10 or more years prior to the survey (Figure 1). There was a large decrease in the percentage of women reporting *pleasure 'mostly'*; down from 70.4% of the regularly menstruating women to 34.3% of the women whose last menstrual bleeding had

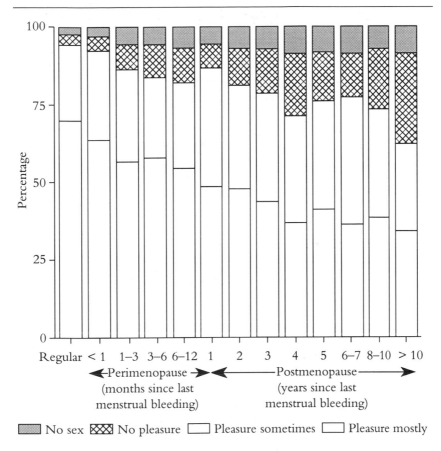

Figure 1 Pleasure in sex according to climacteric status in women with a partner ($n = 4788$)

occurred 10 or more years previously – a decrease by 36.1%. During the premenopausal phase, which had a mean length of 4–5 years (see Table 1), pleasure 'mostly' decreased by 16% and in the following 10 postmenopausal years by a further 20%. 'No pleasure' was reported infrequently (2–3%) by regularly menstruating and early premenopausal women (last menstrual bleeding ≤ 1 month previously). In the other three premenopausal groups (last menstrual bleeding 1–3, 3–6 and 6–12 months previously), 'no pleasure' was reported by 3.8–9.8% of the women, a percentage which slowly increased to 20.4% 10 years after the last menstrual bleeding. These results do not indicate that the climacteric or the absence of menstruation had a liberating or positive effect on the

Table 1 Mean age according to climacteric status ($n = 4788$)

Climacteric status	Age (years)		
	Mean	SD	Range
Regular menstrual pattern	43.9	3.7	39–57
Premenopause			
≤ 1 month	45.7	4.2	39–57
1–3 months	48.9	3.9	39–58
3–6 months	50.2	3.7	39–57
6–12 months	51.0	3.8	40–58
Postmenopause			
1 year	52.3	3.6	39–59
2 years	52.8	3.5	40–59
3 years	54.3	3.2	45–60
4 years	54.6	3.3	42–60
5 years	55.7	3.2	39–60
6–7 years	56.1	2.4	46–60
8–10 years	56.2	3.4	41–60
≥ 10 years	56.3	3.4	41–60

pleasure experience in sex. As shown by Table 1, climacteric status was related to age.

As the correlation between climacteric status and age was high ($r = 0.78$, $p < 0.001$), the correlations between climacteric status or age and pleasure in sex were similar, $r = 0.25$ for climacteric status and $r = 0.22$ for age (both $p < 0.001$). When adjusted for age, the partial correlation between climacteric status and pleasure in sex was $r = 0.10$ ($p \leq 0.001$) and when adjusted for climacteric status, the partial correlation between age and pleasure in sex was $r = 0.08$ ($p \leq 0.001$). Climacteric status was, therefore, a slightly better predictor of 'pleasure in sex' than age, although the small differences between the partial correlations showed that the effects of climacteric status and age were difficult to distinguish from each other.

As Table 1 showed, the greatest difference in the mean ages according to climacteric status were found in the premenopausal groups. The size of the population enabled us to look at the effect of climacteric status within a limited age range. We decided to study, in 733 women aged 45–49 years, the difference in pleasure in sex between women with a regular menstrual pattern ($n = 586$) and those who had not menstruated for at least 6 months ($n = 147$). The results were then adjusted for age within this 5-year age group. Selecting such a limited age range had the additional

Table 2 Pleasure in sex in 733 women aged 45–50 years according to climacteric status (%)

	Mostly	*Sometimes*	*No pleasure*	*No sex*	*n*
Regular menstrual pattern	65.3	28.1	4.5	2.1	586
Last menstrual bleeding $\geq$ 6 months	49.3	33.8	7.7	9.2	147

Cross-tabulation: χ^2 24.61, d.f. = 3, $p < 0.001$
Climacteric status with age as covariate: ANOVA, d.f. = 1, f = 9.56, $p = 0.002$

advantage that it also made some adjustment for the change in attitudes to sexuality since the late 1960s, which may have had a differential influence on women in different age groups.

In women aged 45–49 years, pleasure in sex 'mostly' was reported more frequently by regularly menstruating women (65.3%) than by women who had not menstruated for at least 6 months (49.3%) (Table 2). The difference between the two groups was significant ($p < 0.001$). The 'pleasure in sex' variable was then changed into a two-point scale variable, pleasure 'mostly' vs. the other three answer categories combined (pleasure sometimes, no pleasure, no sex). When adjusted for age, the effect of climacteric status on pleasure in sex was significant (ANOVA, d.f. = 1, f = 9.56, $p = 0.002$). The effect of age on pleasure in sex was also significant (ANOVA, d.f. = 1, f = 4.47, $p < 0.05$). Thus pleasure in sex was influenced more by climacteric status than by age.

Pain during coitus

In the whole population, pain during coitus was reported by 16.2% of the women, specifically as slight pain by 9.2%, moderate pain by 4.8% and severe pain by 2.2%. Some 2–16% of the women reported '*not engaging in sex*' when asked how much pleasure they experienced in sex (see above). These women therefore also faithfully reported that they did not experience pain during coitus. Women not engaging in sex are shown separately (Figure 2). Pain during coitus was reported by approximately 12.5% of the regularly menstruating women and premenopausal women, and by about 25% of the postmenopausal women. The prevalence of pain during coitus (slight to severe) increased from 11% in regularly menstruating women to 12–18% in premenopausal women (last menstrual bleeding $\leq$ 1 month previously, 15%, 1–3 months, 18%, 3–6 months, 12%, and 6–12 months, 13%). In the premenopausal group, women whose last

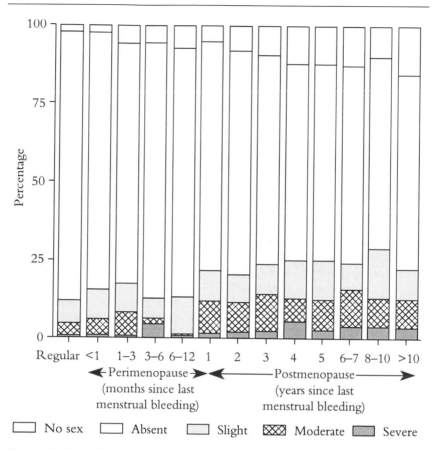

Figure 2 Pain during coitus according to climacteric status in women with a partner (*n* = 4788)

menstrual bleeding was 1–3 months previously reported pain during coitus slightly more often (18%) than regularly menstruating women and women in the three other premenopausal groups. Pain during coitus was reported by 19–28% of the postmenopausal women. Four years after the last menstrual bleeding, the prevalence of pain during coitus had more or less stabilized at 25%. *Severe* pain during coitus was reported relatively infrequently, by 1% of the regularly menstruating women, by 1–3% of the premenopausal women and by 2–6% of the postmenopausal women. Of the regularly menstruating women, 2% did not engage in sex, a percentage which increased to approximately 6% in premenopausal women (last menstrual bleeding < 12 months previously) and stabilized at about 13%

Table 3 Pain during coitus in 733 women aged 45–50 years according to climacteric status (%)

	Absent	*Slight*	*Moderate*	*Severe*	*n*
Regular menstrual pattern	90.6	6.3	2.3	0.9	586
Last menstrual bleeding $\geq$ 6 months	75.9	12.1	9.2	2.8	147

Cross-tabulation: χ^2 26.4, d.f. = 3, $p < 0.001$
Climacteric status with age as covariate: ANOVA, d.f. = 1, $f = 25.2$, $p < 0.001$

in women who had been postmenopausal for 4 or more years. Thus 4 or more years after the last menstrual bleeding, 38% of the women reported either experiencing pain during coitus (25%) or not engaging in sex (13%).

In examining the relative influence of climacteric status and age on the prevalence of pain during coitus in the whole population we excluded from the analysis women who did not engage in sex. The effect of age on the severity of pain during coitus adjusted for climacteric status (the partial correlation with age) was 0.06 ($p \leq 0.001$). The effect of climacteric status on pain during coitus adjusted for age (the partial correlation with climacteric status) was greater, 0.11 ($p \leq 0.001$).

The relative influence of age and climacteric status on pain during coitus was assessed in 733 regularly menstruating women aged 45–49 years and in women in the same age group whose last menstruation had occurred at least 6 months previously. Within this 5-year age range the results were adjusted for age (Table 3). In women aged 45–49 years, slight, moderate or severe pain during coitus was reported less frequently by regularly menstruating women (8.4%) than by women who had not menstruated for at least 6 months (24.1%). The difference between the two groups was significant ($p < 0.001$). When adjusted for age, the effect of climacteric status within this 5-year age group was significant (ANOVA, $p < 0.001$), whereas the effect of age on pain during coitus was not significant (ANOVA, d.f. = 1, $f = 0.62$, $p = 0.43$). Thus climacteric status was a much better predictor of pain during coitus than age.

Vaginal dryness

In the whole population, vaginal dryness was reported as absent by 74%, slight by 12%, moderate by 9% and severe by 5% of the women. There was no significant difference between women who engaged in sex and

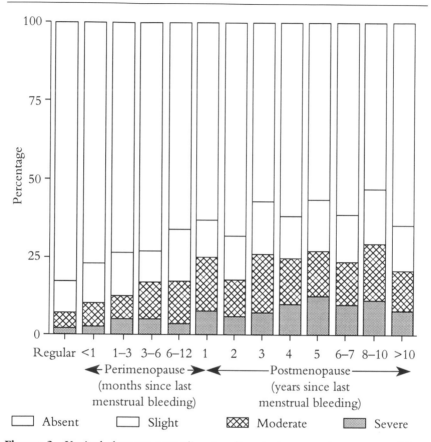

Figure 3 Vaginal dryness according to climacteric status in women with a partner (*n* = 4788)

those who did not. According to climacteric status, the prevalence of vaginal dryness (slight to severe) increased from 16% in regularly menstruating women to 22–33% in premenopausal women (last menstrual bleeding ≤ 1 month previously, 22%; 1–3 months, 27%; 3–6 months, 16%; and 6–12 months, 33%) (Figure 3). Vaginal dryness (slight to severe) was reported by 40–50% of the postmenopausal women. The prevalence of vaginal dryness more or less stabilized at approximately 40–45% 3 years or more after the last menstrual bleeding. *Severe* vaginal dryness was reported infrequently by regularly menstruating women and premenopausal women whose last menstrual bleeding had occurred up to 1 month previously (2%), but its prevalence increased later in the climacteric to stabilize at about 10–12% 4 years or more after the last menstrual bleeding.

Table 4 Vaginal dryness in 733 women aged 45–50 years according to climacteric status (%)

	Absent	*Slight*	*Moderate*	*Severe*	*n*
Regular menstrual pattern	80.6	11.2	5.6	2.6	586
Last menstrual bleeding ≥ 6 months	63.1	18.4	10.6	7.8	147

Cross-tabulation: χ^2 22.0, d.f. = 3, $p < 0.001$
Climacteric status with age as covariate: ANOVA, d.f. = 1, $f = 19.68$, $p < 0.001$

In the whole population the effect of age on the severity of vaginal dryness adjusted for climacteric status (the partial correlation with age) was 0.06 ($p \leq 0.001$). The effect of climacteric status on the severity of vaginal dryness adjusted for age (the partial correlation with climacteric status) was 0.11 ($p \leq 0.001$).

The difference in vaginal dryness according to climacteric status was analyzed in 733 women aged 45–49 years. Within this 5-year age range, the effects of climacteric status were adjusted for age (Table 4). Regularly menstruating women aged 45–49 years reported slight, moderate or severe vaginal dryness less frequently (19.4%) than women of similar age who had not menstruated for at least 6 months (36.9%). The difference between the two groups was significant ($p < 0.001$), as was the effect of climacteric status adjusted for age ($p < 0.001$). The effect of age was not significant (ANOVA, d.f. = 1, $f = 2.0$, $p = 0.16$). Thus climacteric status was a much better predictor of vaginal dryness than age.

DISCUSSION

This study shows that pleasure in sex, vaginal dryness and pain during coitus are influenced more by climacteric status than by age. However, climacteric status was found to have much less effect on pleasure in sex than on vaginal dryness and pain during coitus. In addition, the study showed that there is also a wide variation in pleasure in sex, vaginal dryness and pain during coitus in postmenopausal women. Eight-four percent of the women whose last menstrual bleeding occurred 10 years or more previously still engaged in sex and 34% enjoyed it 'mostly', while the majority (around 60%) reported an *absence* of vaginal dryness or pain during coitus. In future studies attention should be paid to the physical and psychological characteristics of the (aging) partner of the climacteric woman, because for pleasure in sex – apart from masturbation – it required (at least) two persons. Hallström[3] also found a progressive decline in sexual interest according to climacteric status. In that study the effect of climacteric status was greater than that of age. In a small scale prospective study ($n = 16$), there were small but significant decreases in sexual activity, vaginal lubrication and sexual thoughts[4]. From the literature it is known that estrogen levels are relatively independent of sexual interest and enjoyment[5]. Low estrogen levels, however, are associated with vaginal dryness, which may lead to pain during coitus[6]. On the other hand, there is some evidence that regular and continued sexual activity protects against vaginal dryness[7]. In two studies by Hunter[8,9] 80% of women aged 45–56 years felt satisfied with their sexual relationships. Sexual interest did, however, decrease according to climacteric status after adjustment for age. Sexual difficulties were associated with marital problems, stress and ill health as well as menopausal status[8,9]. Since for quite a lot of middle-aged or older women it is difficult to discuss spontaneously vaginal dryness or pain during coitus, it would help them if the physician initiates this topic. If vaginal dryness is primarily caused by the climacteric hormonal changes (and not caused by other sexual problems between the partners or of the male partner), the use of a lubricant or a vaginal estrogen cream or vaginal estrogen ring can be advised. Hysterectomized women in whom the ovaries have been conserved are at a higher risk for vaginal dryness and pain during coitus[10]. Hysterectomized women aged 39–41 years with ovarian conservation, report more vaginal dryness[11] and similarly severe pain during coitus than non-operated women aged 57–60 years[10]. In aging women gynecological examination may be very painful (for the woman) and difficult (for the physician). In some cases it is advisable to do the gynecological examination after a couple of weeks of estrogen therapy.

ACKNOWLEDGEMENTS

The study was financially supported by The International Health Foundation (Brussels, Belgium), The Dutch Ministry of Health and the Dutch van den Bogaard Association Limited.

REFERENCES

1. Deutsch, H. (1984). The menopause. Translation, Roazen, P. (ed.) *Int. J. Psychoanal.*, **65**, 55–62
2. Bachman, G. A. (1990). The impact of vaginal health on sexual function. *J. Clin. Prac. Sexual.*, Special Issue, 18–21

3. Hallström, T. Sexuality in the climacteric. *Clin. Obstet. Gynecol.*, **XX** 4, 227–39
4. McCoy, N. L. and Davidson, J. M. (1985). A longitudinal study of the effects of menopause on sexuality. *Maturitas,* 7, 203–10
5. Bancroft, J. (1983). *Human Sexuality and its Problems.* (Edinburgh: Churchill Livingstone)
6. Hutton, J. D., Jacobs, H. S. and James, V. H. T. (1979). Steroid endocrinology after the menopause – a review. *J. Soc. Med.,* **72**, 835–41
7. Bachman, G. A., Liblum, S. R., Kemman, E., Colburn, D. W., Swatzman, L. and Sheldon, R. (1984). Sexual expression and its determinants in the postmenopausal women. *Maturitas,* **6**, 19–29
8. Hunter, M. S., Battersby, R. and Whitehead, M. (1986). Relationship between psychological symptoms, somatic complaints and menopausal status. *Maturitas,* **8**, 217–28
9. Hunter, M. S. (1990). Psychological and somatic experience of the menopause: a prospective study. *Psychosom. Med.,* **52**, 357–67
10. Oldenhave, A. (1991). Well-being and sexuality in the climacteric. A survey based on 6622 women aged 38–60 years in the Dutch municipality of Ede. Dissertation, Excelsior, Leidschendam, The Netherlands
11. Oldenhave, A., Jaszmann, L. J. B., Everaerd, W. Th. A. M. and Haspels, A. A. (1993). Hysterectomized women with ovarian conservation report more severe climacteric complaints than do normal climacteric women of similar age. *Am. J. Obstet. Gynecol.,* **168**, 765–71

63

Sexuality and the menopause

B. B. Sherwin

It has long been acknowledged that human sexual behavior is multideter-mined and that biological, psychosocial and cultural factors affect its expression and experience. Because of the biological and psychosocial changes that occur around the time of menopause, in addition to changes associated with the aging process itself, it is not surprising that sexual functioning also undergoes change around this time.

Epidemiologic studies of normal population samples have found that between one-third and one-half of women report a decrease in one or more aspects of sexual functioning peri- and postmenopausally compared to premenopausally[1-4]. Not surprisingly, the incidence of sexual dysfunc-tion is even higher in women attending a menopause clinic[5]. Although cause and effect relationships are difficult to establish with complex behaviors, there is considerable evidence to suggest that biological factors, personal psychological factors, socioeconomic and cultural factors are major determinants of sexual functioning in postmenopausal women.

BIOLOGICAL FACTORS

The considerable decrease in estrogen production at the menopause results in atrophy of the vaginal epithelium which, in turn, may lead to a decrease in vaginal lubrication and dyspareunia. These atrophic changes in the genital tissues can understandably decrease sexual interest and activity. In most cases, estrogen replacement therapy reverses this sexual dysfunction if this is causally related to the atrophic changes. On the other hand, there is by now considerable evidence that testosterone is the libido-enhancing hormone in both women and men. The addition of testosterone to the estrogen replacement regimen is frequently successful in restoring libido in both naturally[5] and surgically menopausal women[6-7]. Insomnia caused by severe night sweats may also dampen sexual functioning.

PERSONAL PSYCHOLOGICAL FACTORS

Enjoyment of sex prior to the menopause is a predictor of sexual enjoyment and behavior following the menopause[8]. Equally obvioius is the fact that sexual functioning in postmenopausal women is strongly dependent upon the quality of the marital relationship, although little if any empirical work has been carried out in this area. Moreover, other life stresses that often coincide with the menopause, such as the need to care for one's own elderly parents, financial difficulties and problems associated with raising teenage or young adult children, also negatively affect the sexual life of the couple. An additional important but heretofore neglected factor relates to the sexual interest and potency of the husband or partner. Indeed, in a cross-sectional study, 32% of postmenopausal women cited their partner's disinterest as reason for their celibacy[9]. The fact that divorce now occurs in 50% of married couples and that women outlive men also means that many postmenopausal women are single with few opportunities to engage in sexual relationships.

SOCIOECONOMIC FACTORS

Several studies of sexuality in aging women have served to underline the importance of socioeconomic status and level of education as correlates of sexual behavior later in life. In Hallstrom's study of 800 perimenopausal Swedish women[1], sexual interest was more commonly decreased in low socioeconomic groups. The author suggested that this occurred because education leads to greater freedom from cultural inhibitions and sexual stereotypes. The finding that sexually inactive postmenopausal women were from lower socioeconomic groups was further supported by the results of investigations undertaken on Belgian[10] and American women[9].

CULTURAL FACTORS

Throughout life, psychosexual behavior is influenced to a considerable degree by the cultural mores of a given society. In some non-industrialized societies, the changes in a woman's life brought about by the onset of middle age appear to be mostly positive. In these societies, middle-aged women are freed from cumbersome restrictions which they had to observe when younger, are allowed to exert authority over younger members, and are eligible for special status and for recognition beyond the confines of the household[11]. Although there is greater gender equality among younger people in industrialized societies, it would seem that women experience a disproportionate decrease in status with increasing age; mature men are still perceived as being sexually attractive whereas this is generally not true for mature women. Furthermore, western societies are still coming to terms with the fact that sexual behavior continues into old age. For example, it is only fairly recently that older married couples who enter senior citizen homes or nursing homes have been housed together in the same room and the practice is still prohibited in some settings.

SUMMARY

During the past decade, the increasing liberalization of western societies, in general, and the upsurge in interest in the menopause, in particular, have helped to legitimize both the study of female sexual behavior and the treatment of its dysfunctions. We have learned a great deal in the past 10 years concerning the biological and psychosocial determinants of female sexual behavior. On the other hand, while our database is now richer, it is far from complete. More research is needed on the efficacy of hormonal interventions for complaints of sexual dysfunctions in the postmenopause with respect to which particular women are likely to be helped by them. In the clinical situation, it is critical to evaluate disturbances in sexual functioning in the context of the woman's life, including her marital relationship, concurrent life stresses and her general physical and psychological health. Because sexuality encompasses a complex, multifaceted repertoire of behaviors, it is unlikely that simple cause and effect relationships exist. Finally, it is important to remember that not all women experience troublesome changes in sexual functioning postmenopausally and, of those who do, not all see such changes as problematic. The continuation of an active sexual life into the postmenopausal years is a quality of life issue whose fulfilment depends entirely on the wishes of the individual women.

REFERENCES

1. Hallstorm, T. and Samuelsson, S. (1990). Changes in women's sexual desire in middle life: the longitudinal study of women in Gothenberg. *Arch. Sex. Behav.*, **19**, 259–68

2. McCoy, N. L. and Davidson, J. M. (1985). A longitudinal study of the effects of menopause on sexuality. *Maturitas,* **7**, 203–10

3. Cutler, W. B., Garcia, C. R. and McCoy, N. (1987). Perimenopausal sexuality. *Arch. Sex. Behav.,* **16**, 225–34

4. Hunter, M. S. and Whitehead, M. I. (1989). Psychological experience of the climacteric. In Hunter, M. S. and Whitehead, M. I. (eds.) *Menopause: Evaluation, Treatment and Health Concerns,* pp. 211–24. (New York: Liss)

5. Studd, J. W. W., Collins, W. P. and Chakravarti, S. (1977). Oestradiol and testosterone implants in the treatment of psychosexual problems in the postmenopause. *Br. J. Obstet. Gynaecol.,* **84**, 314–19

6. Sherwin, B. B., Gelfand, M. M. and Brender, W. (1985). Androgen enhances sexual motivation in females: a prospective cross-over study of sex steroid administration in the surgical menopause. *Psychosom. Med.,* **7**, 339–51

7. Sherwin, B. B. and Gelfand, M. M. (1987). The role of androgen in the maintenance of sexual functioning in oophorectomized women. *Psychosom. Med.,* **49**, 397–409

8. Hunter, M. S. (1990). Emotional well-being, sexual behavior and hormone replacement therapy. *Maturitas,* **12**, 299–314

9. Bachmann, G., Leiblum, S. R., Kemmann, E., Colburn, D. W., Swartzman, L. and Shelden, R. (1984). Sexual expression and its determinants in the post-menopausal women. *Maturitas,* **6**, 19–29

10. Busse, E. (1973). Sexual attitudes and behavior in the elderly. *Geriatric Focus,* **12**, 1–7

11. Brown, J. K. and Kerns, V. (eds.) (1985). *In Her Prime,* pp. 1–11. (South Hadley, MA: Bergin & Garvey Publ. Inc.)

Index

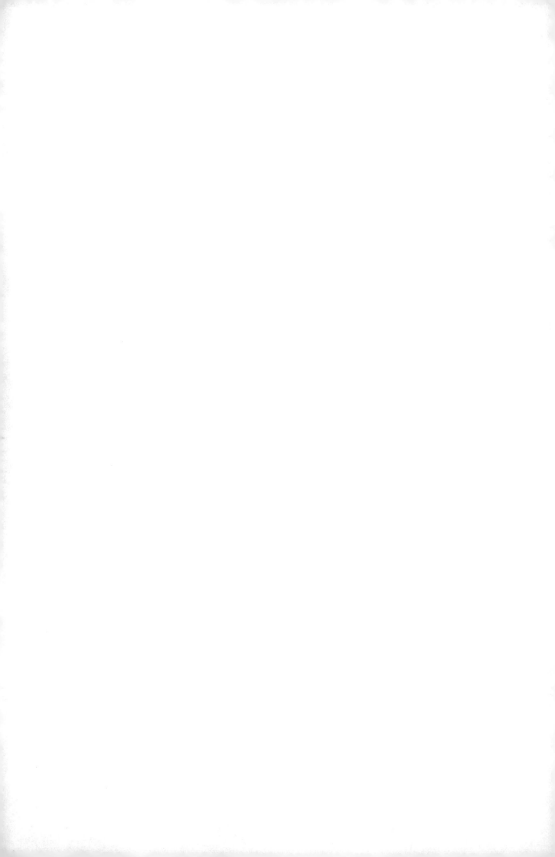

Co-op - IX